DuVries' **Surgery of the foot**

DuVries'
Surgery of the foot

Editor
VERNE T. INMAN, M.D., Ph.D.

THIRD EDITION
with 1,041 *illustrations*

The C. V. Mosby Company

SAINT LOUIS 1973

THIRD EDITION

Copyright © 1973 by The C. V. Mosby Company

All rights reserved. No part of this book may be reproduced in any manner without written permission of the publisher.

Previous editions copyrighted 1959, 1965

Printed in the United States of America

Distributed in Great Britain by Henry Kimpton, London

Library of Congress Cataloging in Publication Data

DuVries, Henri L
  DuVries' Surgery of the foot.

  Bibliography: p.
  1. Foot—Surgery. I. Inman, Verne Thompson,
1905-   ed. II. Title. III. Title: Surgery of
the foot. [DNLM: 1. Foot diseases—Surgery. WE 880
D987s 1973]
RD563.D94 1973   617'.585   73-16
ISBN 0-8016-2332-4

Contributors

Edwin G. Bovill, Jr., M.D.

Professor of Orthopaedic Surgery, Vice Chairman, Department of Orthopaedic Surgery, University of California, San Francisco; Chief, Department of Orthopaedic Surgery, San Francisco General Hospital, San Francisco

Michael W. Chapman, M.D.

Assistant Professor of Orthopaedic Surgery, University of California, San Francisco; Assistant Chief, Department of Orthopaedic Surgery, San Francisco General Hospital, San Francisco

Henri L. DuVries, D.P.M., M.D.

Assistant Clinical Professor of Orthopaedic Surgery (retired), University of California, San Francisco; Chief of Foot Surgery, Highland General Hospital, Oakland; Member, Senior Surgical Staff, Samuel Merritt Hospital, Oakland; Clinical Professor of Surgery, California College of Podiatric Medicine, San Francisco

James M. Glick, M.D.

Assistant Clinical Professor of Orthopaedic Surgery, University of California, San Francisco; Associate Professor of Physical Education and Team Physician, California State University, San Francisco; Active Staff, Mount Zion Hospital and Medical Center, Ralph K. Davies Medical Center, and Unity Hospital, San Francisco

Verne T. Inman, M.D., Ph.D.

Professor of Orthopaedic Surgery and Director, Biomechanics Laboratory, University of California, San Francisco

S. William Levy, M.D.

Clinical Professor of Dermatology, University of California, San Francisco; Active Staff, Children's Hospital and Adult Medical Center, and Mount Zion Hospital and Medical Center, San Francisco; Dermatologic Consultant to the United States Army, Letterman General Hospital, San Francisco; Courtesy Staff, Ralph K. Davies Medical Center, San Francisco

Roger A. Mann, M.D.

Assistant Clinical Professor of Orthopaedic Surgery, University of California, San Francisco; Assistant Surgeon, Shriners Hospital for Crippled Children, San Francisco; Consultant to the Foot Surgery Clinic, University of California, San Francisco; Consultant in Foot Surgery, Highland General Hospital, Oakland.

James M. Morris, M.D.

Associate Professor of Orthopaedic Surgery, University of California, San Francisco; Active Staff, University of California Hospitals, San Francisco; Consultant, Laguna Honda Hospital, San Francisco

William R. Murray, M.D.

Professor of Orthopaedic Surgery, Vice Chairman, Department of Orthopaedic Surgery, and Chief, Orthopaedic Surgery Clinic, University of California, San Francisco; Chief, Orthopaedic Service, University of California Hospitals, San Francisco; Orthopaedic Consultant, Rheumatic Disease Group, University of California, San Francisco, and Langley Porter Neuropsychiatric Institute, San Francisco

Stanford F. Pollock, M.D.

Assistant Clinical Professor of Orthopaedic Surgery, University of California, San Francisco; Research Associate, Veterans Administration Hospital, San Francisco; Active Staff, Mills Memorial Hosppital, San Mateo

Robert L. Samilson, M.D.

Associate Clinical Professor of Orthopaedic Surgery, University of California, San Francisco; President, American Orthopaedic Foot Society; President-elect, American Academy for Cerebral Palsy; Active Staff, Children's Hospital and Adult Medical Center, University of California Hospitals, and Hahnemann Hospital, San Francisco; Consultant, Child Development Center of Children's Hospital

and Adult Medical Center, and Sunshine School, San Francisco

F. Scott Smyth, Jr., M.D.

Assistant Clinical Professor of Orthopaedic Surgery, University of California, San Francisco; Active Staff, Mills Memorial Hospital and Chope Hospital, San Mateo, and Peninsula Hospital, Burlingame

Elmer E. Specht, M.D.

Assistant Professor of Orthopaedic Surgery, University of California, San Francisco; Diplomate, American Board of Orthopaedic Surgery and American Board of Pediatrics

Foreword

Almost fifteen years have elapsed since Dr. DuVries' book on the foot emerged to fill a serious breach in the surgical literature. This it has done nobly and well to provide in a much neglected subject an important guide and reference work for the diagnosis, treatment, and management of pedal disabilities. Foot disabilities not only physically cripple but, even when minor, are among the most psychologically aggravating of disorders, interrupting and irritating men and women in their daily pursuits.

Therefore, it is a great privilege to welcome the third edition. In it the reader will find not only an extensive revision but a new emphasis with the addition of discussions on biomechanics, replacing the anatomic section more fully treated in standard basic texts. The change in emphasis recognizes that the foot is a complex mechanism that participates in the total harmony of the motion of the lower extremity, and is necessary for the fuller understanding of surgical procedures and their prognostic evaluation. In addition, the ankle as the joint of transition from leg to foot of necessity has been given consideration as an integral part affecting many of the problems of the foot. The volume will, I am sure, continue to advance the surgery of the foot as a practical treatise enriched in its new dimension.

J. B. deC. M. Saunders
M.D., LL.D., D.Sc., F.R.C.S.(E)
Regents Professor
University of California, San Francisco

Preface to third edition

When I accepted the job of editing the third edition of *Surgery of the Foot,* I was under the impression that few changes in the book were indicated except that some of the material needed to be updated. However, as I became more familiar with the contents I began to feel that some radical changes should be made. I discussed these changes with my fellow orthopaedists and questioned them, and podiatrists as well, as to what should and should not be incorporated in the new edition. I asked myself and consulted others as to who the purchasers of the third edition of this book would be and what material they would want and need covered in this revision.

Some interesting items evolved from these questions. Orthopaedists and podiatrists felt that they already possessed a good working knowledge of the anatomy of the foot but were woefully lacking in their understanding of the mechanics of the foot. Therefore, purely descriptive anatomy was deleted, and a discussion of the biomechanics of the foot was substituted.

The foot is not an isolated part of the locomotor system and must function through its attachment to the rest of the leg. In particular, definite relationships exist between the foot and the ankle, each affecting the other. Therefore, a discussion of the mechanics of the ankle as it influences the behavior of the foot, together with surgical procedures on the ankle, was added.

But the foot is not only a part of the whole locomotor system, it is a part of the whole body as well and is affected by systemic diseases and disabilities of the rest of the body. I have therefore included chapters on systemic diseases.

My responsibility as editor of the book led me also to take the liberty of rearranging much of the material in the body of the text. Discussions of the clinical disorders were separated from description of the surgical procedures necessary to correct the disorders.

The reason behind this separation of material seemed compelling, since many different surgical procedures have been employed for the same disability, and similar procedures have been employed for different pathologic conditions. Thus, I felt that the third edition could not be simply a book of surgical recipes for specific disorders. Instead, *all* the major surgical procedures performed on the ankle joint (such as open reduction, internal fixation of fractures, ligamentous repairs, arthrodeses, arthrotomies, synovectomies, and stabilization procedures) are discussed in the beginning section of Chapter 19, followed by a discussion of *all* of the major procedures performed on the talus (for example, talectomies and reconstructive procedures), those on the subtalar joint, the calcaneus, and so forth, down through the toes and nails. Procedures that are specific to specific disorders, such as treatment of a ganglion by excision and treatment of hallux rigidus by cheilectomy, will be found in the text preceding Chapter 19. Moreover, to make the book a good reference text, a short historical review of all the various procedures is given, so that surgeons who wish to learn the basic assumptions that led to the development of a particular surgical procedure or who wish to know the details of that procedure can find this information by means of the bibliography. The list of references is being enlarged to provide ready access to the pertinent literature.

I wish to express my appreciation to the members of the Department of Orthopaedic Surgery who have contributed chapters to this revised edition: to Dr. Charles D. Noonan, Associate Professor of Radiology, and Dr. Ronald J. Stoney, Assistant Professor of Surgery, for consultant services; to the residents in Orthopaedic Surgery who reviewed and described some of the surgical procedures; and to my editor, Mrs. Eleanor Haas, who not only worked very hard to make this book a success, but also contributed valuable insights. Finally, I wish to thank Dr. Henri L. DuVries for his continuing concern and important contributions to the work. I might add that if anyone has a copy of the first edition, he should keep it. It is an invaluable record of one man's lifelong experience with surgery of the foot.

Verne T. Inman

Preface to first edition

This book has been written in response to a continuing request by my students and colleagues that I draw together into one place of reference the fundamentals and the recommendations contained in my lectures and clinical demonstrations over a span of 30 years. As Frederic Wood Jones commented, "It is probably the experience of most teachers of anatomy that the student is generally better acquainted with the intimate structure of the hand than with that of the foot."* My friends among orthopaedic surgeons agree that the teaching of their specialty does not allot sufficient time to problems of the foot. They will forgive, therefore, and perhaps welcome as an adjunct to teaching, the elementary portions of the contents and the didactic approach.

Extreme disabilities of the foot, such as the talipes deformities, have received studious attention in published reports. They have on that account been given only a cursory nod of recognition here. This book is directed toward the commoner disabilities, which have been sparsely considered in medical writing and which have been widely neglected in teaching and practice.

The expanding awareness of the diversity of pathologic changes in the feet and of the complexities of treatment represents an advance since the days when all foot disabilities were always attributed to so-called fallen arches and when a prescription of arch supports satisfied the diagnostician that nothing further could be done about the patient whose feet continued to hurt.

This far from definitive effort of mine has reached the printed page through the encouragement and helpfulness, advice, and direction of so many of my friends and colleagues that I hesitate to name them lest by inadvertence one should be overlooked. If that happens, my deepest regret! Certainly I must mention my friends of long standing, Dr. August F. Daro; Dr. William M. Scholl, who turned his collection of photographs and anatomic models over to me for study and selective use and who has been otherwise helpful in so many ways; Dr. Ernest Nora, Sr., a constant friend since our medical school days, who reviewed the chapter on Tumors, Cysts, and Exostoses; so many on the Staff of Columbus Hospital; Dr. Carlo Scuderi, who reviewed the first rough material and then introduced me to my patient and cooperative publishers; Dr. Edwin Hirsch, who made the photographic

*Jones, F. W.: Structure and function as seen in the foot, London, 1944, Baillière, Tindall & Cox, Ltd., p. 3.

facilities of St. Luke's Hospital* available to me; Dr. Karl A. Meyer, my former professor in medical school, who wrote the Foreword as a final expression of years of encouragement. Dr. Edward L. Compere crowned my effort by writing the Introduction, having first reviewed some of the material in its early stages and, later, all in its final form.

Special credit should be given to Miss Ethel H. Davis for superbly editing and organizing the manuscript.

It is tempting to list those who gave me direction in one way or another: Dr. Peter A. Rosi, Dr. Charles N. Pease, Dr. Joseph P. Cascino, Dr. Steven O. Schwartz, Dr. Caesar Portes, Dr. Abe Rubin, and Dr. Harold Wheeler. The skill of my artists, Miss Edith Hodgson, Miss Gloria Jones, and Dr. Allen Whitney, must not go unsung. And to all, mentioned or not, in the measure of their interest, my gratitude!

Only wives whose husbands have attempted the writing of books and the husbands who have known the stamina of their wives during the process can appreciate how much meaning there is in my dedication to Frances DuVries.

*Now Presbyterian-St. Luke's Hospital.

Henri L. DuVries, D.P.M., M.D.
1959

Prefatory note to third edition

I am deeply indebted to Dr. Verne T. Inman for his diligent editing, his original contributions, and the extensive qualitative changes he made in the revision of this text.

It has been very gratifying to observe the tremendous interest and progress the healing arts have made in recent years in both the care and knowledge of the diseases and deformities of the human foot—disorders that, although they have comprised a most common human ailment, have been practically ignored in the past. This marked advancement is evidenced within the fields of orthopaedic surgery and podiatry, and in the quality of training that is presently offered in the colleges of podiatry.

My profound gratitude also goes to the faculty of the University of California School of Medicine in San Francisco for their extensive contributions to this edition. Much credit must be given to Eleanor Haas for her splendid editing of the manuscript, and to the artist Mark Mikulich for his excellent drawings, photographs, and x-ray illustrations.

Henri L. DuVries, D.P.M., M.D.
Oakland, California

Contents

Part one

1   Biomechanics of the foot and ankle, 3
Verne T. Inman and Roger A. Mann

2   Principles of examination of the foot and ankle, 23
Verne T. Inman

3   Ancillary diagnostic procedures, 44
S. William Levy and Verne T. Inman

Part two

4   Minor congenital deformities and anomalies of the foot, 51
Elmer E. Specht

5   Major congenital deformities and anomalies of the foot, 88
Elmer E. Specht

6   Fractures and fracture-dislocations of the foot and ankle, 119
Edwin G. Bovill, Jr., and Verne T. Inman

7   Traumatic injuries to the soft tissues of the foot and ankle, 168
James M. Glick

8   Acquired nontraumatic deformities of the foot, 204
Henri L. DuVries

9   Neuromuscular diseases affecting the foot, 268
Robert L. Samilson and Elmer E. Specht

10   Vascular and metabolic disorders affecting the foot, 282
William R. Murray and Verne T. Inman

11 Infectious disorders and noninfectious inflammatory diseases of the foot, 299
Stanford F. Pollock and James M. Morris

12 Disorders of the skin and toenails, 318
Henri L. DuVries

13 Local affections of the bones and soft tissues of the foot, 371
F. Scott Smyth, Jr.

14 Diseases of the nerves of the foot, 413
Roger A. Mann

Part three

15 Conservative treatment and office procedures, 425
Roger A. Mann

16 Operative principles and requirements, 435
Michael W. Chapman

17 Amputations, 443
Michael W. Chapman

18 Surgical approaches to the deep structures of the foot and ankle, 457
Verne T. Inman

19 Major surgical procedures for disorders of the ankle, tarsus, and midtarsus, 471
Verne T. Inman

20 Major surgical procedures for disorders of the forefoot, 506
Henri L. DuVries

Part one

1

Biomechanics of the foot and ankle

Verne T. Inman
Roger A. Mann

The initial chapters of this text on surgery will be devoted not to anatomy, as was done in the second edition, but to a discussion of the biomechanics of the foot and ankle. Specific relationships will be emphasized and some methods for functional evaluation of the foot will be presented. These alterations were initiated for several reasons.

First, it has been assumed that the orthopaedic surgeon possesses an accurate knowledge of the anatomic aspects of the foot and ankle. If this knowledge is lacking, textbooks of anatomy are available that depict in detail the precise anatomic structures that comprise this part of the human body. It seems redundant to devote space here to what can only be a superficial review of the anatomy of the foot and ankle.

Second, it seems mandatory that any textbook on surgery of the foot should begin with a discussion of the biomechanics of the foot and ankle as an integral part of the locomotor system. The human foot is an intricate mechanism that functions interdependently with other components of the locomotor system. No text is readily available to the surgeon that clearly enunciates the functional interrelationships of the various parts of the foot. Interference with the functioning of a single part may be reflected in altered functions of the re-

maining parts. Yet the surgeon is constantly called upon to change the anatomic and structural components of the foot. When so doing, he should be fully aware of the possible consequences of his actions.

Third, wide variations are known to occur in the component parts of the foot and ankle and these variations are reflected in the degree of contribution of each of these parts to the behavior of the entire foot. Depending on the contributions of an individual component, the loss or functional modification of that component by surgical intervention may result in either minimal or major alterations in the functional behavior of adjacent components. An understanding of basic interrelationships may assist the surgeon in explaining to himself why the same procedure performed on the foot of one person produced a satisfactory result while the result was unsatisfactory in another person.

Fourth, by being alert to the mechanical behavior of the foot, the physician may find that some foot disabilities caused by malfunction of a component part can be successfully treated by nonsurgical procedures rather than attacked surgically as has been customary. Furthermore, some operative procedures that fail to achieve completely the desired result can be further improved by minor alterations in the behavior of adjacent components through

3

shoe modification or the use of inserts. An understanding of the biomechanics of the foot and ankle should, therefore, be an essential aid in surgical decision-making and contribute to the success of postoperative treatment.

THE LOCOMOTOR SYSTEM

The human foot is too often viewed as a semirigid base, the principal function of which is to provide a stable support for the superincumbent body. In reality the foot is poorly designed for this purpose. Standing for prolonged periods of time can result in a feeling of fatigue or can produce actual discomfort in the feet. One always prefers to sit rather than stand. Furthermore, it is far less tiring to walk, run, jump, or dance on normally functioning feet—either barefooted or in comfortable shoes—than it is to stand. It appears, therefore, that the foot has evolved as a dynamic mechanism functioning as an integral part of the locomotor system and should be studied as such rather than as a static structure designed exclusively for support.

Since human locomotion involves all major segments of the body, it is obvious that certain suprapedal movements demand specific functions from the foot and that alterations in these movements from above may be directly reflected below by changes in the behavior of the foot. Likewise, the manner in which the foot functions may be reflected in patterns of movement in the other segments of the body. Therefore, the basic functional interrelationships between the foot and the remainder of the locomotor apparatus must be clearly understood.

To begin a review of the locomotor system, one must recognize that ambulating man is both a physical machine and a biologic organism. The former makes him subject to the physical laws of motion, the latter to the laws of muscular action. All characteristics of muscular behavior are exploited in locomotion; for example, when called upon to perform such external work as initiating or accelerating angular mo-

tion around joints, muscles rarely contract at lengths below their resting lengths (Bresler and Berry, 1951; Ryker, 1952; Close and Inman, 1953). When motion in the skeletal segments is decelerated or when external forces work upon the body, activated muscles become efficient. Activated muscles, in fact, are approximately six times as efficient when resisting elongation as they are when shortening to perform external work (Abbott et al., 1952; Asmussen, 1953; Banister and Brown, 1968). In addition, noncontractile elements in muscles and specific connective-tissue structures assist muscular action. Thus, human locomotion is a blending of physical and biologic forces, which compromise to achieve maximal efficiency at minimal cost.

Man uses a unique and characteristic orthograde bipedal mode of locomotion. This method of locomotion imposes gross similarities in the manner in which all of us walk. However, each of us exhibits minor individual differences that permit us to recognize a friend or acquaintance even when he is viewed from a distance. The causes of these individual characteristics of locomotion are many. Each of us differs somewhat in the length and distribution of mass of the various segments of the body—segments that must be moved by muscles of varying fiber lengths. Furthermore, individual differences occur in the position of axes of movement of the joints, with concomitant variations in effective lever arms. Such factors as these and many more combine to establish in each of us a final idiosyncratic manner of locomotion.

A smoothly performing locomotor system results from the harmonious integration of its many components. This final integration does not require that the specific contribution of a single isolated component be identical in every individual, nor must it even be identical within the same individual. The contribution of a single component varies under different circumstances. Type of shoe, amount of fatigue, weight of load carried, and other such variables can cause diminished functioning of some components with compensatory increased functioning of others. An enormous number of variations in the behavior of individual components is possible; however, the diversely functioning components, when integrated, are found to be complementary and will produce smooth bodily progression.

Average values of single anthropometric observations are in themselves of little value. The surgeon should be alert to the anthropometric variations that occur within the population, but it is more important for him to understand the functional interrelationships among the various components. This is particularly true in the case of the foot, where anatomic variations are extensive. If average values are the only bases of comparison, it becomes difficult to explain why some feet function adequately and asymptomatically, although their measurements deviate from the average, while others function symptomatically, even though their measurements approximate the average. It appears reasonable, therefore, to use average values only to provide a mathematical reference for demonstrating the extent of possible deviations from these averages. For these reasons, emphasis will be placed upon functional interrelationships and not upon descriptive anatomy.

Human locomotion is a learned process; it does not develop as the result of an inborn reflex. This statement is supported by Popova (1935), who studied the changing gait in growing children. The first few steps of an infant holding onto his mother's hand exemplify the learning process that is necessary to achieve orthograde progression. Scott (1969) of the Canadian National Institute for the Blind noted that congenitally blind children never attempt to stand and walk spontaneously but must be carefully taught. The result of this learning process is the integration of the neuromusculoskeletal mechanisms, with their gross similarities and individual variations, into an adequately functioning system of locomotion. Once a person has learned to walk and has attained maximal growth, there appears to be a built-in regulatory mechanism that will work whether the person is an amputee learning to use a new prosthesis, a long distance runner, or a woman wearing high heels. Ralston (1958) has noted that nature's sole aim with all of us seems to be to achieve a system that will take us from one spot to another with the least expenditure of energy.

THE KINEMATICS OF HUMAN LOCOMOTION

Walking is more than merely placing one foot before the other. During walking all major segments of the body are in motion and displacements of the body occur that can be accurately described.

Vertical displacements of the body

The rhythmic upward and downward displacement of the body during walking is familiar to everyone. It is particularly noticeable when someone is out of step in a parade. These displacements in the vertical plane are obviously a necessary concomitant of bipedal locomotion. When the legs are separated, as during the period of transmission of the body weight from one leg to the other (double weight bearing), the distance between the trunk and the floor must be less than when it passes over a relatively extended leg as it does during midstance. Since the nature of bipedal locomotion demands such vertical oscillations of the body, they should occur in a smooth manner for the conservation of energies. Fig. 1-1 shows that the center of gravity (C.G.) of the body does displace in a smooth sinusoidal path; its amplitude is approximately 4 to 5 cm. (Ryker, 1952; Saunders et al., 1953).

While movements of the pelvis and hip modify the amplitude of the sinusoidal pathway, the knee, ankle, and foot are particularly involved in converting what would be a series of intersecting arcs into a smooth, sinusoidal curve (Saunders et al., 1953). This conversion requires both

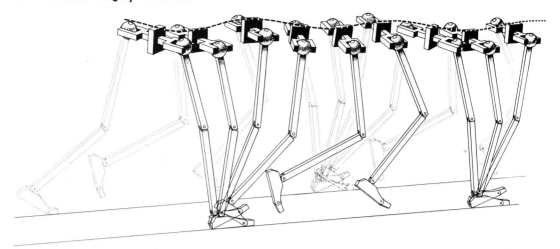

Fig. 1-1. Displacement of center of gravity (C.G.) of body in smooth sinusoidal path. (From Saunders, J. B. deC. M., Inman, V. T., and Eberhart, H. D.: J. Bone Joint Surg. **35-A:**552, 1953.)

simultaneous and precise sequential motions in the knee, ankle, and foot.

The center of gravity of the body reaches its maximal elevation immediately after its passage over the weight-bearing leg; it then begins to fall. This fall must be stopped at the termination of the swing phase of the other leg as the heel strikes the ground. If one were forced to walk stiff-kneed and without the foot and ankle, the downward deceleration of the center of gravity at this point would be instantaneous. The body would be subject to a severe jar and the locomotor system would lose kinetic energy. Actually the falling center of gravity of the body is smoothly decelerated, because relative shortening of the leg occurs at the time of impact against a gradually increasing resistance. The knee flexes against a graded contraction of the quadriceps muscle; the ankle plantar flexes against the resisting anterior tibial muscles. After foot flat position is reached, further shortening is achieved by pronation of the foot to a degree permitted by the ligamentous structures within it. While the occurrence of this pronatory movement is more important in regard to other functions of the foot, it must be mentioned here since

it constitutes an additional factor to that of knee flexion and ankle plantar flexion needed to smoothly decelerate and finally to stop the downward path of the body.

After decelerating to zero, the center of gravity must now evenly accelerate upward to propel it over the opposite leg. While the kinetics of this phenomenon are complex, the kinematics are simple. The leg is relatively elongated by transitory extension of the knee; further plantar flexion of the ankle elevates the heel, and supination of the foot occurs. Elevation of the heel is the major component contributing to upward acceleration of the center of gravity at this time.

Horizontal displacements of the body

In addition to vertical displacements of the body, a series of axial, rotatory movements occur, which can be measured in a horizontal plane. Rotations of the pelvis and the shoulder girdle are familiar to any observant person. Similar horizontal rotations occur in the femoral and tibial segments of the extremities. The tibias rotate about their long axes internally during swing phase and into the first part of stance phase, and rotate externally during the latter part of stance. This motion continues until the toes leave the ground; the degree of these rotations is subject to marked individual variations. Levens and co-workers (1948), in a study of a series of twelve male subjects, recorded the minimal amount of horizontal rotation of the tibia in space at 13 degrees and the maximal at 25 degrees, with an average of 19 degrees. A great portion of this rotation occurs when the foot is firmly placed on the floor; the shoe normally does not slip but remains fixed. The rotations, however, generate a torque of 7 to 8 newton-meters, which is one of considerable magnitude (Cunningham, 1950).

In order for these movements to occur, a mechanism must exist in the foot that will permit the rotations but will offer resistance to them of a magnitude such that they will be transmitted through the foot to the floor and will be recorded on the force plate as torques. The ankle and subtalar joints are such mechanisms and will be described.

Lateral displacement of the body

When a person is walking, his body does not remain precisely in the plane of progression, but oscillates slightly from side to side to keep the center of gravity approximately over the weight-bearing foot. Everyone has experienced this lateral shift of the body with each step but may not have consciously appreciated its cause. Everyone has at some time walked side by side with a companion. If one gets out of step with the other, their bodies are likely to bump (followed by appropriate apologies).

The body is shifted slightly over the weight-bearing leg with each step; therefore, there is a total lateral displacement of the body from side to side of approximately 4 to 5 cm. with each complete stride. This lateral displacement can be increased by walking with the feet more widely separated and decreased by keeping the feet close to the plane of progression (Fig. 1-2). Normally, the presence of

the tibiofemoral angle (slight genu valgum) permits the tibia to remain essentially vertical and the feet close together, while the femurs diverge to articulate with the pelvis. Again the lateral displacement of the body is through a smooth sinusoidal pathway.

THE KINETICS OF HUMAN LOCOMOTION

The only forces that can produce motion in the human body are obviously those created by gravity, by muscular activity, and in a few instances by the elasticity of specific connective tissue structures. A force plate is used to record accurately the gravitational effects upon the whole body while walking (Cunningham, 1950). The principle of the force plate can be demonstrated by the bathroom scale. When one stands on the scale quietly and then flexes and extends the knees to raise and lower the body, the indicator on the dial moves abruptly as vertical floor reaction is being registered.

The force plate records instantaneously the forces imposed by the body upon the foot, which are transmitted through the interface between the sole of the shoe and the walking surface. These measurements include vertical floor reactions, fore-and-aft shears, lateral shears, and horizontal torques. During the stance phase of walking, the floor reactions in all four categories are continuously changing. These changes indicate that the foot is being subjected to varying forces imposed upon it by movements of the superincumbent body.

While floor reactions are important in demonstrating the totality of these forces transmitted through the foot, they give little information concerning the movements in the several articulations of the foot and ankle or about the activity of the muscles controlling these movements. Continuous goniometric recordings and electromyographic studies are required to indicate joint motion and phasic activity of the intrinsic and extrinsic muscles.

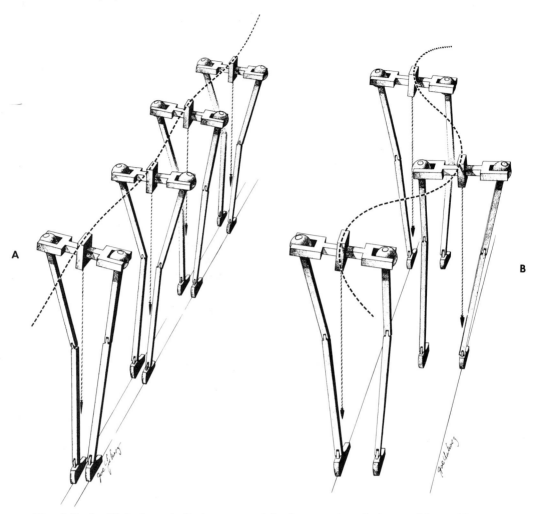

Fig. 1-2. A, Slight lateral displacement of body occurring during walking with feet close together. **B,** Increased lateral displacement of body occurring during walking with feet wide apart. (From Saunders, J. B. deC. M., Inman, V. T., and Eberhart, H. D.: J. Bone Joint Surg. **35-A**:552, 1953.)

From the moment of heel strike to the instant of toe-off, floor reactions, joint motions, and muscular activity are changing constantly. Thus, one cannot summarize this information for the entire period of stance and hope to even approximate what in reality is occurring in the foot and ankle. If, however, the stance phase is roughly divided into three intervals, a reasonably accurate summary of all factors can be presented. The division consists of the first interval, extending from heel strike to foot

flat; the second interval, occurring at the period of foot flat with the body passing over the foot; and the third interval, extending from the moment of heel rise to toe-off. The duration of the second interval is approximately twice as long as either the first or the third interval.

Many of the activities that occur during stance phase have been studied. Cunningham (1950) has recorded shifts in body weight reflected in floor reaction; Ryker (1952), and Wright et al. (1964) have re-

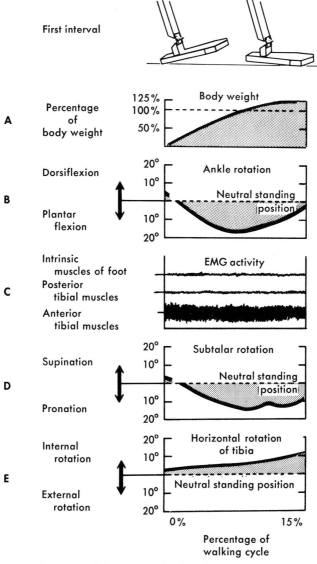

First interval

A   Percentage of body weight

B   Dorsiflexion / Plantar flexion

C   Intrinsic muscles of foot / Posterior tibial muscles / Anterior tibial muscles

D   Supination / Pronation

E   Internal rotation / External rotation

125%
100%
50%

Body weight

20°
10°

Ankle rotation

Neutral standing position

10°
20°

EMG activity

20°
10°

Subtalar rotation

Neutral standing position

10°
20°

20°
10°

Horizontal rotation of tibia

Neutral standing position

10°
20°

0%   15%

Percentage of walking cycle

Fig. 1-3. Composite of events of first interval of walking or period that extends from heel strike to foot flat.

corded ankle rotation; Mann and Inman (1964) have reported on the phasic activity of muscles; Wright et al. (1964) have reported studies of the action of the subtalar and ankle joint complex, which account for the amount of pronation or supination of the foot; and Levens et al. (1948) have recorded the rotation of the tibia during locomotion.

The walking cycle consists of the stance phase of one foot, including the double-weight-bearing period, and the swing phase of the same leg. The weight-bearing period, or stance phase, comprises, within a 5 percent variation, 65 percent of the entire cycle.

The first interval

The first interval occurs during approximately the first 15 percent of the walking cycle. The center of gravity of the body must be decelerated and then immediately accelerated to carry it over the extended leg. The heel's impact and shift of the center of gravity account for a vertical floor reaction that exceeds the body weight by 25 percent (Fig. 1-3, *A*). Characteristically, the first interval begins with plantar flexion of the ankle and continues toward dorsiflexion (Fig. 1-3, *B*).

During this first interval the anterior tibial and extensor muscles of the toes are functioning to prevent foot slap (Fig. 1-3, *C*). The triceps surae, the peroneals, and the tibialis posterior are all electrically quiet, as are the intrinsic muscles in the sole of the foot and the long flexors of the toes. There is no muscular response in those muscles that are usually considered important in supporting the longitudinal arch of the foot.

At this time the foot is being loaded with the weight of the body, and pronation of the foot occurs (Fig. 1-3, *D*). Careful inspection of the feet of individuals during walking will reveal this momentary pronation of the foot as it receives the impact of the body weight. It is interesting to note that this pronation of the foot is recorded as motion originating in the subtalar joint. The amount of pronation appears to depend entirely upon the joints of the foot— upon their capsular and extra-articular ligaments.

Because of the specific linkage of the leg to the foot through the subtalar articulation, pronation of the foot and internal rotation of the leg, as indicated by the direction of the curve in Fig. 1-3, *E*, must occur simultaneously.

The second interval

The second interval extends throughout 15 to 45 percent of the walking cycle. The center of gravity of the body has passed over the weight-bearing leg and has commenced to fall. The force plate records that the foot is now supporting less than the actual body weight. In normal walking, the least load on the foot may be only 50 to 60 percent of the actual body weight (Fig. 1-4, *A*). The second interval is characterized by relative dorsiflexion of the ankle as the body passes over the weight-bearing foot (Fig. 1-4, *B*).

During this second interval important functional changes occur in both the foot and the leg. These changes are the result of muscular action. The triceps surae, peroneals, tibialis posterior, long flexors of the toes, and all the intrinsic muscles in the sole of the foot spring into action (Fig. 1-4, *C*). The combined action of these muscles causes the heel to invert; supination of the foot, recorded as motion in the subtalar joint, begins (Fig. 1-4, *D*).

Since the forefoot is fixed to the floor, inversion of the heel must be accompanied by external rotation of the leg. The direction of the curve in Fig. 1-4, *E*, indicates the beginning of this rotation. The mechanical linkage provided by the subtalar joint makes this effect inevitable. It appears most fortuitous that these skeletal movements, which are produced by muscular effort, should occur while the foot is subjected to a load that is less than the total body weight. Furthermore, inversion of the heel with the forefoot fixed is the very process that transforms a flexible midfoot into a rigid structure. These rearrangements of the skeletal components of the foot, necessary in preparation for heel rise and push-off, can be demonstrated by simple manipulation of the normal foot (Fig. 1-5). Should they not occur at this time, abnormal stresses would be placed on the ligamentous structures of the foot, which could result in pain and disability.

The third interval

The third interval comprises the last third of stance phase, or the period that extends from 45 to 65 percent of the walking cycle. Force-plate recordings reflect an upward acceleration of the center of gravity at the beginning of this interval; the load on the foot again exceeds the body weight by approximately 25 percent. However, the vertical floor reaction promptly

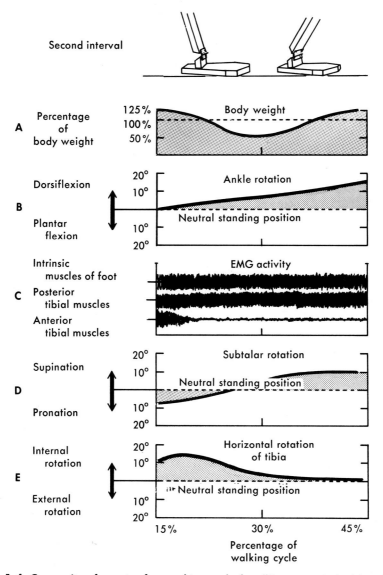

Second interval

Fig. 1-4. Composite of events of second interval of walking or period of foot flat.

falls to zero during this interval, since the body weight is being transferred to the other foot (Fig. 1-6, *A*). Plantar flexion of the foot occurs during this interval (Fig. 1-6, *B*). It is caused primarily by the contraction of the triceps surae and leads to relative elongation of the extremity.

During this phase the long flexors of the toes assist the triceps surae. The peroneals and tibialis posterior assist in plantar flexion but also stabilize the leg upon the foot. Additionally, the tibialis posterior functions to aid the intrinsic muscles in the sole of the foot, which cannot by themselves invert the heel and raise the longitudinal arch (Fig. 1-6, *C*). The inability of the intrinsic muscles to raise the arch is strikingly apparent in those individuals who have lost the function of the tibialis posterior through rupture or paralysis.

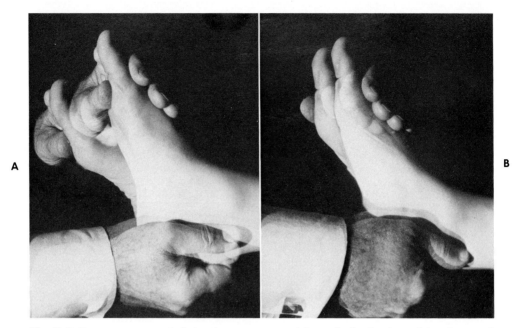

Fig. 1-5. Rearrangement of skeletal components of foot. **A,** Supination of forefoot and eversion of heel permitting maximal motion in all components of foot. **B,** Pronation of forefoot and inversion of heel resulting in locking of all components of foot, producing rigid structure.

During the third interval the foot progressively supinates (Fig. 1-6, *D*), and the leg continues to rotate externally (Fig. 1-6, *E*).

Another mechanism that aids the intrinsic muscles in the inversion of the heel and the raising of the longitudinal arch has been emphasized by Hicks (1954). Since the plantar aponeurosis is attached distally to the base of the proximal phalanges, extension of the metatarsophalangeal joints causes relative shortening of the plantar aponeurosis, which exerts tension upon the calcaneus, thus passively inverting the heel and raising the longitudinal arch. Hicks named this mechanism "windlass action" (Fig. 1-7).

AXES OF ROTATION
The ankle joint

It is easy to visualize that the direction of the ankle axis in the transverse plane of the leg will dictate the vertical plane in which the foot will flex and extend. In the clinical literature this plane of ankle motion in relation to the sagittal plane of the leg is referred to by orthopaedists as the degree of tibial torsion and by podiatrists as malleolar torsion. While it is common knowledge that the ankle axis is directed laterally and posteriorly as projected on the transverse plane of the leg, it is not widely appreciated that the ankle axis is also directed laterally and downward as seen in the coronal plane. Isman and Inman (1969), in anthropometric studies, found that in the coronal plane, the functional axis of the ankle may deviate from 88 to 68 degrees from the vertical axis of the leg (Fig. 1-8). Since the axis of the ankle passes just distally to the tip of each malleolus, the examiner may obtain a reasonably accurate estimate of the position of the axis by placing the ends of his index fingers at the most distal bony tips of the malleoli (Fig. 1-9).

A horizontal axis that remains normal to the vertical axis of the leg can only affect

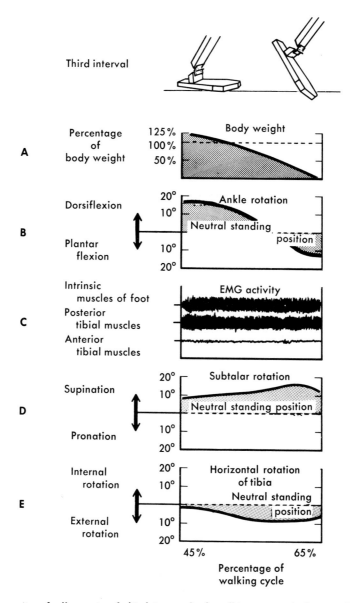

Fig. 1-6. Composite of all events of third interval of walking or period extending from foot flat to toe-off.

the amount of toeing out or toeing in of the foot; it cannot impose any rotatory influence in a transverse plane on either the foot or the leg during flexion and extension of the ankle. However, since the ankle joint axis is an obliquely oriented axis, it allows horizontal rotations to occur in the foot or the leg with movements of the ankle.

These rotations are clearly depicted in Figs. 1-10 and 1-11. With the foot free and the leg fixed, the oblique ankle joint axis causes the foot to deviate outward on dorsiflexion and inward on plantar flexion. The projection of the foot onto the transverse plane, as shown by the shadows in the sketches, reveals the extent of this external and internal rotation of the foot (see Fig. 1-10). The amount of this rotation will vary

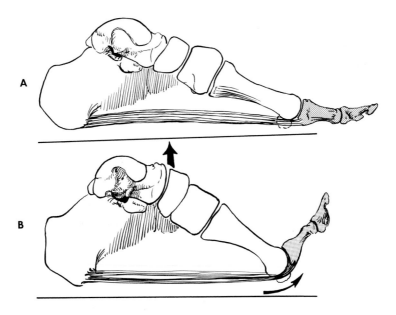

Fig. 1-7. Diagrammatic representation of "windlass action." **A,** Foot flat. **B,** Increased tension of plantar aponeurosis caused by dorsiflexion of toes, with resultant elevation of longitudinal arch.

Fig. 1-8. Variations in inclination of axis of ankle joint. (Derived from anthropometric studies of 107 cadaver ankles at the University of California, San Francisco.)

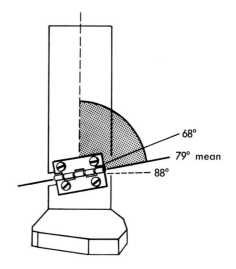

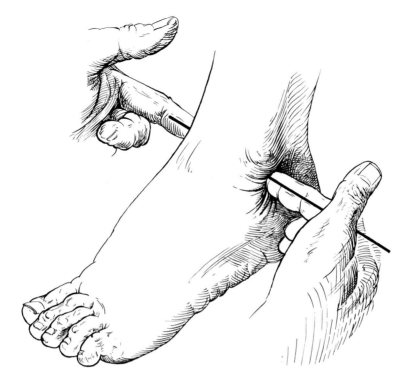

Fig. 1-9. Estimation of obliquity of ankle axis by palpating tips of malleoli.

with the obliquity of the ankle axis and the amount of dorsiflexion and plantar flexion.

With the foot fixed on the ground during midstance, the body passing over the foot produces dorsiflexion of the foot relative to the leg (see Fig. 1-11). The oblique ankle axis then imposes an internal rotation on the leg (Levens et al., 1948). Again, the degree of internal rotation of the leg on the foot will depend upon the amount of dorsiflexion and the obliquity of the ankle axis. As the heel rises in preparation for push-off, the ankle is plantar flexed. This in turn reverses the horizontal rotation, causing the leg to rotate externally.

When the horizontal rotations of the leg are studied independently, it is evident that this sequence of events is precisely what occurs in human locomotion. The lower part of the leg rotates internally during the first half and externally during the last half of stance. The average amount of this rotation is 19 degrees, within a range

of from 13 to 25 degrees (Levens et al., 1948). The recording of torques imposed on a force plate substantiates these rotations. Magnitudes vary from individual to individual but range from 7 to 8 newton-meters (Cunningham, 1950).

In summary, the oblique ankle axis produces the following series of events: from the instant of heel contact to the time the foot is flat, plantar flexion occurs and the foot appears to toe in. The more oblique the axis, the more apparent the toeing in. During midstance, the foot is fixed on the ground; relative dorsiflexion, with resulting internal rotation of the leg, occurs as the leg passes over the foot. As the heel rises, plantar flexion takes place, which results in external rotation of the leg.

Rotations of the leg and movements of the foot caused by an oblique ankle axis, when observed independently, are seen to be qualitatively and temporarily in agreement. However, when the magnitudes of the various displacements are studied, ir-

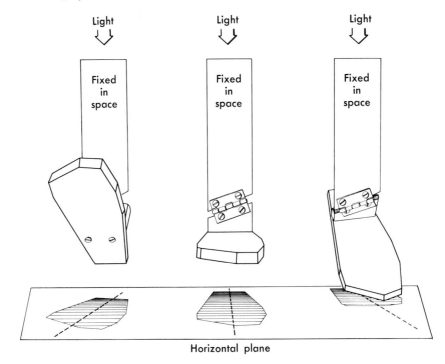

Fig. 1-10. Effect of obliquely placed ankle axis upon rotation of foot in horizontal plane during plantar flexion and dorsiflexion, with foot free. The displacement is reflected in the shadows of the foot.

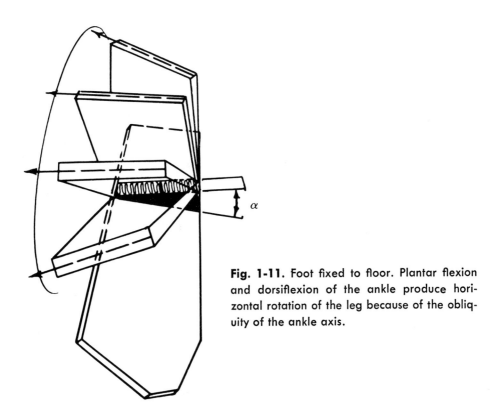

Fig. 1-11. Foot fixed to floor. Plantar flexion and dorsiflexion of the ankle produce horizontal rotation of the leg because of the obliquity of the ankle axis.

reconcilable disparities are evident. In normal locomotion ankle motion ranges from 20 to 36 degrees, with an average of 24 degrees (Ryker, 1952; Berry, 1952). The obliquity of the ankle axis ranges from 68 to 88 degrees, with an average of 78 degrees from the vertical (Isman and Inman, 1969). Even in the most oblique axis and movement of the ankle through the maximal range of 36 degrees, only 11 degrees of rotation of the leg around a vertical axis will occur. This is less than the average amount of horizontal rotation of the leg as measured independently in normal walking. The average obliquity of the ankle, together with the average amount of dorsiflexion and plantar flexion, would yield values for the horizontal rotation of the leg that are much smaller than the degree of horizontal rotation of the leg that actually occurs while the foot remains stationary on the floor and is carrying the superincumbent body weight.

The subtalar joint

It is necessary to examine other articulations in the foot that could, in cooperation with the ankle, allow the leg to undergo the additional amount of internal and external rotation. The mechanism that appears to be admirably designed for this very function is the subtalar joint.

The subtalar joint is a single-axis joint that acts like a mitered hinge connecting the talus and calcaneus. The direction of its axis is backward, downward, and lateral (Close and Inman, 1953; Manter, 1941). It should be noted that individual variations are extensive and imply variations in the behavior of this joint during locomotion. Furthermore, the subtalar joint appears to be a determinative joint of the foot, which influences the performance of the more distal articulations and modifies the forces imposed upon the skeletal and soft tissues. Therefore, it is mandatory to understand the anatomic and functional aspects of this joint.

Based upon the anatomic fact that the subtalar joint moves around a single in-

clined axis and functions essentially like a hinge connecting the talus and calcaneus, the functional relationships that result from such a mechanical arrangement are easily illustrated. Fig. 1-12, *A*, shows two boards joined by a hinge. If the axis of the hinge is at 45 degrees, a simple torque converter has been created. Rotation of the vertical member causes equal rotation of the horizontal member. Those who are mathematically inclined will readily appreciate that changing the angle of the hinge will alter this one-to-one relationship. A more horizontally placed hinge will cause a greater rotation of the horizontal member for each degree of rotation of the vertical member; the reverse holds true if the hinge is placed more vertically. In Fig. 1-12, *B*, to prevent the entire horizontal segment from participating in the rotatory displacement, the horizontal member has been divided into a short proximal and a long distal segment with a pivot in between. Thus, the distal segment remains stationary while only the short segment adjacent to the hinge rotates.

To approach more closely the true anatomic situation of the human foot, in Fig. 1-13, *A* and *B*, the distal portion of the horizontal member has been replaced by two structures. The medial represents the three medial rays of the foot that articulate through the cuneiforms to the talus; the lateral represents the two lateral rays that articulate through the cuboid to the calcaneus. In Fig. 1-13, *C* and *D*, the entire mechanism has been placed into the leg and foot to demonstrate that the mechanical linkages result in specific movements in the leg and the foot. External rotation of the leg causes inversion of the heel, elevation of the medial side of the foot, and depression of the lateral side. Internal rotation of the leg produces the opposite effect on the foot.

It is interesting to note that in persons with flatfoot the axis of the subtalar joint is more horizontal than in persons with "normal" feet, and that therefore the same amount of rotation of the leg imposes a

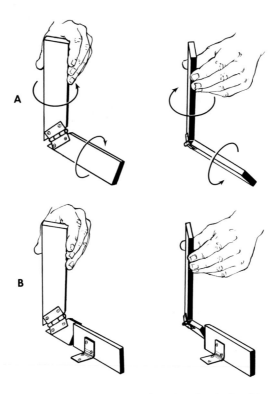

Fig. 1-12. Simple mechanism demonstrating functional relationships. **A,** Action of mitered hinge. **B,** Addition of pivot between two segments of mechanism.

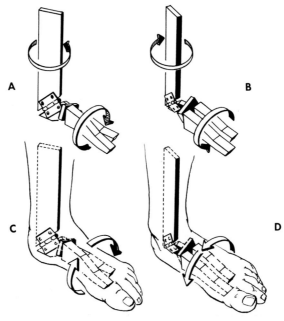

Fig. 1-13. Distal portion of horizontal member replaced by two structures. **A** and **B,** Mechanical analog of principal components of foot. **C** and **D,** Mechanical components inserted into foot and leg.

greater supinatory and pronatory effect upon the foot. This may partially explain why some individuals with asymptomatic and flexible pes planus break down their shoes and frequently prefer to go without shoes, which they find restrictive. Furthermore, the person with asymptomatic flatfoot usually shows a greater range of subtalar motion than does the person with "normal" feet. The reverse holds true for people with pes cavus; here one is often surprised at the generalized rigidity of the foot and the limited motion in the subtalar joint.

The transverse tarsal articulation

The calcaneocuboid and the talonavicular articulations together are often considered to comprise the transverse tarsal articulation. Each possesses some independent motion and has been subjected to intensive study (Elftman, 1960). However, from a functional standpoint they perform together. In most textbooks of anatomy, movement is described in the most general terms and as if the foot did not bear the weight of the body. The following statement is illustrative: Movement in the transverse tarsal articulation "consists of a sort of rotation by means of which the foot may be slightly flexed or extended, the sole being at the same time carried medially (inverted) or laterally (everted)."*

Actually, the importance of the transverse tarsal articulation lies not in its axes of motion while non–weight-bearing, but in how it behaves during the stance phase of motion when the foot is required to support the body weight. Some specific changes occur in the amount of motion sustained by the transverse tarsal articulation with the forefoot fixed and the heel everted or inverted. Everting the heel produces relative pronation of the foot; varying amounts of flexion and extension in the sagittal plane, adduction and abduction in the transverse plane, and rotation between

---

*Goss, C. M., editor: Gray's anatomy, ed. 28, Philadelphia, 1970, Lea & Febiger, p. 368.

the forefoot and the heel now occur. The examiner gets the impression that the midfoot has become "unlocked" and that maximal motion is possible in the transverse tarsal articulation. However, if the forefoot is held firmly in one hand, something happens in the transverse tarsal articulation to make it appear "locked." The previously elicited motions all become suppressed and the midfoot becomes rigid (see Fig. 1-5).

The mechanisms that might produce this dramatic change from flexibility to rigidity in the midfoot have not been adequately studied. Elftman (1960) has described one such mechanism, but others may exist that are as yet unidentified. In any case, inversion of the heel in the normal foot promptly occurs as weight is transferred from heel to forefoot when a person rises on the toes. As previously mentioned, such inversion of the heel causes the midfoot to convert from a mobile structure to a rigid lever. This reorientation of the skeletal components is obviously the result of activity in the intrinsic and extrinsic muscles of the foot, and also in the ligamentous structures.

The metatarsophalangeal break

After wearing a new pair of shoes for a while, one notices the appearance of an oblique crease in the area overlying the metatarsophalangeal articulation (Fig. 1-14). Its obliquity is due, of course, to the unequal forward extension of the metatarsals. The head of the second metatarsal is the most distal head; that of the fifth metatarsal is the most proximal. Although the first metatarsal is usually shorter than the second (because the first metatarsal head is slightly elevated and is supported by the two sesamoids), it often functionally approximates the length of the second.

When the heel is elevated during standing or at the time of push-off, the weight of the body is normally shared by all the metatarsal heads. To achieve this fair division of the body weight among the metatarsals, the foot must supinate slightly and deviate laterally. The oblique crease in the

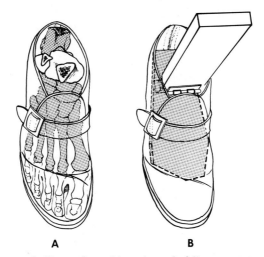

Fig. 1-14. Diagrammatic illustration of location of oblique metatarsophalangeal crease. **A,** Skeletal foot in one shoe. **B,** Wooden mechanism in other shoe.

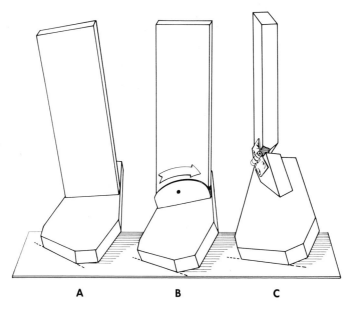

Fig. 1-15. Supination and lateral deviation of foot during raising of heel caused by oblique metatarsophalangeal break. **A,** Wooden mechanism without articulation. If no articulation were present the leg would also deviate laterally. **B,** Wooden mechanism with articulation. The leg remains vertical; hence some type of articulation must exist between the foot and the leg. **C,** Articulation similar to that of subtalar joint. It is fortuitous that in addition to its other complex functions, the subtalar joint also functions to permit the leg to remain vertical.

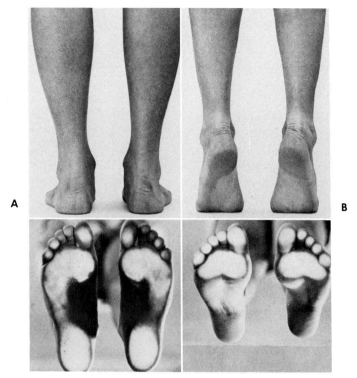

Fig. 1-16. Feet and legs of subject standing on barograph. **A,** Subject bearing weight, with muscles relaxed. **B,** Subject now rising on toes.

shoe gives evidence that these motions occur with every step. It has been demonstrated that the angle between the metatarsophalangeal break and the long axis of the foot may vary from 50 to 70 degrees (Isman and Inman, 1969). Obviously, the more oblique the metatarsophalangeal break the more the foot must supinate and deviate laterally.

If the leg and foot acted as a single rigid member without ankle, subtalar, or transverse tarsal articulations, the metatarsophalangeal break would cause lateral inclination and external rotation of the leg (Fig. 1-15, *A*). However, to permit the leg to remain in a vertical plane during walking, an articulation must be provided between leg and foot (Fig. 1-15, *B*). Such an articulation is supplied by the subtalar joint (Fig. 1-15, *C*). Because of its anatomic arrangement, it is ideally suited to permit the foot to respond to the supinatory

forces exerted by the oblique metatarsophalangeal break and still allow the leg to remain in a vertical plane.

All the essential mechanisms discussed in this chapter are pictorially summarized in Fig. 1-16. The two lower photographs were taken with the subject standing on a barograph; they reveal the distribution of pressure between the foot and the weight-bearing surface. (A barograph records reflected light through a transparent plastic platform; the intensity of the light is roughly proportionate to the pressure the foot imposes on the plate.)

In Fig. 1-16, *A*, the subject was asked to stand with muscles relaxed. Note that the leg is moderately rotated internally and the heel is slightly everted (in valgus position). The body weight is placed upon the heel, the outer side of the foot, and the metatarsal heads.

In Fig. 1-16, *B,* the subject was asked

to rise on the toes. Note that the leg is now externally rotated, the heel is inverted (in varus position), and the longitudinal arch is elevated. The weight is concentrated upon the metatarsal heads and is equally shared by the metatarsal heads and the toes.

Even though such movements cannot be illustrated pictorially, it is easy to imagine the contraction of the intrinsic and extrinsic muscles that is necessary to stabilize the foot and ankle as the subject transfers the body weight to the forefoot and raises the heel. It should also be recalled that dorsiflexion of the toes tightens the plantar aponeurosis and assists in the inversion of the heel. The supinatory twist activates the "locking" mechanism in the foot, thus converting a flexible foot (Fig. 1-16, *A*) into a rigid lever (Fig. 1-16, *B*), an action that is necessary at push-off.

REFERENCES

Abbott, B. C., Bigland, B., and Ritchie, J. M.: The physiological cost of negative work, J. Physiol. (London) 117:380-390, July 1952.

Asmussen, E.: Positive and negative muscular work, Acta Physiol. Scand. 28:364-382, 1953.

Banister, E. W., and Brown, S. R.: The relative energy requirements of physical activity. In Falls, H. B., editor: Exercise physiology, New York, 1968, Academic Press, pp. 292-294.

Berry, F. R., Jr.: Angle variation patterns of normal hip, knee and ankle in different operations. Prosthetic Devices Research Project, Institute of Engineering Research, University of California, Berkeley. Series 11, issue 21. Berkeley, The Project, Feb. 1952.

Bresler, B., and Berry, F. R.: Energy and power in the leg during normal level walking. Prosthetic Devices Research Project, Institute of Engineering Research, University of California, Berkeley. Series 11, issue 15, Berkeley, The Project, May 1951.

Close, J. R., and Inman, V. T.: The Action of the ankle joint. Prosthetic Devices Research Project, Institute of Engineering Research, University of California, Berkeley. Series 11, issue 22, Berkeley, The Project, April 1952.

Close, J. R., and Inman, V. T.: The Action of the Subtalar Joint. Prosthetic Devices Research Project, Institute of Engineering Research, University of California, Berkeley. Series 11, Issue 24, Berkeley, The Project, May 1953.

Cunningham, D. M.: Components of floor reactions during walking. Prosthetic Devices Research Project, Institute of Engineering Research, University of California, Berkeley. Series 11, issue 14, Berkeley, The Project, Nov. 1950.

Elftman, H.: The transverse tarsal joint and its control, Clin. Orthop. 16:41-45, 1960.

Hicks, J. H.: The mechanics of the foot. II. The plantar aponeurosis and the arch, J. Anat. 88:25-30, 1954.

Isman, R. E., and Inman, V. T.: Anthropometric studies of the human foot and ankle, Bull. Prosthetics Res. BPR 10-11: 97-129, Spring 1969.

Levens, A. S., Inman, V. T., and Blosser, J. A.: Transverse rotation of the segments of the lower extremity in locomotion. J. Bone Joint Surg. 30-A:859-872, Oct. 1948.

Mann, R., and Inman, V. T.: Phasic activity of intrinsic muscles of the foot, J. Bone Joint Surg. 46-A:469-481, April 1964.

Manter, J. T.: Movements of the subtalar and transverse tarsal joints, Anat. Rec. 80:397-410, Aug. 1941.

Popova, T.: Quoted in Issledovaniia po biodinamike lokomotsii, chapter 3, vol. 1; Biodinamika khod'by normal'nogo vzroslogo muzhchiny, edited by N. A. Bernshtein. Moscow: Idat. Vsesoiuz. Instit. Eksper. Med., 1935.

Ralston, H. J.: Energy-speed relation and optimal speed during level walking, Int. Z. Angew. Physiol. 17:277-283, 1958.

Ryker, N. J., Jr.: Glass walkway studies of normal subjects during normal level walking. Prosthetic Devices Research Project, Institute of Engineering Research, University of California, Berkeley. Series 11, issue 20, Berkeley, The Project, Jan. 1952.

Saunders, J. B. deC. M., Inman, V. T., and Eberhart, H. D.: The major determinants in normal and pathological gait, J. Bone Joint Surg. 35-A:543-558, July 1953.

Scott, E.: Personal communication.

Wright, D. G., Desai, M. E., and Henderson, B. S.: Action of the subtalar and ankle-joint complex during the stance phase of walking, J. Bone Joint Surg. 46-A:361-382, March 1964.

2

Principles of examination of the foot and ankle

Verne T. Inman

Fortunately, the foot, ankle, and leg are parts of the body that are readily accessible to adequate physical examination. Usually a specific diagnosis can be reached through proper physical examination and ancillary laboratory procedures are confirmatory. The techniques of examination available to the practitioner in his attempt to gather information concerning the foot and to make proper diagnoses vary with the age of the patient. In examining the preambulatory infant the practitioner must rely upon inspection, palpation, and manipulation. In examining the toddler, inspection, palpation, and manipulation may be supplemented with observations on the emerging patterns of locomotion. However, one should be aware that this period is one of experimentation for the child, and that his behavioral patterns are constantly changing. Since they may be based upon transitory findings, definitive surgical procedures at this stage of a child's development should be undertaken with caution. Only in the older child and in the adult can all the anatomic features and the functional behavior of the various components be realistically evaluated.

THE NEWBORN AND PREAMBULATORY INFANT— CONGENITAL ABNORMALITIES

Gross abnormalities of the lower limbs of children are easily recognized at birth or shortly thereafter. These congenital abnormalities present themselves in many different forms. During the past decade several attempts have been made to name and classify congenital limb defects based upon the site and extent of the skeletal abnormality. Universal acceptance and use of such a system of classification with its standardized nomenclature would do much to improve communication and to expedite the development of therapeutic principles. At present the various types of limb deficiencies are reasonably well classified under the general heading of dysmelia, with the subdivisions of ectromelia, phocomelia, and amelia. Other abnormalities of the lower limb are still classified under specific descriptive names.

It is impossible to be encyclopedic in a book of this nature. Therefore, we are providing the reader with an extensive bibliography at the end of this chapter as a vehicle for obtaining information of a more detailed nature than is offered in this book or for acquiring knowledge about deformities that occur infrequently. The following list attempts to be all-inclusive but should serve only as a reminder to the examiner. If more extensive discussions are available in chapters that follow, the chapter containing such discussion is indicated; if the subject is covered minimally or not at all, the reader is referred to the bibliography.

Dysmelia. Under this heading are found all limb deficiencies, including congenital absence of skeletal parts and aplasia. See Bibliography and Chapter 5.

Dimelia. For supernumerary bones and skeletal elements see Chapter 4.

Anterior or posterior bowing of the tibia. See Bibliography.

Length of leg discrepancies. See Bibliography.

Hemihypertrophy and local gigantism. See Bibliography and Chapter 4.

Calcaneovalgus foot. See Bibliography and Chapter 5.

Clubfoot. See Chapter 5.

Congenital metatarsus varus. See Chapter 5.

Congenital hammertoes. See Chapter 4.

Flatfoot. See Chapters 5 and 8.

The appearance of low arches in newborns and infants is primarily caused by the presence of fat deposits in the soles of the feet. However, it is mandatory during an examination to manipulate the feet gently in order to check the motion of the major articulations. There are two general categories of flatfoot—mobile and spastic—and the examiner should discern which type of flatfoot he is observing.

Mobile flatfoot. Mobile flatfoot is a condition in which there is a wide range of motion in the hindfoot and midfoot. The important factor to determine is whether there is a short tendo achillis that may impose abnormal forces on the foot when the child begins to walk.

Rigid flatfoot. In the presence of rigid flatfoot, passive inversion of the heel and pronation of the forefoot will not produce elevation of the longitudinal arch, which is the case in normal feet. Rigid flatfoot occurs in two conditions that should be recognized early: tarsal coalition and congenital vertical talus (see Chapter 5).

THE TODDLER

As the child begins to walk, it becomes possible to examine the behavior of all segments of the lower extremity and to observe the effects of weight-bearing upon them.

The degree of toeing in or toeing out should be observed. The position of the foot during stance is determined by: (1) the degree of anteversion or retroversion of the neck of the femur (see Bibliography); (2) tibial or malleolar torsion (see Bibliography); (3) the mobility of the major joints; and (4) the musculature.

The degree of anteversion or retroversion of the neck of the femur should be checked. This position may be clinically determined by noting the amount of passive internal and external rotation that is possible in the extended leg. Also, as the child walks, the position and degree of horizontal motion of the patellas should be observed.

Tibial or malleolar torsion is still a controversial subject among clinicians; the measurements reported by many investigators vary widely. However, it is clear that when the child sits on the edge of the examining table with the knees flexed and with the patellas and feet facing forward, the plane of the long axes of the feet should not deviate markedly from the sagittal plane.

The degree of pronation of the foot while the child walks or stands barefoot is readily observed by the examiner. By encouraging the child to rise on the toes or to walk on tiptoe, the examiner is quickly able to determine the mobility of the major joints and the adequacy of the musculature.

A rough check of the musculature can often be made by tickling the feet and observing the various displacements of the feet and toes. Possible shortening of the tendo achillis should be investigated.

THE OLDER CHILD AND ADULT

To prevent overlooking pertinent findings, every examiner should follow a rigorous routine. The particular routine adopted will vary depending upon personal preference and arrangement of office facilities. However, it appears appropriate to emphasize that no matter what procedure he adopts, the examiner must consider the foot and ankle from three different points of view.

First, the foot and ankle should be seen as parts of the entire body. Since their examination may reveal the presence of systemic disease, evidence of circulatory, metabolic, and cutaneous abnormalities should be sought.

Second, the foot and ankle should be considered as important constituents of the locomotor system. As has been previously discussed, they play reciprocal roles with the suprapedal segments; abnormal function of any part of the locomotor apparatus is reflected in adaptive changes in the remaining parts. Therefore, it is essential for the examiner to observe the patient walking over an appreciable distance in order to:

1. Detect obvious abnormalities of locomotion (for example, unequal step length or limp must be investigated)
2. Perceive asymmetrical behavior of the two sides of the body (for example, asymmetrical arm swing denotes unequal horizontal rotation of the components of the torso)
3. Observe the position of the patellas, which are indicators of the degree of horizontal rotation of the leg in the horizontal plane
4. Observe the degree of toeing in or out (toeing in or out that is relatively constant during the walking cycle indicates the degree of malleolar torsion; toeing in or out occurring only during the interval between heel strike and foot flat indicates the degree of obliquity of the ankle axis)
5. Observe the amount of pronation of the foot during the first half of stance-phase walking
6. Note the amount of heel inversion and supination of the foot during push-off, together with presence or absence of rotatory slippage of the forefoot on the floor (these motions indicate the amount of movement in the subtalar joint at that moment)

It must be stressed that one only sees what one is looking for. If the implications of the preceding statements are not readily apparent, it is suggested that the reader review Chapter 1 at this time.

Third, the human foot and ankle should be viewed as relatively recent evolutionary acquisitions; as such, they are subject to considerable individual anatomic and functional variation. It is regrettable that in most of the anatomic and orthopaedic literature, average values for the positions of axes of the major articulations and for ranges of motion about these axes are given (see Chapter 1). It so happens that an average individual is difficult to find, particularly among patients seeking help in the busy practitioner's office. The examiner should be aware of these variations and should also be cognizant of their functional implications. Only with such knowledge and insight will he be able to determine the proper therapeutic procedure to use and to evaluate realistically his success or failure with that procedure.

Sequence of examination

When examining the foot and ankle the examiner should follow the procedural sequence taught in courses in introductory physical diagnosis as closely as possible. After taking an adequate history, the examiner first *inspects,* then *palpates,* and finally (in an orthopaedic examination) *manipulates.* This sequence must be modified and repeated several times as the patient performs tasks with and without shoes, while walking, standing, and (for the sake of the examiner) sitting on the edge of the examining table. The following outline for the examination of the foot and ankle has proved adequate in our experience; to increase its value, annotations have been inserted to elucidate the significance of some findings and to explain the use of special diagnostic procedures. Even if one does not wish to adopt the routine as presented here, it may prove useful as a checklist.

The patient generally presents himself dressed in customary street clothes. It is usually convenient at that time for the examiner to observe the patient walking at various speeds, with shoes on, hands empty, and arms hanging freely at the sides. The following observations should be made:

Type of limp, if present. A pathologic condition of the lower extremity may produce a limp that is characteristic of the particular disorder. A patient with a painful hip, for example, will throw himself over the painful side during walking.

Type of shoe and height of heel. Since the type of shoe worn and its heel height affects the way a person walks, it must be noted. When wearing high heels, for example, women will show less ankle-joint motion than they will when wearing flat heels. When walking in tennis shoes, women show little difference from men in their gait.

Symmetry of arm swing. As a rule, the shoulders rotate 180 degrees out of phase with the pelvis; this is a passive response to pelvic rotation. If there are no abnormalities in the spine or upper extremities, rotation of the shoulders is reflected in equal and symmetrical arm swing. If the arm swing is asymmetrical, then horizontal rotation of the pelvis is also asymmetrical. Since such asymmetrical pelvic rotation may be the result of abnormality in any of the components of the lower extremity, it is mandatory that the practitioner take extra care in examining not only the foot and ankle, but the knees and hips as well.

Degree of toe-in or toe-out. At toe-off the leg has achieved its maximal external rotation and the foot toes out slightly. During swing phase the entire leg with its attached foot rotates internally. The average amount of this rotation is about 15 degrees but varies greatly among individuals. It may be almost imperceptible (3 degrees) or considerable (30 degrees) (Levens et al., 1948). At the time of heel strike the long axis of the foot has approached, to a varying degree, the plane of progression. The degree of parallelism between the long axis of the foot and the plane of progression at this point is subject to considerable individual variation. However, the transition from heel strike to foot flat, which occurs rapidly, should be carefully observed. Some individuals will show an increase in toe-in during this very short period of plantar flexion of the ankle, indicating a greater degree of obliquity of the ankle axis (see Chapter 1).

Amount of pronation of the foot during early stance phase. Normally, the foot will pronate as it is loaded with the body weight during the first half of stance phase. The amount of this pronation is subject to extreme individual variation. The important factor, however, is whether the foot remains pronated during the period of heel rise and push-off. In the normally functioning foot, as the heel rises, an almost instantaneous inversion of the heel occurs. If the heel fails to invert at this time, the examiner should check the strength of the intrinsic and extrinsic muscles of the foot, as well as the ranges of motion in the articulations of the hindfoot and midfoot.

Rotatory slippage of the shoe on the floor at push-off. Except on slippery surfaces, the shoe does not visibly rotate externally or slip on the floor at the time of push-off. Failure of the ankle and subtalar joints to permit adequate external rotation of the leg during this phase of walking may result in direct transmission of the rotatory forces to the interface between the sole of the shoe and the walking surface, with resultant rotatory slippage of the shoe on the floor. Upon noting this slippage, the examiner should look for possible muscular imbalance and should check the obliquity of the ankle axis and the range of motion in the subtalar joint.

Examination of shoes. While the patient is disrobing, it is convenient for the examiner to inspect the shoes and note the following:

1. The path of wear from heel to toe
2. Presence of supportive devices or corrections in the shoes (arch supports, Thomas heels, sole wedges, or metal tabs indicate previous difficulties)
3. Obliquity of the angle of the crease in the toe of the shoe (the angle varies from person to person; the greater the obliquity of the crease in the shoe to its long axis, the greater the amount of subtalar motion that is required to distribute the body weight evenly over the metatarsal heads)
4. The impression the forefoot has made on the insole of the shoe, which often gives important information about the patient's symptoms
5. Presence or absence of circular wear

on the sole of the shoe (such wear indicates rotatory slippage of the foot on the floor during push-off from suppressed subtalar motion)

The patient, now barefoot, is requested to walk. The same sequence of observations is repeated. Any gross abnormalities that were obscured by stockings and shoes can now be seen.

For the convenience of the examiner who is seated, the patient is next requested to stand before him upon a raised platform or lift, distributing his weight equally on the two feet. The examiner makes a preliminary evaluation of the patient's posture and a cursory inspection of the lower extremities from both front and back. He notes the following.

Presence of pelvic tilt. To estimate pelvic tilt from the front, the examiner places his index fingers on either the anterior superior iliac spines or the iliac crests; from the back, he observes the gluteal creases. An anatomic or functional shortening of one leg can readily be seen if the shortening is greater than one-quarter of an inch.

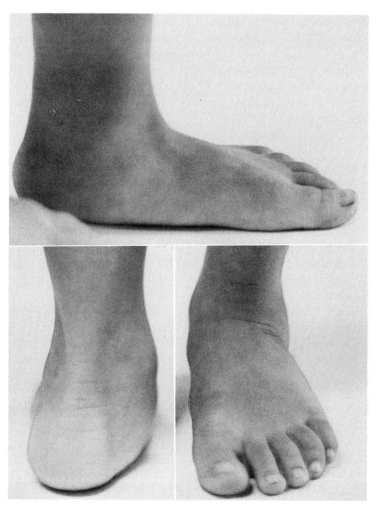

Fig. 2-1. One type of pes planus (flatfoot). Note depression of longitudinal arch, without everted heel, abducted forefoot, or longitudinal rotation of metatarsals and phalanges.

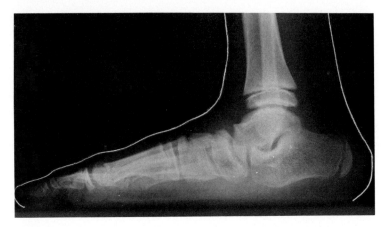

Fig. 2-2. Weight-bearing roentgenogram of foot of Negro youth. Note flatfoot and plantar flexed talus.

Inspection of the popliteal creases will reveal whether major shortening is in the thigh or in the leg.

Gross abnormalities of components of the lower extremity. These abnormalities include differences in circumferences of the thighs and calves, excessive deviations in skeletal alignment, and the degree of pes planus or pes cavus.

There appear to be at least two general categories of pes planus. In one category the longitudinal arch is depressed, without the complicating factors of everted heel, abducted forefoot, or longitudinal rotation of the metatarsals and phalanges (Fig. 2-1). This type of flatfoot is seen typically in individuals with a plantar flexed talus (Fig. 2-2). In the other category the foot appears to have fallen inward like the tilting of a half-hemisphere; the heel is everted, the outer border of the foot shows angulation at the midfoot, and the forefoot is abducted. In addition, there may be varying degrees of rotation of the metatarsals and phalanges around their long axes (Fig. 2-3). In the first category, the tendo achillis remains relatively straight; in the second, the tendo achillis deviates laterally when the patient bears weight upon the relaxed foot. The pathologic implications of these two types of flatfoot are different.

Movements occurring when the patient rises on his toes. When the patient is asked to raise his heels, the heel will promptly invert, the longitudinal arch will rise, and the leg will rotate externally if his foot is functioning normally. Failure of these movements to occur may indicate a weak foot or a specific pathologic process. Since inversion of the heel is achieved through proper performance of the subtalar and transverse tarsal articulations, failure to invert the heel should immediately focus the examiner's attention upon possible malfunction of these structures. Conditions that may limit activity in these joints are muscular weakness, rupture or weakness of the tibialis posterior, arthritic changes in the subtalar joint, and such skeletal abnormalities as vertical talus and tarsal coalition.

Windlass action. Normally, dorsiflexion of the toes increases the tension of the plantar aponeurosis, which causes the longitudinal arch to rise (Fig. 2-4, *A* and *B*). Failure of the longitudinal arch to do so suggests the presence of prolonged pes planus with attendant abnormal stretching and elongation of the plantar aponeurosis (Fig. 2-4, *C* and *D*).

Stability of the subtalar joint. The weight-bearing line of the body normally falls medial to the axis of the subtalar joint; therefore, when the patient stands on one foot with muscles relaxed, the foot pronates. Because of the linkage between the

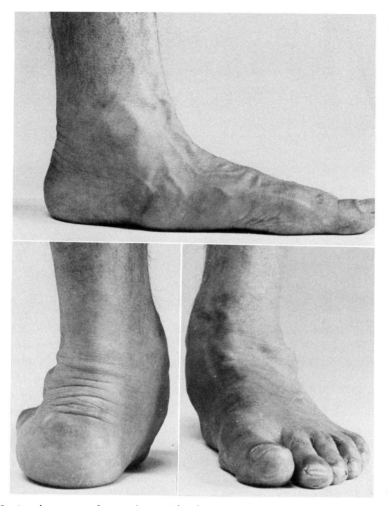

Fig. 2-3. Another type of pes planus. The foot appears to have fallen inward like a half-hemisphere.

foot and the leg provided by the subtalar articulation, when the examiner rotates the leg externally the heel will invert and the weight-bearing line will move laterally. This position creates a metastable state, which, in the normal foot, extends over a moderate range of longitudinal rotation of the leg (10 to 15 degrees). When the examiner exerts minimal external rotatory force upon the leg with his hand, the patient's full body weight can be transmitted through the hindfoot to the floor. However, in some patients this metastable state cannot be achieved even if the examiner applies maximal external rotatory force to the leg. In others, the metastable state is so tenuous that if the examiner exerts a few degrees of internal or external rotatory force upon the leg, the foot will promptly pronate or supinate.

The patient is now instructed to sit on the examining table with his legs and feet hanging over the side. A more detailed examination is now possible:

Examination of the surface of the foot, ankle, and leg. Any vascular abnormalities such as varicosities, areas of telangiectasia, and edema should be noted. The dorsalis pedis and posterior tibial pulses should be palpated. The speed of capillary filling

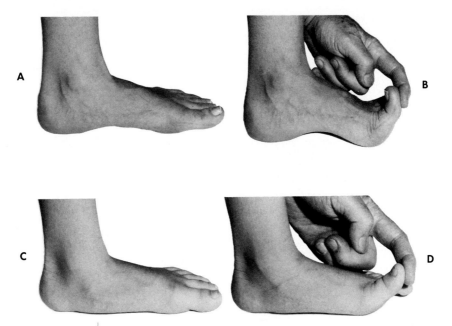

Fig. 2-4. A, "Normal" weight-bearing foot. **B,** Same foot. Dorsiflexion of the great toe causes elevation of the arch because of the windlass action of the aponeurosis. **C,** Flat weight-bearing foot. **D,** Dorsiflexion of great toe. In this foot, dorsiflexion does not cause the arch to rise.

after compression of the nail bed should be checked. The skin over joints is normally cooler than the skin over muscular areas of the extremity; inflammatory processes in or around deep structures result in increased temperature of the overlying skin. The examiner, by gently passing his hand over the extremity, can frequently localize "hot spots" that, when located, should alert him to investigate the underlying components.

Appraisal of skeletal structures. Gross skeletal deformities are readily discernible and can hardly be overlooked even by the most inexperienced examiner. Difficulties in making a diagnosis are more likely to arise in patients whose feet, on casual inspection, appear to be relatively normal.

Ranges of motion

Having described a sequential examination in some detail, it appears appropriate at this juncture to discuss techniques of eliciting other pertinent information.

The passive ranges of motion of all the major articulations of the foot should be rapidly checked for limitation of motion, painful movement, and crepitus. These symptoms may occur separately or in any combination.

The ankle joint should be moved through its full range of motion. Although the ankle is essentially a single-axis joint, its axis is skewed to both the transverse and the coronal planes of the body; it passes downward and backward from the medial to the lateral side. A reasonably accurate estimate of the location of the ankle axis can be obtained by placing the tips of the index fingers just below the most distal projections of the two malleoli (Fig. 2-5). Depending upon the degree of obliquity of the axis, dorsiflexion and plantar flexion produce medial and lateral deviation of the foot. If the examiner has noted previously that the patient tended to toe in during the interval between heel strike and foot flat, an oblique axis of the ankle as projected on the coronal plane of the body

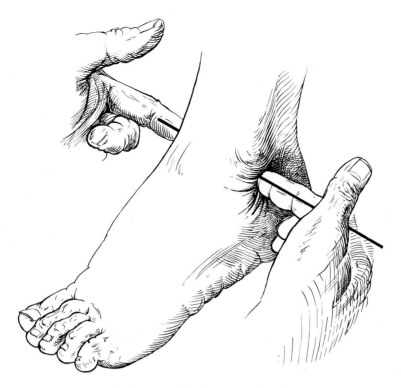

Fig. 2-5. Estimating location of ankle axis.

is to be expected. Since an oblique axis of the ankle will assist in absorbing the horizontal rotation of the leg, its range of motion is related to the range of motion in the subtalar joint. Thus, range of subtalar motion should also be estimated.

It may be recalled that the amount of motion in the subtalar joint varies; however, Isman and Inman (1969) found that in a series of feet in cadaver specimens a minimum of 20 and a maximum of 60 degrees of motion was present. The simplest method of determining the degree of subtalar motion is to apply rotatory force on the calcaneus while permitting the rest of the foot to move passively. When rotatory force is applied to the forefoot, abnormally large displacements may be obtained through movements of the articulations in the midfoot that are additive to subtalar motion. By far the most accurate method of determining the degree of subtalar motion is to place the patient prone and flex his knee

to approximately 135 degrees. The axis of the subtalar joint now lies close to the horizontal plane. The examiner then passively inverts and everts the heel while he measures the extent of motion by attaching a gravity goniometer, or level, to the calcaneus, using a metal spring clip (Fig. 2-6). Lack of subtalar motion should alert the examiner to the possibility of an arthritic process in the subtalar joint, of peroneal spastic flatfoot, or of an anatomic abnormality such as tarsal coalition.

Normally there is no lateral play of the talus in the mortise even when the foot is in full plantar flexion. Any lateral displacement that can be imposed on the talus in its mortise by the examiner is indicative of abnormal widening of the mortise. Frequently the talus can be displaced forward and backward a millimeter or so in the mortise, but this is a normal finding.

Occasionally a degree of lateral talar tilt can be demonstrated in the normal ankle joint in the following manner: The

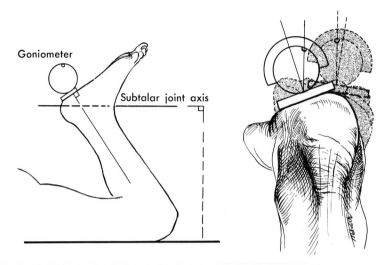

Fig. 2-6. Spherical goniometer attached to calcaneus to measure degree of subtalar motion.

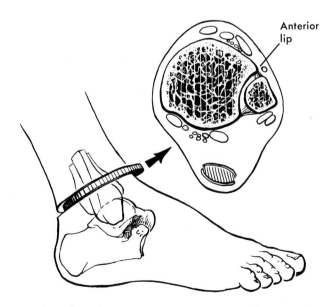

Fig. 2-7. Cross section of leg just proximal to ankle joint, showing fibula nestled in its groove in tibia. Note the prominent anterior lip. (Adapted from Eycleshymer, A. C., and Shoemaker, D. M.: A cross-section anatomy, New York, 1970, Appleton-Century-Crofts.)

examiner places the ankle in full plantar flexion, thus displacing the trochlea anteriorly. He forcibly inverts the foot while placing his thumb just in front of the lateral malleolus and pressing against the anterior portion of the trochlea. He can then feel a slight medial rocking of the talus. Excessive talar tilt should alert the examiner to suspect injury to the lateral ligaments.

Ligamentous and muscular structures

The attachments of the collateral ligaments of the ankle should be palpated for tenderness. The deltoid, anterior talofibular, and calcaneofibular ligaments are readily palpable. The posterior talofibular ligament is too deeply situated to be felt.

Injuries to the distal fibular syndesmosis are too frequently overlooked by orthopaedists, even though patients with such injuries may suffer pain when walking, jumping, and running. The construction of this articulation is such that the fibula is nestled into a groove on the lateral side of the tibia (Fig. 2-7). The anterior lip of the tibial groove is prominent while the posterior lip is much less pronounced. When attempting to displace the fibula anteriorly in an uninjured ankle, the examiner cannot elicit movement. However, even in a normal ankle the examiner frequently can feel movement when he attempts to displace the fibula posteriorly. Rarely can he initiate an increase in anterior displacement of the fibula in patients who have sustained injuries to the ligamentous structures supporting the syndesmosis; only occasionally does the attempt produce an increase in pain. He can, however, usually initiate an increase in posterior displacement and is likely to elicit the particular pain of which the patient complains. In all patients who complain of vague ankle pain when they walk, run, or jump, the stability of the fibular syndesmosis should be investigated.

The ability of the heel to invert adequately determines the effectiveness of the foot to fulfill its role as a rigid lever at the time of push-off. Should inversion of the heel be insufficient to achieve skeletal stability, abnormal stresses may be placed upon the ligamentous and muscular components of the foot. Such stresses may produce areas of tenderness, which should be sought by applying deep pressure upon the following structures:

The plantar aponeurosis. This area should be palpated along its entire surface. Dorsiflexion of the toes will make the fascia more prominent and will facilitate palpation (Fig. 2-8).

The calcaneal tuberosity. The plantar aponeurosis is attached proximally to the calcaneal tuberosity. Tenderness in this area is indicative of abnormal tension in the aponeurosis. The presence of calcaneal spur is confirmatory evidence of this condition.

The plantar calcaneonavicular (spring) ligament. The examiner can most effectively test for tenderness by applying pressure to the area immediately below the head of the talus, with the foot completely relaxed.

The calcaneocuboid, talonavicular, and cuneonavicular articulations

Abnormal stresses are often imposed upon the capsular structures of the joints of the midfoot; hence, these articulations should all be palpated for areas of tenderness and should be stressed for pain.

Of course, no examination is complete without a rough check of the strengths of the various major muscle groups controlling the movements of the foot and ankle. Abnormal shortening of the triceps surae should always be investigated. In patients with pes planus, the examiner frequently finds that a shortened triceps surae will prevent sufficient dorsiflexion of the foot to allow the heel, if held in inversion, to contact the floor. Until the tendon is surgically lengthened or the triceps surae is stretched by assiduous exercise, wedged heels, heel cups, inserts, and arch supports will probably be ineffective. To check the degree of shortening the examiner

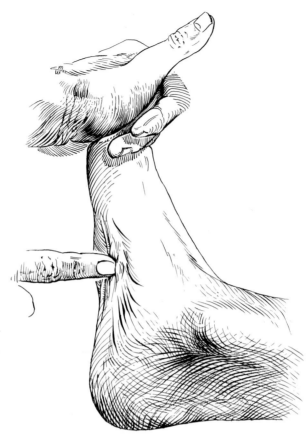

Fig. 2-8. Palpation of plantar aponeurosis facilitated by dorsiflexion of toes.

should initiate forceful dorsiflexion of the foot with the heel in a fully inverted position. He may determine whether the shortening is in the soleus, the gastrocnemius, or both, by checking the amount of dorsiflexion with the knee extended and with the knee flexed. In the latter position, the gastrocnemius is relaxed.

Metatarsalgia

Pain in the region of the metatarsophalangeal articulation is a frequent complaint. When it occurs in the first metatarsophalangeal joint, it is usually caused by: (1) lateral angulation of the first phalanx (hallux valgus), with or without medial exostosis and overlying bunion, (2) injury or degenerative changes with resultant arthritis (hallux rigidus), or (3) arthritic changes in the sesamoid articulation. The latter changes are frequently overlooked, partic-

ularly when hallux valgus is present, in which case the sesamoids may be displaced laterally. Fractures of the sesamoids are infrequent and must be distinguished from bipartite sesamoids. When the patient reacts with pain to pressure or attempted displacement of the sesamoids, an abnormality should be suspected.

The second metatarsal is "dadoed" between the three cuneiform bones, making it relatively immobile in relation to the midfoot. It is usually the longest of the metatarsals. Unless the foot is free to deviate laterally, the second metatarsal takes an undue share of the body weight at pushoff—weight that otherwise would be distributed among the other metatarsals. Frequently the concentration of forces on the second metatarsal head is revealed by the presence of plantar callosities.

Many types of metatarsalgia are commonly seen in women who wear heels that are too high to permit adequate lateral deviation of the foot. Other causes of the concentration of body weight upon the second metatarsal with resultant pain in that area of the foot are: (1) absolute weakness of the intrinsic muscles of the foot, with functional inability to depress adequately the more movable metatarsals and (2) insufficient supination of the forefoot at push-off because of functional abnormality of the midfoot and hindfoot.

Peripheral nerves

When the patient complains of a burning type of pain, often accompanied by a feeling of numbness, he should be given a careful sensory examination. Such complaints are often indicative of peripheral nerve disorder and may be early symptoms of a generalized neuritis or neuropathy. The examiner should check not only for deficits in cutaneous sensation, but also for diminished positional and vibratory sensation.

Two areas exist in the foot where peripheral nerves may be locally entrapped and irritated: (1) the place where the posterior tibial nerve passes posteriorly to the medial malleolus (tarsal tunnel syndrome) and (2) the place where the digital nerves (particularly the second and third digital nerves) pass between the metatarsal heads (Morton's neuralgia). Patients with tarsal tunnel syndrome experience pain when pressure is applied to the back of the medial malleolus; they may respond with a positive Tinel sign to percussion of this area. Patients with Morton's neuralgia experience characteristic pain when pressure is applied to the interspaces between the metatarsal heads. Evidence of delayed conduction time confirms the presence of peripheral nerve abnormality.

REFERENCES

Isman, R. E., and Inman, V. T.: Anthropometric studies of the human foot and ankle, Bull. Prosthetics Res. BPR 10-11:97-129, Spring 1969.
Levens, A. S., Inman, V. T., and Blosser, J. A.: Transverse rotation of the segments of the lower extremity in locomotion, J. Bone Joint Surg. 30-A:859-872, Oct. 1948.

BIBLIOGRAPHY
Classifications and general discussion
Burtch, R. L.: Nomenclature for congenital skeletal limb deficiencies: A revision of the Frantz and O'Rahilly classification, Artif. Limbs 10:24-35, Spring 1966.
Frantz, C. H., and O'Rahilly, R.: Congenital skeletal limb deficiencies, J. Bone Joint Surg. 43-A:1202-1224, Dec. 1961.
Henkel, L., and Willert, H. G.: Dysmelia: A classification and a pattern of malformation in a group of congenital defects of the limbs, J. Bone Joint Surg. 51-B:399-414, Aug. 1969.
O'Rahilly, R.: Morphological patterns in limb deficiencies and duplications, Amer. J. Anat. 89:135-187, Sept. 1951.
Wiedemann, H. R.: Derzeitiges Wissen über Exogenese von Missbildungen im Sinne von Embryopathien beim Menschen. Med. Welt. 24:1343-1349, June 1962.

Congenital absence of the fibula and tibia
Aitken, G. T.: Amputation as a treatment for certain lower-extremity congenital anomalies, J. Bone Joint. Surg. 41-A:1267-1285, Oct. 1959.
Coventry, M. B., and Johnson, E. W.: Congenital absence of the fibula, J. Bone Joint Surg. 34-A:941-956, Oct. 1952.
Dankmeijer, J.: Congenital absence of the tibia, Anat. Rec. 62:179-194, June 1935.
Dennison, W. M.: Delayed ossification of the tibia in apparent congenital absence, Brit. J. Surg. 28:101-105, July 1940.
Duraiswami, P. K.: Experimental causation of congenital skeletal defects and its significance in orthopaedic surgery, J. Bone Joint Surg. 34-B:646-698, Nov. 1952.
Evans, E. L., and Smith, N. R.: Congenital absence of tibia, Arch. Dis. Child. 1:194-229, 1926.
Farmer, A. W., and Laurin, C. A.: Congenital absence of the fibula, J. Bone Joint Surg. 42-A:1-12, Jan. 1960.
Frantz, C. H., and O'Rahilly, R.: Congenital skeletal limb deficiencies, J. Bone Joint Surg. 43-A:1202-1224, Dec. 1961.
Gaenslen, F. J.: Congenital defects of tibia and fibula, Amer. J. Orthop. Surg. 12:453-481, 1914.
Gray, J. E.: Congenital absence of the tibia, Anat. Rec. 101:265-273, July 1948.
Harmon, P. H., and Fahey, J. J.: The syndrome of congenital absence of the fibula: Report of three cases with special reference to pathogenesis and treatment, Surg. Gynec. Obstet. 64:876-887, May 1937.

Harris, R. I.: The history and development of Syme's amputation, Artif. Limbs 6:4-43, April 1961.

Kruger, L. M., and Talbott, R. D.: Amputation and prosthesis as definitive treatment in congenital absence of the fibula, J. Bone Joint Surg., 43-A:625-642, July 1961.

Nutt, J. J., and Smith, E. E.: Total congenital absence of the tibia, Amer. J. Roentgenol. Radium Ther. Nucl. Med. 46:841-849, Dec. 1941.

Ollerenshaw, R.: Congenital defects of the long bones of the lower limbs: A contribution to the study of their causes, effects, and treatment, J. Bone Joint Surg. 7:528-552, July 1925.

Putti, V.: The treatment of congenital absence of the tibia or fibula, Int. Abstr. Surg. 50:42, Jan. 1930.

Thompson, T. C., Straub, L. R., and Arnold, W. D.: Congenital absence of the fibula, J. Bone Joint Surg. 39-A:1229-1237, Dec. 1957.

Wood, W. L., Zlotsky, N., and Westin, G. W.: Congenital absence of the fibula: Treatment by Syme amputation—indications and technique, J. Bone Joint Surg. 47-A:1159-1169, Sept. 1965.

Congenital bowing and pseudarthrosis of the tibia

Aegerter, E. E.: The possible relationship of neurofibromatosis, congenital pseudarthrosis, and fibrous dysplasia, J. Bone Joint Surg. 32-A:618-626, July 1950.

Aegerter, E. E., and Kirkpatrick, J. A., Jr.: Orthopedic diseases, ed. 2, Philadelphia, 1963, W. B. Saunders Co.

Badgley, C. E.: Primary and secondary congenital deformities. In American Academy of Orthopaedic Surgeons, Instructional Course Lectures, vol. 10, Ann Arbor, 1953, J. W. Edwards, pp. 158-160.

Badgley, C. E., O'Connor, S. J., and Kudner, D. F.: Congenital kyphoscoliotic tibia, J. Bone Joint Surg. 34-A:349-371, April 1952.

Barber, C. G.: Congenital bowing and pseudarthrosis of the lower leg: Manifestations of von Recklinghausen's neurofibromatosis, Surg. Gynec. Obstet. 69:618-626, Nov. 1939.

Birkett, A. N.: Note on pseudarthrosis of the tibia in childhood, J. Bone Joint Surg. 33-B:47-49, July 1941.

Boyd, H. B., and Fox, K. W.: Congenital pseudarthrosis: Follow-up study after massive bone grafting, J. Bone Joint Surg. 30-A:274-283, April 1948.

Crenshaw, A. H., editor: Campbell's operative orthopaedics. vol. 2, ed. 5, St. Louis, 1971, The C. V. Mosby Co., pp. 1947-1953.

Charnley, J.: Congenital pseudarthrosis of the tibia treated by the intramedullary nail, J. Bone Joint Surg. 38-A:283-290, April 1956.

Compere, E. L.: Localized osteitis fibrosa in the new-born and congenital pseudarthrosis, J. Bone Joint Surg. 18:513-523, April 1936.

Duraiswami, P. K.: Experimental causation of congenital skeletal defects and its significance in orthopaedic surgery, J. Bone Joint Surg. 34-B:646-698, Nov. 1952.

Eyre-Brook, A. L., Baily, R. A. J., and Price, D. H. G.: Infantile pseudarthrosis of the tibia: Three cases treated successfully by delayed autogenous by-pass graft, with some comments on the causative lesion, J. Bone Joint Surg. 51-B:604-613, Nov. 1969.

Freund, E.: Congenital defects of femur, fibula, and tibia, Arch. Surg. 33:349-376, Sept. 1936.

Green, W. T., and Rudo, N.: Pseudarthrosis and neurofibromatosis, Arch. Surg. 46:639-651, May 1943.

Hallock, H.: The use of multiple small bone transplants in the treatment of pseudarthrosis of the tibia of congenital origin or following osteotomy for the correction of congenital deformity, J. Bone Joint Surg. 20:648-660, July 1938.

Henderson, M. S.: Congenital pseudarthrosis of the tibia, J. Bone Joint Surg. 10:483-491, July 1928.

Heyman, C. H., and Herndon, C. H.: Congenital posterior angulation of the tibia, J. Bone Joint Surg. 31-A:571-580, July 1949.

Heyman, C. H., Herndon, C. H., and Kingsbury, G. H.: Congenital posterior angulation of the tibia with talipes calcaneus, J. Bone Joint Surg. 41-A:476-488, April 1959.

Jaffe, H. L.: Tumors and tumorous conditions of the bones and joints, Philadelphia, 1958, Lea & Febiger.

Kite, J. H.: Congenital pseudarthrosis of tibia and fibula: Report of fifteen cases, South. Med. J. 34:1021-1032, Oct. 1941.

Kite, J. H.: Congenital deformities of lower extremity. In Bancroft, F. W., and Marble, H. C., editors: Surgical treatment of the motor-skeletal system, ed. 2, vol. 1, Philadelphia, 1951, J. B. Lippincott Co., pp. 55-62.

Krida, A.: Congenital posterior angulation of the tibia: A clinical entity unrelated to congenital pseudarthrosis, Amer. J. Surg. 82:98-102, July 1951.

Madsen, E. T.: Congenital angulation and fractures of extremities, Acta Orthop. Scand. 25:242-280, 1956.

McElvenny, R. T.: Congenital pseudo-arthrosis of the tibia, Northwestern Univ. Med. School Quart. Bull. 23:413-423, Winter 1949.

McFarland, B.: "Birth fracture" of the tibia, Brit. J. Surg. 27:706-712, April 1940.

McFarland, B.: Pseudarthrosis of the tibia in childhood, J. Bone Joint Surg. 33-B:36-46, Feb. 1951.

Middleton, D. S.: Studies on prenatal lesions of striated muscle as a cause of congenital deformity, Edinburgh Med. J. 41:401-442, July 1934.

Milgram, J. E.: Impaling (telescoping) operation for pseudarthrosis of long bones in childhood, Bull. Hosp. Joint Dis. 17:152-172, Oct. 1956.

Moore, B. H.: Some orthopaedic relationships of neurofibromatosis, J. Bone Joint Surg. 23:109-140, Jan. 1941.

Moore, J. R.: Delayed autogenous bone graft in the treatment of congenital pseudarthrosis, J. Bone Joint Surg. 31-A:23-39, Jan. 1949.

Moore, J. R.: Congenital pseudarthrosis of the tibia. In American Academy of Orthopaedic Surgeons, Instructional Course Lectures, vol. 14, Ann Arbor, 1957, J. W. Edwards, pp. 222-237.

Nicoll, E. A.: Infantile pseudarthrosis of the tibia, J. Bone Joint Surg. 51-B:589-592, Nov. 1969.

Purvis, G. D., and Holder, J. E.: Dual bone graft for congenital pseudarthrosis of the tibia: Variations of technic, South. Med. J. 53:926-931, July 1960.

Sofield, H. A., and Millar, E. A.: Fragmentation, realignment, and intramedullary rod fixation of deformities of the long bones in children. A ten-year appraisal, J. Bone Joint Surg. 41-A:1371-1391, Dec. 1959.

Williams, E. R.: Two congenital deformities of the tibia. Congenital angulation and congenital pseudarthrosis, Brit. J. Radiol. 16:371-376, Dec. 1943.

Wilson, P. D.: A simple method of two-stage transplantation of the fibula for use in cases of complicated and congenital pseudarthrosis of the tibia, J. Bone Joint Surg. 23:639-675, July 1941.

Congenital vertical talus

Axer, A.: Into-talus transposition of tendons for correction of paralytic valgus foot after poliomyelitis in children, J. Bone Joint Surg. 42-A:1119-1142, Oct. 1960.

Dickson, J. W.: Congenital vertical talus, J. Bone Joint Surg. 44-B:229, Feb. 1962.

Eyre-Brook, A. L.: Congenital vertical talus, J. Bone Joint Surg. 49-B:618-627, Nov. 1967.

Grice, D. S.: The role of subtalar fusion in the treatment of valgus deformities of the feet. In American Academy of Orthopaedic Surgeons, Instructional Course Lectures, vol. 16, St. Louis, 1959, The C. V. Mosby Co., pp. 127-150.

Hark, F. W.: Rocker-foot due to congenital subluxation of the talus, J. Bone Joint Surg. 32-A:344-350, Apr. 1950.

Harrold, A. J.: Congenital vertical talus in infancy, J. Bone Joint Surg. 49-B:634-643, Nov. 1967.

Herndon, C. H., and Heyman, C. H.: Problems in the recognition and treatment of congenital convex pes valgus, J. Bone Joint Surg. 45-A:413-429, Mar. 1963.

Heyman, C. H.: The diagnosis and treatment of congenital convex pes valgus or vertical talus. In American Academy of Orthopaedic Surgeons, Instructional Course Lectures, vol. 16, St. Louis, 1959, The C. V. Mosby Co., pp. 117-126.

Hughes, J. R.: On congenital vertical talus, J. Bone Joint Surg. 39-B:580, Aug. 1957.

Lamy, L., and Weissman, L.: Congenital convex pes valgus, J. Bone Joint Surg. 21:79-91, Jan. 1939.

Lloyd-Roberts, G. C., and Spence, A. J.: Congenital vertical talus, J. Bone Joint Surg. 40-B:33-41, Feb. 1958.

Mead, N. C., and Nast, G.: Vertical talus (congenital talonavicular dislocation), Clin. Orthop. 21:198-203, 1961.

Osmond-Clarke, H.: Congenital vertical talus, J. Bone Joint Surg. 38-B:334-341, Feb. 1956.

Outland, T., and Sherk, H. H.: Congenital vertical talus, Clin. Orthop. 16:214-218, 1960.

Silk, F. F., and Wainwright, D.: The recognition and treatment of congenital flat foot in infancy, J. Bone Joint Surg. 49-B:628-633, Nov. 1967.

Steindler, A.: Orthopedic operations, Springfield, 1940, Charles C Thomas, Publisher, p. 458.

Stone, K. H.: Congenital vertical talus: A new operation, Proc. Roy. Soc. Med. 56:12-14, Jan. 1963.

Thompson, J. E. M.: Treatment of congenital flatfoot, J. Bone Joint Surg. 28:787-790, Oct. 1946.

Townes, P. L., DeHart, G. K., Hecht, F., and Manning, J. A.: Trisomy 13-15 in a male infant, J. Pediat. 60:528-532, Apr. 1962.

Uchida, I. A., Lewis, A. J., Bowman, J. M., and Wang, H. C.: A case of double trisomy: Trisomy No. 18 and triplo-x, J. Pediat. 60:498-502, Apr. 1962.

Wainwright, D.: The recognition and cure of congenital flat foot, Proc. Roy. Soc. Med. 57:357-364, May 1964.

White, J. W.: Congenital flatfoot: A new surgical approach, J. Bone Joint Surg. 22:547-554, July 1940.

Whitman, A.: Astragalectomy and backward displacement of the foot: An investigation of its practical results, J. Bone Joint Surg. 4:266-278, Apr. 1922.

Hemihypertrophy and gigantism

Bryan, R. S., Lipscomb, P. R., and Chatterton, C. C.: Orthopedic aspects of congenital hypertrophy, Amer. J. Surg. 96:654-659, Nov. 1958.

Charters, A. D.: Local gigantism, J. Bone Joint Surg. 39-B:542-547, Aug. 1957.

Goidanich, I. F., and Campanacci, M.: Vascular hamartomata and infantile angioectatic osteohyperplasia of the extremities: A study of ninety-four cases, J. Bone Joint Surg. 44-A:815-842, July 1962.

Hutchison, W. J., and Burdeaux, B. D., Jr.: The influence of stasis on bone growth, Surg. Gynec. Obstet. 99:413-420, Oct. 1954.

Peabody, C. W.: Hemihypertrophy and hemiatrophy: Congenital total unilateral somatic asymmetry, J. Bone Joint Surg. 18:466-474, Apr. 1936.

Pease, C. N.: Local stimulation of growth of long bones, J. Bone Joint Surg. 34-A:1-24, Jan. 1952.

Peremans, G.: An unusual case of congenital asymmetry of the pelvis and of the lower extremities, J. Bone Joint Surg. 5:331-338, Apr. 1923.

Sabanas, A. O., and Chatterton, C. C.: Crossed congenital hemihypertrophy, J. Bone Joint Surg. 37-A:871-874, July 1955.

Strobino, L. J., French, G. O., and Colonna, P. C.: The effect of increasing tensions on the growth of epiphyseal bone, Surg. Gynec. Obstet. 95:694-700, Dec. 1952.

Thomas, H. B.: Partial gigantism: Overgrowth and asymmetry of bones and skeletal muscle, Amer. J. Surg. 32:108-112, Apr. 1936.

Trueta, J.: The influence of the blood supply in controlling bone growth, Bull. Hosp. Joint Dis. 14:147-157, Oct. 1953.

Ward, J., and Lerner, H. L.: A review of the subject of congenital hemihypertrophy and a complete case report, J. Pediat. 31:403-414, Oct. 1947.

Inequality of length of leg

Abbott, L. C.: The operative lengthening of the tibia and fibula, J. Bone Joint Surg. 9:128-152, Jan. 1927.

Aitken, A. P.: Overgrowth of the femoral shaft following fracture in children, Amer. J. Surg. 49:147-148, July 1940.

Anderson, M. S., Green, W. T., and Messner, M. B.: Growth and predictions of growth in the lower extremities, J. Bone Joint Surg. 45-A:1-14, Jan. 1963.

Arkin, A. M., and Katz, J. F.: The effects of pressure on epiphyseal growth, J. Bone Joint Surg. 38-A:1057-1076, Oct. 1956.

Barfod, B., and Christensen, J.: Fractures of the femoral shaft in children with special references to subsequent overgrowth, Acta Chir. Scand. 116:235-250, 1958-1959.

Barr, J.: Growth and inequality of leg length in poliomyelitis, N. Eng. J. Med. 238:737-743, May 1948.

Barr, J. S., Lingley, J. R., and Gall, E. A.: The effect of roentgen irradiation on epiphyseal growth. I. Experimental studies upon the albino rat, Amer. J. Roentgenol. Radium Ther. Nucl. Med. 49:104-115, Jan. 1943.

Barr, J. S., Stinchfield, A. J., and Reidy, J. A.: Sympathetic ganglionectomy and limb length in poliomyelitis, J. Bone Joint Surg. 32-A:793-802, Oct. 1950.

Bell, J. S., and Thompson, W. A. L.: Modified spot scanography, Amer. J. Roentgenol. Radium Ther. Nucl. Med. 63:915-916, June 1950.

Bisgard, J. D.: Longitudinal bone growth: The influence of sympathetic deinnervation, Ann. Surg. 97:374-380, March 1933.

Bisgard, J. D., and Bisgard, M. E.: Longitudinal growth of long bones, Arch. Surg. 31:568-578, Oct. 1935.

Blount, W. P.: Unequal leg length in children, Surg. Clin. N. Amer. 38:1107-1123, Aug. 1958.

Blount, W. P.: Unequal leg length. In American Academy of Orthopaedic Surgeons, Instructional Course Lectures, vol. 17, St. Louis, 1960, The C. V. Mosby Co., pp. 218-245.

Blount, W. P., and Clarke, G. R.: Control of bone growth by epiphyseal stapling: A preliminary report, J. Bone Joint Surg. 31-A:464-478, July 1949.

Blount, W. P., and Zeier, F.: Control of bone length, J.A.M.A. 148:451-457, Feb. 1952.

Bohlman, H. R.: Experiments with foreign materials in the region of the epiphyseal cartilage plate of growing bones to increase their longitudinal growth, J. Bone Joint Surg. 11:365-384, Apr. 1929.

Bost, F. C., and Larsen, L. J.: Experiences with lengthening of the femur over an intramedullary rod, J. Bone Joint Surg. 38-A:567-584, June 1956.

Brockway, A., Craig, W. A., and Cockrell, B. R., Jr.: End-result of sixty-two stapling operations, J. Bone Joint Surg. 36-A:1063-1069, Oct. 1954.

Brodin, H.: Longitudinal bone growth, the nutrition of the epiphyseal cartilages and the local blood supply, Acta Orthop. Scand. (Suppl.) 20:1-92, 1955.

Brookes, M.: Femoral growth after occlusion of the principal nutrient canal in day-old rabbits, J. Bone Joint Surg. 39-B:563-570, Aug. 1957.

Cameron, B. M.: A technique for femoral-shaft shortening: A preliminary report, J. Bone Joint Surg. 39-A:1309-1313, Dec. 1957.

Carpenter, E. B., and Dalton, J. B.: A critical evaluation of a method of epiphyseal stimulation, J. Bone Joint Surg. 38-A:1089-1094, Oct. 1956.

Compere, E. L., and Adams, C. O.: Studies of longitudinal growth of long bones. I. The influence of trauma to the diaphysis, J. Bone Joint Surg. 19:922-936, Oct. 1937.

Dalton, J. B., Jr., and Carpenter, E. B.: Clinical experiences with epiphyseal stapling, South. Med. J. 47:544-550, June 1954.

David, V. C.: Shortening and compensatory overgrowth following fractures of the femur in children, Arch. Surg. 9:438-449, Sept. 1924.

Doyle, J. R., and Smart, B. W.: Stimulation of bone growth by short-wave diathermy, J. Bone Joint Surg. 45-A:15-24, Jan. 1963.

Duthie, R. B.: The significance of growth in orthopaedic surgery, Clin. Orthop. **14:**7-19, Summer 1959.

Ferguson, A. B.: Surgical stimulation of bone growth by a new procedure: Preliminary report, J.A.M.A. **100:**26-27, Jan. 1933.

Ferguson, A. B.: Growth as a factor in relation to deformity and disease. In American Academy of Orthopaedic Surgeons, Instructional Course Lectures, vol. 9, Ann Arbor, 1952, J. W. Edwards, pp. 97-103.

Ford, L. T., and Key, J. A.: A study of experimental trauma to the distal femoral epiphysis in rabbits, J. Bone Joint Surg. **38-A:**84-92, Jan. 1956.

Gardner, E.: The development and growth of bones and joints. In American Academy of Orthopaedic Surgeons, Instructional Course Lectures, vol. 13, Ann Arbor, 1956, J. W. Edwards, pp. 235-246.

Gatewood and Mullen, B. P.: Experimental observations on the growth of long bones, Arch. Surg. **15:**215-221, Aug. 1927.

Geiser, M., and Trueta, J.: Muscle action, bone rarefaction and bone formation: An experimental study, J. Bone Joint Surg. **40-B:**282-311, May 1958.

Gelbke, H.: The influence of pressure and tension on growing bone in experiments with animals, J. Bone Joint Surg. **33-A:** 947-954, Oct. 1951.

Gill, G. G., and Abbott, L. C.: Practical method of predicting the growth of the femur and tibia in the child, Arch. Surg. **45:**286-315, Aug. 1942.

Goetz, R. H., Du Toit, J. G., and Swart, B. H.: Vascular changes in poliomyelitis and the effect of sympathectomy on bone growth, Acta Med. Scand. (Suppl.) **306:**56-83, 1955.

Goff, C. W.: Growth determinations, In American Academy of Orthopaedic Surgeons, Instructional Course Lectures, vol. 8, Ann Arbor, 1951, J. W. Edwards, pp. 160-168.

Goff, C. W.: Surgical care of unequal extremities: Measuring and predicting growth. In American Academy of Orthopaedic Surgeons, Instructional Course Lectures, vol. 16, St. Louis, 1959, The C. V. Mosby Co., pp. 219-231.

Goff, C. W.: Surgical treatment of unequal extremities, Springfield, 1960, Charles C Thomas, Publisher.

Green, W. T.: Discussion following prediction of unequal growth of the lower extremities in anterior poliomyelitis, J. Bone Joint Surg. **31-A:** 485, July 1949.

Green, W. T., and Anderson, M.: Experiences with epiphyseal arrest in correcting discrepancies in length of the lower extremities in infantile paralysis, J. Bone Joint Surg. **29:**659-675, July 1947.

Green, W. T., and Anderson, M.: Discrepancy in length of the lower extremities, In American Academy of Orthopaedic Surgeons, Instructional Course Lectures, vol. 8, Ann Arbor, 1951, J. W. Edwards, pp. 295-305.

Green, W. T., and Anderson, M.: The problem of unequal leg length, Pediat. Clin. N. Amer. **2:**1137-1155, Nov. 1955.

Green, W. T., and Anderson, M.: Epiphyseal arrest for the correction of discrepancies in length of the lower extremities, J. Bone Joint Surg. **39-A:**853-872, July 1957.

Green, W. T., and Anderson, M.: Skeletal age and control of bone growth. In American Academy of Orthopaedic Surgeons, Instructional Course Lectures, vol. 17, St. Louis, 1960, The C. V. Mosby Co., pp. 199-217.

Green, W. T., Wyatt, G. M., and Anderson, M. S.: Orthoroentgenography as a method of measuring the bones of the lower extremities, J. Bone Joint Surg. **28:**60-65, Jan. 1946.

Gruelich, W. W., and Pyle, S. I.: Radiographic atlas of skeletal development of the hand and wrist, Stanford, 1950, Stanford University Press.

Greville, N. R., and Ivins, J. C.: Fractures of the femur in children. An analysis of their effect on the subsequent length of both bones of the lower limb, Amer. J. Surg. **93:**376-384, Mar. 1957.

Greville, N. R., and Janes, J. M.: An experimental study of overgrowth after fractures, Surg. Gynec. Obstet. **105:**717-721, Dec. 1957.

Gullickson, G., Jr., Olson, M., and Kottke, F. J.: The effect of paralysis of one lower extremity on bone growth, Arch. Phys. Med. Rehabil. **31:**392-400, June 1950.

Haas, S. L.: The relation of the blood supply to the longitudinal growth of bone, Amer. J. Orthop. Surg. **15:**157, 305, 1917.

Haas, S. L.: Interstitial growth in growing long bones, Arch. Surg. **12:**887-900, April 1926.

Haas, S. L.: Retardation of bone growth by a wire loop, J. Bone Joint Surg. **27:**25-36, Jan. 1945.

Haas, S. L.: Restriction of bone growth by pins through the epiphyseal cartilaginous plate, J. Bone Joint Surg. **32-A:**338-343, 350, Apr. 1950.

Haas, S. L.: Femoral shortening in subtrochanteric region combined with angulation at site of resection, Amer. J. Surg. **80:**461-463, Oct. 1950.

Haas, S. L.: Stimulation of bone growth, Amer. J. Surg. **95:**125-131, Jan. 1958.

Harris, H. A.: The growth of the long bones in childhood. (With special reference to certain bony striations of the metaphysis and to the role of vitamins.) Arch. Intern. Med. **38:**785-806, Dec. 1926.

Harris, H. A.: Lines of arrested growth in the long bones in childhood: The correlation of histological and radiographic appearances in clinical and experimental conditions, Brit. J. Radiol. 4:561-588, 1931.

Harris, H. A.: Bone growth in health and disease, London, 1933, Oxford University Press.

Harris, R. I., and McDonald, J. L.: The effect of lumbar sympathectomy upon the growth of legs paralyzed by anterior poliomyelitis, J. Bone Joint Surg. 18:35-45, Jan. 1936.

Hayes, J. T., and Brody, G. L.: Cystic lymphangiectasis of bone, J. Bone Joint Surg. 43-A:107-117, Jan. 1961.

Herndon, C. H., and Spencer, G. E.: An experimental attempt to stimulate linear growth of long bones in rabbits, J. Bone Joint Surg. 35-A:758-759, July 1953.

Hiertonn, T.: Arteriovenous anastomoses and acceleration of bone growth, Acta Orthop. Scand. 26:322, 1956.

Hutchison, W. J., and Burdeaux, B. D.: The influence of stasis on bone growth, Surg. Gynec. Obstet. 99:413-420, Oct. 1954.

James, C. C. M., and Lassman, L. P.: Spinal dysraphism: The diagnosis and treatment of progressive lesions in spina bifida occulta, J. Bone Joint Surg. 44-B:828-840, Nov. 1962.

Janes, J. M., and Musgrove, J. E.: Effect of arteriovenous fistula on growth of bone: An experimental study, Surg. Clin. N. Amer. 30:1191-1200, 1950.

Kruger, L. M., and Talbott, R. D.: Amputation and prosthesis as definitive treatment in congenital absence of the fibula, J. Bone Joint Surg. 43-A:625-642, July 1961.

Maresh, M. M.: Linear growth of long bones of extremities from infancy through adolescence, Amer. J. Dis. Child. 89:725-742, 1955.

Marino-Zuco, C.: Treatment of length discrepancy of the lower limbs, J. Bone Joint Surg. 38-B:934, Nov. 1956.

Moore, B. H.: A critical appraisal of the leg lengthening operation, Amer. J. Surg. 52:415-423, June 1941.

Morgan, J. D., and Somerville, E. W.: Normal and abnormal growth at the upper end of the femur, J. Bone Joint Surg. 42-B:264-272, May 1960.

Neer, C. S., II, and Cadman, E. F.: Treatment of fractures of the femoral shaft in children, J.A.M.A. 163:634-637, Feb. 1957.

Park, E. A., and Richter, C. P.: Transverse lines in bone: Mechanism of their development, Johns Hopkins Med. J. 93:234-248, 1953.

Pearse, H. E., and Morton, J. J.: The stimulation of bone growth by venous stasis, J. Bone Joint Surg. 12:97-111, Jan. 1930.

Pease, C. N.: Local stimulation of growth of long bones: A preliminary report, J. Bone Joint Surg. 34-A:1-24, Jan. 1952.

Phemister, D. B.: Operative arrestment of longitudinal growth of bones in the treatment of

deformities, J. Bone Joint Surg. 15:1-15, Jan. 1933.

Ratliff, A. H. C.: The short leg in poliomyelitis, J. Bone Joint Surg. 41-B:56-69, Feb. 1959.

Reidy, J. A., Lingley, J. R., Gall, E. A., and Barr, J. S.: The effect of roentgen irradiation on epiphyseal growth. II. Experimental studies upon the dog, J. Bone Joint Surg. 29:853-873, Oct. 1947.

Richards, V., and Stofer, R.: The stimulation of bone growth by internal heating, Surgery 46:84-96, July 1959.

Ring, P. A.: Shortening and paralysis in poliomyelitis, Lancet 2:980-983, Nov. 1957.

Ring, P. A.: Experimental bone lengthening by epiphyseal distraction, Brit. J. Surg. 46:169-173, Sept. 1958.

Ring, P. A.: Congenital short femur: Simple femoral hypoplasia, J. Bone Joint Surg. 41-B:73-79, Feb. 1959.

Ring, P. A.: The influence of the nervous system upon the growth of bones, J. Bone Joint Surg. 43-B:121-140, Feb. 1961.

Ring, P. A., and Lee, J.: The effect of heat upon the growth of bone, J. Pathol. 75:405-412, Apr. 1958.

Schneider, M.: Experimental epiphyseal arrest by intra-osseous injection of papain, J. Bone Joint Surg. 45-A:25-35, Jan. 1963.

Siffert, R.: The effect of staples and longitudinal wires on epiphyseal growth, J. Bone Joint Surg. 38-A:1077-1088, Oct. 1956.

Siffert, R. S.: The effect of juxta-epiphyseal pyogenic infection on epiphyseal growth, Clin. Orthop. 10:131-139, 1957.

Sofield, H. A., Blair, S. J., and Millar, E. A.: Leg-lengthening, J. Bone Joint Surg. 40-A:311-321, Apr. 1958.

Sofield, H. A., and Millar, E. A.: Fragmentation, realignment, and intramedullary rod fixation of deformities of the long bones in children, J. Bone Joint Surg. 41-A:1371-1391, Dec. 1959.

Stewart, S. F.: Effect of sympathectomy on the leg length in cortical rigidity, J. Bone Joint Surg. 19:222, Jan. 1937.

Stinchfield, A. J., Reidy, J. A., and Barr, J. S.: Prediction of unequal growth of the lower extremities in anterior poliomyelitis, J. Bone Joint Surg. 31-A:478-484, July 1949.

Straub, L. R., Thompson, T. C., and Wilson, P. D.: The results of epiphyseodesis and femoral shortening in relation to equilization of limb length, J. Bone Joint Surg. 27:255-266, Apr. 1945.

Strobino, L. J., Colonna, P. C., Brodey, R. S., and Leinbach, T.: The effect of compression on the growth of epiphyseal bone, Surg. Gynec. Obstet. 103:85-93, July-Dec. 1956.

Strobino, L. J., French, G. O., and Colonna, P. C.: The effect of increasing tensions on the growth of epiphyseal bone, Surg. Gynec. Obstet. 95:694-700, July-Dec. 1952.

Thompson, T. C., Straub, L. R., and Arnold, W. D.: Congenital absence of the fibula, J. Bone Joint Surg. **39-A**:1229-1236, Dec. 1957.

Thompson, T. C., Straub, L. R., and Campbell, R. D.: An evaluation of femoral shortening with intramedullary nailing, J. Bone Joint Surg. **36-A**:43-56, Jan. 1954.

Truesdell, E. D.: Inequality of the lower extremities following fracture of the shaft of the femur in children, Ann. Surg. **74**:498-500, Aug. 1921.

Trueta, J.: Stimulation of bone growth by redistribution of the intra-osseous circulation, J. Bone Joint Surg. **33-B**:476, Aug. 1951.

Trueta, J.: The influence of the blood supply in controlling bone growth, Bull. Hosp. Joint Dis. **14**:147-157, Oct. 1953.

Trueta, J., and Amato, V. P.: The vascular contribution to osteogenesis, J. Bone Joint Surg: **42-B**:571-587, Aug. 1960.

Tupman, G. S.: Treatment of inequality of the lower limbs, J. Bone Joint Surg. **42-B**:489-501, Aug. 1960.

Tupman, G. S.: A study of bone growth in normal children and its relationship to skeletal maturation, J. Bone Joint Surg. **44-B**:42-67, Feb. 1962.

White, J. W.: A simplified method for tibial lengthening, J. Bone Joint Surg. **12**:90-96, Jan. 1930.

White, J. W.: Femoral shortening for equalization of leg length, J. Bone Joint Surg. **17**:597-604, July 1935.

White, J. W.: A practical graphic method of recording leg length discrepancies, South. Med. J. **33**:946-948, Sept. 1940.

White, J. W.: A method of subtrochanteric limb shortening, J. Bone Joint Surg. **31-A**:86, Jan. 1949.

White, J. W.: Leg-length discrepancies. In American Academy of Orthopaedic Surgeons, Instructional Course Lectures, vol. 6, Ann Arbor, 1949, J. W. Edwards, pp. 201-211.

White, J. W., and Stubbins, S. G.: Growth arrest for equalizing leg lengths, J.A.M.A. **126**:1146-1148, Dec. 1944.

White, J. W., and Warner, W. P.: Experiences with metaphyseal growth arrests. South. Med. J. **31**:411-413, Apr. 1938.

Wilson, C. L., and Percy, E. C.: Experimental studies on epiphyseal stimulation, J. Bone Joint Surg. **38-A**:1096-1104, Oct. 1956.

Wise, C. S., Castleman, B., and Watkins, A. L.: Effect of diathermy (short wave and microwave) on bone growth in the albino rat, J. Bone Joint Surg. **31-A**:487-500, July 1949.

Wu, Y. K., and Miltner, L. J.: A procedure for stimulation of longitudinal growth of bone, J. Bone Joint Surg. **19**:909-921, Oct. 1937.

Tarsal coalitions

Anderson, R. J.: The presence of an astralago-scaphoid bone in man, J. Anat. **14**:452-455, 1879-1880.

Austin, F. H.: Symphalangism and related fusions of tarsal bones, Radiology **56**:882-885, June 1951.

Badgley, C. E.: Coalition of the calcaneus and the navicular, Arch. Surg. **15**:75-88, July 1927.

Bersani, F. A., and Samilson, R. L.: Massive familial tarsal synostosis, J. Bone Joint Surg. **39-A**:1187-1190, Oct. 1957.

Boyd, H. B.: Congenital talonavicular synostosis, J. Bone Joint Surg. **26**:682-686, Oct. 1944.

Bullitt, J. B.: Variations of the bones of the foot: Fusion of the talus and navicular, bilateral and congenital, Amer. J. Roentgenol. Radium Ther. Nucl. Med. **20**:548-549, Dec. 1928.

Harris, B. J.: Anomalous structures in the developing human foot (abstract), Anat. Rec. **121**:399, Feb. 1955.

Harris, R. I.: Rigid valgus foot due to talocalcaneal bridge, J. Bone Joint Surg. **37-A**:169-183, Jan. 1955.

Harris, R. I.: Peroneal spastic flatfoot. In American Academy of Orthopaedic Surgeons, Instructional Course Lectures, vol. 15, Ann Arbor, 1958, J. W. Edwards, pp. 116-134.

Harris, R. I.: Follow-up notes on articles previously published in this journal, J. Bone Joint Surg. **47-A**:1657-1667, Dec. 1965.

Harris, R. I., and Beath, T.: Etiology of peroneal spastic flat foot, J. Bone Joint Surg. **30-B**:624-634, Nov. 1948.

Harris, R. I., and Beath, T.: John Hunter's specimen of talocalcaneal bridge, J. Bone Joint Surg. **32-B**:203, May 1950.

Hodgson, F. G.: Talonavicular synostosis, South. Med. J. **39**:940-941, Dec. 1946.

Holl, M.: Beiträge zur chirurgischen Osteologie des Fusses, Arch. klin. Chir. **25**:211-223, 1880.

Illievitz, A. B.: Congenital malformations of the feet: Report of a case of congenital fusion of the scaphoid with the astragalus, and complete absence of one toe, Amer. J. Surg. **4**:550-552, May 1928.

Jack, E. A.: Bone anomalies of the tarsus in relation to "peroneal spastic flat foot," J. Bone Joint Surg. **36-B**:530-542, Nov. 1954.

Kendrick, J. I.: Treatment of calcaneonavicular bar, J.A.M.A. **172**:1242-1244, March 1960.

Lapidus, P. W.: Congenital fusion of the bones of the foot: With a report of a case of congenital astragaloscaphoid fusion, J. Bone Joint Surg. **14**:888-894, Oct. 1932.

Lapidus, P. W.: Bilateral congenital talonavicular fusion: Report of a case, J. Bone Joint Surg. **20**:775-777, July 1938.

Lapidus, P. W.: Spastic flat-foot, J. Bone Joint Surg. **28**:126-136, Jan. 1946.

Mahaffey, H. W.: Bilateral congenital calcaneocuboid synostosis: A case report, J. Bone Joint Surg. **27**:164-165, Jan. 1945.

Nievergelt, K.: Positiver Väterschaftnachweis auf Grund erblicher Missbildungen der Extremitäten, Arch. Julius Klaus Stift. Vererbungsforsch. **19**:157-159, 1944.

O'Donoghue, D. H., and Sell, L. S.: Congenital talonavicular synostosis: A case report of a rare anomaly, J. Bone Joint Surg. **25**:925-927, Oct. 1943.

Outland, T., and Murphy, I. D.: Relation of tarsal anomalies to spastic and rigid flatfeet, Clin. Orthop. **1**:217-224, 1953.

Pearlman, H. S., Edkin, R. E., and Warren, R. F.: Familial tarsal and carpal synostosis with radial-head subluxation (Nievergelt's syndrome), J. Bone Joint Surg. **46-A**:585-592, April 1964.

Pfitzner, W.: Beiträge zur Kenntnis des menschlichen Extremitätenskelets. VII. Die Variationen im Aufbau des Fussskelets. In Schwalbe, G.: Morphologische Arbeiten, vol. 6, Jena, 1896, Gustav Fischer.

Schreiber, R. R.: Talonavicular synostosis, J. Bone Joint Surg. **45-A**:170-172, Jan. 1963.

Seddon, H. J.: Calcaneo-scaphoid coalition, Proc. R. Soc. Med. **26**:419-424, 1932-1933.

Shands, A. R., Jr., and Wentz, I. J.: Congenital anomalies, accessory bones, and osteochondritis in the feet of 850 children, Surg. Clin. N. Amer. **33**:1643-1666, 1953.

Simmons, E. H.: Tibialis spastic varus foot with tarsal coalition, J. Bone Joint Surg. **47-B**:533-536, Aug. 1965.

Slomann: On coalitio calcaneo-navicularis, J. Orthop. Surg. **3**:586, Nov. 1921.

Vaughan, W. H., and Segal, G.: Tarsal coalition, with special reference to rotentgenographic interpretation, Radiology **60**:855-863, June 1953.

Wagoner, G. W.: A case of bilateral congenital fusion of the calcanei and cuboids, J. Bone Joint Surg. **10**:220-223, Apr. 1928.

Waugh, W.: Partial cubo-navicular coalition as a cause of peroneal spastic flat foot. J. Bone Joint Surg. **39-B**:520-523, Aug. 1957.

Webster, F. S., and Romerts, W. M.: Tarsal anomalies and peroneal spastic flatfoot, J.A.M.A. **146**:1099-1104, July 1951.

Weitzner, I.: Congenital talonavicular synostosis associated with hereditary multiple ankylosing arthropathies, Amer. J. Roentgenol. Radium Ther. Nucl. Med. **56**:185-188, Aug. 1946.

Wray, J. B., and Herndon, C. N.: Hereditary transmission of congenital coalition of the calcaneous to the navicular, J. Bone Joint Surg. **45-A**:365-372, March 1963.

Torsional deformities of the lower extremities

Appleton, A. B.: Postural deformities and bone growth, Lancet **1**:451-454, 1934.

Arkin, A. M., and Katz, J. F.: Effects of pressure on epiphyseal growth, J. Bone Joint Surg. **38-A**:1056-1076, Oct. 1956.

Backman, S.: The proximal end of the femur: Investigations with special reference to the etiology of femoral neck fractures, Acta Radiol. (Stockh.) (Suppl.) **146**:1-166, 1957.

Badgley, C. E.: Correlation of clinical and anatomical facts leading to a conception of the etiology of congenital hip dysplasias, J. Bone Joint Surg. **25**:503-523, July 1943.

Badgley, C. E.: Etiology of congenital dislocation of the hip, J. Bone Joint Surg. **31-A**:341, Apr. 1949.

Baker, L. D., and Hill, L. M.: Foot alignment in the cerebral palsy patient, J. Bone Joint Surg. **46-A**:1-15, Jan. 1964.

Bergmann, G. A.: Die Bedeutung der Innendrehung der Unterschenkel für die Entwicklung des Senk-Knickfusses, mit der Angabe einer Messmethode der Unterschenkeltorsion und Mitteilung von Messergebnissen, Z. Orthop. **96**:177-186, July 1962.

Billing, L.: Roentgen examination of the proximal femur end in children and adolescents, Acta Radiol. (Stockh.) (Suppl.) **110**:1-80, 1954.

Blount, W. P.: Bow leg, Wis. Med. J. **40**:484-487, June 1941.

Blumel, J., Eggers, G. W. N., and Evans, E. B.: Eight cases of hereditary bilateral medial tibial torsion in four generations, J. Bone Joint Surg. **39-A**:1198-1202, Oct. 1957.

Böhm, M.: The embryologic origin of club-foot, J. Bone Joint Surg. **11**:229-259, Apr. 1929.

Böhm, M.: Infantile deformities of the knee and hip, J. Bone Joint Surg. **15**:574-578, July 1933.

Browne, D.: Congenital deformities of mechanical origin. Proc. R. Soc. Med. **29**:1409-1431, May 1936.

Chapple, C. C., and Davidson, D. T.: A study of the relationship between fetal position and certain congenital deformities, J. Pediat. **18**:483-493, Apr. 1941.

Crane, L.: Femoral torsion and its relation to toeing-in and toeing-out, J. Bone Joint Surg. **41-A**:421-428, Apr. 1959.

Doyle, M. R.: Sleeping habits of infants, Phys. Ther. Rev. **25**:74-75, Mar.-Apr. 1945.

Dunlap, K., Shands, A. R., Hollister, L. C., Gahl, J. S., and Streit, H. A.: A new method for determination of torsion of the femur, J. Bone Joint Surg. **35-A**:289-311, Apr. 1953.

Dunn, D. M.: Anteversion of the neck of the femur, J. Bone Joint Surg. **34-B**:181-186, May 1952.

Durham, H. A.: Anteversion of the femoral neck in the normal femur and its relation to congenital dislocation of the hip, J.A.M.A. **65**:223-224, July 1915.

Elftman, H.: Torsion of the lower extremity, Amer. J. Phys. Anthropol. **3**:255-265, Sept. 1945.

Fitzhugh, M. L.: Faulty alignment of the feet and legs in infancy and childhood, Phys. Ther. Rev. **21**:239-245, Sept.-Oct. 1941.

Garden, R. S.: The structure and function of the proximal end of the femur, J. Bone Joint Surg. **43-B**:576-589, Aug. 1961.

Geist, E. S.: An operation for the after treatment of some cases of congenital club-foot, J. Bone Joint Surg. **6**:50-52, Jan. 1924.

Howorth, M. B.: A textbook of orthopedics, Philadephia, 1952, W. B. Saunders Co.

Hutter, C. G., and Scott, W.: Tibial torsion, J. Bone Joint Surg. **31-A**:511-518, July 1949.

Irwin, C. E.: The iliotibial band: Its role in producing deformity in poliomyelitis, J. Bone Joint Surg. **31-A**:141-146, Jan. 1949.

Kaplin, E. B.: The iliotibial tract: Clinical and morphological significance, J. Bone Joint Surg. **40-A**:817-832, July 1958.

Kingsley, P. C., and Olmstead, K. L.: A study to determine the angle of anteversion of the neck of the femur, J. Bone Joint Surg. **30-A**:745-751, July 1948.

Kite, J. H.: Torsion of the lower extremities in small children, J. Bone Joint Surg. **36-A**:511-520, June 1954.

Kite, J. H.: Torsion of the legs in small children, Med. Assoc. Georgia **43**:1035-1038, Dec. 1954.

Kite, J. H.: Torsional deformities of the lower extremities, West Va. Med. J. **57**:92-97, March 1961.

Knight, R. A.: Developmental deformities of the lower extremities, J. Bone Joint Surg. **36-A**:521-527, June 1954.

Lanz-Wachsmuth: Praktische Anatomie, Berlin, 1938, Springer.

LeDamany, P.: La torsion du tibia, normale, pathologique, expérimentale, J. Anat. Physiol. **45**: 598-615, 1909.

Lowman, C. L.: Rotation deformities, Boston Med. Surg. J. **21**:581-584, May 1919.

Lowman, C. L.: The sitting position in relation to pelvic stress, Phys. Ther. Rev. **21**:30-32, Jan.-Feb. 1941.

MacKenzie, I. G., Seddon, H. J., and Trevor, D.: Congenital dislocation of the hip, J. Bone Joint Surg. **42-B**:689-705, Nov. 1960.

Milch, H.: Subtrochanteric osteotomy, Clin. Orthop. **22**:145-156, 1962.

Morgan, J. D., and Somerville, E. W.: Normal and abnormal growth at the upper end of the femur, J. Bone Joint Surg. **42-B**:264-272, May 1960.

Nachlas, I. W.: Medial torsion of the leg, Arch. Surg. **28**:909-919, Apr. 1934.

Nachlas, I. W.: Common defects of the lower extremity in infants, South. Med. J. **41**:302-307, Apr. 1948.

O'Donoghue, D. H.: Controlled rotation osteotomy of the tibia, South. Med. J. **33**:1145-1149, Nov. 1940.

Rabinowitz, M. S.: Congenital curvature of the tibia, Bull. Hosp. Joint Dis. **12**:63-74, Apr. 1951.

Rosen, H., and Sandick, H.: The measurement of tibiofibular torsion, J. Bone Joint Surg. **37-A**: 847-855, July 1955.

Sell, L. S.: Tibial torsion accompanying congenital club-foot, J. Bone Joint Surg. **23**:561-566, July 1941.

Sterling, R. I.: "Derotation" of the tibia, Brit. Med. J. **1**:581, Mar. 1936.

Swanson, A. B., Green, P. W., and Allis, H. D.: Rotational deformities of the lower extremity in children and their clinical significance, Clin. Orthop. **27**:157-175, 1963.

Thelander, H. E., and Fitzhugh, M. L.: Posture habits in infancy affecting foot and leg alignments, J. Pediat. **21**:306-314, July 1942.

Yount, C. C.: The role of the tensor fasciae femoris in certain deformities of the lower extremities, J. Bone Joint Surg. **8**:171-193, Jan. 1926.

3

Ancillary diagnostic procedures

S. William Levy
Verne T. Inman

A tentative diagnosis made by the clinician as a result of his examination of the patient may require confirmation through specific laboratory procedures. Since this text is concerned essentially with surgery, it is not appropriate to incorporate in it detailed descriptions of these techniques. They must be noted, however, because knowledge of such special procedures and the indications for using them should be available to every surgeon. The following section contains a listing of such procedures. Only essential information is presented.

ROENTGENOGRAPHIC EXAMINATION OF THE FOOT

The most important ancillary procedure in diagnosing mechanical disorders of the foot is roentgenographic examination. However, one must not lose sight of the two-dimensional limitation of an x-ray film. Since it is almost impossible to visualize some areas of the foot adequately from standard anteroposterior and lateral views alone, additional views may be necessary to delineate clearly the particular skeletal relationships and bony abnormalities. Special views may be obtained and unique techniques such as tomography are available to the radiologist. To obtain maximal value from a roentgenographic examination, the practitioner should adhere to the following principles:

1. The radiologist should be provided with both an adequate clinical history of the patient and a tentative physical diagnosis.
2. The ankle joint should be considered an integral part of the foot. In any roentgenographic study of the foot, anteroposterior and lateral views of the ankle must be included.
3. In cases of functional disability, weight-bearing views of the foot must be taken.
4. If the clinician has focused upon a specific anatomic structure as a possible source of disability, he must give the radiologist this information.

If possible, a continuing working arrangement should be established between the clinician and radiologist so that agreements can be reached as to which basic views should be obtained routinely for various clinical conditions, when "stressed" views are necessary, and when arthrography should be performed. The abilities of the radiologist should be exploited to the fullest by the clinician, who should use the radiologist as a true and valuable consultant.

For the practitioner who maintains x-ray equipment in his own office or who does not have available to him the expertise of the diagnostic radiologist, a bibliography of standard texts and pertinent articles on roentgenographic examination is provided at the end of this chapter.

DERMATOLOGIC PROCEDURES

In dealing with abnormalities of the skin, the practitioner has one distinct advantage: He is able to see and feel the skin lesions. However, interpretation of the clinical picture is sometimes difficult, since lesions that are identical in appearance may occur upon the skin from causes that are widely different. Conversely, the same causative factor may give rise to a great diversity of eruptions.

Fortunately, various tests are available to assist the clinician in making his evaluation. Smears and cultures may be readily made for bacteria and fungi. Excisional biopsies and microscopic examinations of lesions are easily performed. The pathologic picture can, in fact, be studied in relation to its clinical appearance in the skin much more readily than it can be studied in the deeper tissues.

The objective of this section is to describe some laboratory procedures that may be used to confirm or to alter the clinical impression the practitioner receives during his examination of the patient.

Scraping for fungus

One of the most valuable and most frequently performed examinations in cutaneous disease is the examination to determine the presence of a fungus. This examination should be done routinely when lesions are present on the lower legs, around the ankles, or on the feet. Although one fungus may be responsible for a single dermatologic entity, a fungus will often produce several clinical manifestations. Conversely, one cutaneous condition may be caused by any of several fungi.

Direct microscopic examination. The lesion to be examined is gently cleansed of debris with either benzalkonium chloride, U.S.P. (Zephiran solution) or alcohol. A light scraping of the area with a Bard-Parker No. 15 blade removes the superficial scales at the periphery of the lesion. These scales are placed on a glass slide, one or two drops of 10 percent sodium or potassium hydroxide are added, and a coverglass is placed over the area. The material is allowed to clear and react with the hydroxide agent for 10 to 15 minutes. When the slide is clear, the specimen is examined under low-power magnification; the substage condenser is lowered to produce a contrast of the elements in the field. The appearance of little lace-like or tube-like branching mycelia or hyphae, with slight double-refringent walls, points to the presence of a fungus. Examination under a higher power of magnification will confirm the finding even more specifically. This examination is about 70 percent efficient; the more experienced and skillful the technician, the higher the rate of efficiency.

Culture. At the time the specimen is taken from the skin of the foot for direct microscopic examination, scales are also removed for culture. The material is inoculated onto Sabouraud's medium (dextrose agar). The specimen is kept at room temperature for the incubation period; growth begins in 3 or 4 days for the yeast fungi (*Candida* species) and in 10 to 14 days for other organisms productive of onychomycosis and tinea pedis (*Trychophyton* and *Epidermophyton* species). Diagnosis of the specific fungus that causes a given disease is made by gross and microscopic examination of the culture growth. For those who are untrained, present-day laboratories have facilities for the diagnosis of these cultures.

The biopsy

It is sometimes necessary to study the cutaneous tissue in order to corroborate a clinical diagnosis. If the lesions are small, they may be totally excised for the purpose of microscopic examination. In other instances one may remove a specimen with a cutaneous punch or obtain a specimen by partial wedge excision or by scissor excision of the lesions. Under some circumstances a curettage biopsy is acceptable. It is important to select the proper lesion and to obtain a representative specimen for biopsy. In most instances the lesion selected should be one that is well developed, rather than one that has just appeared or is disappearing. If the lesion is large, the specimen is ordinarily taken from the margin, not from a crater or an ulcer. Lidocaine or procaine hydrochloride should be injected into the skin around the lesion and not directly into the lesion, as injection into the lesion may distort the structure of the cells. Wounds on the lower legs and on the feet heal more slowly than those on the upper parts of the body; it is important to inform the patient of this fact.

Generally, it is inadvisable to include normal tissue in the biopsy specimen because improper cutting by the technician could produce a section in which only normal skin can be seen. Because the characteristic features of many dermatoses are found in the lower dermis or in the subcutaneous fat, some subcutaneous fat should be included in the specimen.

In our experience a specimen obtained with a 3- or 4-mm. cutaneous punch is adequate for the biopsy. Suturing is optional but is usually not required after using a 3-mm. punch; adhesive tape is sometimes sufficient to approximate the wound edges. After using a 4-mm. biopsy punch, we have found that one suture is adequate to close the wound.

Every specimen submitted to the dermal pathologist for examination should be accompanied by detailed clinical information and a differential diagnosis. The possession of such information enables the dermal pathologist to be of optimal use to the clinician.

The patch test

Scratch tests are particularly valuable in diagnosing pollen allergies and other inhalant allergies; intracutaneous tests are useful for determining allergies to foodstuffs. The patch test, because it reproduces the epidermal reaction, is of the greatest value for determining sensitivity to contactants. This simple technique is a method of testing the skin for its sensitization to various substances. It is particularly useful in diagnosing eruptions of contact dermatitis that occur in the lower extremities and in the feet, especially when the suspected causes of the dermatitis or eczema are products applied to the feet or contacted by them, such as wearing apparel, chemicals, medicinal products, or cosmetic agents.

The patch test consists of application to uninjured skin (usually of the upper arms or the back) of these substances. A tiny piece of gauze or blotting paper is saturated with one of the substances in a concentration that will not cause irritation. It is placed on the skin, covered with a piece of plastic or other protective material, which is then affixed with adhesive tape. Ready-made patches are now available. Unless pronounced irritation occurs, the patch is allowed to remain in place for 48 hours. Readings should be taken after the patch has been removed for at least 20 minutes, as a positive reaction may not be evident immediately. It may even take 2 or 3 days for a positive reaction to appear; it is therefore important to watch for any delayed reaction. Wide variations in response occur, but the most important reactions are diffuse redness and small vesicles, or blisters. These reactions may later be followed by crusting and scaling.

The Tzanck test

In vesicular and bullous diseases examination of the cells on the floor of the blister may show cytologic variations characteristic of such disorders as varicella (chickenpox), herpes simplex, herpes zoster, and pemphigus. A young blister is selected and the top is removed with a scalpel. Fluid contents are blotted away, while care is taken to avoid touching the base. The lesion is then pinched while its floor is scraped with a sharp curet. The scrapings are spread on a clean glass slide and are air-dried and stained with Giemsa's or Wright's stain. Characteristic cells are frequently found in the fluid of the blister, and detection of these cells may be helpful in differentiating one disease from another. The appearance of the cell of pemphigus vulgaris seen in such a preparation is different from that of cells of the viral disorders.

Any of the foregoing procedures can be carried out to diagnose a variety of diseases with manifestations on the legs and feet, including lichen planus, prurigo, pruritus, erythema nodosum, erythema induratum, varicose ulcers, varicose eczema, purpura, syphilis, elephantiasis, psoriasis, Kaposi's sarcoma, leprosy, flea bites, and dermatitis caused by a variety of contactants. In addition, dermatophytosis, plantar warts, arsenical keratoses, hyperhidrosis or dyshidrosis, frostbite, eczema, callus, corn, melanoma, dermatitis from shoe dyes, and scabies can be diagnosed on the feet. Erythema multiforme, granuloma annulare, radiodermatitis, carcinoma, and a variety of benign and malignant tumors commonly occur on the feet.

Tests for bacteria

Many types of bacteria are found in diseases of the skin. In some instances they are primary invaders, but in others they are secondary invaders and may influence the disease process. These bacteria can be checked by using the smear technique on a microscopic slide or by culturing the bacterial organism in an appropriate medium.

Capillary fragility is important in some lower leg conditions and may manifest itself in purpura.

TESTS FOR OTHER DISEASE PROCESSES

When the foot and ankle show evidence of a nontraumatic inflammatory process, the examiner should secure a blood count (which should include a differential leukocyte count and a sedimentation rate) and a urinalysis, whether he believes the pathologic process to be degenerative, pyogenic, or metabolic in origin.

Rheumatoid arthritis

Patients with rheumatoid arthritis often suffer from anemia. Leukocytosis and an elevated sedimentation rate usually accompany rheumatoid arthritis, gout, and bacterial infection, but are not present in degenerative arthritis. Most adult patients with active rheumatoid arthritis possess an unusual macroprotein in their serum, which is capable of reacting with gamma globulin. The presence of this 19S globulin (rheumatoid factor) can be demonstrated by several serologic methods. Patients with chronic rheumatoid arthritis may develop amyloidosis; the presence of protein in the urine will confirm the existence of this condition.

Diabetes

If clinical evidence of circulatory insufficiency exists (manifested by a decrease in the arterial pulse and a history of claudication) or if persistant infection and indolent ulcers occur, diabetes mellitus should be suspected. Even if glycosuria is not present, a test to determine the level of blood sugar is indicated.

Gout

A clinical diagnosis of acute gout should be confirmed by a laboratory procedure to test for the level of blood uric acid. The level is almost always elevated in this disease. The presence of urate crystals in joint fluid aspirates provides further confirmation of this condition.

Cryoglobulinemia

Raynaud-like manifestations, which may consist of cyanosis, cutis marmorata (mottling), petechiae, purpura, thrombosis, hemorrhage, ulceration, and gangrene, may appear in some patients when their extremities are exposed to cold. The cause of these disorders is the presence in the blood of an abnormal globulin which, on exposure to cold, precipitates in the small vessels. An increase in viscosity is produced, which may lead to stasis and thrombosis.

A test for the presence of cryoglobulins is readily performed. In a warm syringe 10 ml. of venous blood is collected; the serum is separated at 37° C and is then cooled in a refrigerator to 5° C. If the test is positive, a gelatinous precipitate will form, which dissolves when the serum is rewarmed.

REFERENCES

Roentgenographic examination of the foot

Antonsen, W.: An oblique projection for roentgen examination of the talo-calcanean joint, particularly regarding intra-articular fracture of the calcaneus, Acta Radiol. (Stockh.) **24**:306-310, 1943.

Broden, B.: Roentgen examination of the subtaloid joint in fractures of the calcaneus, Acta Radiol. (Stockh.) **31**:85-91, Jan.-June 1949.

Freiberger, R. H., Hersh, A., and Harrison, M. O.: Roentgen examination of the deformed foot, Semin. Roentgenol. **5**:341-353, Oct. 1970.

Gamble, F. O., and Yale, I.: Clinical foot roentgenology: An illustrated handbook, Baltimore, 1966, The Williams & Wilkins Co.

Rubin, G., and Witten, M.: The talar-tilt angle and the fibular collateral ligaments: A method for the determination of talar tilt, J. Bone Joint Surg. **42-A**:311-326, Mar. 1960.

Dermatologic procedures

Andrews, G. C., and Domonkos, A. N.: Diseases of the skin: For practitioners and students, ed. 5, Philadelphia 1963, W. B. Saunders Co.

Lever, W. F.: Histopathology of the skin, ed., 3, Philadelphia, 1954, J. B. Lippincott Co.

Pillsbury, D. M., Shelley, W. B., and Kligman, A. M.: Dermatology, Philadelphia, 1956, W. B. Saunders Co.

Part two

4

Minor congenital deformities and anomalies of the foot

Elmer E. Specht

Anomalies of the foot may be inherited through autosomal dominant or autosomal recessive genes; they may be acquired; or they may be transmitted through genetic factors that are poorly delineated. Anomalies may occur as specific syndromes, either alone or in association with malformations of other parts of the body, or they may be manifestations of a generalized syndrome reflected in the feet.

McKusick (1968) attributes the following specific syndromes in which the foot is involved to autosomal dominant transmission: accessory navicular; os tibiale externum, os paranaviculare, and talonavicular fusion; three types of syndactyly (zygodactyly, synpolydactyly; and syndactyly with metatarsal fusion); split hand, split foot, or both, with and without cleft lip and palate; postaxial polydactylia with median cleft of the upper lip; misshapen toes; and two phalanges in the fifth toe. Relative length of the first and second toes is also genetically determined.

Generalized syndromes with manifestations reflected in the feet exist which must be viewed as possible indicators of serious anomalies elsewhere in the body. Myositis ossificans progressiva (short hallux) and acrocephalosyndactyly of Apert (broad distal thumb and toe, syndactyly) are such syndromes; their transmission is attributed to autosomal dominant genes. Chondroectodermal dysplasia (short distal phalanges), Laurence-Moon-Biedl syndrome (polydactylia), and acrocephalosyndactyly of Carpenter (synpolydactyly) are generalized syndromes with manifestations in the feet whose transmission is attributed to autosomal recessive genes. Smith (1970) categorized the following as generalized syndromes that either are transmitted through poorly delineated genetic factors or are nonhereditary in origin: (1) Cornelia de Lange syndrome (small or malformed hands and feet); (2) Rubinstein Taybi syndrome (broad toes); Mohr's syndrome (partial duplication of the hallux); Forney's syndrome (fusion of some tarsals and carpals); Prader-Willi syndrome (small hands and feet); Smith-Lemli-Opitz syndrome (syndactyly of the second and third toes); and Sotos' cerebral gigantism (large hands and feet).

Other syndromes may be related to chromosomal abnormality and, although such syndromes occur rarely, they should nonetheless be borne in mind. They are regularly associated with developmental retardation and frequently with other serious anomalies and early death. Taylor (1967) noted that in 119 cases of Edwards' syndrome with trisomy of an E chromosome, 79 percent of the infants had short

51

dorsiflexed hallux and 63 percent had calcaneovalgus feet. In fifty-five cases of Patau's syndrome with trisomy of a D chromosome, 76 percent of the infants had polydactylia and 65 percent had prominent calcaneus.

In spite of the impressive list of anomalies that are known to be genetically determined, the majority of anomalies are probably nonhereditary in origin. Many minor abnormalities occur with such frequency that they must be considered to be normal variants. Trolle (1948), for example, found os sesamoideum interphalangeale digiti I in 56 percent and os sesamoideum metatarsophalangeale V in 26 percent of 254 pairs of carefully examined embryonic feet. Furthermore, O'Rahilly (1953) and others agree that minor anomalies do not warrant such phylogenetic speculations as they have often received.

ACCESSORY BONES

Both O'Rahilly and Trolle have studied accessory bones. O'Rahilly (1953) catalogued thirty-eight tarsal and sesamoid bones of the foot ("ossa tarsalia et sesamoidea") and stated that they may have been incomplete fusions, accessoria, or bipartitions. Trolle (1948) studied serial microscopic sections from the 508 feet of 254 embryos between 6 and 27 weeks of fetal age and found that in nearly 80 percent of them accessory bones preformed in hyaline cartilage were present. The high incidence of such bones in embryonic feet did not correlate well with their incidence in adult feet. He was unable to find os trigonum in any of the embryonic feet he studied, although it occurs frequently in adults. Conversely, in 13 percent of the embryonic feet he found anlagen of the os paracuneiforme, in spite of its much lower incidence in adult feet. He concluded that accessory bones may: (1) develop from an independent element preformed in hyaline cartilage; (2) develop from an inconstant ossification center; (3) be explained as tendon bones; (4) be due to unrecognized pathologic lesions. Thus it would seem that

there are several explanations for the presence of these abnormalities. Henderson (1963) and Wildervanck et al., (1967) have shown hereditary causation in some instances. From the clinical standpoint only two, the os trigonum and the accessory navicular (prehallux), become symptomatic with any frequency.

Os trigonum

The os trigonum varies greatly in size and shape and appears at the posterior process of the talus. It may be an actual part of the body of the talus (Fig. 4-1, A) or a separate bone that may or may not adhere to the talus by a cartilaginous plate (Fig. 4-2). These ossicles are usually asymptomatic and are detected only during routine roentgenography. They have been mistaken for fracture of the posterior process of the talus. The ossicle arises from a separate ossification center and appears between 8 and 11 years of age (McDougall, 1955). It is present in 7 percent of roentgenograms of normal feet (Bizarro, 1921). The ossicles that are separated from the talus may become loose, producing pain on plantar flexion of the foot; those that are part of the talus may be fractured.

Diagnosis. The os trigonum may cause pain in the retrocalcaneal space that is aggravated on walking, especially when the foot is in plantar flexion. When pressure is applied with the thumb and index finger against the posterior lip of the talus, pain is sharp. The onset of symptoms is gradual except in sudden fracture of an attached os trigonum. The symptoms become progressively worse, and the condition must be differentiated from retrocalcaneal bursitis. In bursitis the symptoms are acute, generally with swelling and tenderness over the retrocalcaneal space, usually posteriorly and just above the insertion of the tendo achillis instead of at the anterior part of the retrocalcaneal space. Symptomatic cases require surgical removal of the os trigonum.

Procedure for removal of the os trigonum. By the procedure for removal of the os trigonum outlined here, ambulation may

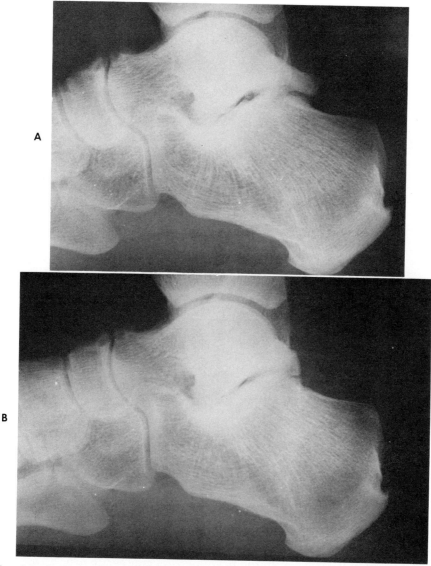

Fig. 4-1. A, Os trigonum as actual part of posterior part of talus; painful. **B,** Same foot 1 year after removal of os trigonum; completely asymptomatic.

begin in 4 days. Healing is uneventful in most cases (Fig. 4-1, *B*).

1. Make a linear incision, about 8 cm. long, over the retrocalcaneal space just behind the lower end of the fibula.
2. Retract the skin and make a similar incision in the fascia; deflect the margins. The anterior margin of the fascia will be contiguous with the sheath of the peroneal tendons, which are readily retracted to expose the retrocalcaneal space.
3. Denude the os trigonum of all attachments with small scissors. The separated os trigonum can usually be brought out of the wound. The adherent type may be amputated by means of a nasal saw or an osteotome.
4. Smooth the cut surface with a rasp.

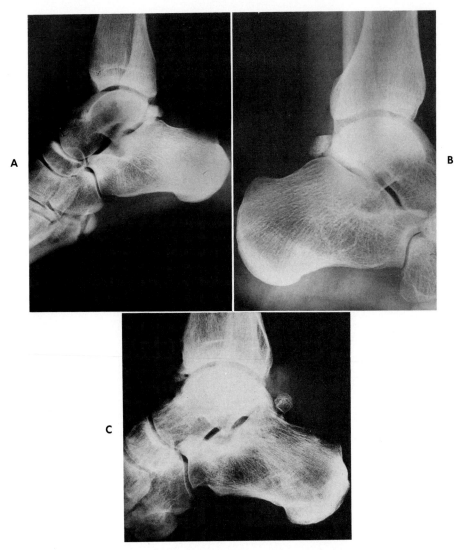

Fig. 4-2. A, Os trigonum attached to talus by cartilaginous plate. Note the os vesalianum at the base of the fifth metatarsal. **B,** Os trigonum attached to talus by cartilaginous plate. **C,** Os trigonum completely detached from body of talus.

5. Suture the fascia and skin in layers.
6. If there is indication that the dead space in the wound should be occluded, it may be accomplished by placing a button over both sides of the retrocalcaneal space and passing a wire through the space and the holes of the button.

Accessory navicular (tarsal scaphoid)

Accessory navicular is a congenital anomaly wherein the tuberosity develops from a second center of ossification. McKusick (1968) lists this ossicle with those that are inherited as an autosomal dominant trait. McKusick reports an incidence of 5 percent. However, Geist (1925) reported a 14 percent incidence in supposedly normal feet and Harris and Beath (1947) reported a 4 percent incidence in young men. There are two distinct types. One is a typical, usually small, accessory bone without attachment to the body of the navicular but with a well-defined round or oval outline

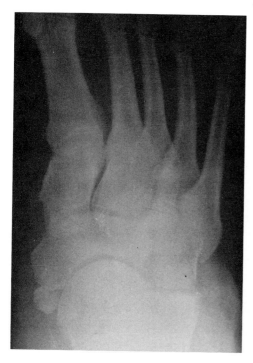

Fig. 4-3. Accessory navicular.

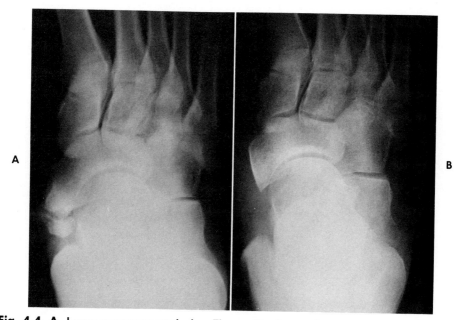

Fig. 4-4. A, Large accessory navicular. The cartilaginous plate is loosened and painful. **B,** Same foot, 1 year postoperatively.

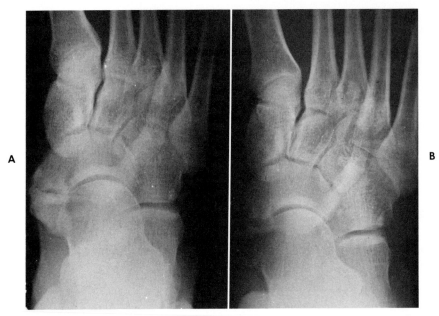

Fig. 4-5. A, Preoperative accessory navicular. B, Same foot postoperatively.

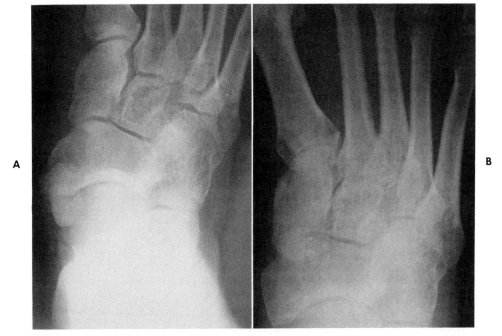

Fig. 4-6. A, Large accessory navicular extending under body of navicular, resulting in abduction of forefoot. B, Two years postoperatively.

of demarcation (Fig. 4-3). The other type is a definite part of the body of the navicular, but the tuberosity is separated by a fibrocartilaginous plate of irregular outline (Figs. 4-4 to 4-6). The first type is the true os tibiale externum or navicular secundarium, which seldom produces symptoms. The second type often has an elongated neck articulating with the tibial side of the head of the talus and fits the description of prehallux or bifurcated navicular. It may become symptomatic and be mistaken for fracture of the neck of the navicular; therefore, the discussion concerns this type.

Zadek (1926) studied fourteen cases of symptomatic accessory navicular. Roentgenographically he observed definite fusion with the body of the navicular in five cases. In three cases there was partial fusion, and in six cases there was complete separation. In 1948 Zadek and Gold studied microscopically the structures connecting the accessory bone to the body of the navicular. They recorded that these structures were variously composed of a soft-tissue plate of hyaline cartilage, dense fibrocartilage, or both, and sometimes showed ossification as well.

Kidner (1929) called attention to the altered line of the pull caused by the insertion of the tendon of the tibialis posterior into the prehallux. The altered line of pull results in loss of normal eversion and suspensory action of the tendon. Thus it is transformed into an adductor of the forefoot instead of an elevator of the tarsus and longitudinal arch. This crowds the medial side of the talonavicular joint and causes pain, which can be alleviated when the foot is forced in abduction. Chater (1962) supported Kidner's contention in a study of twenty patients between the ages of 7 and 40 years, all of whom had accessory navicular ossicles. Twelve were cured by nonoperative treatment; of the eight remaining patients, six (children) had excision of the ossicles and two (adults) had the Kidner operation. Chater believed that the Kidner technique appeared to have two advantages over simple excision. It rein-

forced the buttress mechanism of the spring ligament and it helped counteract and correct talonavicular sag. Giannestras (1967), on the other hand, stated that in his experience only occasionally was the accessory navicular associated with pes planovalgus; he advocated simple excision if pressure symptoms occurred. Leonard and associates (1965) reported thirteen patients (twenty-five feet) who had prehallux associated with pes planovalgus in whom the Kidner operation was performed for correction of the deformity.

In roentgenographic examination Harris and Beath (1947) found accessory tarsal navicular in the feet of 4 percent of 3,619 recruits of the Canadian army. Moreover, the results of a follow-up study of 77 men throughout their training showed that only 4 developed symptoms after prolonged marching. They concluded that except in rare instances neither accessory bones nor prominence of the navicular tuberosity produces significant symptoms.

Symptoms. Symptomatic cases may occasionally occur in early adulthood, especially in women. The anomaly appears equally in the two sexes, but women's shoes undoubtedly cause symptoms. As a rule, the anomaly is bilateral, but symptoms appear only in one foot. Patients state that the protrusion was always present over the medial side of both navicular bones and that one foot gradually became progressively painful and swollen, even at rest. Palpation of the navicular bone elicits sharp, deep pain, especially when the foot is adducted and inverted. Roentgenograms verify the diagnosis.

Treatment. In early cases of moderate symptoms, conservative expectant measures relieve pain. Such measures include a shoe that exerts little or no pressure over the navicular, wedging of the heel for added support under the talonavicular joint, strapping, and an elastic ankle support for partial immobilization of the joint. The intractable case requires surgical intervention. A modified Kidner procedure usually alleviates symptoms.

1. Make a slightly curved incision convex dorsally and centered over the talonavicular joint from a point just in front of and just below the medial malleolus to the base of the first metatarsal.
2. Incise the ligament and fascia along the anterior border of the tibialis posterior tendon throughout the length of the incision. By sharp periosteal dissection, reflect the fascial ligamentous tendinous flap inferiorly and superiorly to expose the accessory bone, the body of the navicular, and the anterior talus.
3. Excise the accessory navicular. The plane of excision can be detected by manual motion of the accessory bone.
4. Remove the roughened tuberosity of the navicular with the talus and first cuneiform, using osteotomes and a rasp.
5. Transpose the whole tendon outward and downward to the plantar surface of the navicular to assure reconstitution of the suspensory activity of the tibialis posterior tendon.
6. Close ligaments, fascia, and skin in layers, and apply a supportive compression dressing.
7. Do not permit weight bearing for seven to ten days, at which time remove sutures and apply a short leg walking cast with the forefoot slightly adducted and inverted.
8. Maintain the extremity in a short leg walking cast in the corrected position for five weeks, after which time instruct the patient to wear a well-fitted oxford with an extended counter for six months.

Uncommon accessory ossicles; bifurcated medial cuneiform

The rare accessory medial cuneiform (os paracuneiforme) may present a problem. The procedure for removal of this bone is comparable to that described for removal of an accessory navicular.

Henderson (1963) reported four cases of os intermetatarseum between the first and second metatarsal heads bilaterally. All were associated with hallux valgus and three were familial.

Harris (1965) implicated the os sustentaculare and the os calcaneus secundarius in tarsal coalition and peroneal spastic flatfoot. Wildervanck and co-workers (1967) reported a family with eight members in three generations who had ossa tibiale, ossa paranaviculare, tarsal coalition, and proximal symphalangism of the fingers.

Osteochondritis dissecans of any of the accessory ossicles may rarely be encountered (Fig. 4-7).

Any of the uncommon accessory ossicles may occasionally become diseased and produce symptoms. Horizontal bifurcation of the medial cuneiform is rare. Fig. 4-8 shows an asymptomatic case. Fig. 4-9 shows an asymptomatic anomalous medial cuneiform.

ABNORMALITIES OF THE TOES
Polydactylia

Accessory toes are seen frequently and occur more commonly among Negroes than Caucasians (Lamy and Frézal, 1961). The extra digit is often rudimentary and bilateral and it may become a major handicap. Aside from cosmetic offensiveness, the problem varies from discomfort as a result of crowding the shoe to complete inability to wear a standard shoe. The variations of polydactylia are numerous, the most common being a sixth toe or an additional hallux. Syndactylism may be associated with the anomaly. Supernumerary toes often are accompanied by accessory metatarsals that are fused with the adjacent metatarsal at the base (Figs. 4-10 and 4-11); or the metatarsal bone may assume a bizarre shape (Figs. 4-12 and 4-13). Hereditary tendency seems apparent. In some cases, other persons in the immediate family or ancestry had a similar deformity (Fig 4-14). Hurwitz encountered an accessory hallux in a little girl whose mother and maternal grandmother had a similar anomaly (Fig. 4-15).

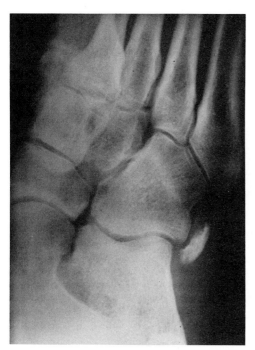

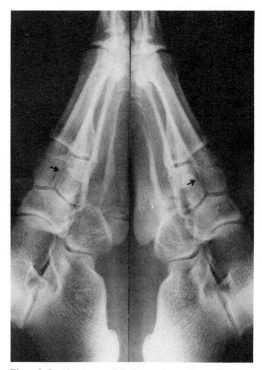

Fig. 4-7. Osteochondritis dissecans of os peroneum.

Fig. 4-8. Horizontal bifurcation of medial cuneiform.

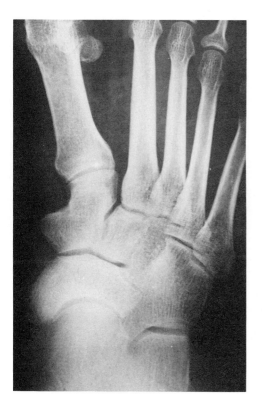

Fig. 4-9. Anomalous medial cuneiform; asymptomatic.

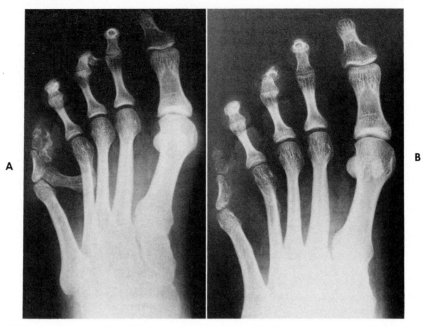

Fig. 4-10. **A,** Polydactylia with accessory metatarsal lying transversely. **B,** Same case postoperatively.

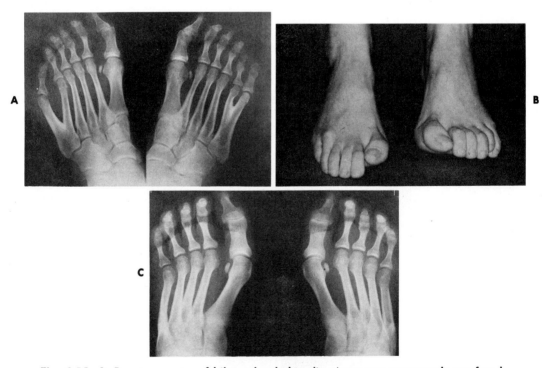

Fig. 4-11. **A,** Roentgenogram of bilateral polydactylia. Accessory metatarsals are fused at the base. **B,** Clinical appearance in same case. **C,** Sixteen months postoperatively.

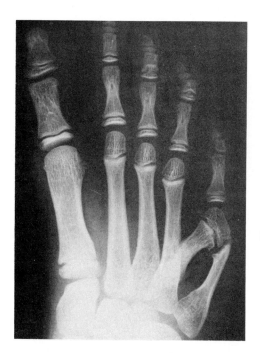

Fig. 4-12. Bizarre accessory metatarsal.

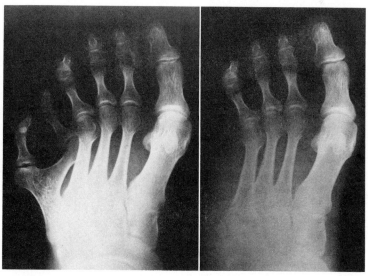

Fig. 4-13. Roentgenograms of foot of 28-year-old man, showing polydactylia, Y-shaped deformity of fifth metatarsal and accessory toe. A good functional result was obtained postoperatively.

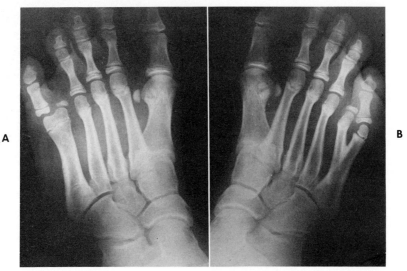

Fig. 4-14. Roentgenogram of foot of brother of patient represented in Fig. 4-11. Note fifth digits amputated in infancy without the reshaping of metatarsals. Remaining epiphyses of the bases of the proximal phalanges and the accessory metatarsals became constant pressure points.

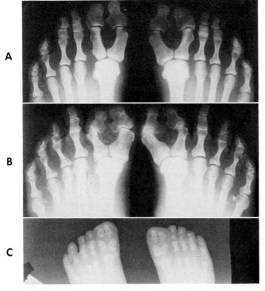

Fig. 4-15. Accessory hallux and syndactyly in three generations. **A,** Mother's; **B,** grandmother's; **C,** child's. (Courtesy Dr. Lester H. Hurwitz.)

Delta phalanx (Fig. 4-16) is a manifestation of polydactylia in which there is a duplication of a portion of a digit with a common proximal epiphysis shared by both the supernumerary and the normal ray. Angular deformity requiring surgical intervention may develop (Watson and Boyes, 1967). Polydactylia of the fifth toe included in a web of syndactyly of the fourth and fifth toes was reported to be transmitted as an autosomal dominant trait (McKusick, 1968) and was associated with similar synpolydactyly of the third and fourth fingers. Synpolydactyly of hands and feet with symphalangia of the thumb has been reported by Savarinathan and Centerwall (1966) as being transmitted as a dominant trait. Simopoulos et al. (1967) reported the occurrence in three siblings of polydactylia of both hands and feet, internal hydrocephalus, polycystic kidneys, premature birth, and neonatal death.

Treatment for polydactylia. Extreme deformity is an operative problem. The technique chosen must meet the requirement of the presenting case. The selection of the structures to be removed must be made

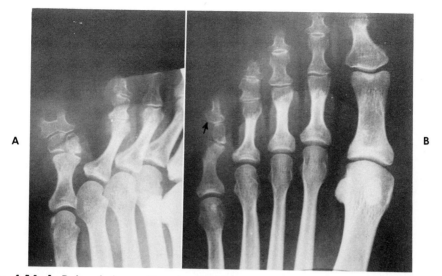

Fig. 4-16. A, Delta phalanx with extra phalanges incorporated into one toe. **B,** Same case postoperatively.

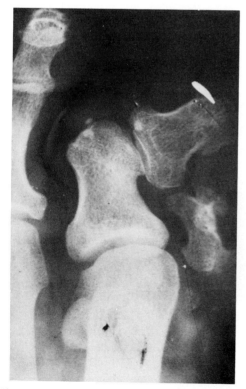

Fig. 4-17. Accessory distal phalanx of the hallux.

with the idea of providing normal contour to the foot as well as of retaining normal muscle function. Treatment is usually sought during childhood, because serious cases are self-evident from infancy. It is therefore important to consider the results of the operation on the growth of the foot.

Accessory hallux

An accessory hallux (Figs. 4-17 to 4-20) presents a formidable problem because of muscular attachments to the base of the proximal phalanx and because of multiple-type deviations. The tibialmost toe should always be the one amputated unless the fibularmost toe is grossly deformed or abnormal in size. In that case, the adductor hallucis, which is inserted into the base of the proximal phalanx of the fibularmost hallux, must be sutured to the proximal phalanx of the remaining hallux; otherwise, in a growing child the remaining abductor hallucis will gradually pull the toe into a serious hallux varus (Fig. 4-19). By the same token, when the tibialmost hallux is removed, the abductor must be reattached to the remaining hallux.

An unusual instance of "true prehallux" with a polydactylous hallux arising from

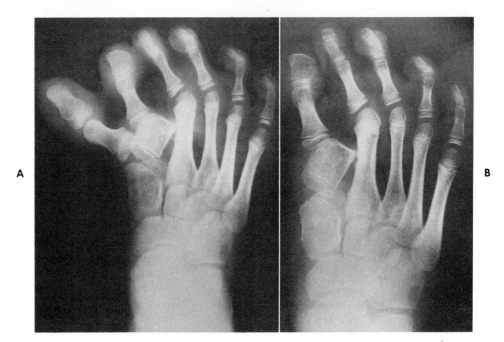

Fig. 4-18. **A,** Bizarre type of accessory hallux of the first metatarsal. **B,** Same case postoperatively.

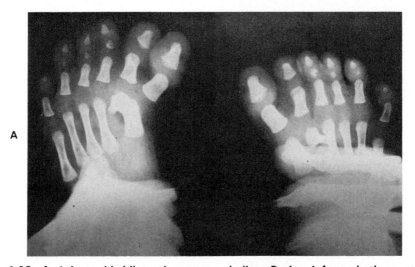

Fig. 4-19. **A,** Infant with bilateral accessory hallux. During infancy both great toes on the fibular side of the accessory hallux had been amputated. **B,** Same patient at 6 years of age. Note extreme hallux varus caused by loss of adductor hallucis insertion. **C,** Clinical appearance of left foot shown roentgenographically in **B.** Note extreme contracture of the abductor hallucis and skin over the tibial side of the first metatarsophalangeal joint. Extensive repair was required to reduce deformity. **D,** Roentgenogram of same patient at age 19, who has became a basketball star.

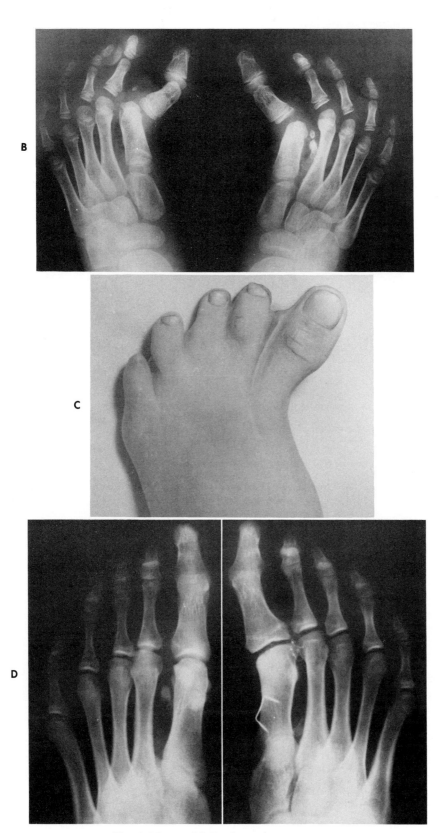

Fig. 4-19, cont'd. For legend see opposite page.

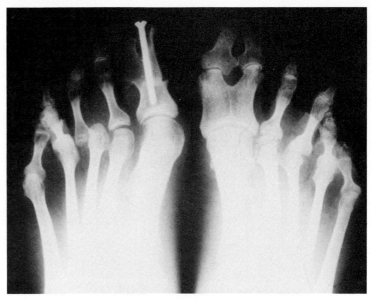

Fig. 4-20. Mother of patient in Fig. 4-19.

the navicular in an otherwise normal foot has been described by Cobey and Covey (1966).

Syndactyly

McKusick (1968) classified five hereditary types of syndactyly of the hands and feet, all transmitted as autosomal dominant traits. Three types manifest abnormalities in the feet:

1. Type I (zygodactyly)—partial or complete webbing of the second and third toes; hands also involved at times
2. Type II (synpolydactyly)—syndactyly of the lateral two toes and polydactylia of the fifth toe in the syndactyly web
3. Type V—associated with metatarsal and metacarpal fusion (see p. 74)

Syndactylism, with ectodermal dysplasia and congenital deafness, was also reported and was classified as an autosomal dominant trait.

Laurin et al. (1964) and Sharma et al. (1965) described an extreme type of synpolydactyly that suggests a mirror-image duplication of the tibia, the tarsals, the metatarsals, and the phalanges, with sim-

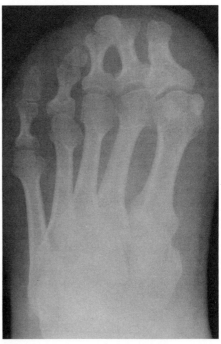

Fig. 4-21. Complete syndactyly of all toes. (Courtesy Dr. C. Ormond.)

ilar anomalies in the arm and hand. In Sharma's cases a mother and six children were all similarly affected.

Treatment. In the more usual types of syndactyly, treatment is seldom functionally indicated because webbed toes rarely become symptomatic (Fig. 4-21). Intervention for cosmetic reasons is generally inadvisable. When surgical treatment is re-

quired, the same technique as is used in separating webbed fingers should be used in the separation of webbed toes. The correct techniques all require skin grafting. Methods that utilize linear incisions along the volar aspect of one toe and up the dorsal aspect of the adjacent toe are contraindicated, since scar contracture will convert the long V to a short U, restoring the web

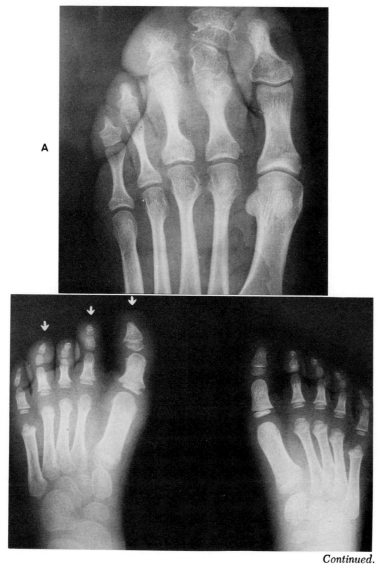

Continued.

Fig. 4-22. A, Megalodactylia of second and third toes. **B,** Megalodactylia of first, second, and fourth toes of left foot. **C,** Megalodactylia of second toe of left foot (seen at right in illustration).

C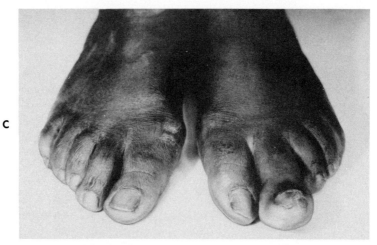

Fig. 4-22, cont'd. For legend see p. 67.

and distorting the digit in rotation, flexion, and contracture (Bunnell, 1964). The Bunnell technique is advised.

This technique fixes the depth of the cleft by outlining a dorsal and a volar-pointed skin flap, with the bases proximal. The web is then slipped through, and the two flaps are crossed through the cleft and are sutured side to side. The denuded side of each toe is then covered by three-split thickness skin, which should be thick enough to keep contracture to a minimum.

Megalodactylia or macrodactyly

Local gigantism of one or more toes is sometimes encountered (Fig. 4-22). The condition may interfere with wearing ordinary shoes, and it may be unsightly. Partial amputation of the toe or excision of the middle phalanx or part of the distal half of the proximal phalanx reduces the toe to almost normal size. Charters (1957) presented an excellent discussion in conjunction with a report of a case regarding the possible relation between neurofibromatosis and macrodactyly as well as other etiologic theories.

Congenital hammertoe

Congenital hammertoes are rare. They are usually multiple and are associated with the different types of talipes equinus or clawfoot. Occasionally a single toe may be congenitally hammered; in that case the condition is bilateral and is ordinarily located in the second toe or in the hallux (Fig. 4-23). The distal interphalangeal joint is the one most commonly involved. (For surgical treatment of hammertoes, see Chapter 20.)

Overlapping toes

Overlapping is a condition in which one toe lies on the dorsum of an adjacent toe, commonly the fifth toe lying over the fourth and, next in order of frequency, the second toe lying over the great toe. Fifth toe overlapping (Fig. 4-24) is usually congenital but may be acquired as a result of flaccid feet, square feet (the toes of which are nearly equal in length) and the wearing of pointed shoes. Contracture of the tendon of the extensor digitorum longus, of the dorsal capsule of the fifth metatarsophalangeal joint, and especially of the dorsal skin maintains the deformity. Lantzounis (1940) and Lapidus (1940) stated that this condition may be hereditary. Giannestras (1967) feels that an infant with overlapping toes should be treated beginning at the age of 6 months by applying an adhesive strapping to the overlapping toes placed in corrected position to the adjacent toes.

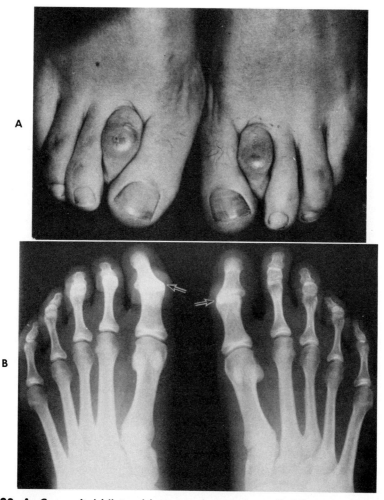

Fig. 4-23. A, Congenital bilateral hammered second toe. **B,** Bilateral congenital hammered great toes in a 14-year-old girl. The metatarsophalangeal joints are normal.

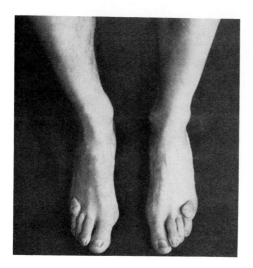

Fig. 4-24. Bilateral congenital overlapping of fifth toe.

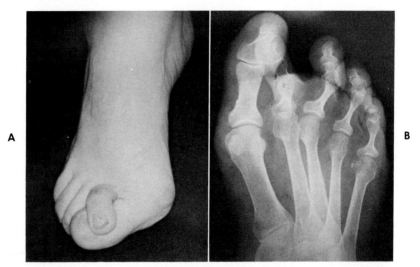

Fig. 4-25. A, Overlapping second toe with hallux valgus. **B,** Overlapping second toe without hallux valgus.

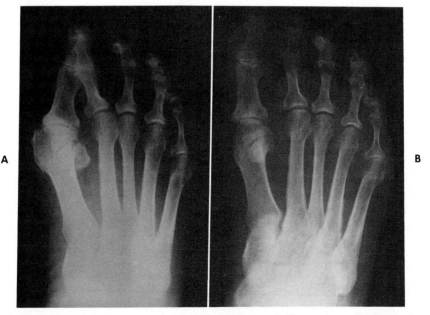

Fig. 4-26. A, Overlapping second toe with moderate hallux valgus. **B,** Same foot 2 years postoperatively, with correction.

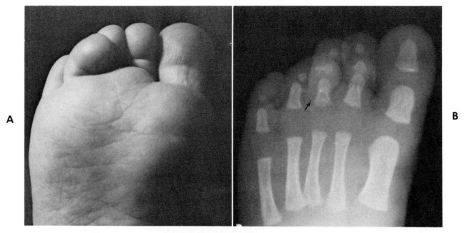

Fig. 4-27. A, Plantar surface of underlapping fourth toe. **B,** Roentgenogram of same foot. Note the distal phalanx underlapping the third toe.

In second toe overlapping, in which the second toe lies over the great toe, hallux valgus is usually present (see Figs. 4-25 and 4-26). The second toe normally is maintained in a slightly dorsiflexed attitude, whereas the great toe normally is maintained in a straight line. When a great toe is forced into a valgus position, it glides under the second toe. The deformity frequently is coupled with dislocation of the second metatarsophalangeal joint. Overlapping toes produce a cosmetic rather than a functional problem; plastic techniques involving skin and tendon revision are available to correct it. (For surgical treatment of overlapping toes, see Chapter 20.)

Congenital underlapping toes

The term "underlapping toe" is applied to a common occurrence in which one of the lesser toes curves from its natural course, usually tibialward, under the adjacent toe (Fig. 4-27). Usually the condition is congenital, and, as a rule, advice is sought by the parents during the patient's childhood. Most commonly both interphalangeal joints are involved. Generally it is the third or fourth toe which is involved, but the second or third may also be afflicted. No specific cause for this peculiar deformity has been found, and it must be included in the idiopathic group of congen-

ital deformities. This deformity may be acquired (see mallet toe p. 241) and in that instance it is ascribed to the same factors as are the more common acquired toe deformities; that is, footwear unsuited to the peculiar variation in the anatomy of the foot, which causes the restraining forces to incurvate the toe instead of the usual buckling. (See hammertoe and mallet toe procedures, Chapter 20.) Treatment is usually unnecessary, but in instances in which pressure symptoms develop, wedge excision of the bony prominence will allow realignment of the toe:

1. Make a spindle-shaped incision over the angle of curvature, usually on the fibular side.
2. Remove all the integuments within the incision.
3. Excise a wedge of the bony prominence within the exposure.
4. The distal end of the toe will now fit into a neutral position.
5. Insert a vertical mattress suture incorporating bolsters, as is done in the procedure for hammertoes.

Abnormalities of the great toe

Congenital hallux varus. Congenital hallux varus is uncommon (Figs. 4-28 and 4-29). Only about twenty-eight cases had been reported up to 1937 (Sloane, 1935;

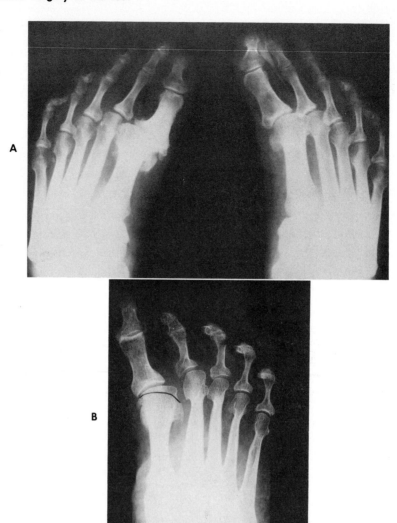

Fig. 4-28. A, Bilateral congenital hallux varus in adult. Secondary osteoarthritic changes are present in the left first metatarsophalangeal joint. **B,** Congenital hallux varus. Note sloping of the first metatarsal head on the tibial side (possibly secondary to congenital overpowering of the abductor hallucis). The black line over the first metatarsal head indicates the amount of articular surface to be removed for the hallux to assume a normal position.

Haas, 1938). A comparable condition is sometimes seen in the hallux interphalangeal joint (Fig. 4-30).

According to McElvenny (1941), medial angulation of the great toe at the metatarsophalangeal joint is usually unilateral and is associated with one or more of the following abnormalities: (1) short, thick first metatarsal; (2) accessory bones or toes;

(3) varus deformity of one or more of the lateral four metatarsals; and (4) a firm, fibrous band (perhaps the residuum of an accessory hallux that has failed to develop) which gradually draws the toe into varus. Thompson (1960) concluded that the primary type (that which is unassociated with other anomalies) was twice as common in males as in females and resulted from

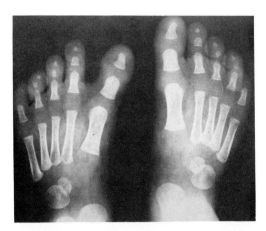

Fig. 4-29. Congenital hallux varus of left foot caused by hyperactive abductor hallucis muscle without metatarsus adductus.

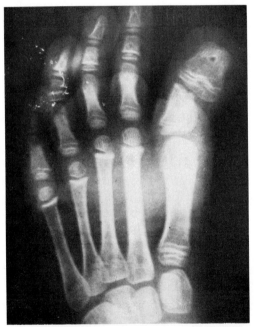

Fig. 4-30. Hallux varus at interphalangeal joint as a result of malformation of head of proximal phalanx.

overpull of the abductor hallucis. He advocated total resection of this muscle.

Treatment. Congenital hallux varus presents individual problems. True hallux varus when seen in childhood is unaccompanied by metatarsus adductus (see p. 99). Tenotomy of the abductor hallucis followed

by maintenance of the hallux in a moderate valgus attitude for a few months will afford correction in most cases.

Congenital hallux rigidus. The congenital type of hallux rigidus is very rare. An anomalous joint surface creates an imperfect ball-and-socket relationship of the first metatarsophalangeal articulation, which causes a predisposition to hallux rigidus. In children, the articular surface of the metatarsal head is almost always flattened, ill-shaped, or angulated plantarward so that the normal excursion of dorsiflexion of the great toe is limited or absent. Each step the child takes is mildly traumatic and over a long period, osseous proliferation occurs. Treatment of symptomatic cases consists of some type of arthroplasty.

Interphalangeal valgus of the great toe. Lateral angulation of the distal phalanx of the hallux may cause painful callosities that overlie the convexity of the deformity and require osteotomy or arthrodesis in later life.

ABNORMALITIES OF THE METATARSALS
Metatarsus primus varus

In this deformity the first metatarsal lies in an excessively adducted position in relation to the lateral four metatarsals, and this positioning may be responsible for the development of hallux valgus in later life. Harris and Beath (1947) concluded, on the basis of a roentgenographic study of the feet of over 3,000 young men, that the mean angle of divergence between the longitudinal axes of the first and second metatarsals was 7.5 degrees, whereas the mean angle in cases of severe hallux valgus was 11.3 degrees. Some degree of hallux valgus showed in over 40 percent of those feet in which this angle was more than 14.5 degrees. They were unable, however, to demonstrate that increased medial obliquity of the first metatarsocuneiform joint was associated with hallux valgus. During childhood, the deformity responds to plaster cast correction and sometimes to soft-tissue stretching by manipulation. For adults with significant symptoms, corrective osteotomy is necessary. Tachdjian (1967) feels that during infancy this condition should be treated similarly to congenital metatarsus varus, with serial plaster casts.

Metatarsal fusion

Metatarsal fusion may occur as part of a syndrome described by Nievergelt (1944) in which there are dominantly transmitted multiple synostoses of the hands and feet, including tarsal and carpal coalitions and radial head subluxations (Pearlman et al., 1964). Metatarsal and metacarpal fusion, most commonly of the fourth and fifth or third and fourth rays and associated with soft-tissue syndactyly of both fingers and toes, has also been reported in five generations of one family by Kemp and Ravn (1932).

Congenital short metatarsals

Shortness of the first metatarsal, posterior displacement of the sesamoids, and hypertrophy of the shaft of the second metatarsal was described by Morton (1935) as a syndrome causing pain at the base of the second metatarsal and calluses under the second and third metatarsal heads. He attributed this syndrome to atavistic regression of the human foot to a more primitive form; since that time numerous authors have supported his contention. Subsequent studies would indicate, however, that relative shortness of the first metatarsal should not be considered to be an abnormality; such shortness is hereditarily determined and probably is not connected with significant foot symptoms.

The hereditary aspects of relative lengths of the great and second toes in Caucasian twins were studied by Kaplan (1964). He concluded that the gene for longer hallux (than second toe) is recessive but has a greater gene frequency (87 percent for longer hallux, 13 percent for longer second toe); therefore longer second toe, although dominant, has a lesser frequency and occurred in only 24 percent of phenotypes in the population studied. Harris and Beath (1947) studied shortness of the first metatarsal (defined as being at least 1 mm. shorter than the second) and found that 33 percent of 3,619 Canadian recruits had relatively short first segments. However, even in instances where the first metatarsal was markedly shorter than the second, there was no resultant functional incapacity.

Shortness of other metatarsals (brachymetapody) may occur, and occasionally this condition results in excessive loading of the adjacent segments, with consequent plantar callus. Most cases are probably nonhereditary, but shortness of the first and fifth metatarsals was reported in persons with pseudohypoparathyroidism, and Steggerda (1942) reported the case of a family with apparently dominant transmission. One or many of the metatarsals may be congenitally short (Figs. 4-31 to 4-33) and occasionally they may produce disability. Therapy cannot be standardized.

Metatarsus proximus

Normally the second and third metatarsal heads are adjacent to each other, with little space in between them. They are occasionally situated so close to each other that the wearing of ordinary shoes squeezes them together and causes pain from friction, which may necessitate excision of the side of one of the heads (Fig. 4-34).

ABNORMALITIES OF THE SESAMOIDS
Distorted and hypertrophied sesamoids

The sesamoids vary widely in size and shape. Some may have projections that become weight-bearing points, thereby producing a deep-seated callus, usually under the tibial sesamoid.

Congenital variations of the sesamoids may become a problem if the whole or part of the plantar surface of the sesamoid is not smooth or evenly shaped. The types vary extensively. They may be extraordinarily large or thick or have a sharp projection on the plantar surface. Acquired irregularities of a sesamoid may be secondary to a

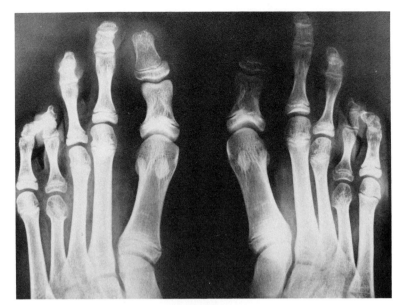

Fig. 4-31. Bilateral congenital short fourth metatarsal.

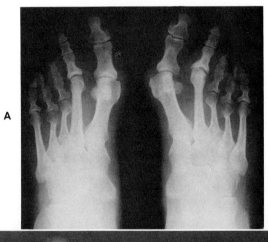

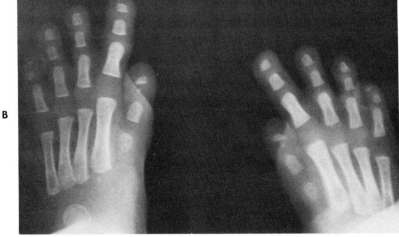

Fig. 4-32. A, Bilateral congenital short third and fourth metatarsals. **B,** Bilateral congenital underdevelopment of first metatarsal.

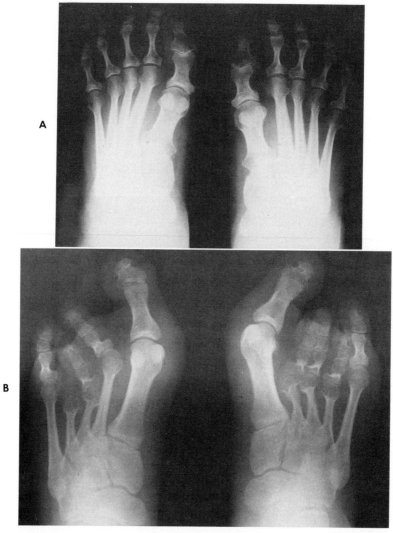

Fig. 4-33. A, Bilateral congenital short first metatarsals in adult. **B,** Bilateral short multiple lesser metatarsals.

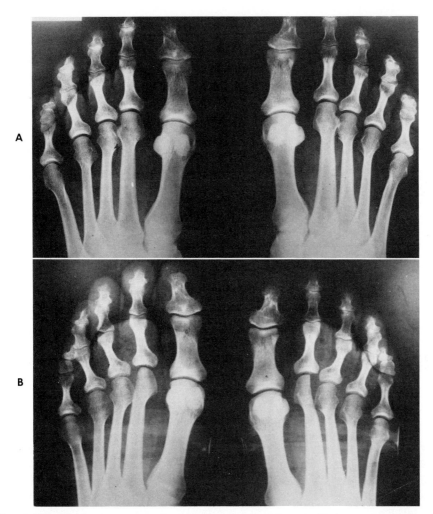

Fig. 4-34. **A,** Metatarsus proximus between second and third metatarsal heads. **B,** Same case postoperatively.

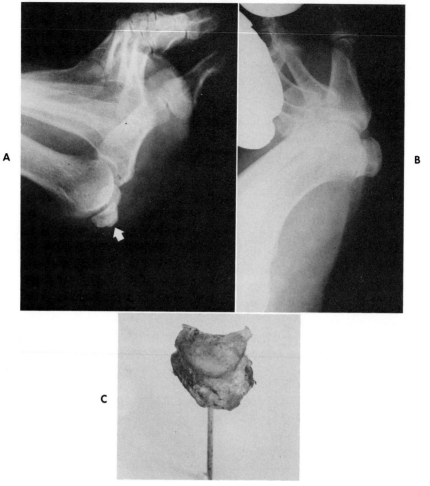

Fig. 4-35. A, Hypertrophic ridge on plantar surface of tibial sesamoid that produced hyperkeratosis in skin beneath it. **B,** Unusually thick tibial sesamoid that induced deep-seated callus beneath. **C,** Extensive hypertrophy of excised sesamoid. It had caused a chronic ulcer under the first metatarsal head.

congenitally anomalous-shaped sesamoid or to rotation of the sesamoid secondary to deformity of the great toe joint. Because the sesamoids normally fit into a groove on the plantar surface of the first metatarsal head (see hallux valgus, p. 209), any rotation or abduction of the first metatarsal tends to rotate the sesamoids. Their distorted shape also may be the result of hypertrophy. If hypertrophy is plantarward, the excess bone will induce a deep-seated callus and ultimately may ulcerate the soft tissue beneath it because of the pressure of weight bearing (Figs. 4-35 and 4-36).

Bipartite and multipartite sesamoids are common (Apley, 1965). Giannestras (1967) states that the medial sesamoid of the hallux may consist of two, three, or even four bones, whereas the lateral sesamoid divides rarely and then only into a bipartite configuration.

Symptoms. Constant pain on weight bearing is the symptom that makes the patient seek relief. A deep-seated callus is typically present under the pivotal area. The callus may be mistaken for a verruca plantaris. The soft tissue under the sesamoid, debilitated by chronic irritation,

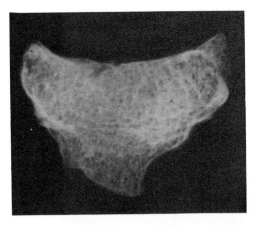

Fig. 4-36. Medial-lateral roentgenogram of tibial sesamoid after removal. Exostotic enlargement on its plantar aspect caused a keratotic lesion and chronic ulcer in the foot after 15 years' duration.

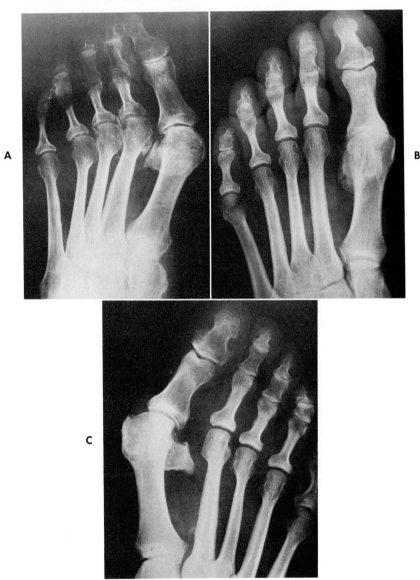

Fig. 4-37. Hypertrophic changes of fibular sesamoid resulting in pain in first metatarsal interspace.

may ulcerate and resist all palliative treatment. Misshapen or hypertrophied fibular sesamoids seldom produce keratotic changes of the skin, because normally they do not bear weight. The pain experienced between the first and second metatarsal heads may be the result of irritation (Fig. 4-37). Occasionally an exostosis develops on the fibular sesamoid (Fig. 4-38).

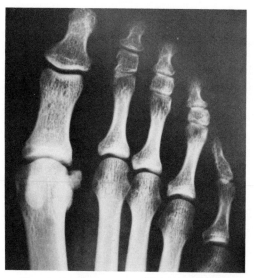

Fig. 4-38. Exostosis of fibular sesamoid.

Treatment. In mild cases proper weight distribution alleviates symptoms. In protracted cases sesamoidectomy is indicated.

Congenital absence of the tibial sesamoid

Two cases of congenital absence of the tibial sesamoid, in each case on one foot only, were reported by Inge (1936). The anomaly is probably more prevalent than is realized and goes unnoticed because ordinarily it is symptomless. Such an anomaly, however, can produce a painful callus under the first metatarsal head when there is a hammertoe deformity of the great toe. The absence of the sesamoid weakens the flexor hallucis brevis and predisposes the great toe to a clawed shape. Bilateral absence of the tibial sesamoid also may produce such deformity and intractable callus under the first metatarsal head as to require reduction of the hammered toe with lengthening of the extensor hallucis longus for relief of symptoms (Fig. 4-39).

Inconstant sesamoids

Accessory, or inconstant, sesamoids may occur under any weight-bearing surface of the foot (Figs. 4-40 to 4-42), especially un-

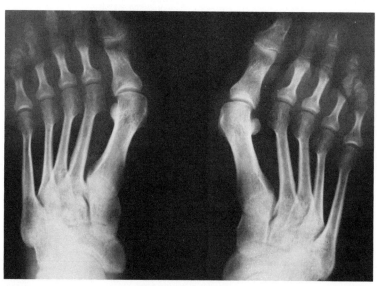

Fig. 4-39. Congenital absence of both tibial sesamoids. Hammered great toe with resulting pain under first metatarsal head occurred.

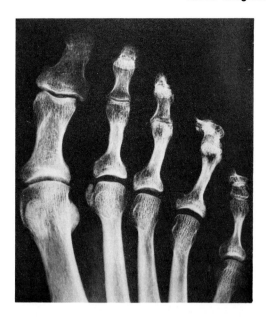

Fig. 4-40. Accessory sesamoid in short flexor of second toe. It had rotated into the first metatarsal interspace and caused chronic pain.

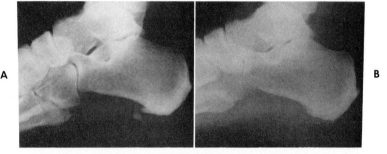

A   B

Fig. 4-41. Pain under calcaneal tuberosity caused by accessory sesamoid in plantar fascia. Symptoms were relieved by excision of the sesamoid.

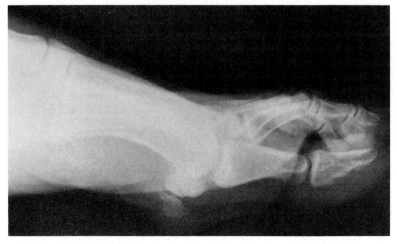

Fig. 4-42. Accessory tibial sesamoid immediately under normal tibial sesamoid.

der the heads of the lesser metatarsals (Fig. 4-43) or any of the phalanges and at times under all the metatarsal heads. Patterson (1937) and Lapidus (1940) each reported such a case. The accessory sesamoids vary widely in size and shape. Ordinarily they are asymptomatic, but they may become

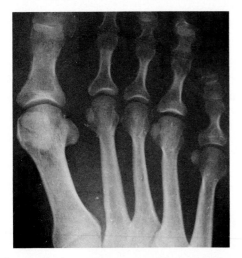

Fig. 4-43. Inconstant sesamoids under lesser metatarsals.

painful when the ossicle is extraordinarily large or when the metatarsal above it rotates. They are more likely to produce symptoms under the second or fifth metatarsal head. Sesamoids under the second metatarsal head can be excised through an incision over the first metatarsal interspace. Under the fifth metatarsal head they are best excised through an incision along the lateral plantar border of the fifth metatarsophalangeal joint.

Sesamoid under the head of the first proximal phalanx

Sesamoids occur often as accessory bones under the head of the first proximal phalanx. Typically they occur singly, but they may appear in pairs. When a sesamoid is unusually large, or when the phalanx rotates so that the sesamoid acts as a pivot, it can become disabling. This can happen in cases of hallux valgus.

Characteristics. The fibular side of the phalanx (Fig. 4-44) is more often involved than is the tibial side. The first evidence of

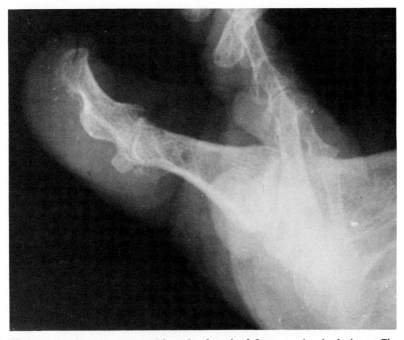

Fig. 4-44. Large accessory sesamoid under head of first proximal phalanx. The sesamoid caused a chronic ulcer beneath it.

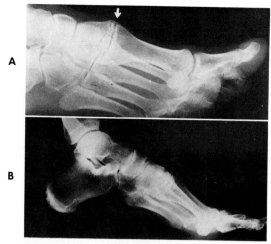

Fig. 4-45. A, High dorsum of base of first metatarsal–first cuneiform articulation. **B,** Postoperative appearance.

the disorder is a deep-seated callus, which may break down and ulcerate.

Treatment. The treatment of choice is excision. Through an incision on that side of the toe with the offending ossicle, the sesamoid under the head of the first proximal phalanx can be excised readily.

MISCELLANEOUS MINOR CONGENITAL ANOMALIES
High dorsum of the base of the first metatarsal–first cuneiform joint

Congenital enlargement of the dorsum of the first metatarsal–first cuneiform joint is common (Fig. 4-45). It becomes symptomatic only from friction and pressure of the shoe, usually in early adult life and mostly in women. Some of the resulting problems are: (1) Acute cellulitis over the dorsum of the joint, which may or may not extend down to the bone, producing osteomyelitis (the infection enters through a hair follicle in the skin over the bony prominence) (2) tenosynovitis of the extensor hallucis longus tendon, which lies immediately over this enlargement. (3) constant friction and pressure over the area, gradually producing a fibrotic mass which may break down and form a chronic drain-

ing sinus, and (4) osteophytic changes in the form of lipping at the base of the first metatarsal and medial cuneiform.

Treatment. In moderate cases, avoidance of shoes that exert pressure and friction over the area ameliorates symptoms. In protracted cases, especially when lipping has formed, removal of the bony prominence is indicated.

The following technique makes ambulation possible in 48 hours. Healing is usually uneventful and complete in from 6 to 8 weeks.

1. Make a longitudinal incision along the dorsomedial aspect of the base of the first metatarsal–first cuneiform.
2. Retract the lateral skin margin and make a longitudinal incision in the ligaments and capsule over the middle of the joint. This will obviate having two lines of sutures in the same plane.
3. Retract the fascial margins to expose the bony prominence, which is removed with an osteotome. Smooth with a rasp. Removal of the bony prominence should leave a moderate depression, which allows for some new bone formation that may result from surgical irritation. Place additional dressing material over the depressed area to prevent subdermal bleeding into a pocket.
4. Close the fascia and skin in layers and apply a compression bandage.

Rare minor anomalies

Some rare anomalies are illustrated in Figs. 4-46 through 4-51. These include (1) aseptic necrosis in the base of the second metatarsal as a result of grating of the base of the first metatarsal into the second; (2) a bifurcated first cuneiform with an abnormal hallux and proximal phalanges; (3) synostosis of the shafts of the left second and third metatarsals; (4) polydactylia, syndactyly, and anomalous lesser metatarsals in the same foot; (5) syndactyly of both feet with symphalangism of the left third toe and absence of all of the right third toe except for the epiphysis of the

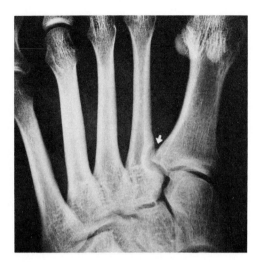

Fig. 4-46. Base of first metatarsal grating into base of second metatarsal. Note secondary aseptic necrosis in the base of the second metatarsal.

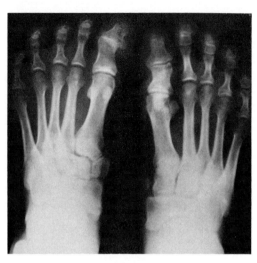

Fig. 4-47. Bifurcated first cuneiform; abnormal hallux and proximal phalanges.

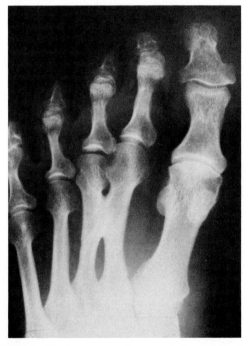

Fig. 4-48. Asymptomatic synostosis of shafts of left second and third metatarsals.

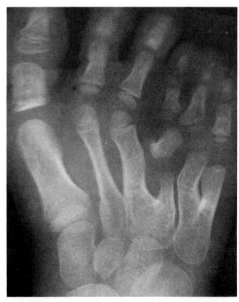

Fig. 4-49. Polydactylia, syndactyly, and anomalous lesser metatarsals in same foot.

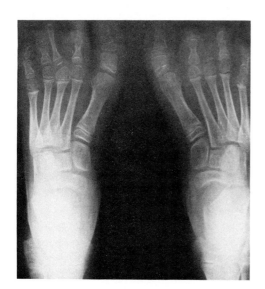

Fig. 4-50. Syndactyly of both feet with symphalangism of left third toe and absence of all of right third toe except for epiphysis of proximal phalanx. This child had a hypoplastic external ear, hypoplastic thumbs, and was also mentally retarded.

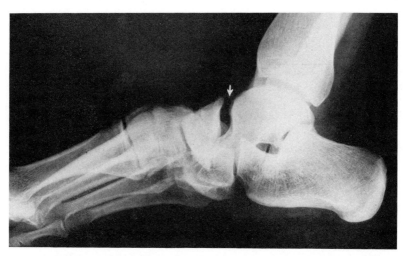

Fig. 4-51. Congenital deformity of talonavicular joint resulting in unstable foot. The talus appears to be vertically aligned, and the talonavicular findings may represent adaptive changes.

proximal phalanx; and (6) a congenital deformity of the talonavicular joint.

REFERENCES

General

Giannestras, N. J.: Foot disorders: Medical and surgical management. Philadelphia, 1967, Lea & Febiger.

Harris, R. I.: Retrospect—peroneal spastic flat foot (rigid valgus foot), J. Bone Joint Surg. **47-A:**1657-1667, Dec. 1965.

Harris, R. I., and Beath, T.: Army foot survey: An investigation of foot ailments in Canadian soldiers, (forms no. 1574, Rep. Nat. Res. Counc., Canada) Ottawa, 1947.

Leonard, M. H., Gonzales, S., Breck, L. W., Basom, C., Palafox, M., and Kosicki, Z. W.: Lateral transfer of the posterior tibial tendon in certain selected cases of pes plano valgus (Kidner operation), Clin. Orthop. **40:**139-144, May-June 1965.

McKusick, V. A.: Mendelian inheritance in man: Catalogues of autosomal dominant, autosomal recessive, and X-linked phenotypes, ed. 2, Baltimore, 1968, Johns Hopkins Press.

Smith, D. W.: Recognizable patterns of human malformation: Genetic, embryologic, and clinical aspects, Philadelphia, 1970, W. B. Saunders Co.

Taylor, A. I.: Patau's, Edward's and cri du chat syndromes: Tabulated summary of current findings, Dev. Med. Child Neurol. **9:**78-86, 1967.

Accessory bones

Bizarro, A. H.: On sesamoid and supernumerary bones of the limbs, J. Anat. **55:**256-268, 1921.

Chater, E. H.: Foot pain and the accessory navicular bone, Irish J. Med. Sci. **442:**471-475, 1962.

Geist, E. S.: The accessory scaphoid bone, J. Bone Joint Surg. **7:**570-574, July 1925.

Henderson, R. S.: Os intermetatarseum and a possible relationship to hallux valgus, J. Bone Joint Surg. **45-B:**117-121, Feb. 1963.

Kidner, F. C.: The prehalux (accessory scaphoid) in its relation to flat-foot, J. Bone Joint Surg. **11:**831-837, Oct. 1929.

McDougall, A.: The os trigonum. J. Bone Joint Surg. **37-B:**257-265, May 1955.

O'Rahilly, R.: A survey of carpal and tarsal anomalies, J. Bone Joint Surg. **35-A:**626-642, July 1953.

Trolle, D.: Accessory bones of the human foot (Translated by E. Aagesen) Copenhagen, 1948, Munksgaard.

Wildervanck, L. S., Geodhard, G., and Meiier, S.: Proximal symphalangism of fingers associated with fusion of os naviculare and talus and occurrence of two accessory bones in the feet (os paranaviculare and os tibiale externum) in an European-Indonesian-Chinese family, Acta Genet. (Basel) **17:**166-177, 1967.

Zadek, I.: The significance of the accessory tarsal scaphoid, J. Bone Joint Surg. **8:**618-626, 1926.

Zadek, I., and Gold, A. M.: Accessory tarsal scaphoid, J. Bone Joint Surg. **30-A:**957-968, Oct. 1948.

Abnormalities of the toes

Bunnell, S.: Surgery of the hand, ed. 4, revised by J. H. Boyes, Philadelphia, 1964, J. B. Lippincott Co., pp. 81-90.

Charters, A. D.: Local gigantism, J. Bone Joint Surg. **39-B:**542-547, Aug. 1957.

Cobey, M. C., and Covey, J. C.: A true prehallux, J. Bone Joint Surg. **48-A:**953-954, July 1966.

Hurwitz, L. H.: Personal communication.

Lamy, M., and Frézal, J.: The frequency of congenital malformations. In First International Conference on Congenital Malformations, Philadelphia, 1961, J. B. Lippincott, pp. 34-44.

Lantzounis, L. A.: Congenital subluxation of the fifth toe and its correction by a periostocapsuloplasty and tendon transplantation, J. Bone Joint Surg. **22:**147-150, Jan. 1940.

Lapidus, P. W.: Transplantation of the extensor tendon for correction of overlapping fifth toe, J. Bone Joint Surg. **24:**555-559, July 1942.

Laurin, C., Favreau, M., and Labelle, P.: Bilateral absence of the radius and tibia with bilateral reduplication of the ulna and fibula, J. Bone Joint Surg. **46-A:**137-142, Jan. 1964.

Savarinathan, G., and Centerwall, W. R.: Symphalangism: A pedigree from south India. J. Med Genet. **3:**285-289, Dec. 1966.

Sharma, N., Singh, R., and Anand, J.: Polydactylosyndactylism with unusual skeletal anomalies in a mother and her six children, Indian J. Pediat. **32:**233-237, July 1965.

Simopoulis, A., Brennan, G., Alwan, A., and Fidis, N.: Polycystic kidneys, internal hydrocephalus and polydactylism in newborn siblings, Pediatrics **39:**931-934, June 1967.

Watson, H. K., and Boyes, J. H.: Congenital angular deformity of the digits: Delta phalanx, J. Bone Joint Surg. **49-A:**333-338, Mar. 1967.

Abnormalities of the great toe

Haas, S. L.: An operation for the correction of hallux varus, J. Bone Joint Surg. **20:**705-708, July 1938.

McElvenny, R. T.: **Hallux varus,** Quart. Bull. Northwestern Univ. Med. School **15:**277-280, Winter Quarter 1941.

Sloane, D.: Congenital hallux varus, J. Bone Joint Surg. **17:**209-211, Jan. 1935.

Thompson, S. A.: Hallux varus and metatarsus varus: A five-year study (1954-1958), Clin. Orthop. **16:**109-118, 1960.

Abnormalities of the metatarsals

Kaplan, A. R.: Genetics of relative toe lengths, Acta Genet. Med. Gemellol. (Roma) 13:295-304, 1964.

Kemp, T., and Ravn, J.: Über erbliche Hand- und Fussdeformitäten in einem 140-köpfigen Geschlecht, nebst einigen Bemerkungen über Poly- und Syndaktylie beim Menschen, Acta Psychiatr. Neurol. 7:275-296, 1932.

Morton, D. J.: The human foot: Its evolution, physiology, and functional disorders, New York, 1935, Columbia University Press.

Nievergelt, K.: Positiver Väterschaftsnachweis auf Grund erblicher Missbildungen der Extremitäten, Arch. Julius Klaus Stift. Vererbungsforsch. 19:157-159, 1944.

Pearlman, H. S., Edkin, R. E., and Warren, R. F.: Familial tarsal and carpal synostosis with radial-head subluxation (Nievergelt's syndrome), J. Bone Joint Surg. 46-A:585-592, Apr. 1964.

Steggerda, M.: Inheritance of short metatarsals, J. Hered. 33:233-234, June 1942.

Tachdjian, M. O.: Diagnosis and treatment of congenital deformities in the musculoskeletal system in the newborn and the infant, Pediat. Clin. N. Amer. 14:307-358, May 1967.

Abnormalities of the sesamoids

Apley, A. G.: Open sesamoid! A re-appraisal of the medial sesamoid of the hallux, Proc. Roy. Soc. Med. 59:120, Feb. 1966.

Inge, G. A. L.: Congenital absence of the medial sesamoid bone of the great toe: A report of two cases, J. Bone Joint Surg. 18:188-190, Jan. 1936.

Lapidus, P. W.: Sesamoids beneath all the metatarsal heads of both feet, J. Bone Joint Surg. 22:1059-1062, Oct. 1940.

Patterson, R. F.: Multiple sesamoids of the hands and the feet, J. Bone Joint Surg. 19:531-532, Apr. 1937.

5

Major congenital deformities and anomalies of the foot

Elmer E. Specht

*Thou knowest not . . . how the bones
do grow in the womb of her that is
with child . . ."*

ECCLESIASTES 11:5

CONGENITAL DEFORMITIES AND ANOMALIES OF THE FOOT DURING INFANCY AND CHILDHOOD

The infant foot

At birth the infant's foot may seem to be deformed because the longitudinal arch is lacking and the foot appears abducted and flat. Only the most obvious deformities and not these initial deficiencies should cause concern, for the foot may continue to appear abducted and flat until the child is 2 years old. During the first year the infant's muscles develop through his kicking, twisting, and crawling activities. The age at which children begin to stand or walk varies within widely normal limits, but a child should not be urged to stand or walk until he is naturally ready. Between the ages of 2 and 4 a longitudinal arch develops and the child assumes a normal gait. Running and jumping develop the structure of the foot and leg further; but it is during this period that the normal attitude of the foot may deviate. Flatfoot accompanied by abduction of the forefoot and internal tibial torsion (pigeon toe) may become evident at this time. Correction is possible in most instances through the use of shoe appliances, padding, and wedging of the shoe. Plaster casts or surgical intervention will be required only in extreme cases.

Congenital deformities and anomalies of the foot in infancy and childhood are usually self-evident, but some types are unnoticed until static deformities develop. Shands and Wentz (1953) reviewed 4,230 cases of disorders of the foot in children treated at the Alfred I. du Pont Institute and selected for study those in which roentgenograms had been taken, 850 in all. Of the selected cases, they found that 231, or 27 percent, showed significant congenital anomalies.

The prognosis in cases of congenital deformities of the foot is in direct relation to early diagnosis and treatment.

The foot during childhood

Problems encountered in the feet of children are different from those encountered in the feet of adults, because during childhood changes in the foot are taking place while the immature foot is growing and developing. Activities normal to childhood probably play an additional role in the growth of the foot during the process of maturation. Ossification of the epiphyses takes place during adolescence, but at varying years. The degree of ossification of the different bones of the foot and ankle varies according to the year in which ossification takes place. Slight injuries or the wearing of poorly fitted shoes predisposes the child to osteochondritis or fracture of the epiphyseal plate. Although children have a high potential for injuries incurred at play, healing capability of the child and adolescent is superior to that of the adult.

Age of ossification centers. The only bones seen in roentgenograms of the foot at birth are the diaphyses of the phalanges and metatarsals and the nuclei of the calcaneus, talus, and sometimes the cuboid. The nuclei of the calcaneus and talus show the typical shape of the bone at birth. The calcaneus is formed by the fusion of two nuclei that are present in the early embryonic stage.

During the first few months the nucleus of the cuboid begins to ossify; ossification of the third cuneiform follows during the sixth postnatal month. At the beginning of the second year the nuclei of the first cuneiform and of the epiphyses of the phalanges are observable. Toward the end of the second year all the tarsal nuclei may be present as well as the epiphyses of the metatarsals and phalanges. In the male the nucleus of the middle cuneiform may not appear until the end of the fourth year, and the nucleus of the navicular may not be seen until the fourth year (Fig 5-1).

TYPES OF MAJOR CONGENITAL DEFORMITIES

The terms clubfoot and talipes are generally used to mean a deformed or distorted foot. Medical usage of the term clubfoot, however, tends to limit the meaning to talipes equinovarus. Talipes (from the Latin *talus,* meaning ankle, and *pes,* mean-

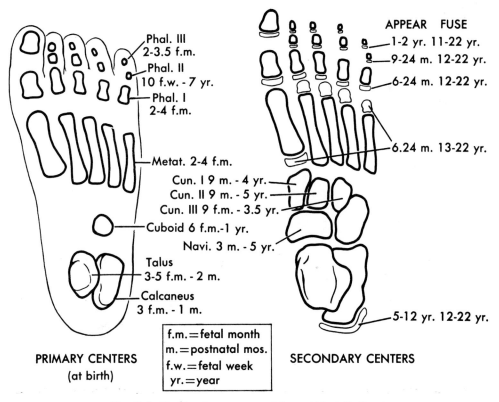

Phal. III
2-3.5 f.m.
Phal. II
10 f.w. - 7 yr.
Phal. I
2-4 f.m.

APPEAR   FUSE
1-2 yr. 11-22 yr.
9-24 m. 12-22 yr.
6-24 m. 12-22 yr.

6.24 m. 13-22 yr.

Metat. 2-4 f.m.
Cun. I 9 m. - 4 yr.
Cun. II 9 m. - 5 yr.
Cun. III 9 f.m. - 3.5 yr.
Cuboid 6 f.m.-1 yr.
Navi. 3 m. - 5 yr.
Talus
3-5 f.m. - 2 m.
Calcaneus
3 f.m. - 1 m.

5-12 yr. 12-22 yr.

| f.m.=fetal month |
| m.=postnatal mos. |
| f.w.=fetal week |
| yr.=year |

PRIMARY CENTERS
(at birth)

SECONDARY CENTERS

Fig. 5-1. Ossification centers of foot. (After Caffey.)

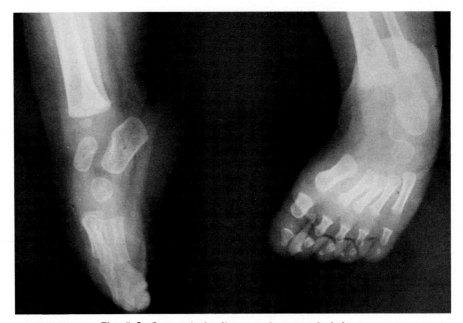

Fig. 5-2. Congenital talipes equinovarus in infant.

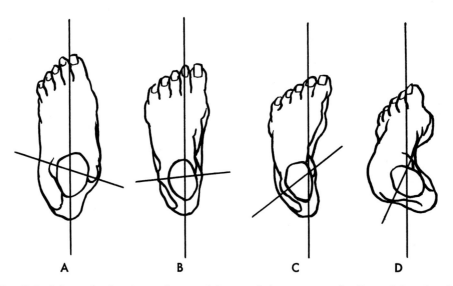

A   B   C   D

Fig. 5-3. Schematic drawings of normal foot and three types of talipes deformity. **A,** Talipes valgus. **B,** Normal. **C,** Metatarsus adductus. **D,** Talipes varus.

ing foot), without other modification, retains its general meaning; it will be used in this discussion to indicate any foot deformity.

Talipes is generally thought of as being congenital in origin; however, the term is often applied to acquired and paralytic deformities (Whitman, 1930). Many of these deformities overlap; for instance, clawfoot, which is generally considered congenital in origin, and peroneal spastic flatfoot, which is often caused by congenital tarsal coalition or talonavicular anomalies, do not appear until early childhood. The deformities may be (1) congenital, as in talipes equinovarus; (2) acquired, as in talipes planovalgus; and (3) neurologic, as in paralytic talipes equinus.

The major deformities of the foot may be classified as (1) equinus (plantar flexion of the ankle and foot), (2) calcaneus (dorsiflexion of the ankle and foot), (3) varus (inversion and adduction of the foot), and (4) valgus (eversion and abduction of the foot). Deformities of the foot more commonly occur as combinations of these than as isolated deformities, whether congenital or acquired. Types of deformity found in congenital talipes, according to Whitman, appear in the following order of frequency (from highest to lowest): equinovarus, valgus, varus, calcaneovalgus, equinus, and calcaneus.

In talipes equinus the foot is held in plantar flexion, the calf muscles are contracted, and the toes are contracted and hammered (clawtoes). When the child begins to walk, he bears weight only on the ball of the deformed foot. In talipes calcaneus the anterior muscles are contracted, the foot is held in dorsiflexion, and the weight is borne primarily on the heel. In talipes calcaneovalgus the foot is in dorsiflexion and eversion. The lateral toe extensors and the peroneal muscles are contracted. Talipes equinovarus is characterized by contracture of the calf muscles, resulting in equinus; the toes are flexed and the forefoot is adducted (Fig. 5-2). The heel is in varus, and the tibia is in-

ternally rotated. When the child stands, the weight is borne by the shaft and base of the fifth metatarsal (Fig. 5-3, *D*).

Swann et al. (1969) have challenged the general belief that the tibia is medially rotated in uncorrected clubfoot. They posit that the hindfoot and ankle mortise are in fact laterally rotated on an unrotated tibia. Thus in lateral roentgenograms of the uncorrected deformity, the talus will appear flat-topped, and there will be an apparent anteroposterior projection of the ankle mortise; medial rotation of the leg (from 30 to 60 degrees) will project the talus and ankle mortise into normal lateral configuration. The authors concede, however, that premature forced dorsiflexion is a cause of osteochondral compression, which flattens the dome of the talus.

In talipes valgus the foot is abducted and pronated, the peroneal muscles are contracted, and the weight is borne by the shaft of the first metataral, first cuneiform, and navicular bones (see Fig. 5-3, *A*). Talipes equinovalgus is characterized by contracted calf and peroneal musculature; the forefoot is abducted.

From the standpoint of treatment, one may classify the major foot deformities into two groups: (1) congenital and acquired deformities that may be altered during the growth period (making use of Wolff's and Davis' laws, on the basis of which alteration of bone and soft tissue structure and function through orthotic or surgical measures will take place) and (2) paralytic deformities whose basic cause makes them incurable. In both instances, if the deformities are left untreated, there is a tendency for bones and soft tissues to conform to the deforming forces. In general it is best to undertake treatment as early as possible.

Congenital talipes equinovarus

In civilized countries congenital talipes in the adult has become a rarity, because the adage, "the time to treat a congenital clubfoot is immediately after tying the natal cord," is followed in modern medical practice. Most clubfeet are now reversed in infancy before they become static. It is only the irreversible type and the type that does not appear until early childhood, such as clawfoot, that is now encountered.

Etiology. The cause of congenital clubfoot is generally conjectural and has been theorized upon for centuries. Many hypotheses advanced are speculative; research is based upon embryologic studies and studies of postnatal incidence, but there are no direct scientific means of investigation. The causes of congenital clubfoot noted in the historical literature are (1) heredity, (2) mechanical or intrauterine pressure, (3) prenatal neuromyic maldevelopment, (4) arrest of development, (5) primary germ plasm defects, and (6) retarded rotation or nonrotation of the extremities.

Heredity. Polygenic inheritance may account for the definite familial occurrence of talipes equinovarus; however, Palmer (1964) believes that in some families transmission is by autosomal dominant genes with 40 percent penetrance. The probability of recurrence in subsequently born children is about 10 percent in this group, whereas overall risk of the occurrence of clubfoot in the sibling of a child with this deformity is one in thirty-five. In identical twins it is one in three. Males are affected twice as commonly as females.

Abnormal intrauterine pressure. Hippocrates, who described clubfoot in 400 B.C., suggested that abnormal pressure on the developing fetal foot might cause deformity in a foot that was otherwise developing normally. This theory still has its modern adherents. Another cause of constraint and thus of ultimate deformity may be the interlocking of the fetal feet. Many museum specimens show the feet in this position. In some cases of talipes seen in the first weeks of life the feet are placed in the attitude in which they had been fixed before birth.

Prenatal musculoneurogenesis. That alteration of the muscles, with or without a central nervous lesion, caused clubfoot was a speculation supported by many early writers. One popular theory was that the deformity was caused by a contracture of specific leg muscles. Bechtol and Mossman (1950) and Stewart (1951) supported the theory that the imbalance of opponent muscles and the abnormal differentiation of tendons play an important role in the etiology of clubfoot. During an infant mortality survey Wiley (1959), in an anatomic study of infants with clubfoot, compared these findings with findings based on studies of experimental rabbits in which muscle changes were produced. He believed the evidence indicated that in clubfoot the primary cause of deformity was an inherent factor that maintained the foot in a deformed position and caused growth deficiency in the long muscles. Fried (1959), after making surgical dissections of fifty-six clubfeet, concluded that the primary pathology was the thickening and abnormal insertion of the posterior tibial tendon. Garceau and Palmer (1967) felt that the most common deforming element in recurrent clubfoot was the anterior tibial muscle, while Dwyer (1963) emphasized that the deforming vector was the medially directed pull of the tendo achillis on the inverted heel. Knight (1954) believed that postural habits in infants and children during sleeping, sitting, and playing were often directly or indirectly a cause of later developmental deformities of the foot. One is thus forced to conclude that differentiation between primary and adaptive changes is impossible in our present state of knowledge.

Arrest of development. Many early writers suggested that the cause of arrest in development was the persistence of the feet in the physiologic position of the sixth or seventh week of fetal life, with the sole turned inward.

Primary germ plasm defect. Irani and Sherman (1963) have postulated that a primary germ plasm defect in the cartilaginous anlage of the anterior part of the talus causes clubfoot. The neck of the talus is always short so that the head seems to fuse directly with the body, and the head deviates medially and plantarward. They could find no primary abnormalities of soft-tissue structures, including tendons, in eleven dissected fetal specimens with equinovarus deformities.

Retarded rotation or nonrotation. About the third month of intrauterine life the thighs of the fetus are abducted, flexed, and rotated outward. The legs are crossed and the feet are plantar flexed and adducted so that the inner surfaces of the thighs, the tibial borders of the legs, and the plantar surfaces of the feet are held in close apposition to the fetal abdomen and pelvis. Later there is inward rotation of the limb, with the feet gradually being turned outward until the soles are brought into contact with the uterine wall. The feet are then in the attitude of abduction and dorsiflexion. According to this theory there is a regular succession of attitudes during intrauterine life. If, for some reason, the inward rotation of the lower extremity is prevented, or if it is incomplete, the foot that remains in the original position becomes deformed.

Conservative treatment of talipes equinovarus. Conservative treatment in infancy and early childhood is effective in most instances. The basic step in correction of a foot deformity in early childhood is to place the components of the deformity in an exact opposite or overcorrected position by continuous retentive leverage by splints or casts until a normal attitude of the foot has been attained. It must be stressed that treatment of a foot that demonstrates a fixed deformity must be started early in the life of the infant, preferably in the newborn nursery. Treatment must be continuous until all elements of the deformity have been overcorrected, and retention devices such as splints or braces are required until such time as careful follow-up leads to the certainty that correction will be maintained. A growth deformity is being treated, and this fact should be borne in mind constantly: Recurrence of the deformity can occur until growth of the foot is complete. Kite (1932, 1939, 1964) has reported extensively on his method of plaster

correction and his results. In a review in 1964 of the results of treating nearly a thousand patients early in life who were followed afterward for 5 years, Kite claimed successful correction in 92 percent of cases by casting and wedging alone.

By Kite's method a padded cast is applied to the extremity from the toes to the midthigh. The knee is flexed in a 90-degree angle, and the foot is held in mild correction without undue strain on the deformity. The cast is changed once or twice a week, increasing the correction as rapidly as it can be tolerated. The forefoot adduction and heel varus are first overcorrected before the equinus deformity is corrected. Unless the adduction deformity is corrected first, a rocker foot may result if dorsiflexion correction is attempted. The head of the calcaneus is rotated laterally from under the neck of the talus. Roentgenograms of the foot should demonstrate a divergence of the long axes of the calcaneus and the talus. One of the disadvantages of this technique is that the calf contracture and resultant equinus deformity are allowed to remain and the deformity becomes more resistant. Failure to correct the forefoot, however, frequently results in recurrence of the deformity (Bechtol and Mossman, 1950).

When the deformity has been completely corrected, a retentive cast is applied for several months. The retentive cast should be changed every few weeks, depending upon the rate of growth of the extremity.

Some practitioners prefer splints (Browne, 1933; Thomson, 1942, Blumenfeld et al., 1946; Blockey and Smith, 1966). The Denis Browne splint works on the principle that it is possible to control the position of one foot by the other. In an infant this is accomplished by bandaging and strapping both feet to metal footplates, which are fastened to a horizontal crossbar (Fig. 5-4, A). The foot must be protected by sufficient padding from skin irritation and pressure points. The strapping and bandaging are changed every 5 to 8 days. Correction of the deformities takes place

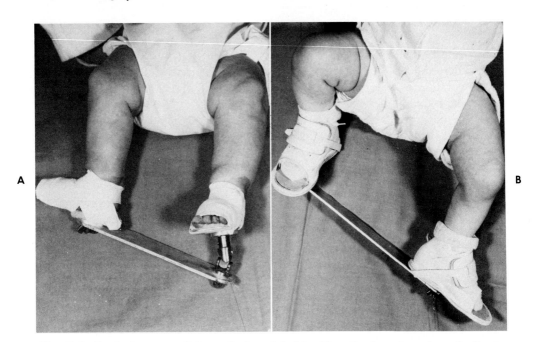

A

B

Fig. 5-4. Denis Browne splint applied and held with adhesive strapping. **B,** Denis Browne splint with shoes. (Courtesy Dr. S. A. Thomson.)

in from 6 to 8 weeks; however, the foot must be held in a normal position for many months, even for as long as a year, to prevent recurrence. When the child can be fitted with a firm high-top shoe, the sole of the shoe can be fastened to the footplate (Fig. 5-4, *B*) and the appliance is worn day and night. Occasionally the splint may be removed for a few hours. In mild cases firm high-top shoes may be worn during the day and the splints at night. In severe cases the splint should be worn continuously for a year or longer with only short rest periods.

Relapsed or partly corrected cases have followed both methods of treatment. Perhaps most failures are the result of hasty evaluation of the deformity or inadequate subsequent treatment.

Surgical treatment of talipes equinovarus. Some authorities differ (e.g., Goldner, 1970) but in general, surgical intervention should be undertaken only after adequate casting or splinting measures have failed. An exception to this statement is the judicious use of tendo achillis lengthening or tenotomy, combined with posterior

capsulotomy, if necessary, in correcting the equinus portion of the deformity (having first corrected the adduction and varus components by conservative means). It is better to resort to such releases than to risk crushing the dome of the talus by forceful dorsiflexion of the ankle against unyielding posterior structures. Tendon transfers should be reserved for relapsing cases in which a definite deforming influence can be localized to a particular muscle. The use of osteoplastic procedures may be indicated in the older child with recurrent deformity. Triple arthrodesis and the Lambrinudi procedure (Bényi, 1960) essentially should be regarded as salvage procedures in the mature or nearly mature foot. They should seldom be performed on a child under the age of 9, and then only with recognition of the inevitable growth loss that will follow. Furthermore, arthrodesis of the hindfoot joints in the immature foot may lead to the development of a ball-and-socket tibiotalar joint.

Abnormal insertions and attachments of the opponent abductors and adductors of the forefoot may produce imbalance of their function and cause recurrence of the deformity. Scherb (1930) explained how abnormality of tendinous attachment, particularly of the peroneus brevis to the extensor digitorum brevis, causes recurrence of the adduction deformity. Garceau and Manning (1947) have shown how abnormal attachments of the tibialis anterior tendon lead to recurrence.

Lengthening of the tendo achillis. Residual contracture of the tendo achillis with resultant uncorrected equinus deformity is the most common unyielding deformity encountered. The equinus is usually the first deformity to recur in the relapsed clubfoot. The contracted tendo achillis may be lengthened by subcutaneous tenotomy, or by tendo achillis lengthening under direct vision.

A number of lengthening procedures are in common use. They differ in position and number of incisions into the tendon, such as triple hemisection and double hemisection. Lengthening by open tenotomy is generally preferable, since tendon lengthening alone does not allow adequate release of the contracture in many resistant equinus deformities. Division of the posterior ankle joint capsule can then be performed to gain necessary dorsiflexed overcorrection without the use of force.

Subcutaneous tendo achillis tenotomy is a safe procedure in some surgeons' hands. Ponseti and Smoley (1963) advocated subcutaneous tendo achillis tenotomy as a primary treatment to attain complete correction of the equinus deformity. Correction of severe equinus deformity can be shortened radically by subcutaneous section of the heel cord, followed by application of a plaster cast. After this procedure the tendon always heals with little scarring, and, if done early, a posterior capsulotomy of the ankle joint is unnecessary. Rocker-bottom foot and flattening of the upper articular surfaces of the talus are prevented as well. An unyielding contracture in the hindfoot should not be allowed to remain if conservative correction is not progressing. A posterior capsulotomy should be performed if tendo achillis lengthening is not followed by complete correction of the equinus contracture. A thickened posterior ankle capsule is always found to be the cause for unyielding equinus after unsuccessful tendo achillis lengthening. The tendon sheaths of the posterior calf muscles are also contracted and require sectioning. These may be expected in a foot with a comparatively fat, small heel in which the lines of the calcaneus are not easily identifiable.

Medial release. Failure to correct the original adduction and inversion contracture of the foot caused by soft-tissue contracture may necessitate surgical release of the medial and plantar aspect of the arch of the foot. The principles of surgical correction of this deformity have been described and emphasized by Brockmann (1930) and Turco (1971). The aim of these procedures is directed toward release of contracted ligamentous, capsular, tendon sheath, and tendinous structures, which prevent overcorrection of the deformity. In the performance of such a surgical release, the surgeon may expect to encounter a variety of abnormalities. A thorough understanding of the principles upon which such operations are based is imperative. The ability to improvise to meet the situation of the movement is invaluable.

Tendon transposition. The fundamentals of tendon transposition in the surgical treatment of the clubfoot deformity must be considered in the same light as the treatment of paralytic deformities. Tendon transposition usually involves the tibialis anterior tendon, which produces a supinating and adducting effect, and the tibialis posterior tendon, which produces a varus and equinus deformity. Transposition of the tendons to the dorsum or to the dorsolateral or lateral aspects of the foot not only removes a deforming force, but also creates a correcting force by its new point of insertion. Weakness of the dorsiflexors and evertors of the foot has been shown to be present. This is especially true of the peroneal group. Transposition of the tibialis anterior muscle and tendon insertion has been utilized to help overcome some of this weakness. The technique of rerouting the muscle and its tendons is well known. The point of insertion of the tendon into the foot must be determined by the surgeon so that the effective pull will create a correcting force. Whether this is in the midfoot, the dorsolateral aspect of the foot, or the cuboid or styloid of the fifth metatarsal is a matter the surgeon must decide. The principle of insertion of the tendon into bone must be emphasized.* (See description of the technique under metatarsus varus, p. 101.) Garceau, however, has pointed out that the purpose is to prevent recurrence and not to correct deformity. In 1967, Garceau and Palmer reported satisfactory or better results in 17 out of 22 feet in which tibialis anterior tendon transfers had been done 5 or more years previously. After tibialis anterior tendon transplantation to the midfoot or laterally, a dropping of the first metatarsal head with a resultant cocking up of the first toe is usually encountered. In the presence of residual contracture behind the ankle joint, clawing of all the toes is encountered. Clawtoe deformity procedures are necessary sometimes to correct these deformities.

POSTERIOR TIBIAL TRANSPOSITION. Reports in the literature indicate that the forward transposition of the posterior tibial tendon has been utilized in the treatment of deformities resulting from causes other than congenital (Watkins et al., 1954; Gunn and Molesworth, 1957). Fried (1959), Singer (1961), and Gartland (1964) share the opinion that the most consistent deforming force in recurrent clubfoot is the tibialis posterior muscle. They advocate transfer of its insertion to the dorsolateral foot. Both Singer and Gartland have reported satisfactory results following this transfer in over 90 percent of cases. Ober

*Garceau, 1940; Garceau and Manning, 1947; Critchley and Taylor, 1952; Carpenter and Huff, 1953.

(1933) transferred the tibialis posterior tendon by detaching its origin through a medial plantar incision, withdrawing the tendon and muscle belly proximally through a medial linear incision in the lower leg, and then rerouting the tendon anteriorly around the medial aspect of the tibia. The tendon and the belly of the muscle are passed through the anterior compartment, and a new insertion is developed in the second and third metatarsals. We believe that techniques which allow a direct line of pull from the muscle belly to the tendon insertion through a window in the interosseous membrane are better.

Osteotomy. A deformity of the foot that does not respond to wedging techniques, and in some instances soft-tissue release, may require correction by reshaping after osteotomy. In general, the metatarsal adduction and varus components yield to wedging, and in some instances capsulotomy (Kendrick et al., 1970). However, in neglected deformities osteotomy of the metatarsal bases may be utilized to correct the condition (Berman and Gartland, 1971). Osteotomy for correction of the forefoot adduction is described in the treatment of congenital metatarsus varus.

CALCANEAL OSTEOTOMY FOR TREATMENT OF UNCORRECTED OR RELAPSED HEEL VARUS. Dwyer (1959) has outlined the effects of osteotomy through the calcaneus to correct the varus of the heel in clubfoot deformity. In clubfoot the force of the tendo achillis is directed toward the inner border of the small inverted heel and from there to the medial part of the plantar fascia. A combination of deforming influences results: (1) a small inverted heel never reaches the ground properly; (2) the medially inserted calcaneal tendon is spread over the inner edge of the bone to become continuous with the plantar fascia (Stewart, 1951), and thus force is transmitted directly to the inner border of the already adducted and supinated forefoot, to tether it and drag it toward the heel; and (3) because the heel is high, the adducted forefoot strikes its outer border first in walking and is thrust medially toward the heel; thus the plantar fascia is not properly stretched by weight bearing.

We feel that the calcaneus can be effectively realigned, without the need for taking a bone graft, by using the lateral closing wedge osteotomy that Dwyer (1959) first described for pes cavus correction. Skin closure problems that may occur when the bulk of the calcaneus is increased by the graft are avoided in using this procedure, although there is some shortening of the heel. Calcaneal osteotomy is particularly useful during the years of active growth; if properly done, it does not interfere with the growth of the foot.

Evans (1961) and Abrams (1969) held that wedge resection and fusion of the calcaneocuboid joint, combined with medial release, are more logical procedures to use for uncorrected heel varus because they limit the relative overgrowth of the lateral column (calcaneus, cuboid, and fifth metatarsal) and allow for reduction of the medially dislocated navicular.

ROTATIONAL OSTEOTOMY FOR TREATMENT OF UNCORRECTED TIBIAL TORSION. After complete correction of all the elements of the clubfoot deformity, there may be a residual tibial deformity. Proximal tibial osteotomy to correct this rotatory deformity is required in some older children. It is usually noted that the torsional deformity is resolved with growth after complete correction of the clubfoot deformity. Several techniques of controlled rotational osteotomy have been developed to correct the residual deformity.

Reshaping procedures for treatment of severe or neglected talipes equinovarus deformities. The older patient who has a severely deformed foot may not respond adequately to wedging techniques or soft-tissue releases. It becomes necessary to reshape the foot by wedge resections through the midtarsal joint and through the hindfoot and the talocalcaneal joint. Many reconstructive operations have been described in the orthopaedic literature. The principles of re-

shaping and rebalancing the foot in performing triple arthrodesis are applicable. Before such reshaping procedures are performed, as much correction as is possible should be accomplished by plaster of paris casting. In this way less wedging resection will be required to accomplish the desired correction and less shortening of the foot will occur. The age at which osseous reshaping is advisable varies. Some feet develop maturity at the age of 8; others may not mature sufficiently until the age of 11 or 12.

Talectomy has also been reported by some surgeons (e.g., Menelaus, 1970) to give good results in old, neglected cases. Our experience is insufficient to draw valid conclusions.

For surgical procedures used in the correction of talipes equinovarus, see Chapter 19.

Talipes calcaneovalgus

In this common deformity of the newborn foot, the dorsum of the foot approximates the anterior distal tibia, the posterior ankle structures are lax, and the anterior ankle structures are somewhat contracted. It is probably caused in almost all cases by intrauterine position, and it is essentially self-limited (Wetzenstein, 1970). Most cases of talipes calcaneovalgus are corrected easily. The mother is asked to stretch out the contracted dorsal structures of her infant's foot; growth and active exercise on the part of the infant will do the rest. There is no bony abnormality in the calcaneovalgus foot, and it must be distinguished from the much less common and more serious congenital vertical talus since both give the appearance of flatfoot. It must also be differentiated from the paralytic calcaneus foot (see Chapter 9), which it does not resemble clinically but which is similarly named.

Treatment. In rare instances an unusually rigid deformity may require casting in equinus position for a few weeks after birth. It will sometimes be found that when the child begins to walk, he has developed

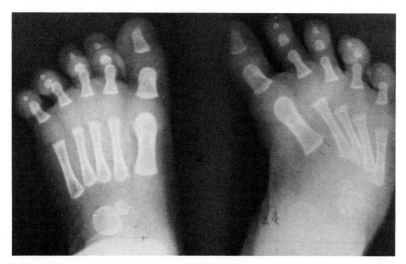

Fig. 5-5. *Left,* Normal foot. *Right,* Congenital metatarsus varus in infant.

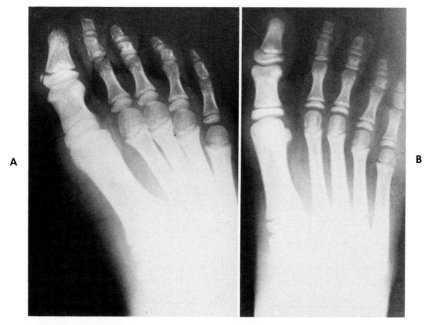

A

B

Fig. 5-6. **A,** Metatarsus adductus in 12-year-old boy. **B,** Nine months after transferring tibialis anterior into cuboid.

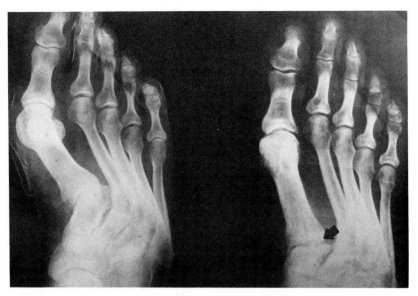

Fig. 5-7. A, Metatarsus adductus in adult. **B,** Same foot after stabilizing first metatarsal and first cuneiform joints.

a pronated heel and valgus flatfoot. This condition should be treated with medial heel wedges.

Metatarsus adductus and metatarsus varus

Metatarsus varus (Fig. 5-5) is nearly ten times as common as talipes equinovarus. The tarsus is normal or in moderate valgus position (Ponseti and Becker, 1966), although there may be an associated internal rotation of the tibia. Some authorities distinguish between metatarsus varus and metatarsus adductus, in which there is only adduction without inversion at the tarsometatarsal joint (Figs. 5-6; 5-7). The distinction is academic, however, as treatment is the same in both conditions. The longitudinal arch is higher than normal; the weight is borne by the base of the fifth metatarsal. The deformity is more common than is realized, and it would appear to be increasing in frequency.

Etiology. Usually the deformity is congenital, but it is not always recognized at birth. In some cases recognition of the deformity takes place when the child begins to walk, in other cases not until the age

of 3 or 4 years. Often treatment is not sought until adulthood.

The tibialis anterior muscle may be overactive in metatarsus adductus, and the abnormal insertion of this muscle is often a basic cause for the condition. Normally this muscle inserts equally into the base of the first metatarsal and the first cuneiform. Sometimes insertion is primarily into the base of the first metatarsal and may even give off tendinous slips to the head of the first metatarsal. When this occurs, an opponent muscle to keep the forefoot in alignment is lacking, and thus the forefoot assumes the varus position.

Treatment. Many milder cases of metatarsus varus, if recognized early in infancy, can be managed adequately by performing passive stretching exercises against the deformity four to six times daily. The hindfoot must be stabilized with one hand while the other hand exerts pressure along the medial surface of the first metatarsal until resistance is met, thus abducting the forefoot. Care must be taken not to put pressure on the great toe and to avoid overstretching the medial structures, but most intelligent parents can be taught this

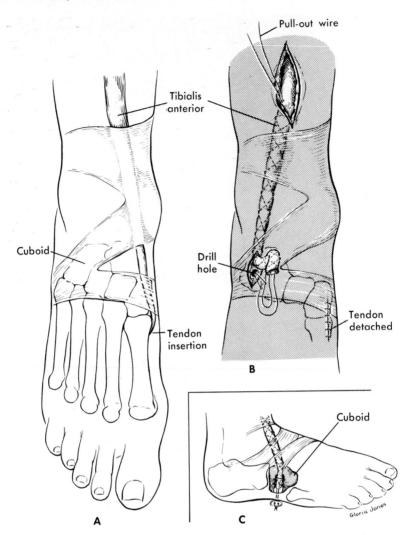

Fig. 5-8. Transference of tibialis anterior tendon into cuboid.

technique in a few minutes. When the infant's deformity fails to respond to manipulation in a few weeks or seems especially rigid, treatment with serial plaster casting for 6 to 12 weeks will usually correct the deformity. Relapse is common, however, and recasting may be necessary (McCauley et al., 1964). Passive stretching should be continued after the casts are discontinued. Abductor shoes may be helpful in maintaining the correction. During adolescence the transfer of the tibialis anterior into the lateral aspect of the foot corrects the deformity in most cases. In adulthood the deformity has become static and requires osteotomy and arthrodesis of the first metatarsal and the first cuneiform articulation, with correction of an abnormal insertion of the tibialis anterior muscle. Capsulotomy of the tarsometatarsal joint during childhood frequently accomplishes satisfactory correction. Basilar osteotomies have been utilized. Peabody and Muro (1933) performed excision of the bases of the second, third, and fourth metatarsals and capsulotomy of the first cuneiform joint. Somewhat similar procedures are described by Lange (1962).

Technique for transference of the tibialis

anterior into the cuboid for treatment of metatarsus adductus and metatarsus varus (Fig. 5-8).

1. Make a horizontal incision over the plantar aspect of the first cuneiform. Detach the tibialis anterior tendon from its insertion.
2. Make a second linear incision about 1½ inches long on the lateral side of the crest of the tibia, at the junction of the middle and lower thirds; pull the tendon out through this incision.
3. Make a third horizontal incision medially over the cuboid.
4. Make a tunnel with a long firm probe or a straight uterine forceps and connect the second and third incisions. Be certain that this tunnel underscores the transverse crural and cruciate crural ligaments.
5. Thread a stainless steel wire through the entire length of the exposed tibialis anterior tendon, and insert a pullout wire through the most proximal loop of the threaded wire.
6. Attach the terminal end of the threaded wire to a Bunnell tendon guide; thread the guide through the cuboid.
7. Close the first and second incisions, and leave the pullout wire on the skin surface of the second incision.
8. Drill a 6 mm. dorsoplantar hole through the posterior aspect of the cuboid to clear the peroneus longus tendon.
9. Attach the terminal ends of the threaded wire to a Keith needle and guide it through the drill hole and through the plantar surface.
10. Remove the threaded wires from the Keith needle, and pass it through the hole of a button and tie while the foot is held in eversion.
11. Immobilize the foot and leg in a plaster cast.
12. After wound healing has been accomplished, apply a walking plaster boot.

13. Remove the plaster and pullout wires at the eighth postoperative week. Gradually the foot assumes the normal attitude (Fig. 5-6).

Technique for arthrodesis of first metatarsal–first cuneiform joint (Fig. 5-7).

1. Make a semielliptical incision over the medial side of the first metatarsal–medial cuneiform joint. The crest should be dorsally placed.
2. Dissect the skin margins and retract.
3. Detach the tibialis anterior tendon from its insertion and free for about 6 cm. proximally. Lay it aside.
4. Incise the ligaments and capsule horizontally over the base of the first metatarsal and first cuneiform and retract the margins.
5. Make a wedge osteotomy with its base fibularward at the first metatarsal–first cuneiform articulation. Make the wedge so that the two bones will fuse in a straight line. A pin, screw, or staple may be used to maintain the bones in coaptation.
6. Suture the ligaments and fascia. Suture the free end of the tibialis anterior to the covering of the medial side of the first metatarsal–first cuneiform articulation.
7. Close the skin. While holding the foot in abduction and eversion, apply a plaster mold to the foot and leg. Bivalve the mold in 24 hours.
8. Remove the skin sutures in 10 days; apply a walking plaster boot with the foot held in mild abduction and eversion for 6 weeks.
9. Maintain correction by a sturdy walking oxford, which the patient wears for 6 months.

Mobilization of tarsometatarsal and intermetatarsal joints (Heyman, Herndon, and Strong technique, Fig. 5-9).

1. Make a curved incision across the dorsum of the foot, beginning on the medial side of the first tarsometatarsal joint, and extend this incision to the base of the fifth metatarsal.
2. Retract the skin flaps to expose the

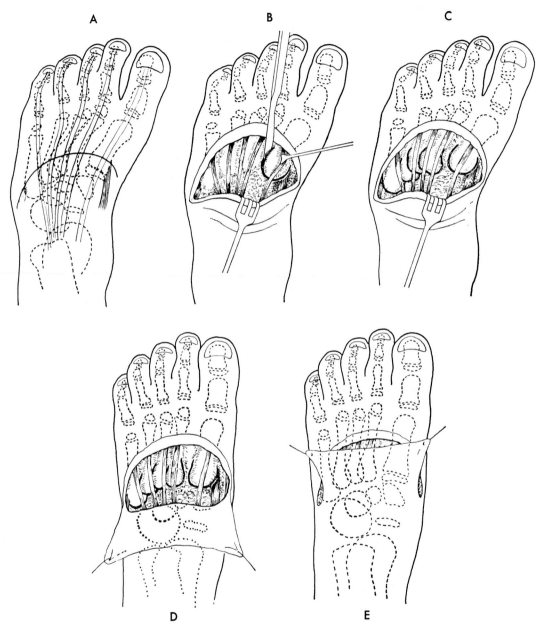

Fig. 5-9. Technique of Heyman, Herndon, and Strong for correcting congenital metatarsus varus. **A,** Skin incision. **B,** Freeing of base of the first metatarsal. **C,** Freeing of bases of all five metatarsals. **D,** Abduction of forefoot into normal position. **E,** Closing of wound. Note that the overlapping and the varus deformity of the three middle metatarsals have been greatly decreased when compared with **A.** (From Heyman, C. H., Herndon, C. H., and Strong, J. M.: J. Bone & Joint Surg. **40A:**299, 1958.)

deep fascia that covers the tarsometatarsal articulation. Identify the tibialis anterior tendon, paying careful attention to its insertion. It is necessary to identify and protect the extensor tendons as well.

3. Make a longitudinal incision over the deep fascia of the first tarsometatarsal joint. Cut the dorsal and interosseous ligaments and the joint capsule freely around the base of the first metatarsal. The joint should be flexed sufficiently so that the capsular ligaments in the anterior aspect of the joint can be cut.

4. Make incisions over the base of the first and second metatarsals and carry out capsulotomies of these joints in a similar fashion.

5. A third longitudinal incision should be made through the bases of the fourth and fifth metatarsals and corresponding ligaments and capsules. Cut these articulations (Fig. 5-9).

6. After ligaments and joint capsules of the intermetatarsal and tarsometatarsal articulations have been cut thoroughly, the forepart of the foot will swing outward at the tarsometatarsal joint.

7. Close the skin and apply a well-molded cast, with the forepart of the foot held in as much abduction as is possible.

8. Remove the cast 2 weeks after operation. Stretch the forefoot to improve and reduce deformity.

9. Maintain the foot in the corrected position in plaster for at least 3 months.

Treatment for resistant metatarsus varus. Wedging techniques are not satisfactory to overcome metatarsus varus deformities in the older child. Soft-tissue releases or transference of the tibialis anterior into the third cuneiform or cuboid give better results. Osteotomy and capsulotomy can be combined to mobilize the adducted forefoot.*

*Peabody and Muro, 1933; Lange, 1962; Steytler and Van der Walt, 1966; Kendrick et al., 1970; Berman and Gartland, 1971.

Congenital clawfoot (pes cavus, pes cavovarus)

Clawfoot, also known as hollow foot, pes cavus, or pes arcuatus, is a distinct deformity (Fig. 5-10) that begins after the age of 3 and differs from congenital talipes equinus or calcaneus as well as from paralytic pes calcaneocavus ("posterior pes cavus"). Characteristics of the typical condition are (1) an exaggeration in the height of the longitudinal arch, (2) slight shortening of the foot, (3) prominence of the metatarsal heads in the sole, (4) distal migration of the pad of the ball of the foot, (5) clawing of the toes, (6) loss of flexibility in all the joints of the foot, (7) reduction of the treading surface, and (8) often a limited dorsiflexion capability at the ankle joint. Dorsal contracture and dislocation of the metatarsophalangeal joints are typical. The apex of the deformity on the inner border of the foot is usually the naviculocuneiform joint. The degree of the cavus is varied, ranging from a simple high arch and dorsally elevated midfoot area to an extreme concavity of the longitudinal arch. Often the forefoot is dropped, and the deformity may be accompanied by a true equinus attitude brought about by contracture of the calf muscles; it may also be combined with varying degrees of malposition of the calcaneus as a result of lengthening of the heel cord.

A varus component to the deformity of the hindfoot may also be present (hence the name pes cavovarus), so that too much weight is thrown on the outer border, often causing the base of the fifth metatarsal to become a weight-bearing, pressured point. In clawfoot the base of the metatarsals is so high that the heads of the metatarsals strike the ground pointedly; consequently, most patients have heavy callosities and sometimes traumatic ulcers under one or more of the heads.

Etiology. The pathomechanics of cavus foot are poorly understood. The deformity has been ascribed to (1) imbalance of the intrinsic muscles, a theory first proposed by Duchenne in 1867; and (2) imbalance

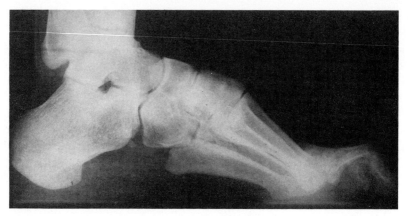

Fig. 5-10. Clawfoot. Note the high longitudinal arch and the contracture of all the toes.

of various extrinsic muscles (Bentzon, 1933; Hallgrímsson, 1939).

Brewerton et al. (1963), in studying the causes of cavus feet, found that in 66 percent of their seventy-seven cases, neurologic signs could be detected during clinical examination. The most commonly made diagnosis in this series was peroneal muscular atrophy (Charcot-Marie-Tooth disease), which was found in one-third of their patients. Myelodysplasia and poliomyelitis were next in frequency. Friedreich's ataxia, although much less common, must also be kept in mind as a cause of clawfoot, as must the absence of ankle jerks and progressive disturbance of balance. In Brewerton's "idiopathic" group, eleven of twenty-six gave a family history of cavus feet. Seven of the twenty-six showed electromyographic and nerve conduction abnormalities, thus pointing up the importance of a thorough neurologic evaluation. Clawfoot may be caused by any of a large number of neurologic diseases, of both the central and peripheral nervous systems; it may be the result of infectious and traumatic diseases as well. A certain percentage of cases undoubtedly represents formes frustes of hereditary conditions such as peroneal muscular atrophy and Friedreich's ataxia.

Symptoms. The degree of deformity is variable. Symptoms of the condition are inability to walk or stand for long periods, easily tiring feet, severe calluses (which may ulcerate) on the ball of the foot and on any or all of the toes, and often a heavy callosity under the base of the fifth metatarsal as a result of foot inversion.

Treatment. The aim in treatment should be to relieve symptoms, correct the deformity, and prevent recurrence. Every foot should be treated as an individual problem. Inasmuch as a method applicable to all cases cannot be offered, an outline of treatment based on the degree of deformity is herewith suggested.

Slight deformity. In mild cases (especially in early cases in which the feet remain flexible, with moderate cavus that disappears on weight bearing), permanent contracture of the plantar structures can sometimes be prevented. The cavus and clawing of the toes can be kept to a minimum by the wearing of carefully fitted shoes with low heels. A metatarsal bar and wedging appliances should be employed if callosities are present. Exercises are recommended to increase flexibility of the foot and to stretch the toes and muscles of the calf.

Moderate to severe deformity. Suggested procedures for the operative correction of clawfoot include tendon relocation and lengthening, fasciotomy, plantar muscle denervation, anterior tarsal wedge osteotomy, and triple arthrodesis. In 1919, Hibbs suggested transferring the extensor hallucis longus and extensor digitorum longus into the cuneiforms. Steindler (1917) advocated stripping of the plantar fascia from the plantar surface of the calcaneus to dispose of its bowstring action on the longitudinal arch. In moderate cases Cole (1940) employed Steindler's fasciotomy, followed by the use of a Thomas wrench and the Hibbs relocation procedure. Alvik (1954) extended the wedge osteotomy forward to include a wedge resection of the first and second cuneiforms and the base of the first and second metatarsals. It is questionable whether such soft-tissue operations as Steindler's fasciotomy or tendon transference, or both combined, ever correct any of the clawfoot deformities. Steindler himself recommended the procedure only in the mildest of cases. Brockway (1940), in discussing Steindler's operation, stated that it was surprising how little correction can be obtained and how frequently relapse occurs. It is of value, however, when combined with other procedures.

Garceau and Brahms (1956) and Garceau (1961), in the belief that clawfoot is the result of intrinsic muscle imbalance, recommended selective plantar neurectomy if (1) the foot is flail, except for functioning plantar muscles which cause the cavus; (2) there is dorsal bunion with cavus; (3) poorly opposed flexor muscles in calcaneocavus deformity are present; and (4) there is cavoadductus deformity due to cerebral palsy. Results are best when procedures are performed before the development of the foot is complete.

McElvenny and Caldwell (1958) described a procedure in which elevation and supination of the first metatarsal are carried out, along with fusion of the tarsometatarsal and, if necessary, the naviculo-cuneiform joints. This procedure is employed in cases in which the deformity is primarily of the medial portion of the foot; however, they combine this procedure with plantar fasciotomy, triple arthrodesis, and first metatarsocuneiform fusion to correct severe deformities.

Dwyer's calcaneal osteotomy (1959) is useful in children in whom a varus deformity of the hindfoot is present; it should be combined with plantar fasciotomy. He reported having attained good results in forty-one children from 3 to 16 years of age. Dwyer's calcaneal osteotomy is probably the procedure of choice for children with deformities in which heel varus in prominent. Dwyer feels that this correction of the weight-bearing alignment of the foot will result in progressive improvement of the deformity.

When the hindfoot is not deformed, anterior tarsal wedge osteotomy (Cole, 1940; Japas, 1968) is indicated for severe deformity in the skeletally mature foot. For older patients, Dwyer also used the calcaneal osteotomy, combined with removal of a dorsally based wedge from the tarsometatarsal region. If the hindfoot is also involved, stabilization of the foot by the use of the Dunn or Hoke arthrodesis procedures may be indicated in severe cases in which skeletal maturity has been reached. (For procedures, see Chapter 19.)

Congenital vertical talus (congenital convex pes valgus, congenital rigid flatfoot)

Congenital vertical talus is an uncommon deformity characterized by a rigid, dorsiflexed, everted forefoot that is associated with an equinus position of the talus and, to a lesser degree, of the calcaneus (Figs. 5-11 and 5-12). The sole of the foot is convex, resembling the rocker-bottom foot of maltreated talipes equinovarus. The head of the talus can be palpated in the sole of the foot; the entire deformity cannot be passively corrected, as can the much more common and self-limited talipes calcaneovalgus, which also appears as flatfoot in the newborn period. Patterson et al. (1968) have described the only anatomic dissection of this deformity. They found that the anterior crural muscles as well as the peroneus brevis were tight, and the posterior tibial and both peroneal tendons were dislocated anteriorly. The talus lay in equinus, as did the calcaneus,

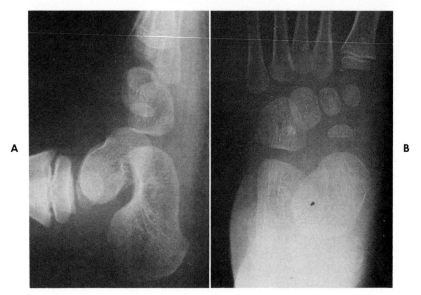

A   B

Fig. 5-11. Congenital vertical talus. Note the equinus position of both the talus and calcaneus in the lateral view and medial deviation of the head of the talus in an anteroposterior view.

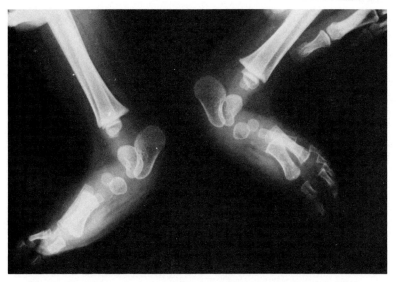

Fig. 5-12. Bilateral congenital vertical talus in 2-year-old child.

which was also more laterally directed than is normal. The navicular was dislocated dorsally onto the neck of the talus. In their opinion the term vertical talus focuses attention on only one aspect of a complex malformation. It is commonly associated with other congenital anomalies (Lloyd-Roberts and Spence, 1958; Eyre-Brook, 1967).

Lateral roentgenograms of the foot show the talus to be in marked equinus, with its long axis corresponding to the long axis of the tibia. Most authors feel that the calcaneus also lies in excessive equinus, but others dispute this notion (e.g., Eyre-Brook). When the primary ossification center of the navicular becomes radiopaque, it is seen to be dorsally dislocated. Anteroposterior views of the foot show abnormal divergence of the long axes of the talus and calcaneus.

Treatment. Management of congenital vertical talus is difficult. Essentially, the forefoot must first be aligned with the hindfoot (which entails reducing the navicular dislocation) and then the entire foot must be brought out of equinus. Closed manipulation of the forefoot with serial plaster casts that maintain the foot in equinus may be successful in aligning the foot if this treatment is started in the first few weeks of life (Henssge and Allmeling, 1966; Harrold, 1967). However, it is frequently necessary to perform tendo achillis lengthening and posterior capsulotomy to allow the hindfoot to be brought into the neutral position without redislocating the forefoot (Wainwright, 1963; Silk and Wainwright, 1967). If closed reduction has not been accomplished after the first few months of life, open reduction is necessary. Hark (1950) described a method of open reduction. Osmond-Clarke (1956) added transfer of the insertion of the peroneus brevis into the neck of the talus. Herndon and Heyman (1963) felt that open reduction was preferable; Eyre-Brook (1967) has advocated partial excision of the navicular to relieve tension in the medial pillar of the foot, thus facilitating maintenance of the reduction. Relapse in the older child may be managed satisfactorily through the use of a subtalar fusion procedure (Grice, 1959).

Deformities resulting from arthrogryposis multiplex congenita

In *Campbell's Operative Orthopaedics,*[*] arthrogryposis is described as a perplexing disease of unknown cause. The muscle tissue becomes replaced by fibrous tissue

---

[*]Crenshaw, A. H., editor, ed. 5, vol. 2, St. Louis, 1971, The C. V. Mosby Co.

with varying degrees of severity. The fibrotic and, therefore, contracted muscles restrict the motions of joints; contracture, atrophy, and weakness (or sometimes absence of function) of muscles ensues, with ankylosis and postural deformity. This condition may be localized to the feet, producing extremely resistant clubfoot or calcaneovalgus deformities; but most often it is generalized, affecting many joints.

Conservative treatment, which includes repeated stretching exercises or wedging casts to correct contracture, should be started soon after birth; but even if correction is possible, the deformities will probably recur. Surgical treatment is often necessary, consisting of soft-structure releases, tendon transfers, and stabilization procedures after growth is complete. The success of either kind of treatment is unlikely, although with many operations the lower extremities may be made stable enough to bear weight. The feet are generally more amenable to treatment than the hands.

Tarsal coalition

Tarsal coalition, an anomalous fusion of two or more tarsal bones, is a condition that has long been recognized. A specimen was prepared by John Hunter (Harris and Beath, 1948); Pfitzner (1896) described nine anatomic specimens of partial or complete bridging of the talus or calcaneus and fifteen specimens of calcaneonavicular bridging. Slomann (1921) reported the first clinical case of calcaneonavicular fusion. O'Rahilly (1953) reviewed the records of tarsal and carpal anomalies. Since then there have been many reports on the clinical aspects of this group of anomalies.

Although most cases of tarsal coalition appear to be nonhereditary, some hereditary instances have been reported. Calcaneonavicular coalition occurring in three generations was described by Wray and Herndon (1963), and massive synostosis of the tarsal bones appearing in a mother and her two children was described by Bersani and Samilson (1957). Pearlman et al.

(1964) described the occurrence of multiple carpal and tarsal synostoses, in addition to other skeletal anomalies, in a mother and daughter. Harris and Beath (1950) suggested that a large number of spastic flatfeet were caused by tarsal bridges. This concept, which they explored studiously, has since been supported by many investigators, notably Webster and Roberts (1951), Jack (1954), de Marchi and coworkers (1955), and Waugh (1957).

The types of fusion reported most are talocalcaneal, talonavicular, sustentaculonavicular, and calcaneocuboid. Fusion of other tarsal bones undoubtedly occurs, preventing any movement of that joint and often resulting in static foot deformities. When fusion occurs, the anomaly may appear as a narrow bar or as partial or complete fusion of two bones; it may be osseous (synostosis), cartilaginous (synchondrosis), or fibrous (syndesmosis). The cause is an error in the differentiation in mesenchyme during formation of the tarsal bones. Such an error may lead to formation of a small accessory bone or to complete fusion of two adjacent bones (Jack, 1954).

Symptoms. A rigid tarsal joint caused by tarsal coalition probably exists from birth; however, in early childhood the condition causes few if any symptoms. Foot discomfort is likely to appear first during adolescence or early in adulthood. Sometimes symptoms do not appear until middle life, and trauma may be the trigger mechanism. A single injury, such as a fall, a jump, or repeated daily stress from occupations requiring standing for prolonged periods or marching may give rise to symptoms. Different types of anomalies produce both similar and varied symptoms and deformities. The coalition may be painful, with concomitant deformity or rigidity of all subtalar joints. Pain is caused by compensatory excessive strain on other tarsal joints because of the rigidity of the fused joints, often resulting in spasm of the leg muscles, especially in the peroneal group. Rigidity of the subtalar joints is soon apparent with

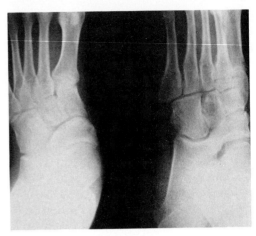

Fig. 5-13. Calcaneonavicular synostosis.

attempts at inversion of the foot. In flaccid flatfoot there is a wide range of movement in the tarsus, whereas in the rigid foot there is little if any movement of the subtalar joint.

Talocalcaneal, talonavicular, and calcaneonavicular fusion often become symptomatic (Fig. 5-13). These are frequent, perhaps the most common, causes of rigid flatfoot or peroneal spastic flatfoot (Webster and Roberts, 1951). (See Chapter 8.) Jack (1954) reviewed sixty-eight cases of rigid flatfoot, of which thirty were his own and showed talocalcaneal bars, twenty-three showed calcaneonavicular bars, and two showed both types of bar. Sixteen were without bony abnormalities. Harris (1955), whose contributions to the literature on disorders of the feet are notable, has also discussed the problem of failure to demonstrate roentgenographically talocalcaneal bridges in the rigid valgus foot. He ascribes this failure to the position of the bone blocks.

Diagnosis. Bony coalition can be demonstrated roentgenographically; however, views other than the usual routine are often necessary to disclose the anomaly (Conway and Cowell, 1969). Vaughan and Segal (1953) advised a lateral and external oblique (eversion) view of the ankle as most valuable in demonstrating the calcaneonavicular coalition. The subtalar joint

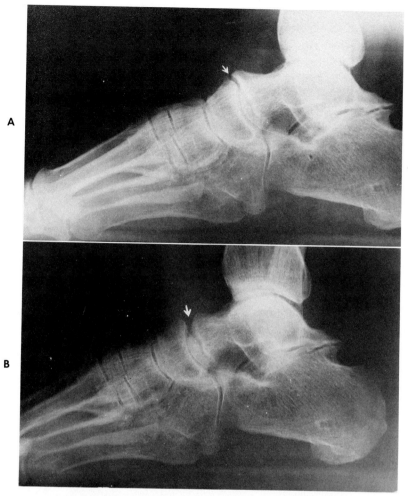

Fig. 5-14. A, Lipping on dorsum of talonavicular joint with pain on dorsiflexion. **B,** Same case as shown in **A** after removal of lipping.

is best visualized by a lateral and modified plantar view (Sante, 1944). Cartilaginous or fibrous union can be suggested only by clinical observation.

Treatment. Asymptomatic cases should be treated expectantly. Mild cases call for relief by shoe wedging or by inlay support. In moderately severe cases, especially those in which there is some mobility in the subtalar articulation and in which pain is localized about the bridge, excision of the bar may relieve symptoms. Mitchell and Gibson (1967) feel that treatment by excision should be limited to younger patients who have painful spasmodic flatfoot of recent origin, before adaptive joint

changes have occurred. In long-standing serious cases of complete rigid flatfoot with extreme eversion, triple arthrodesis is necessary (see Chapter 19).

Lipping on dorsum of the talonavicular joint

Lipping at the talonavicular joint is not uncommon. Because the hypertrophied joint margins collide when the foot is dorsiflexed, the condition is painful (Fig. 5-14, A). It may or may not be associated with rigid or semirigid flatfoot. The lipping is always more pronounced on the dorsum of the head of the talus than on the navicular.

Etiology. The etiology is obscure. Possibly a congenital defect of the joint occurs in which the surfaces are flat where the talus and navicular meet at the dorsum. Normally the surface is an elliptical paraboloid. If the surfaces are not congruous, the two bones collide each time the foot is dorsiflexed. The gradual osteophytic changes are a reaction to this trauma. The etiologic mechanism is presumed to be comparable to that which causes hallux rigidus.

Symptoms. Lipping is usually unilateral; when it is bilateral, ordinarily only one side produces symptoms. The condition may be asymptomatic and disclosed only during routine roentgenographic examination. Symptomatic cases begin in middle life and occur more often in women.

The disability is a mild or severe painful

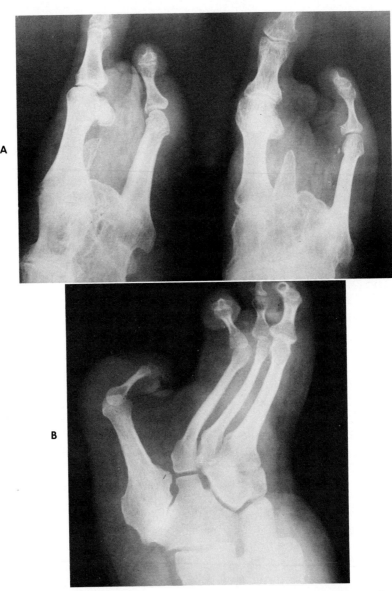

Fig. 5-15. A and **B,** Congenital cleft foot. **C,** Clinical appearance of case shown in **B.** (**B** and **C,** Courtesy Dr. Charles Brooks.)

swelling over the talonavicular joint. The patient cannot bear weight because of pain, which is aggravated when the foot is dorsiflexed. Routine roentgenographic views of the talonavicular joint verify the diagnosis.

Congenital cleft foot (split foot, lobster-claw foot) and absence of part of the foot

Congenital cleft foot and absence of part of the foot are troublesome deformities that vary in type and degree. Usually one or more toes and some or all of the metatarsal bones are absent; often part of the tarsus is also missing. The first and fifth rays are often present (Figs. 5-15 to 5-17). Cleft foot is frequently transmitted as an autosomal dominant trait and may be associated with cleft lip and palate (McKusick, 1968). It sometimes occurs in association with triphalangeal thumb (Phillips, 1971).

Barsky (1964), in describing cleft hand, ascribed to Lange (1962) the recognition of two types: a unilateral deformity without foot involvement or evidence of familial inheritance (atypical) and a bilateral deformity, often with split feet and a family history of deformity (typical).

Treatment. Treatment must be directed toward improving function and only secondarily toward cosmetic improvements. In most instances function can be preserved with the use of specially constructed and molded shoes. Surgical treatment includes excision of useless bony remnants and the creation of suitable skin flaps for closure of the cleft. Metatarsal osteotomies may be required to narrow the feet (Phillips, 1971). A deep suture around adjacent metatarsals is necessary to reduce tension on the skin flaps (Peet and Patterson, 1963). All superfluous tissue that interferes with function should be removed, even to the point of amputation of the deformed foot, since a properly constructed Syme or below-the-knee prosthesis may permit more nearly normal function than repair of a painful foot.

Congenital amputations (Fig. 5-18) occur most commonly at the metatarsophalangeal, tarsometatarsal, or midtarsal levels and are rarely functionally disabling. Frantz and O'Rahilly (1961), in a series of 300 children with congenital skeletal anomalies, reported four cases in which there was absence of all metatarsals and phalanges associated with acheiria, harelip, and cleft

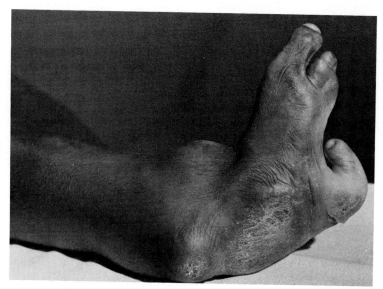

C

Fig. 5-15, cont'd. For legend see opposite page.

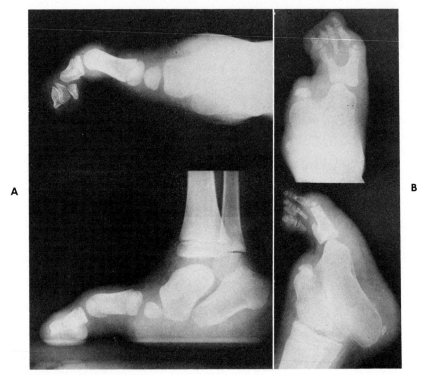

Fig. 5-16. A, Congenital absence of most of foot. Only the first cuneiform–first metatarsal and hallux are present. **B,** Congenitally bizarre foot.

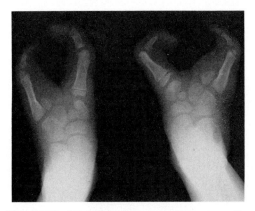

Fig. 5-17. Bilateral cleft foot. (Courtesy Dr. R. Jacobs.)

palate; they suggested hereditary occurrence through autosomal recessive transmission.

Congenital absence of the navicular

Congenital absence of the navicular is a rare anomaly, which is disabling because the talonavicular joint is a highly important element in the biomechanics of the foot. Little can be done about the resultant poorly functioning foot (Fig. 5-19). Congenital absence of the navicular, or possibly congenital talonavicular synostosis in the foot of a 10-year-old boy is shown in Fig. 5-20. The ball-and-socket ankle joint undoubtedly developed because abduction and adduction of the foot took place between the head of the talus and the cuneiforms, causing a rotatory force upon the trochlear surface of the talus. In addition, there appears to be a talocalcaneal coalition, which may have contributed to the development of this deformity. Fig. 5-21 illustrates several anomalies, including absence of the navicular in the right foot.

Congenital ligamentous and muscular weakness

Deficiency of the lateral ligaments of the hindfoot and ankle may be seen (Fig. 5-

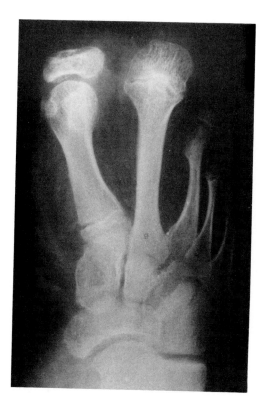

Fig. 5-18. Congenital absence of all toes and dwarfism of third, fourth, and fifth metatarsal. (Courtesy Dr. T. Mason.)

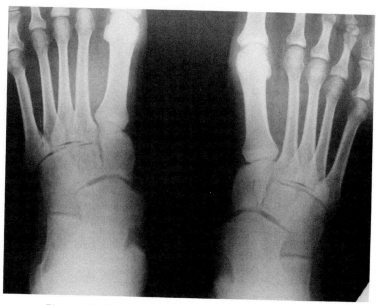

Fig. 5-19. Bilateral congenital absence of navicular.

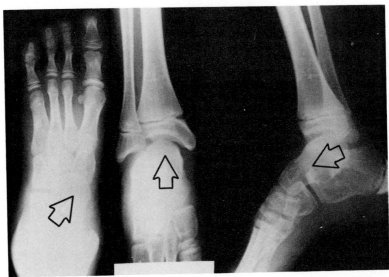

Fig. 5-20. Congenital absence of navicular in foot of 10-year-old boy (possibly congenital talonavicular synostosis). There are only four metatarsals and a ball-and-socket ankle joint.

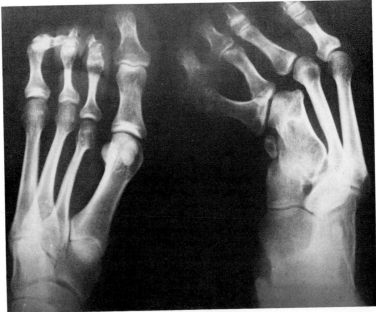

Fig. 5-21. *Right foot,* Rare anomaly. The first three metatarsals are one deformed bone, the navicular is absent, and there are four toes (the first three are syndactylized). *Left foot,* Absence of fifth ray.

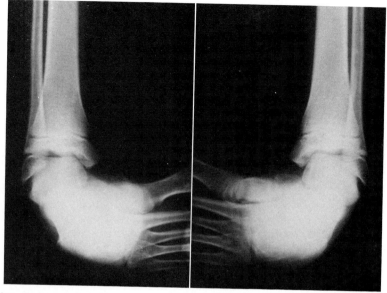

Fig. 5-22. Congenital deficiency of collateral ligaments of ankle and hindfoot combined with peroneal muscle weakness. These were stress films; the foot could be placed in a plantigrade position at will.

22). In our experience this deficiency may occasionally result in recurrent inversion sprain and has responded to the peroneus brevis tenodesis of Watson-Jones.

REFERENCES

Abrams, R. C.: Relapsed club foot, J. Bone Joint Surg. **51-A:**270-282, Mar. 1969.

Alvik, I.: Operative treatment of pes cavus, Acta Orthop. Scand. **23:**137-141, 1954.

Barsky, A. J.: Cleft hand: Classification, incidence, and treatment, J. Bone Joint Surg. **46-A:**1707-1720, Dec. 1964.

Bechtol, C. O., and Mossman, H. W.: Club-foot: An embryological study of associated muscle abnormalities, J. Bone Joint Surg. **32-A:**827-836, Oct. 1950.

Bentzon, P. G. K.: Pes cavus and the M. peroneus longus, Acta Orthop. Scand. **4:**50-52, 1933.

Bényi, P.: A modified Lambrinudi operation for drop foot, J. Bone Joint Surg. **42-B:**333-335, May 1960.

Berman, A., and Gartland, J. J.: Metatarsal osteotomy for the correction of adduction of the fore part of the foot in children, J. Bone Joint Surg. **53-A:**498-505, Apr. 1971.

Bersani, F. A., and Samilson, R. L.: Massive familial tarsal synostosis, J. Bone Joint Surg. **39-A:**1187-1190, Oct. 1957.

Blockey, N. J., and Smith, M. G. H.: The treatment of congenital club foot, J. Bone Joint Surg. **48-B:**660-665, Nov. 1966.

Blumenfeld, I., Kaplan, N., and Hicks, E. O.: The conservative treatment of congenital talipes equinovarus, J. Bone Joint Surg. **28:**765-777, Oct. 1946.

Brewerton, D. A., Sandifer, P. H., Sweetnam, D. R.: "Idiopathic" pes cavus: An investigation into its aetiology, Brit. Med. J. **2:**659-661, Sept. 1963.

Brockmann, E. P.: Congenital club foot, London, 1930, John Wright & Sons, Ltd.

Brockway, A.: Surgical correction of talipes cavus deformities, J. Bone Joint Surg. **22:**81-91, Jan. 1940.

Browne, D.: Congenital malformations, Practitioner **131:**20-32, July 1933.

Carpenter, E. B., and Huff, S. H.: Selective tendon transfers for recurrent clubfoot, South. Med. J. **46:**220-224, Mar. 1953.

Cole, W. H.: The treatment of claw-foot, J. Bone Joint Surg. **22:**895-908, Oct. 1940.

Conway, J. J., and Cowell, H. R.: Tarsal coalition: Clinical significance and roentgenographic demonstration, Radiology **92:**799-811, Mar. 1969.

Crenshaw, A. H., editor: Campbell's operative orthopaedics, ed. 5, vol 2, St. Louis, 1971, The C. V. Mosby Co., pp. 2033-2034.

Critchley, J. E., and Taylor, R. G.: Transfer of the tibialis anterior tendon for relapsed clubfoot, J. Bone Joint Surg. **34-B:**49-52, Feb. 1952.

de Marchi, E., Gambier, R., and Vespignani, L.: Les synostoses tarsiennes dans le pied plat valgus douloureux, J. Radiol. Electrol. Med. Nucl. 36:665-674, 1955.

Duchenne, G. B.: Physiology of motion (Translated and edited by E. B. Kaplan), Philadelphia, 1949, J. B. Lippincott Co. (Original French edition appeared in 1867.)

Dwyer, F. C.: Osteotomy of the calcaneum for pes cavus, J. Bone Joint Surg. 41-B:80-86, Feb. 1959.

Dwyer, F. C.: The treatment of relapsed clubfoot by the insertion of a wedge into the calcaneum, J. Bone Joint Surg. 45-B:67-75, Feb. 1963.

Evans, D.: Relapsed club foot, J. Bone Joint Surg. 43-B:722-733, Nov. 1961.

Eyre-Brook, A. L.: Congenital vertical talus, J. Bone Joint Surg. 49-B:618-627, Nov. 1967.

Frantz, C. H., and O'Rahilly, R.: Congenital skeletal limb deficiencies, J. Bone Joint Surg. 43-A:1202-1224, Dec. 1961.

Fried, A.: Recurrent congenital club-foot, J. Bone Joint Surg. 41-A:243-252, March 1959.

Garceau, G. J.: Anterior tibial tendon transposition in recurrent congenital club-foot, J. Bone Joint Surg. 22:932-936, Oct. 1940.

Garceau, G. J.: Pes cavus. In American Academy of Orthopaedic Surgeons: Instructional Course Lectures, vol. 18, St. Louis, 1961, The C. V. Mosby Co., pp. 184-186.

Garceau, G. J., and Brahms, M. A.: A preliminary study of selective plantar-muscle denervation for pes cavus, J. Bone Joint Surg. 38-A:553-562, June 1956.

Garceau, G. J., and Manning, K. R.: Transposition of the anterior tibial tendon in the treatment of recurrent congenital club-foot, J. Bone Joint Surg. 29:1044-1047, Oct. 1947.

Garceau, G. J., and Palmer, R. M.: Transfer of the anterior tibial tendon for recurrent club foot, J. Bone Joint Surg. 49-A:207-231, Mar. 1967.

Gartland, J. J.: Posterior tibial transplant in the surgical treatment of recurrent club foot, J. Bone Joint Surg. 46-A:1217-1225, Sept. 1964.

Goldner, J. L.: Congenital talipes equinovarus: Analysis of the basic pathology and results of surgical treatment, J. Bone Joint Surg. 52-B:783, Nov. 1970.

Grice, D. S.: The role of subtalar fusion in the treatment of valgus deformities of the feet. In American Academy of Orthopaedic Surgeons: Instructional Course Lectures, vol. 16, St. Louis, 1959, The C. V. Mosby Co., pp. 127-150.

Gunn, D. R., and Molesworth, B. D.: The use of tibialis posterior as a dorsiflexor, J. Bone Joint Surg. 39-B:674-678, Nov. 1957.

Hallgrímsson, S.: Pes cavus, seine Behandlung und einige Bemerkungen über seine Ätiologie Acta Orthop. Scand. 10:73-118, 1939.

Hark, F. W.: Rocker-foot due to congenital sub-

luxation of the talus, J. Bone Joint Surg. 32-A:344-350, Apr. 1950.

Harris, R. I.: Rigid valgus foot due to talocalcaneal bridge, J. Bone Joint Surg. 37-A:169-183, Jan. 1955.

Harris, R. I., and Beath, T.: Etiology of peroneal spastic flat foot, J. Bone Joint Surg. 30-B:624-634, Nov. 1948.

Harris, R. I., and Beath, T.: John Hunter's specimen of talocalcaneal bridge,, J. Bone Joint Surg. 32-B:203, May 1950.

Harrold, A. J.: Congenital vertical talus in infancy, J. Bone Joint Surg. 49-B:634-643, Nov. 1967.

Henssge, J., and Allmeling, W.: Therapeutische Erfahrungen beim angeborenen Plattfuss mit vertikalem talus, Arch. Orthop. Unfallchir. 59:74-78, 1966.

Herndon, C. H., and Heyman, C. H.: Problems in the recognition and treatment of congenital convex pes valgus, J. Bone Joint Surg. 45-A:413-429, Mar. 1963.

Heyman, C. H., Herndon, C. H., and Strong, J. M.: Mobilization of the tarsometatarsal and intermetatarsal joints for the correction of resistance of the fore part of the foot in congenital club-foot or congenital metatarsus varus, J. Bone Joint Surg. 40-A:299-309, Apr. 1958.

Hibbs, R. A.: An operation for "claw foot," J.A.M.A. 73:1583-1584, Nov. 1919.

Irani, R. N., and Sherman, M. S.: The pathological anatomy of club foot, J. Bone Joint Surg. 45-A:45-52, Jan. 1963.

Jack, E. A.: Bone anomalies of the tarsus in relation to "peroneal spastic flatfoot," J. Bone Joint Surg. 36-B:530-542, Nov. 1954.

Japas, L. M.: Surgical treatment of pes cavus by tarsal V-osteotomy, J. Bone Joint Surg. 50-A:927-944, July 1968.

Kendrick, R. E., Sharma, N. K., Hassler, W. L., and Herndon, C. H.: Tarsometatarsal mobilization for resistant adduction of the fore part of the foot, J. Bone Joint Surg. 52-A:61-70, Jan. 1970.

Kite, J. H.: The treatment of congenital clubfeet: A study of the results in two hundred cases, J.A.M.A. 99:1156-1162, Oct. 1932.

Kite, J. H.: Principles involved in the treatment of congenital club-foot, J. Bone Joint Surg. 21:595-606, July 1939.

Kite, J. H.: The clubfoot, New York, 1964, Grune and Stratton.

Knight, R. A.: Developmental deformities of the lower extremities, J. Bone Joint Surg. 36-A:521-527, June 1954.

Lange, M.: Orthopädisch-chirurgische Operationslehre, München, 1962, J. F. Bergmann.

Lloyd-Roberts, G. C., and Spence, A. J.: Congenital vertical talus, J. Bone Joint Surg. 40-B:33-41, Feb. 1958.

McCauley, J., Jr., Lusskin, R., and Bromley, J.: Recurrence in congenital metatarsus varus, J. Bone Joint Surg. 46-A:525-532, Apr. 1964.

McElvenny, R. T., and Caldwell, G. D.: A new operation for correction of cavus foot: Fusion of first metatarsocuneiformnavicular joints, Clin. Orthop. 11:85-92, Spring 1958.

McKusick, V. A.: Mendelian inheritance in man, ed. 2, Baltimore, 1968, The Johns Hopkins Press.

Menelaus, M. B.: Excision of the talus for equino-varus deformity of the feet, J. Bone Joint. Surg. 52-B:790-791, Nov. 1970.

Mitchell, G. P., and Gibson, J. M. C.: Excision of calcaneo-navicular bar for painful spasmodic flat foot, J. Bone Joint Surg. 49-B:281-287, May 1967.

Ober, F. R.: Tendon transplantation in the lower extremity, New Eng. J. Med. 209:52-59, July 1933.

O'Rahilly, R.: A survey of carpal and tarsal anomalies, J. Bone Joint Surg. 35-A:626-642, July 1953.

Osmond-Clarke, H.: Congenital vertical talus, J. Bone Joint Surg., 38-B:334-341, Feb. 1956.

Palmer, R. M.: The genetics of talipes equino-varus, J. Bone Joint Surg. 46-A:542-556, Apr. 1964.

Patterson, W. R., Fitz, D. A., and Smith, W. S.: The pathologic anatomy of congenital convex pes valgus, J. Bone Joint Surg. 50-A:458-466, Apr. 1968.

Peabody, C. W., and Muro, F.: Congenital meta-tarsus varus, J. Bone Joint Surg. 15:171-189, 1933.

Pearlman, H. S., Elkin, R. E., and Warren, R. F.: Familial tarsal and carpal synostosis with ra-dial-head subluxation (Nievergelt's syndrome), J. Bone Joint Surg. 46-A:585-592, Apr. 1964.

Peet, E. W., and Patterson, T. J. S.: The essen-tials of plastic surgery, Oxford, 1963, Blackwell Scientific Publications Ltd.

Pfitzner, W.: Beiträge zur Kenntnis des menschli-chen Extremitätenskelets. VII. Die Variationen im Aufbau des Fussskelets. In Schwalbe, G.: Morphologischen Arbeiten, vol. 6. Jena, 1896, Gustav Fischer, p. 235.

Phillips, R. S.: Congenital split foot (lobster claw) and triphalangeal thumb, J. Bone Joint Surg. 53-B:247-257, May 1971.

Ponseti, I. V., and Becker, J. R.: Congenital meta-tarsus adductus: The results of treatment. J. Bone Joint Surg. 48-A:702-711, June 1966.

Ponseti, I. V., and Smoley, E. N.: Congenital clubfoot: The results of treatment, J. Bone Joint Surg. 45-A:261-275, Mar. 1963.

Sante, L. R.: Principles of roentgenological inter-pretation, ed. 5, Ann Arbor, Michigan, 1944, Edwards Brothers, Inc., pp. 154-155.

Scherb, R.: Zur Ätiologie kongenitaler and kon-genital bedingter Fussdeformitäten mit besond-erer Berücksichtigung des Pes equino-varus congenitus, Acta Chir. Scand. 67:717-750, 1930.

Shands, A. R., Jr., and Wentz, I. J.: Symposium on orthopedic surgery: Congenital anomalies, accessory bones, and osteochondritis in the feet of 850 children, Surg. Clin. N. Amer. 33:1643-1666, Dec. 1953.

Silk, F. F., and Wainwright, D.: The recogni-tion and treatment of congenital flat foot in infancy, J. Bone Joint Surg. 49-B:628-633, Nov. 1967.

Singer, M.: Tibialis posterior transfer in congen-ital club foot, J. Bone Joint Surg. 43-B:717-721, Nov. 1961.

Slomann, H. C.: On coalitio calcaneo-navicularis, J. Orthop. Surg. 3:586-602, 1921.

Steindler, A.: Operative treatment of pes cavus: Stripping of the os calcis, Surg. Gynec. Obstet. 24:612-615, 1917.

Stewart, S. F.: Club-foot: Its incidence, cause, and treatment: An anatomical-physiological study, J. Bone Joint Surg. 33-A:577-588, July 1951.

Steytler, J. C. S., and Van der Walt, I. D.: Cor-rection of resistant adduction of the forefoot in congenital club-foot and congenital meta-tarsus varus by metatarsal osteotomy, Brit. J. Surg. 53:558-560, June 1966.

Swann, M., Lloyd-Roberts, G. C., and Caterall, A.: The anatomy of uncorrected club feet: A study of rotation deformity, J. Bone Joint Surg. 51-B:263-269, May 1969.

Thomson, S. A.: Treatment of congenital talipes equinovarus with a modification of the Denis Browne method and splint, J. Bone Joint Surg. 24:291-298, April 1942.

Turco, V. J.: Surgical correction of the resistant clubfoot, J. Bone Joint Surg. 53-A:477-497, Apr. 1971.

Vaughan, W. H., and Segal, G.: Tarsal coalition, with special reference to roentgenographic in-terpretation, Radiology 60:855-863, 1953.

Wainwright, D.: The recognition and cure of con-genital flat foot. Proceedings and Reports of Universities, Colleges, Councils, and Associa-tions, J. Bone Joint Surg. 45-B:210, Feb. 1963.

Watkins, M. B., Jones, J. B., Ryder, C. T., Jr., and Brown, T. H., Jr.: Transplantation of the posterior tibial tendon, J. Bone Joint Surg. 36-A: 1181-1189, Dec. 1954.

Waugh, W.: Partial cubo-navicular coalition as a cause of peroneal spastic flat foot, J. Bone Joint Surg. 39-B:520-523, Aug. 1957.

Webster, F. S., and Roberts, W. M.: Tarsal anom-alies and peroneal spastic flatfoot, J.A.M.A. 146:1099-1104, July 1951.

Wetzenstein, H.: Prognosis of pes calcaneo-valgus

congenitus, Acta Orthop. Scand. **41**:122-128, 1970.

Whitman, R.: A treatise on orthopaedic surgery, ed. 9, Philadelphia, 1930, Lea & Febiger.

Wiley, A. M.: Club foot: An anatomical and experimental study of muscle growth, J. Bone Joint Surg. **41-B**:821-835, Nov. 1959.

Wray, J. B., and Herndon, C. N.: Hereditary transmission of congenital coalition of the calcaneus to the navicular, J. Bone Joint Surg. **45-A**:365-372, Mar. 1963.

6

Fractures and fracture-dislocations of the foot and ankle

Edwin G. Bovill, Jr.
Verne T. Inman

CRITERIA FOR TREATMENT

To obtain the best functional result in the treatment of all fractures, particularly those involving joints, four criteria must be fulfilled:

1. *The fracture must be accurately reduced as soon after diagnosis as possible.* Reduction is easier to obtain before swelling occurs around the injury and before blood clots appear between the fragments. Furthermore, a disturbance of the distal circulation often occurs when displacement is prolonged; early reduction decreases the risk of circulatory impairment.

2. *All joint surfaces must be precisely reconstituted.* Uneven surfaces may lead to the development of arthritic changes in the joints.

3. *Reduction of the fracture must be maintained during the period of healing.* External splints or plaster casts constitute the traditional method of maintaining reduction. Such means of immobilization, however, have definite deleterious effects upon the soft-tissue components of the injured part. The extent of these undesirable effects is largely dependent upon the age of the patient. The older the patient, the more adverse the effects of long-term immobilization.

An appreciation of the iatrogenic effects of immobilization has prompted many surgeons to employ open reduction, rigid internal fixation, and early mobilization as their treatment of choice, in spite of the possible increased risks of nonunion and infection.

4. *Motion of joints should be instituted as early as possible.* Any organ or organ system, in order to maintain itself in a state of health, obviously must be used. Suppression of the normal functioning of the musculoskeletal system by immobilization of any of its parts is attended by many evils, including muscular atrophy, myostatic contracture, decreased joint motion, increased acidity of the synovial fluid, proliferation of the connective tissue in the capsular structures, internal synovial adhesions, cartilaginous degeneration, and bone atrophy. In addition, vascular changes occur during the period of immobilization, and these changes often result in edema after the external support is removed. Early mobilization obviates or decreases the possibility of the occurrence of these abnormal processes.

The most ardent protagonist for early motion after the reduction of fracture was Lucas-Championnière (1910), who based his beliefs upon clinical experience. Subse-

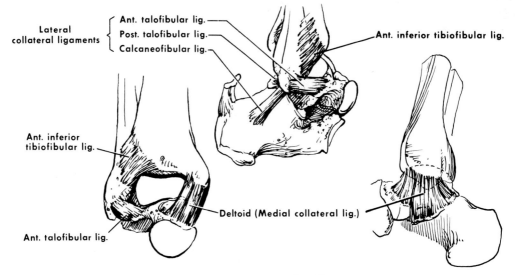

Lateral collateral ligaments { Ant. talofibular lig. — / Post. talofibular lig. — / Calcaneofibular lig. —

Ant. inferior tibiofibular lig.

Ant. inferior tibiofibular lig.

Deltoid (Medial collateral lig.)

Ant. talofibular lig.

Fig. 6-1. Anatomy of ankle.

quent experimental evidence has gradually appeared in the medical literature to support his contentions (1910-1971).

For surgical procedures for the treatment of fractures and dislocations discussed in this chapter, see Chapter 19.

FRACTURES AND FRACTURE-DISLOCATIONS OF THE ANKLE JOINT
Classification

Many classification systems for fractures and fracture-dislocations about the ankle joint exist which, for the most part, are based on the mechanism of injury.[*] Jergesen (1959) has stated that these classifications are of academic interest; however, since an almost infinite variety of malleolar and ligamentous injuries can occur separately or in combination, a functional view of the problem is a more useful one.

When assessing fractures about the ankle within a functional framework, the practitioner will consider two concepts: (1) Anatomic reduction is desirable because the restoration of normal anatomy to a

weight-bearing joint is of primary importance. (2) Stability of the ankle is related to the integrity of the malleolar ligaments.

The foot is securely bound to the leg by two osseous-ligamentous shrouds consisting of the medial malleolus and the corresponding medial collateral ligament on one side, and of the lateral malleolus and the lateral collateral ligaments on the other. In addition, the intermalleolar space is maintained by the inferior tibiofibular ligaments (Fig. 6-1). Any number of fracture and ligamentous disruption combinations can occur that may destroy the normal stability of the ankle. Many such combinations that may result from an eversion-abduction stress are illustrated in Fig. 6-2; they involve lateral malleolar fracture with subluxation of the ankle. Inversion-adduction stress, shear stress, or both combined will produce other combinations of injury. Whatever the mechanism of injury, however, and whatever the method selected to treat the injury, the goal is accurate, stable reconstitution of the ankle mortise.

Soft-tissue injury frequently accompanies fracture; the surgeon should be alert to the interposition of soft tissue, which could prevent accurate reduction. He should also pay particular attention to the possibility

[*]Ashhurst and Bromer, 1922; Bonin, 1950; Kleiger, 1956; Lauge-Hansen, 1948, 1950, 1952, 1954; and Mayer and Pohlidal, 1953.

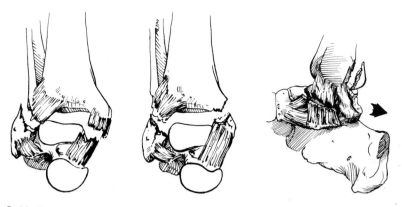

Fig. 6-2. Various types of malleolar fractures and ligamentous tears, with displacement of talus within mortise.

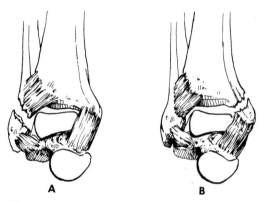

A   **B**

Fig. 6-3. Isolated fractures of malleoli. **A,** Fibular malleolus. **B,** Tibial malleolus.

of injury to the distal tibiofibular ligaments that support the tibiofibular syndesmosis and the medial collateral ligament of the ankle (see Chapter 7). Failure to repair these ligaments may lead to ankle instability and subsequent degenerative changes.

Fractures of one malleolus. It is apparent that a fracture of one malleolus without the involvement of the opposite malleolus (or its ligamentous component) permits using the uninjured side as a buttress to immobilize the part until healing takes place (Fig. 6-3). If only the malleolar tip is injured, simple protection from forced inversion (in the case of the lateral malleolus) or eversion (in the case of the medial

malleolus) suffices, and these injuries will require, at most, a short leg cast to be worn for 6 weeks. Roentgenographic evidence of the fracture of just one malleolus does not guarantee stability, however; clinical evaluation of the ligamentous apparatus at the distal tibiofibular junction and on the opposite side of the ankle is necessary in order to assess the stability of the injury. Isolated fractures of the lateral malleolus are seldom associated with nonunion, even though small avulsion phenomena may occur. Isolated fractures of the medial malleolus are reputed to have a higher incidence of delayed union and nonunion, although the evidence for this characteristic is principally retrospective and is of doubtful statistical significance. Fractures of the medial malleolus, particularly if they occur below the level of the superior surface of the talus, may be asymptomatic even though they heal with fibrous union. Aufranc (1960) and Portis and Mendelsohn (1953) have found little evidence to suggest that the isolated malleolar fracture, if not displaced, requires internal fixation. Fractures of the medial malleolus at the level of the plafond, however, result in complete functional loss of internal support provided by the medial collateral ligament. This fracture must be accurately reduced in order for the ankle to regain stability. Most surgeons feel that the most

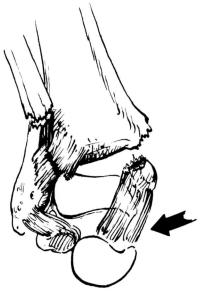

Fig. 6-4. Common type of bimalleolar fracture.

effective treatment for this fracture is open reduction and internal fixation.

Bimalleolar types of fracture and fracture-dislocation. The terms "bimalleolar types of fracture" and "fracture-dislocation" are used to include fractures of both malleoli; fractures of one malleolus plus complete disruption of the ligament on the opposite side; or a fracture of the medial malleolus and rupture of the tibiofibular ligaments (Glick, 1964), with a fracture in the shaft of the fibula proximal to the tibiofibular ligament (Fig. 6-4). Fibular fracture can occur at the proximal end of the fibula. When it does, and if it is accompanied by ankle injury, one can assume that some disruption of the interosseous membrane will occur anywhere from the distal tibiofibular syndesmosis to the level of the fibular fracture and that division of

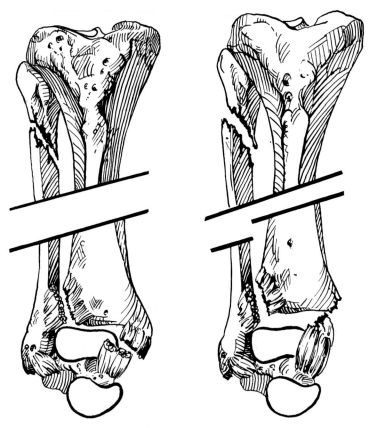

Fig. 6-5. Fracture of medial malleolus, with accompanying proximal fracture of fibula and disruption of tibiofibular syndemosis.

the distal tibiofibular ligaments will also occur (Fig. 6-5). Occasionally this injury will manifest itself as a rupture of the deltoid ligament, with the line of dehiscence passing across the ankle capsule and continuing upward through the distal tibiofibular ligaments and interosseous membrane to the level of the proximal neck of the fibula. This particular combination is easy for the unwary examiner to miss, since the ankle may be relocated when the technician positions it for roentgenographic examination. No fracture will be seen unless a full-length roentgenogram of the leg, which includes the upper end of the fibula, is taken. For this reason, assessment of any ankle injury with severe lateral and medial swelling, pain, and tenderness should include examination for a proximal fibular fracture by both roentgenogram and clinical evaluation of mortise stability. Again, it must be emphasized that accurate reduction of the medial malleolus or repair of the deltoid ligament is critical. The possibility of an accompanying diastasis of the distal tibiofibular syndesmosis in these injuries should always be considered.

Trimalleolar fractures and fracture-dislocations. Trimalleolar fractures and fracture-dislocations include all the combinations described in the bimalleolar types of fracture and dislocation plus fractures of the posterior lip of the tibia. The size of the fragment may vary: It may communicate with the medial malleolar fragment or, if it is laterally placed, it may carry the posterior tibiofibular ligament with it. If the fragment carries with it one-third or more of the articular surface of the tibia, a high risk of posterior subluxation of the talus exists unless the fracture is internally fixed (Fig. 6-6). Fortunately, most posterior lip fragments are small and do not, in themselves, compromise the stability of the ankle (Aufranc, 1960).

Fractures of the anterior lip of the distal tibia. Fracture of the anterior lip of the distal tibia may accompany malleolar fracture as a mirror image of the posterior trimalleolar fracture-dislocation; occasionally it occurs as an isolated injury.

This injury is not usually associated with fracture of the fibular shaft or disruption of the distal tibiofibular ligaments. The anterior lip of the tibia is more commonly comminuted than is the posterior lip; thus, internal fixation techniques may be compromised (Fig. 6-7).

Compound fractures and fracture-dislocations of the ankle. The same principles of wound management with debridement apply to compound fractures and fracture-dislocations of the ankle as apply to compound fractures and injuries of the joints elsewhere in the body. The compound wound in this area almost always communicates with the ankle joint. Joint closure, either as a primary or a delayed primary procedure, is essential (Jergesen, 1959). The skin wound can be closed by primary closure, delayed primary closure, or secondary closure, depending upon the degree of soft-tissue damage and contamination and the amount of elapsed time since the occurrence of the injury.

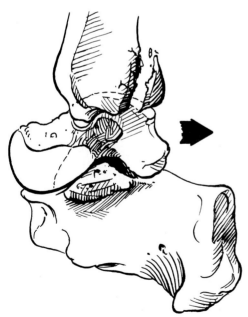

Fig. 6-6. Common type of trimalleolar fracture, with posterior displacement of talus.

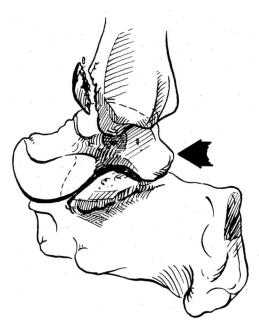

Fig. 6-7. Fracture of anterior lip of tibia.

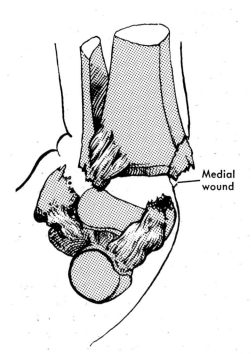

Medial
wound

Fig. 6-8. Compound fracture-dislocation, with transverse wound at level of medial malleolus centered on medial side of leg.

The most commonly seen compound fracture-dislocation about the ankle is one in which a transverse wound occurs at the level of the medial malleolus, centered on the medial side of the leg (Fig. 6-8). The foot is dislocated posterolaterally; frequently the proximal surface of the avulsed medial malleolus and the articular surface of the tibia appear in the wound. In the treatment of compound wounds internal fixation is usually avoided. However, in these injuries the wound is so close to the surface of the fracture and to the joint that rigid internal fixation is employed in order to protect the overlying soft tissues from pressure and recurrent tension. Since the compound wound lies directly over the medial malleolus, internal fixation of the medial malleolar side can usually be accomplished with one screw; little, if any, additional dissection is necessary after the wound has been debrided and irrigated and the dislocation has been reduced.

Fractures with severe comminution and instability. Closed, severely comminuted fractures of the ankle may not be amenable to internal fixation. These injuries can usually be managed with external skeletal traction through the calcaneus or, following manipulation, with fixed traction, produced by placing a pin in the calcaneus and a pin in the tibia proximally (Fig. 6-9). Occasionally, a combination of comminution and a complex-compound wound about the ankle creates a situation in which it is impossible to employ the usual methods of malleolar fixation, yet in order to assure the survival of the foot and to permit management of the surrounding soft tissue, stability must be achieved. In this situation, the technique of driving a vertical Steinmann pin through the calcaneus and the talus into the distal tibia (Fig. 6-10) can be used in order to preserve the foot (Childress, 1965; Dieterle, 1935).

Fractures of the lateral malleolus with posterior displacement of the proximal fibular fragment. Bosworth (1947), Fleming and Smith (1954), and Meyers (1957) have described bimalleolar types of frac-

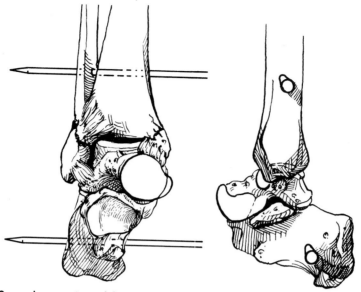

Fig. 6-9. Severely comminuted fracture managed by fixed traction, with pin in calcaneus and pin in tibia.

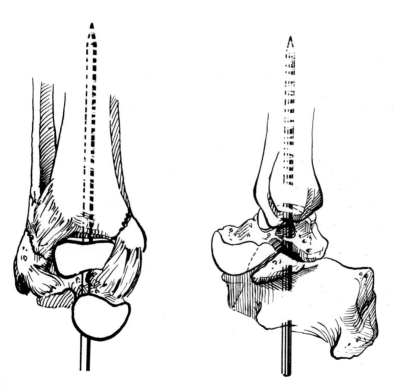

Fig. 6-10. A method of maintaining normal relationships of components of ankle in severe compound comminuted fractures.

ture that are accompanied by displacement of the proximal fibula at the fracture site posteriorly on the tibia in a position that usually makes reduction by closed manipulation impossible. The ligamentous support to the syndesmosis apparently remains intact and holds the fibula in its dislocated position. In these types of fracture, open reduction is necessary and a posterolateral approach is appropriate.

Closed reduction of malleolar fractures

Bimalleolar and trimalleolar fracture-dislocation types of injury (abduction–external rotation mechanisms). These injuries are accompanied by posterolateral subluxation or dislocation of the foot on the leg, and the foot is usually externally rotated with reference to the leg. To achieve reduction, the foot must be brought anteriorly and medially into position, and it must be internally rotated on the tibia. The malleoli are attached to the foot by the collateral ligaments; the "distal fragment" is in reality the foot with the attached malleoli. Hence, reduction entails replacement of the foot in proper relation to the tibia. If the deltoid ligament rather than the medial malleolus is disrupted, or if the medial malleolar fragment is small, a shoulder or buttress exists medially against which the foot (talus) can be reduced. If the medial malleolar fragment is large, internal fixation of the medial malleolus is necessary to produce stability of the joint. A convenient way to carry out manipulative reduction, if an assistant is available, is to flex the patient's hip and knee approximately 30 degrees and to allow the extremity to rotate externally approximately 30 degrees. The assistant holds the limb in this position by supporting the thigh with one hand while he holds the first two toes in order to maintain the foot in the vertical plane. Gravity produces medial and anterior replacement of the foot, and when the foot is held in a vertical position, an attitude of internal rotation of the foot with respect to the leg is achieved. A cast with appropriate molding can then be applied.

Bimalleolar fracture-dislocation types of injury (adduction–inversion mechanisms). In these injuries the reverse of the maneuvers described for the abduction–external rotation injury is required. There is less often a lateral butress against which to reduce the joint, and the medial malleolar fracture line frequently runs proximally from the level of the joint.

Anterior lip fractures. It is difficult to avoid anterior subluxation in this injury when the patient is recumbent with his limb supported in the usual fashion at the foot and knee. Here again, the force of gravity can be used to assist the surgeon to reduce the fracture. The patient suspends his leg over the end of the treatment table, where an assistant can carry out a posterior thrust of the foot against the leg. Or, more simply, the patient may lie prone on the table with his knee on the injured side flexed approximately 60 degrees. An assistant supports the foot in this position, which permits the weight of the leg against the supported foot to reduce the subluxation. Reduction is maintained in this position while the surgeon applies the cast.

Internal fixation of malleolar fractures

In the majority of malleolar types of fracture about the ankle the goal is anatomic reduction and rigid fixation of one or more of the four areas contributing stability to the ankle mortise. Although almost limitless combinations of anatomic disruptions occur in fractures and fracture-dislocations about the ankle, internal fixation will be directed toward the medial malleolus and its associated collateral ligament, the lateral malleolus and its associated collateral ligaments, the distal tibiofibular syndesmosis, and the anterior or posterior lip of the tibia. The surgeon must weigh the goal of maximum stability against such risks as increased soft-tissue trauma from multiple or larger incisions and the ill effects of prolonged surgery. Varying degrees of stability may be achieved (Fig. 6-11); the surgeon may frequently elect to accept the intermediate level of relative stability, since plaster protection will be

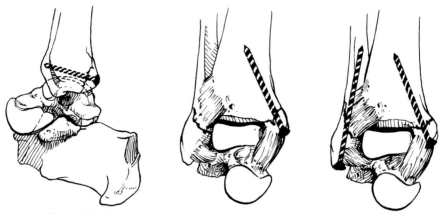

Fig. 6-11. Methods to achieve varying degrees of stability of ankle.

necessary in any case and can be depended upon in most bimalleolar-trimalleolar types of injury to control reduction once the level of relative stability has been reached. One area in which internal fixation is obligatory (soft-tissue conditions permitting) is the posterior lip of the tibia when one-third or more of the articular surface is involved and the fragment is displaced; posterior subluxation is possible in this instance even if both the medial and the lateral malleoli are securely fixed. Internal fixation is also indicated where there is evidence of soft-tissue interposition (Coonrad and Bugg, 1954). In their series of patients in whom a stable situation was produced at the time of internal fixation, Burwell and Charnley (1965) described a minor modification of the usual postoperative care for internal fixation of ankle fractures. In the patient's early postoperative period, the injured limb was removed from the protective plaster cast for active non–weight-bearing exercise, and a long leg cast was replaced by a short leg plaster cast. These authors reported an early recovery of maximum range of motion in patients who were treated in this fashion.

Medial malleolar fractures can be internally fixed with a screw. Comminuted medial malleolar fractures may be fixed with one or more Kirschner wires, or with a Zuelzer hookplate (Zuelzer, 1968).

Frequently the lateral malleolar fracture can be internally fixed with an intramedullary screw or Rush pin. Syndesmosis separation may be repaired with a screw placed horizontally from the fibula to the tibia.

Fractures of the ankle in children are rare. Trauma in this region, if affecting the skeleton proper, usually produces epiphyseal separation. Treatment for these injuries is the same as treatment for epiphyseal separation injuries of the long bones.

FRACTURES AND FRACTURE-DISLOCATIONS OF THE TALUS

While the literature on fractures and fracture-dislocations of the talus is relatively extensive, major fractures of this bone are encountered infrequently. Davidson and colleagues (1967), in a statistical review of 25,000 fractures, found only fifty-six involving the talus. Because fractures and fracture-dislocations of this bone are uncommon, a series of cases reported in a single article is apt to be small. Furthermore, these series often include a variety of fractures, each one of them requiring a different therapeutic approach. Thus it is impossible to enunciate standardized and universally applicable procedures for all fractures of the talus. Excellent reviews of this subject are contained in the literature. Anderson (1919), Coltart (1952), Watson-Jones (1955), Mindell et al. (1963), Pennal (1963), Dunn et al. (1966), and Kenwright and Taylor (1970) provide classifications, discussions about mechanism of injury, and reports of the results of treatment of fractures and fracture-dislocations of the talus.

Complications

Fractures of the talus are complicated by two factors, aseptic necrosis and multiple articular surfaces.

Aseptic necrosis. It is estimated that in approximately one-third of cases of fractures of the talus, aseptic necrosis results because of the vulnerability of the blood supply to the talus. Sneed (1925) demonstrated that the bone had no single nutrient artery. Subsequently others[*] have reported results of their investigations of the blood supply to the talus. All essentially agree that the principal sources of blood supply are through the artery in the sinus tarsi and through the secondary vessels that enter the bone through the dorsum of the neck of the talus. A limited number of vessels enter the talus through the posterior tuberosity and through small inconstant vessels in the region of the collateral ligaments of the ankle. Since the major vessels enter through the neck, fracture in this area may seriously jeopardize the blood supply to portions of the talus and may result in avascular necrosis.

Multiple articular surfaces. The talus, in its articulation with continuous structures, possesses eight well-defined articular facets. Smooth and precise motion over each of these articular surfaces is necessary for normal functioning of the ankle, subtalar, and talonavicular articulations. It appears obvious that if arthritic changes are to be avoided, the articular surfaces must be preserved and the correct anatomic relationships between them must be restored. In treating fractures of the talus, precise repositioning of the parts should be the objective. Boyd and Knight (1942), Taylor (1962), and McKeever (1963) concur that

---

[*]Wildenauer (1950), Haliburton et al. (1958), Kelly (1964), and Mulfinger and Trueta (1970).

open reduction and internal fixation may be the best method of treatment.

Classification

Fractures of the talus are customarily divided into three groups: those of the head, neck, and body. The precise frequency of each type of fracture is not certain.

Fractures of the head of the talus (Figs. 6-12 and 6-13) are less common than fractures of the neck. Both may occur when force is transmitted through the navicular; for example, when a person falls from a height and lands on a plantar flexed foot. The displacement is not usually marked; immobilization of the foot for from 4 to 6 weeks in a well-molded walking cast and subsequent weight bearing without support is usually adequate to ensure the return of normal function.

Next to these small chip or avulsion fractures, fractures through the neck of the talus occur most commonly (Fig. 6-14). Ray (1967) reported a series of thirty-four fractures of the talus; seventeen of them were fractures of the neck. In Coltart's review of over 200 cases, this fracture occurred twice as frequently as fractures of the body of the talus (1952). These fractures deserve particular attention, since they have the potential of healing without disability but may lead to avascular necrosis of the body of the talus.

Hawkins (1970), in an excellent review of fifty-seven fractures of the neck of the talus, classified these fractures into three groups. Group I consisted of six cases of linear vertical fractures that were undisplaced. In these cases the fracture entered the sinus tarsi between the middle and posterior facets. The body of the talus retained its normal position in the ankle and subtalar joints. Treatment consisted of simple immobilization. Aseptic necrosis did not occur in any of the six cases. Group II consisted of twenty-four cases in which the vertical fractures through the neck were displaced and the subtalar joint was luxated. The ankle joint remained normal.

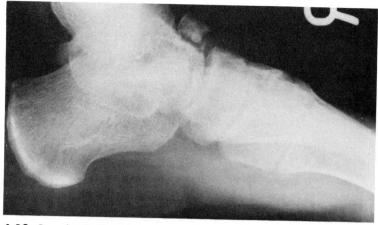

Fig. 6-12. Completely detached fragment of bone from dorsum at head of talus.

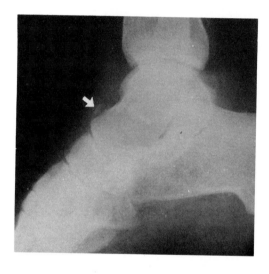

Fig. 6-13. Chip fracture over dorsum of head of talus.

Open reduction was necessary in fourteen of these cases. Avascular necrosis occurred in ten of the twenty-four cases. Group III included twenty-seven cases of displaced vertical fractures of the neck, complicated by dislocations of both subtalar and ankle joints. Primary talectomies were performed in five of the cases, and open reduction was necessary in twenty of them. Avascular necrosis occurred in twenty of the twenty-two cases.

Fractures of the body of the talus may occur in varying degrees. Marginal fractures are easily overlooked but may pro-duce disabling symptoms (Fig. 6-15). The prognosis in fractures of the body of the talus is not as good as that in fractures of the neck. Frequently even a slight disruption of the congruity of the joint surface causes a step deformity and subsequent arthritis of the ankle joint. An equally severe disability occurs when the fracture causes incongruity of the subtalar joint with resulting subtalar motion, which may necessitate subtalar arthrodesis. In these cases of fracture of the body of the talus anatomic reduction should be attempted. Coltart points out that even though reduc-

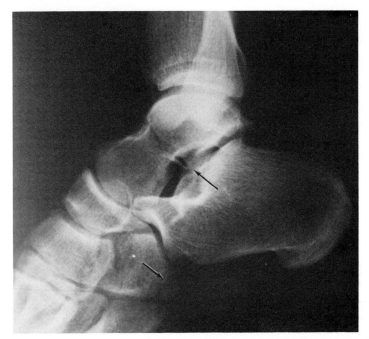

Fig. 6-14. Fracture at neck of talus in 25-year-old man. Note the fractured cuboid. The left foot was on the clutch at the time of a collision.

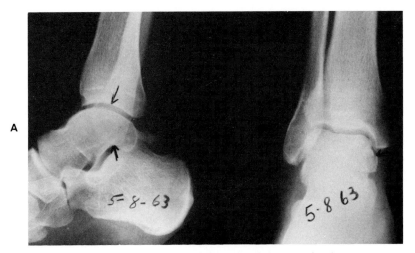

Fig. 6-15. A, Roentgenograms of foot of 30-year-old man. The foot was on an auto brake at the time of a collision. Anteroposterior and lateral views show a comminuted fracture of the body of the talus. **B,** Roentgenograms of same patient 1 year later. Anteroposterior, lateral, and tomogram views show aseptic necrosis of part of the trochlear surface of the talus.

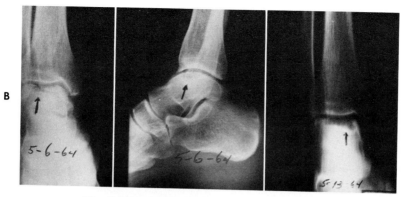

B

Fig. 6-15, cont'd. For legend see opposite page.

tion is achieved, a good painless range of motion may not be restored. Massive comminuted and destructive fractures of the body, of course, require arthrodeses, talectomies, and reconstructive procedures.

Osteochondral fracture of the talus

Thorough clinical and roentgenographic evaluation of painful ankles after injury may uncover osteochondral fractures. These small chip or avulsion fractures of the edges of the articular surfaces are the most frequent ones. To avoid prolonged disability, the fragments should be removed immediately.

Treatment

All surgeons agree that prompt reduction of fractures of the talus should be carried out in order to reduce the possibility of compromising the circulation to the distal portions of the foot and to prevent the occurrence of skin necrosis as a result of swelling.

FRACTURES OF THE CALCANEUS

Fractures of the calcaneus are the most common fractures of the bones of the tarsus and comprise 60 percent of all fractures in this region of the foot. Since these fractures are usually caused by a fall from a considerable height, fractures of other skeletal parts may occur at the same time, which frequently complicate treatment. One out of ten patients with fractures of

the calcaneus also has fractures of the spine; one out of four has other fractures of the extremities.

Approximately 25 to 30 percent of fractures of the calcaneus fortunately do not involve the posterior facet of the subtalar joint. However, the possibility of this involvement should not be overlooked, since it may be a source of residual disability.

Anatomy

The anatomy of the calcaneus is shown in Fig. 6-16. The superior surface of the calcaneus climbs upward from the front and back toward the middle. The angle between these two inclinations is referred to as the tuber angle and according to Böhler (1957) normally varies between 20 and 40 degrees. Decrease in this angle in relation to the normal opposite foot implies upper displacements of the tuberosity.

Classification

Clinical observations have led to various classifications of fractures of the calcaneus. The value of such classifications is greater than merely that of satisfying an academic interest. Since the types of therapeutic procedure employed and the types of fracture sustained are independent variables, final evaluation of any treatment will depend on the control of one of these variables. This control can be partially accomplished by classifying the types of fracture.

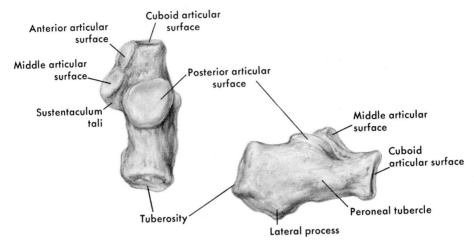

Fig. 6-16. Anatomy of calcaneus.

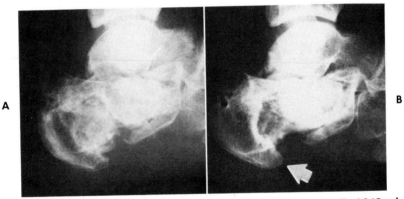

Fig. 6-17. A, Lateral view of foot of 30-year-old male taken Oct. 7, 1969, showing comminuted ("smash") fracture of calcaneus, with multiple vertical and horizontal breaks. The injury occurred on April 28, 1969. **B,** Same view taken 1 year later (Nov. 9, 1970). The posterior part of the calcaneus has lifted dorsally. The arrow points to a sharp prominence on the plantar tuberosity, which is the only point of contact with the ground during weight bearing.

Over 50 years ago Cotton and Henderson (1916) described comminuted fractures of the calcaneus in these general terms:

What we see are *smashes* of the os calcis. . . . The lines of fracture, as sketched by the x-rays, are *not* uniform. In general, there is a smash below the weight-bearing vertical line of the tibia, running more or less (mostly less) vertically, and various radiating lines running down and forward, and backward. The heel is driven up and often is driven outward. The whole bone is compressed vertically and expanded laterally; there is often a pushing of fragments inward, under the ankle, and almost uniformly a considerable pushing outward of bone-fragments, capped by the usually intact outer lamella of the calcis out under the external malleolus. This is *the* type lesion.[*]

_____

[*]Cotton, F. J., and Henderson, F. F.: Results of fracture of the os calcis, Amer. J. Orthop. Surg. 14:290, 1916.

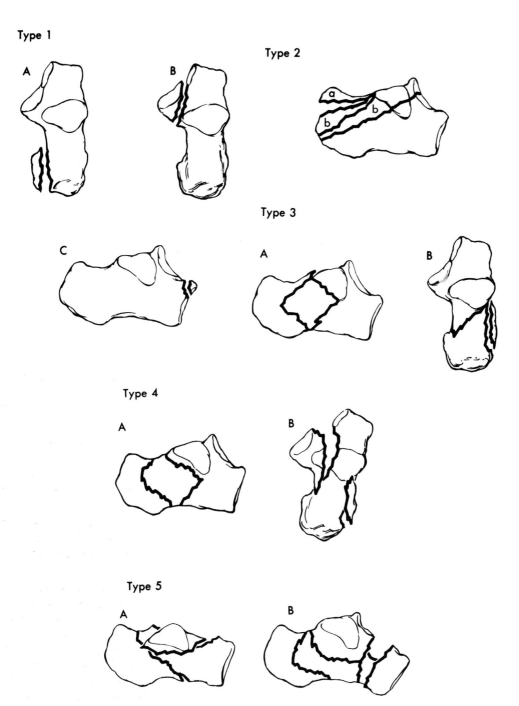

Fig. 6-18. Rowe's classification of fractures of calcaneus. (From J.A.M.A. **184**:922, June 1963.)

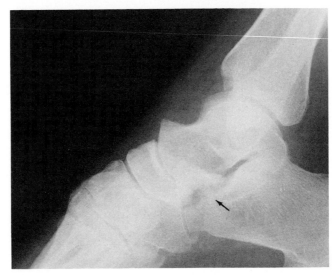

Fig. 6-19. Roentgenogram of large fracture of anterior process of calcaneus in 40-year-old woman. Conservative treatment produced good results.

Fig. 6-17 illustrates a comminuted ("smash") fracture of the calcaneus.

Subsequently, more precise classifications have been proposed. We have used the classification suggested by Rowe et al. (1963), who combine their ideas with those of Watson-Jones and Warrick and Bremner (1953) (Fig. 6-18).

Type 1   (A)   Fracture of the tuberosity
        (B)   Fracture of the sustentaculum
        (C)   Fracture of the anterior process
Type 2   (a)   Beak fracture
        (b)   Avulsion of the tendo achillis insertion
Type 3   Oblique fracture not involving the subtalar joint
Type 4   Fracture involving the subtalar joint
Type 5   Central depression fracture with communition

Fractures involving the upper part of the tuberosity, with displacement of the fragments, usually are not avulsion fractures, because the fracture line is superior to the attachment of the tendo achillis. The fracture can usually be approximated by manipulation. Should displacement recur, the fragments may be secured with a single screw.

Gellman (1951) believes that fracture of the anterior process of the calcaneus is commonly overlooked (Figs. 6-19 and 6-20). The mechanism of this injury is probably forceful adduction of the forepart of the foot in combination with plantar flexion. The bifurcate calcaneonavicular-calcaneocuboid ligament may play a part in the avulsion of the anterior process of the calcaneus. Pain in the region of the calcaneocuboid joint warrants oblique roentgenograms of the foot to rule out this fracture (Fig. 6-20). If there is gross displacement, treatment is directed toward reduction of the fragment and immobilization for 4 to 6 weeks, after which physical therapy treatments should be given. In his four cases Gellman reported the average convalescence to be 13 weeks, with mild residual discomfort and swelling remaining at the end of that time. Piatt (1956) has named the anterior process of the calcaneus the promontory of the calcaneus and describes ten cases of fracture: One case of nonunion occurred with minimal residual disability. Hunt (1970) agrees with Gellman that the significance of this fracture has been underestimated. He states that although not enough cases have been reported to set

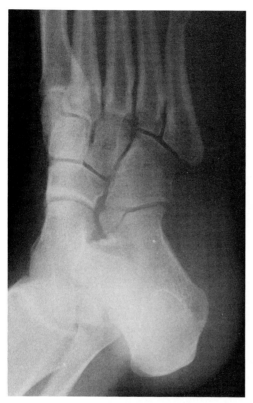

Fig. 6-20. Fracture of anterior process of calcaneus.

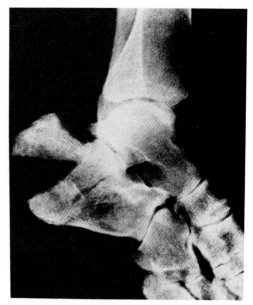

Fig. 6-21. Typical beak fracture of the calcaneus. (From Conwell, H. E., and Reynolds, F. D.: Key and Conwell's management of fractures, dislocations and sprains, ed. 7, St. Louis, 1961, The C. V. Mosby Co., p. 1084.)

forth a definite program of therapy, initial treatment should extend beyond simple immobilization.

Beak fractures may occur, with interruption of the bony attachment of the tendo achillis to the distal fragment (Fig. 6-21). Failure to approximate the fragments may result in deformity and functional loss (Figs. 6-22 and 6-23). Avulsion of the tendo achillis with minimal elevation of the periosteum may be overlooked in the roentgenogram.

Minimally displaced fractures should be treated conservatively. Interesting cases of avulsion fracture of the calcaneus have been reported by Mooney (1935) and Rothberg (1939).

Oblique fractures not involving the subtalar joint (Fig. 6-24) have the same mechanism of injury, such as landing on the heel after a fall or receiving a severe blow from below during standing, as do the more severe fractures that involve the joint. The oblique fracture that extends from the posteromedial aspect to the anterolateral aspect does not enter the joint. The problem of traumatic arthritis is therefore nonexistent, although soft-tissue injury and the problems of associated thickening and broadening of the calcaneus can occur. In these cases, if the displacements are corrected by manipulation, a good functional recovery usually can be expected.

It appears that there is general agreement about the treatment of fractures of the anterior process, beak fractures, and minimally displaced fractures not entering the subtalar joint. For the treatment of comminuted fractures that enter the subtalar joint, however, no such agreement

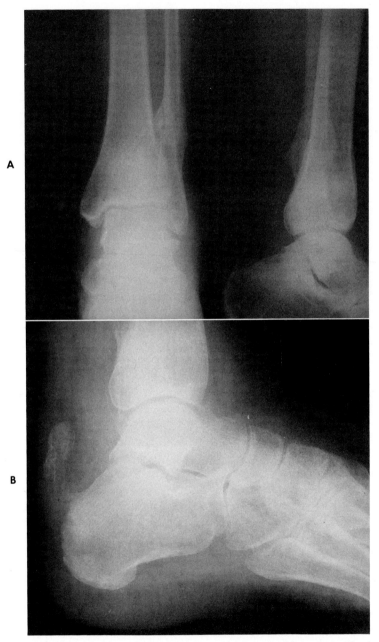

Fig. 6-22. A, Roentgenograms of leg and foot of 60-year-old woman. The leg was immobilized in a short leg walking cast because of pain from an old fracture of the fibula. **B,** After removal of cast. The patient had taken a sudden step and the tendo achillis pulled off a part of the calcaneus.

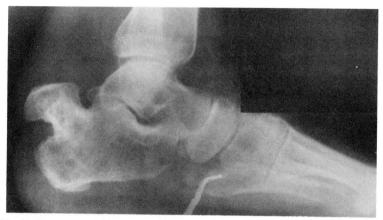

Fig. 6-23. Horizontal fracture of posterior tuberosity of calcaneus with rupture of inserted portion of tendo achillis in 48-year-old woman. Unsuccessful open reduction was performed 4 days after the injury. A roentgenogram taken 6 months later showed a dorsal fragment united with the body of the calcaneus and the tendo achillis attached only to this fragment. (Courtesy Dr. R. J. Westwater.)

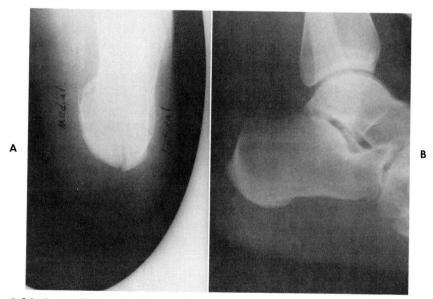

Fig. 6-24. A, Axial view of calcaneus showing horizontal fracture. **B,** Lateral view; fracture not visible.

exists. It is this type that has given fracture of the calcaneus a bad reputation, for it results in a high rate of residual disability. Diverse methods of treatment exist, and each of them has its strong personal advocates. The literature is largely composed of reports of the results of different types of therapy and is so voluminous that it is inadvisable to analyze, evaluate, and summarize here all the therapeutic methods that have been proposed.

A historical approach to treatment

A historical approach appears appropriate, since it defines the problem and orients the practitioner to the origin of the various therapeutic procedures.

Prior to the improvement of roentgenographic techniques, the practitioner could do little more for fractures of the calcaneus than to prescribe bed rest, elevation, and immobilization. The results of this treatment were inevitably poor. Cotton and Wilson (1908) pointed out that loss of subtalar motion appeared to be crucial in permanent residual disabilities from fracture of the calcaneus; they insisted that attempts be made to manipulate the fragments into better alignment. These authors emphasize the need to compress the displaced lateral fragment from under the lateral malleolus, even if beating it with a mallet was necessary. A decade later, Cotton and Henderson (1916), in reviewing their cases, concluded that conservative treatment yielded incredibly poor results. Bankart (1942), in an introductory remark of an article, stated: "The results of the treatment of crush fractures of the os calcis are rotten."* Goff (1938) reviewed the status of the treatment of fractures of the calcaneus in a classic article. In pen-and-ink sketches he depicted forty-one methods of treatment that were being used at the time.

During the past 25 years, clinicians have investigated the problem of fractures of

the calcaneus. Using improved roentgenographic techniques, they have initiated experimental studies and have evaluated the results of treatment in many series of cases. However, unanimity of opinion as to the best method of treatment has not been reached over the years. Treatment is varied and each method has its proponents. Recommended procedures range from no reduction and immediate mobilization to open reduction, bone grafting, and plaster immobilization; a multitude of suggested procedures lie between these extremes. In reviewing the literature, two conclusions seem inescapable: Accurate reduction is desirable, and prolonged immobilization is to be condemned.

Treatment

At present, there are four kinds of treatment of comminuted fractures of the calcaneus: (1) conservative treatment; (2) treatment with pins, traction, or both; (3) treatment by open reduction; and (4) treatment using primary arthrodesis. The decision as to which method to employ should be made immediately upon seeing the patient, keeping in mind that the sole object of corrective treatment is to preserve motion in the disrupted joints. To attain this goal, all procedures to reduce swelling, relieve pain, and obtain early motion should be used.

Conservative treatment. Strictly speaking, conservative treatment excludes reduction, the use of pins, skeletal traction, and surgical procedures (Fig. 6-25). Elevation of the foot, placement of ice packs around the heel, bed rest, massage, exercise, and medication for pain comprise the treatment. The techniques and results of conservative treatment of comminuted fractures of the calcaneus are reported by a number of investigators.*

---

*Bankart, A. S. B.: Fractures of the os calcis, Lancet 2:175, Aug. 15, 1942.

*See Bertelsen and Hasner, 1951; Carothers and Lyons, 1952; Essex-Lopresti, 1952; Dautry, 1961; Lance et al., 1963; Morretti and Piovani, 1967; Dragonetti, 1969, Nosny et al., 1969; and Barnard and Odegard, 1970.

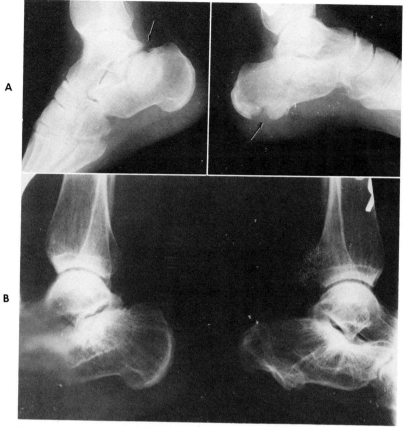

Fig. 6-25. Roentgenograms of bilateral fracture of calcaneus in 40-year-old man. He fell 15 feet from a telephone pole. **A,** X-ray films of both calcanei at time of injury. **B,** Films taken 1 year later. The fracture was treated with elevation, enzymes, compression dressings, and early weight bearing in equinus casts. The patient returned to his job climbing poles in 6 months.

Treatment with pins, traction, or both. The use of pins to improve anatomic relationships was pioneered by Böhler, who found that treatment consisting of postreduction immobilization in plaster casts yielded unsatisfactory results. Reduction by traction, followed by early mobilization, has decreased residual disability (Gossett, 1969; Nosny et al., 1969).

Open reduction. The current method of open reduction that is widely used was described by Palmer (1948) and extended by Widén (1954). Maxfield and McDermott (1955) and Maxfield (1963) reported favorably on their continuing use of open

reduction and grafting. These authors immobilized the patients' limbs in plaster casts for 8 weeks. Vestad (1968) and Hazlett (1969) have reported further encouraging results after using open reduction, maintaining the reduction by bone grafts or metallic fixation. It should be noted that Hazlett, in his treatment of fractures, avoided postoperative immobilization and encouraged immediate motion of the ankle and subtalar joints and the toes.

Primary arthrodesis. Based upon the assumption that comminuted fractures involving the articular surfaces cause irreparable damage and that a painless rigid foot is preferable to a painful movable one, many surgeons have advocated primary subtalar or triple arthrodesis. Leriche (1922) reported having obtained a satisfactory result in a single case. Wilson (1927) strongly advocated immediate arthrodesis, and Kiaer and Anthonsen (1942) reported obtaining "satisfactory" results in eighteen out of twenty-two patients. A number of investigators[*] have reported results of treatment of severe fractures of the calcaneus by immediate arthrodesis. A high percentage of patients treated by this method were able to return to work.

From the voluminous literature concerning fractures of the calcaneus, it is impossible to state the precise manner in which all fractures should be treated. The following recommendations are derived from essentially intuitive deductions we have gained from a study of the various publications:

1. A thorough roentgenographic examination is an absolute necessity.
2. Conservative treatment is preferable for fractures that are not displaced.
3. Isolated displaced fractures not involving articular surfaces should be reduced. If necessary, reduction and internal fixation may be employed; early mobilization is essential.
4. Anything short of exact alignment of joint surfaces is apt to lead to disability. Precise reduction should always be attempted. Such alignment may require pins with traction and open reduction, with or without bone grafting.
5. In markedly comminuted fractures where reconstitution of the joint surfaces is impossible, primary arthrodesis may be the method of choice.

FRACTURES OF THE CUBOID

Isolated fractures of the cuboid are rare. Fractures of the cuboid accompanied by

---

[*]See Gallie, 1943; Brattström, 1953; Moberg and Erfors, 1953; Thompson and Friesen, 1959; Hall and Pennal, 1960; Harris, 1963; and Zagra and Bellistri, 1970.

fractures of the adjacent cuneiforms or of the base of the lateral metatarsals or both are more common, but even these combinations are encountered infrequently. Wilson (1933), in a series of approximately 5,000 fractures, found only ten cases of isolated fracture of the cuboid. Hermel and Gershon-Cohen (1953) reported five cases of compression fracture of the cuboid in which the cuboid was compressed between the fourth and fifth metatarsals and the calcaneus. Fig. 6-26, A shows a comminuted compression fracture of the cuboid of a youth 21 years of age who fell asleep and drove his car into a tree. His fracture was treated during the acute phase by casting; he now wears a shoe insert and walks with minimal disability. Fig. 6-26, B shows a comminuted fracture of the cuboid of a young man 17 years of age who fell from a motorcycle.

Jackson and Dickson (1965) reported having seen three cases of fracture of the cuboid (Fig. 6-27). Watson-Jones (1955) does not discuss the problem; Böhler (1958) and Conwell and Reynolds (1961) both stated that fractures of this bone rarely show major displacements and need be treated only by immobilization.

FRACTURES OF THE NAVICULAR

Although fractures of the navicular occur twice as frequently as fractures of the cuboid (Wilson, 1933), they are still uncommon. Watson-Jones (1955) divides these fractures into three types: (1) fractures of the tuberosity; (2) chip fractures of the dorsal lip; and (3) transverse fractures, with or without separation and displacement of the dorsal fragment(s).

Fracture of the tuberosity of the navicular must be distinguished from congenital os tibiale externum. The line of separation in os tibiale externum is usually smooth and regular, whereas in a fracture it is rough; and unlike the fracture, os tibiale externum commonly occurs bilaterally. Small, persistently painful fractures that fail to heal with immobilization may require excision of the fragments (Figs. 6-28 and 6-29).

Text continued on p. 145.

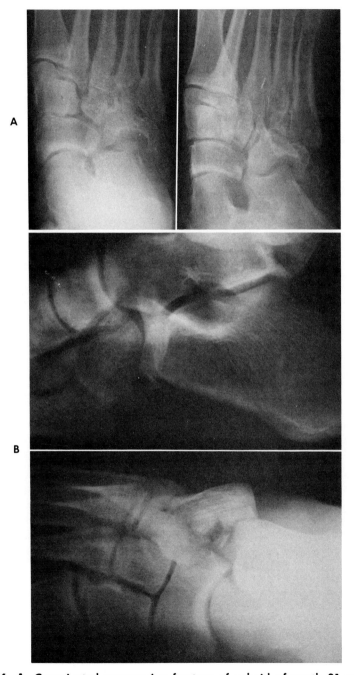

Fig. 6-26. A, Comminuted compression fracture of cuboid of youth 21 years of age.
B, Comminuted fracture and dislocation of left cuboid of youth 17 years of age.

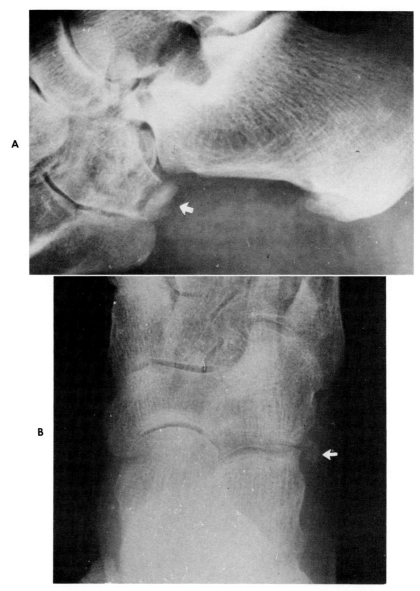

Fig. 6-27. A, Fracture and displacement of plantar surface of the cuboid. **B,** Chip fracture of lateral side of the cuboid.

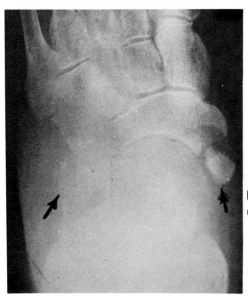

Fig. 6-28. Avulsion fracture of neck of navicular and fracture of head of calcaneus.

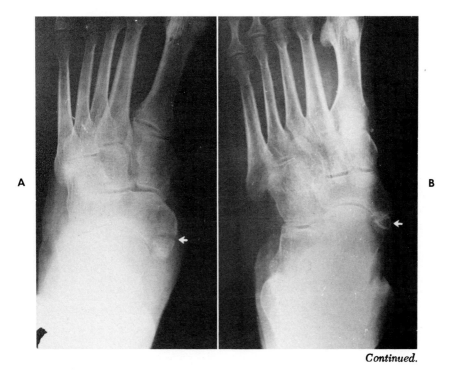

Continued.

Fig. 6-29. A, Fracture of neck of navicular without displacement. **B,** Roentgenogram taken 1 year later. The fractured fragment is tilted on its end, producing a peroneal spastic flatfoot. Note rarefaction at the head of the talus. **C,** Roentgenogram taken after removal of fractured fragment. The peroneal spasm has disappeared.

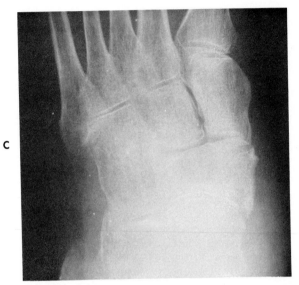

c

Fig. 6-29, cont'd. For legend see p. 143.

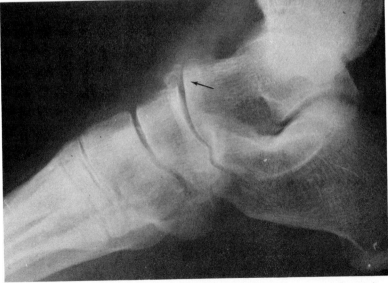

Fig. 6-30. Chip fracture over dorsum of navicular. The chip was removed to relieve pain.

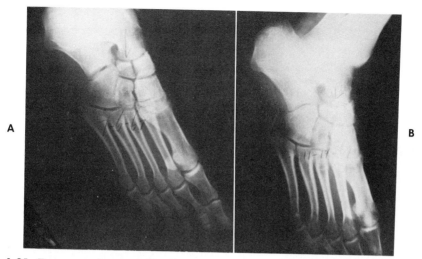

Fig. 6-31. Transverse fracture through body of navicular. It was treated conservatively with casting and non–weight bearing. **B,** Roentgenogram taken 1 year later. The fracture has healed, resulting in minimal disability.

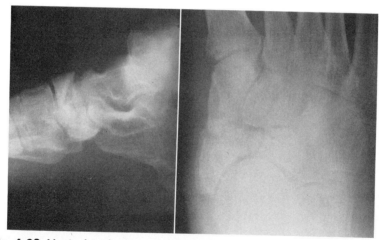

Fig. 6-32. Vertical and transverse views of comminuted fracture of navicular.

Dorsal chip fractures may be treated conservatively; only a short period of immobilization is required and usually little disability results. If pain persists, however, the fragment may be excised (Fig. 6-30).

Transverse fractures through the body of the navicular are more serious. The literature dealing with this type of fracture is not extensive and consists mainly of reports of single cases or small series of cases (1908-1970). No consensus as to preferred treatment seems to have been reached. In general, simple linear fractures without displacement may be treated conservatively; a good functional result is to be anticipated (Fig. 6-31). Displaced fractures should be reduced and fixed by pins or screws. If the articular surfaces are malaligned or destroyed (Fig. 6-32), degenerative changes are to be expected and some type of arthrodesis may be required at a later date.

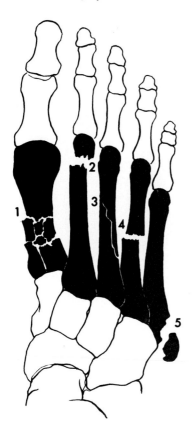

Fig. 6-33. Types of fractures of the metatarsals: **1**, comminuted; **2**, transverse with displacement; **3**, oblique or spiral; **4**, transverse; and **5**, avulsion fracture of tuberosity. (After Netter.)

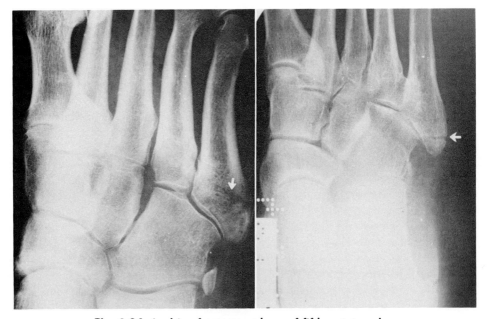

Fig. 6-34. Avulsion fractures at base of fifth metatarsal.

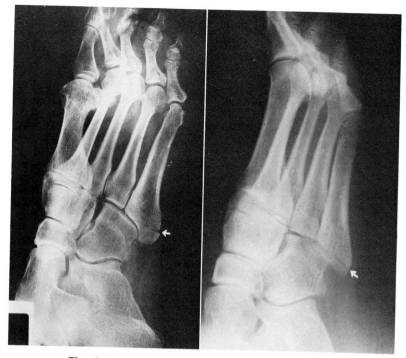

Fig. 6-35. Fractures of tip of fifth metatarsal base.

FRACTURE OF THE METATARSAL BONES

The metatarsals are vulnerable to all types of fractures (Fig. 6-33) due to such causes as the dropping of heavy objects on the foot, muscle pull, and severe twists.

The base of the fifth metatarsal bone is a frequent site of fracture (Figs. 6-34 and 6-35), which can produce complications because the peroneus brevis tendon inserts into it and the peroneus longus tendon is held by it in the cuboid groove. Among children, fracture of the base of the fifth metatarsal bone must be differentiated from fracture of the epiphyseal line. Ordinarily there is no displacement.

The only treatment required in most undisplaced fractures of the base of the metatarsals is to strap the foot by binding the bases and heads of all metatarsals with adhesive tape. Usually, little or no disability results (Fig. 6-37). Sometimes a walking cast is needed for about 6 weeks. In cases of severe avulsion of the broken fragment, open reduction may be required in which

the fragment is pinned through the shaft and maintained while the patient wears a walking cast for 6 weeks.

Fractures of the lateral lesser metatarsal bones resulting from injury are, for the most part, multiple (Figs. 6-36 to 6-38) and usually occur at the neck, the weakest part of the metatarsal bones. Such fractures may be serious when displacement of the heads is extensive. If displacement is plantarward and not reduced, disability may result because of abnormal pressures on weight bearing.

Fractures of the shafts of the metatarsals may require traction. At times, when manipulative reduction fails, it may be necessary to correct the displacement by open reduction and the use of pins or wire to maintain apposition.

Fracture of the first metatarsal bone is rare because of the strength of this bone. When the bone does fracture, displacement is slight (Fig. 6-39); immobilization for 6 weeks suffices. Displacement can be re-

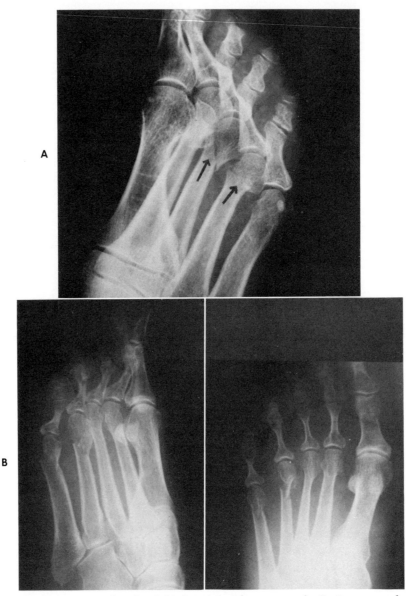

Fig. 6-36. A, Fracture of neck of third and fourth metatarsals. **B,** Fractures of neck of fourth and fifth metatarsals.

duced by closed reduction and, if necessary, maintained by a pin.

FRACTURES OF THE PHALANGES
Fifth proximal phalanx

The most common fracture of the forefoot is that of the fifth proximal phalanx. Stubbing the fifth toe is the usual cause.

Among children the fracture may be at the epiphyseal plate (Fig. 6-40, *A* and *B*); among adults the fracture is likely to be at the base and neck (Fig. 6-40, *C* and *D*).

Phalanges of the middle toes

Fracture of any of the three middle toes is uncommon; when it does occur,

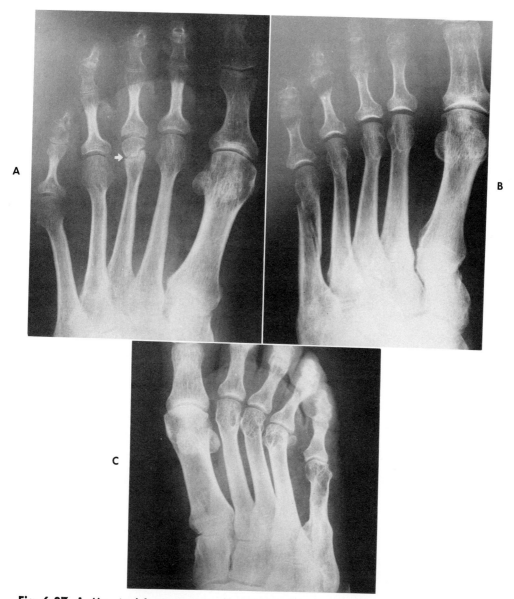

Fig. 6-37. A, Ununited fracture of head of third metatarsal. **B,** Oblique fracture of fifth metatarsal shaft. **C,** Malunited fracture of fifth metatarsal shaft.

it is usually the proximal phalanx, a relatively long bone, that is broken. The middle and distal phalanges are seldom fractured.

Displacement is rare in fracture of the phalanges of the three middle toes; when it does occur, it can be readily reduced, often without an anesthetic.

The adjacent toes may serve as a splint. Adhesive tape, ½ inch wide, is wound around the fractured toe as well as around the two or three adjacent toes so that none can move independently. Strips of adhesive tape wound around the metatarsophalangeal joints will limit motion. Immobilization is maintained for about 4 weeks. Ambula-

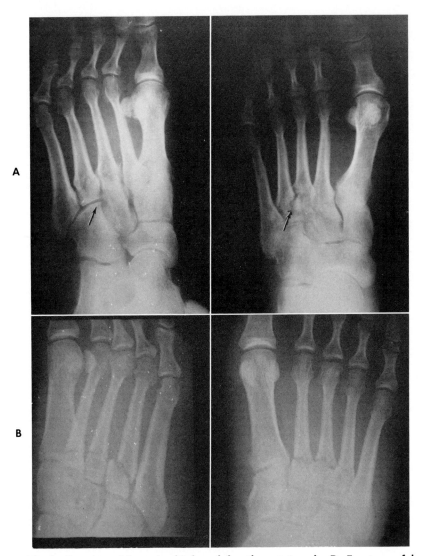

Fig. 6-38. A, Fracture of base in third and fourth metatarsals. **B,** Fracture of base in second, third, and fourth metatarsals treated by immobilization with plaster boot.

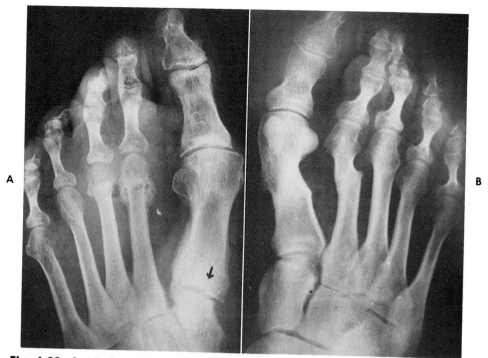

Fig. 6-39. A, Neglected fracture at base of first metatarsal; concomitant fracture of neck of second metatarsal. **B,** Old fracture of first and second metatarsals.

tion is permitted immediately, provided the sole of the shoe is semirigid.

Hallux phalanges

Fractures of the hallux phalanges present a more difficult problem than do fractures of the other phalanges. The hallux phalanges are comparatively large, and their function is as important as that of all the other phalanges put together. The proximal phalanx of the hallux is broken most frequently (Fig. 6-41). However, the distal phalanx may be fractured; when this occurs, the fracture is often comminuted or dislocated (Figs. 6-42 and 6-43). A rare type of injury encountered frequently in the fingers but seldom in the toes is an avulsion fracture of the distal phalanx of the hallux (Fig. 6-44).

If there is no displacement, the hallux should be bound to the two adjacent toes and a walking cast extending beyond the toes should be applied and maintained for 4 weeks. When displacement is present but cannot be reduced by manipulation, open reduction is indicated.

FRACTURES OF THE SESAMOIDS

The tibial sesamoid is more likely to fracture because normally it receives most of the weight transmitted by the first metatarsal. The fracture is usually transverse or comminuted (Fig. 6-45). The condition must always be differentiated from a normal bifurcation: In a true fracture the line of division is jagged and irregular, whereas in bifurcation the outline is regular and the division is smooth. Fracture of the fibular sesamoid is rare (Fig. 6-46).

Direct trauma, injury incurred by jumping from heights or by excessive dancing of any type, may cause the fracture. In rare instances fracture of the sesamoid is spontaneous.

The onset of symptoms is sudden, but the patient may not seek professional help

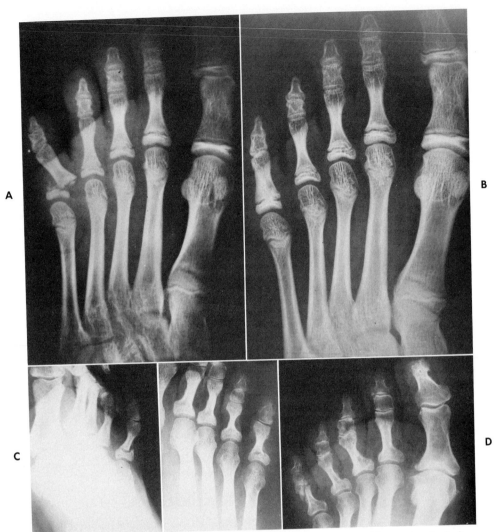

Fig. 6-40. A, Fracture-dislocation at epiphyseal plate at base of fifth proximal phalanx. **B,** Same as **A** after closed reduction and healing. **C,** Fracture at base of fifth proximal phalanx. **D,** Fracture at neck of fifth proximal phalanx. Neglect resulted in nonunion.

for days or weeks after the accident. On palpation of the sesamoid, especially on dorsiflexion of the great toe, pain is sharp. In some cases pain may be mild and gradually become severe. The periarticular structures on the plantar surface of the first metatarsophalangeal joint become swollen.

A recent fracture should be immobilized completely for 3 weeks. In many cases palliative measures fail because of delayed treatment. Surgical removal of the sesamoid is then inevitable.

FATIGUE (MARCH, STRESS) FRACTURES

Fatigue fractures have been recognized by military surgeons for over a century, and the literature about them is voluminous. A critical review of this subject and an exhaustive bibliography may be found in the monograph by Morris and Blickenstaff (1967).

Since 80 percent of all fatigue fractures occur in the bones of the feet, a short discussion of them in this book seems pertinent. The metatarsals are the most fre-

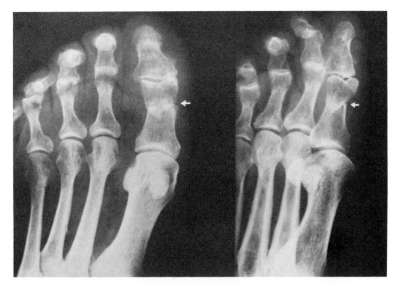

Fig. 6-41. Impacted fracture of proximal phalanx of hallux.

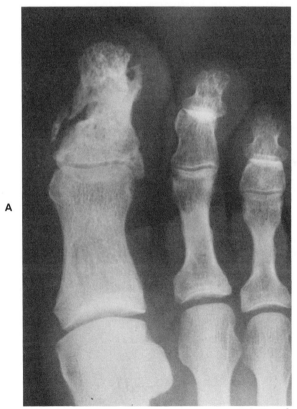

A

Continued.

Fig. 6-42. A, Comminuted fracture of distal phalanx of great toe. Amputation was necessary because of nonhealing of the fragmentation. **B,** Dislocation of hallux interphalangeal joint with chip fracture of head of proximal phalanx. **C,** Same as **B,** after closed reduction. Arthritis may develop in this joint, requiring arthrodesis.

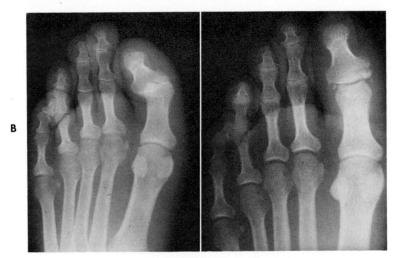

Fig. 6-42, cont'd. For legend see p. 153.

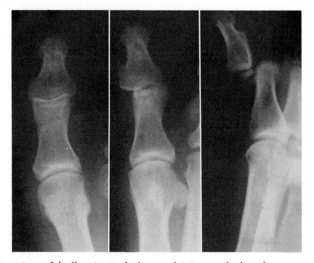

Fig. 6-43. Dislocation of hallux interphalangeal joint and chip fracture of head of the proximal phalanx. It was reduced by closed reduction.

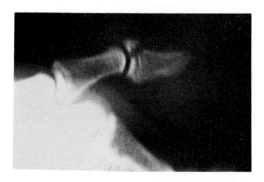

Fig. 6-44. Avulsion fracture of distal phalanx of hallux in young man. He stubbed his toe while he was walking barefoot along a city street.

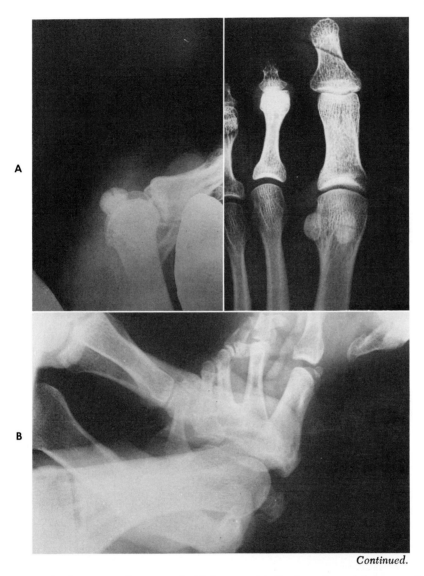

Continued.

Fig. 6-45. A, Transverse fracture of tibial sesamoid. **B,** Comminuted fracture of tibial sesamoid. **C,** Fracture of proximal portion of tibial sesamoid.

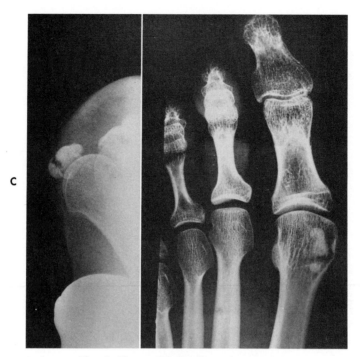

C

Fig. 6-45, cont'd. For legend see p. 155.

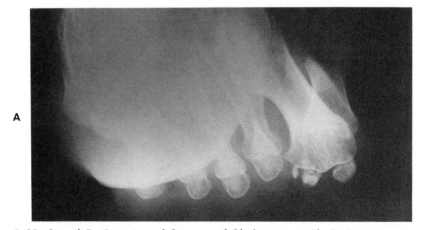

A

Fig. 6-46. A and **B,** Comminuted fracture of fibular sesamoid. **C,** Roentgenograms of feet of 20-year-old woman. She had pain in the left great toe joint for about a year. Routine roentgenograms did not give a definite explanation of pain. **D,** Tangential view showing old fractured fibular sesamoid. Excision of the ossicle gave complete relief.

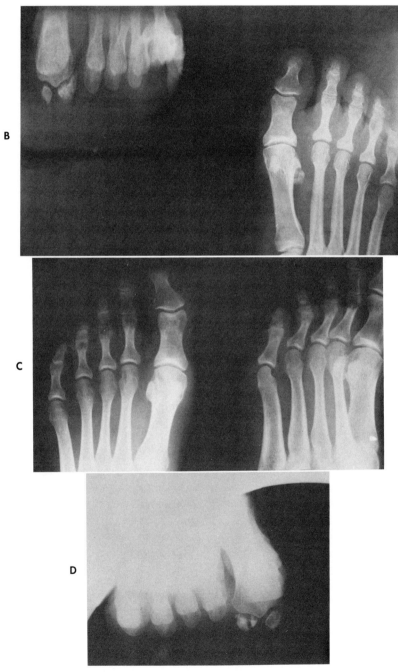

Fig. 6-46, cont'd. For legend see opposite page.

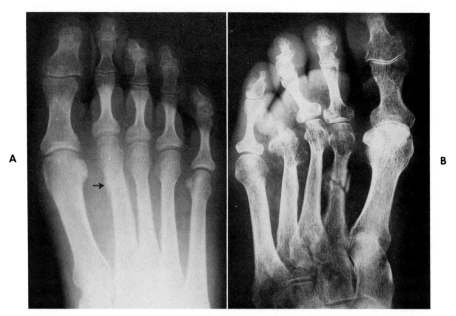

A

B

Fig. 6-47. A, Fatigue fracture at neck of second metatarsal. **B,** Fatigue fracture, comminuted with extensive formation of callus and coincidental aseptic necrosis of fourth digit.

quently involved bones and account for more than 50 percent of all fatigue fractures. Of these, fractures of the second metatarsal occur most frequently (Fig. 6-47), followed by fractures of the third (Fig. 6-48, *A*) and then the fourth metatarsal (Fig. 6-48, *B*). The first metatarsal and the fifth metatarsal (Fig. 6-48, *C*) are rarely affected. The only other bone of the foot about which there are reports of fatigue fractures is the calcaneus (Fig. 6-49). Fracture of this bone occurs only half as frequently as fracture of the metatarsals.

The patient's history often provides diagnostic evidence of this condition. Fatigue fractures occur in people who subject the bones of their feet to prolonged, continued, cyclical stresses (e.g., athletes, joggers, and military personnel). History of specific trauma is lacking; insidious onset of pain is usual. Rest relieves the acute pain, but a residual dull ache may occasionally persist. Activity increases the pain.

Examination reveals sharply localized tenderness that is restricted to the bone;

there is no pain in the ligamentous structures. Swelling and increased local heat may occur over the site of fracture.

Roentgenograms obtained shortly after the onset of symptoms may appear normal. A lapse of 2 or 3 weeks may be necessary before endosteal callus or periosteal callus or both are evident.

When a patient with this condition is seen promptly, the treatment is avoidance of those activities that produced the condition; if the symptoms are more acute, rest and immobilization may be required. If the activity that led to the onset of symptoms is continued, complete fracture with or without displacement may ensue. In such a situation, treatment is similar to that of any acute fracture.

DISLOCATIONS
Dislocations of the subtalar joint

A complete dislocation of the talus onto the calcaneus necessarily involves the talonavicular joint. Basically, this uncommon type of injury may be described as a dis-

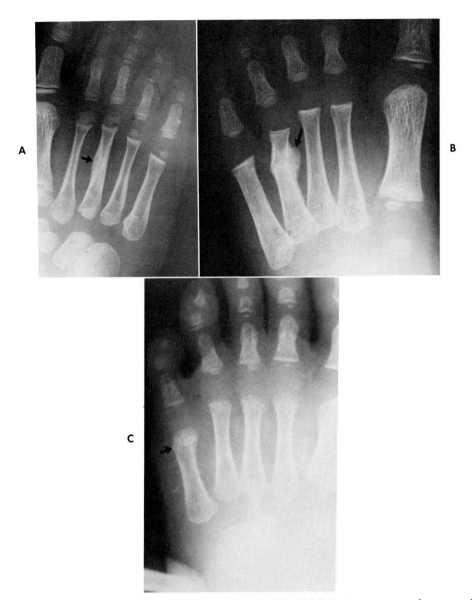

Fig. 6-48. A, Fatigue fracture of third metatarsal in child. **B,** Spontaneous fracture of fourth metatarsal in child. **C,** Spontaneous fracture of neck of fifth metatarsal in infant. (**A,** Courtesy Dr. Jack Stern; **B,** courtesy Dr. Frank Weinstein.)

placement of all the components of the foot from the talus. Leitner (1952) researched the world literature thoroughly and found fewer than 300 reported cases of this type of dislocation. He added fifty-four cases of his own (forty-two were fresh injuries, twelve were old unreduced dislocations) for the review he published. These injuries comprised 1 percent of all of the dislocations that were encountered over a twenty-five year period in his service for the treatment of traumatic injuries. Since Leitner's review, Vogt (1959) has added three cases and Soustelle et al. (1964) have noted one additional case. Since the articles of Leitner (1952, 1954)

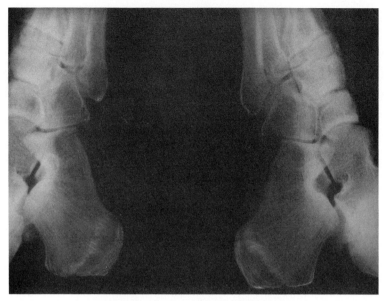

Fig. 6-49. Bilateral fatigue fractures of calcaneus in 22-year-old Army recruit. (Courtesy Dr. David Hunt.)

constitute the most comprehensive studies dealing with this injury, it seems appropriate to summarize them here:

Medial displacements of the foot on the talus occurred six to seven times more frequently than lateral displacements of the foot on the talus. Only one case of posterior displacement was reported. In fresh dislocations closed manipulative reduction was accomplished in 90 percent of cases. In 10 percent of cases open reduction was necessary because of the interposition of soft tissue or the displacement of tendons.

Dislocations of the midtarsal (Chopart's) joint

Dislocations of the midtarsal joints (the talonavicular and calcaneocuboid articulations), unaccompanied by fractures, appear to be rare. Standard textbooks dealing with injuries to the skeletal system give them only passing mention (Watson-Jones, 1955; Böhler, 1958; Conwell and Reynolds, 1961). Individual dislocations of the navicular or the cuboid occur more frequently, but the literature on these dislocations is also sparse. Reports of a few cases have

been published intermittently and student theses have appeared in the French and German literature (Boidard, 1939; Gilland, 1936; Weh, 1939; and Willigens, 1936). Dewar and Evans (1968) reported several cases of subluxed cuboid that were first diagnosed as sprains. They intimated that reduction was accomplished easily enough in those cases that were seen promptly; however, in those that were not, open reduction and internal fixation or limited arthrodesis was necessary.

Dislocations of the cuboid

Drummond and Hastings (1969) reported one case of medial and inferior dislocation of the cuboid that was initially overlooked. They stated that no similar case could be found in the literature. The dislocation, treated by open reduction, was fixed by means of two cross wires, one to the calcaneus and one to the lateral cuneiform.

Dislocations of the tarsometatarsal (Lisfranc's) joint

Dislocations of the tarsometatarsal joint, with or without accompanying fractures be-

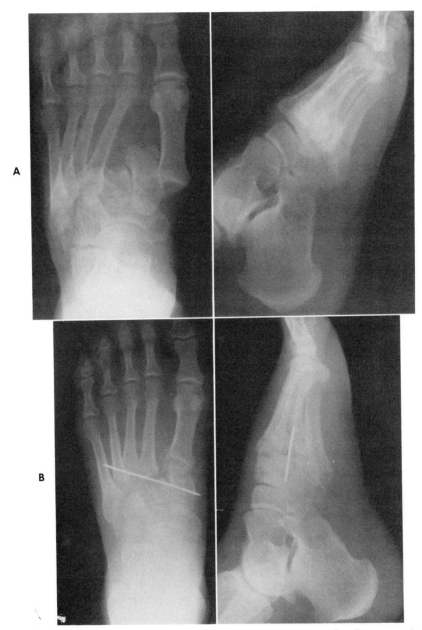

Fig. 6-50. A, Tarsometatarsal fracture-dislocation. **B,** After closed reduction and internal fixation with Kirschner wires.

tween the tarsus and the metatarsus, constitute a special category of injuries to the foot (Fig. 6-50). Although these dislocations exhibit a wide range of individual variation, they share a similar general pattern and have many elements in common. They occur as a result of abrupt force applied to the forefoot, usually in falls from great heights or in automobile accidents. They have also been described as typical injuries sustained by motorcyclists (Detlefsen, 1968). These dislocations can be serious, since the disruption may be complicated by arterial injury, which results in the interruption of the blood supply to the distal portions of the foot. Gissane (1951) reported three cases, and Groulier and Pinaud (1970) reported four others that required amputation. Fortunately, this injury occurs relatively infrequently, but prompt diagnosis and reduction are essential.

Since the monumental study of Quénu and Küss (1909) of thirty-two dislocations of the tarsometatarsal joint, reports of small series of cases or single cases have appeared sporadically in the literature. Schiller and Ray (1970) reported a case of an unusual dislocation of the medial cuneiform bone, which could have been overlooked because of its deceptive roentgenographic appearance. The only comprehensive studies of these injuries, which include case reports, descriptions of the mechanisms of injury, classification of the types of injury, descriptions of treatment, and the evaluation of results are those of Aitken and Poulson (1963), Taussig et al. (1969), Cherkes-Zade (1969), and Perriard et al. (1970). Groulier and Pinaud (1970) reviewed 120 cases in the literature, added ten of their own, and included an exhaustive bibliography in their article on this subject.

The importance of prompt realignment of the joints and reduction of fractures is emphasized in all of these articles. If manipulation is carried out immediately, reduction may be accomplished easily; thereafter, only immobilization in plaster casts is necessary. Arenberg (1969) reported a case in which an excellent reduction was achieved by manipulation within 50 minutes after the initial injury occurred.

Often dislocations or fracture-dislocations or both are unstable; in these cases, several methods have been described to maintain alignment. Fitte and Garacotche (1940) employed traction with pins through the calcaneus and metatarsals. Collett et al. (1958) used toe traction and attached the toes to an outrigger type of appliance to maintain alignment. The majority of authors, however, report the need for open reduction and internal fixation. Huet and Lecoeur (1946) and Ballerio (1953) described the role of the peroneus longus tendon in preventing successful treatment of these injuries by closed reduction and advocated treatment by open reduction. Geckeler (1949), del Sel (1955), Collett et al. (1958), Tondeur (1961), Taussig et al. (1969), and Groulier and Pinaud (1970) all advise open reduction, accurate alignment, and internal fixation with pins or staples.

Dislocations of the metatarsophalangeal joints and the phalanges

Although dislocations of these joints (chronic, progressive, or sometimes both) are common deformities of the forefoot, acute traumatic dislocations are rare. The majority of these chronic dislocations occur between the proximal phalanges and the metatarsals. Dislocation of the first metatarsophalangeal articulation (frequently compound) is the most common dislocation in this area. The usual deformity is one in which the phalanx is displaced onto the dorsum of the metatarsal. The diagnosis is readily made and manipulation will usually reduce the dislocation.

Traction, a usual adjunct in the manipulative reduction of most dislocations, frequently fails to accomplish reduction in dislocations of the metatarsophalangeal articulations because of the peculiar arrangements of the connective-tissue structures in the vicinity of these joints. The inferior capsule may be torn and lie against the metatarsal head, or the capsule may be torn and be displaced around the metatarsal head like a buttonhole, or the flexor tendons may be displaced around the neck of the metatarsal. In these situations traction only tightens the soft tissues around the metatarsal, thus preventing reduction. To achieve reduction, the phalanx should be hyperextended and angled plantarward so that the inferior edge of the articular surface contacts the superior aspect of the articular surface of the metatarsal head. Pressure (not traction) is applied, which keeps the edge of the articular surface of the phalanx against the articular surface of the metatarsal. As the phalanx is replaced, its inferior edge will wipe any soft tissue from the head of the metatarsal.

These dislocations are usually stable and require only minimal external fixation with strapping.

REFERENCES
Effects of immobilization

Akeson, W. H.: An experimental study of joint stiffness, J. Bone Joint Surg. 43-A:1022-1034, Oct. 1961.

Clark, D. D., and Weckesser, E. C.: The influence of triamcinolone acetonide on joint stiffness in the rat, J. Bone Joint Surg. 53-A:1409-1414, Oct. 1971.

Collins, D. H., and McElligott, T. F.: Sulphate ($^{35}SO_4$) uptake by chondrocytes in relation to histological changes in osteoarthritic human articular cartilage, Ann. Rheum. Dis. 19:318-330, 1960.

Davenport, H. K., and Ranson, S. W.: Contracture resulting from tenotomy, Arch. Surg. 21:995-1014, Nov. 1930.

Dziewiatkowski, D. D., Benesch, R. E., and Benesch, R.: On the possible utilization of sulfate sulfur by the suckling rat for the synthesis of chondroitin sulfate as indicated by the use of radioactive sulfur, J. Biol. Chem. 178:931-938, Mar. 1949.

Ely, L. W., and Mensor, M. C.: Studies on the immobilization of the normal joints, Surg. Gynec. Obstet. 57:212-215, Aug. 1933.

Evans, E. B., Eggers, G. W. N., Butler, J. K., and Blumel, J.: Experimental immobilization and remobilization of rat knee joints, J. Bone Joint Surg. 42-A:737-758, July 1960.

Frankshteyn, S. I.: Experimental studies on mechanism of development of contractures due to immobilization in casts, Khirurgiia 8:44-47, 1944.

Frugone, J. E., Thomsen, P., and Luco, J. V.: Changes in weight of muscles of arthritic and immobilized arthritic joints, Proc. Soc. Exper. Biol. Med. 61:31-41, Jan. 1946.

Gasser, H. S.: Contractures of skeletal muscle, Physiol. Rev. 10:35-109, 1930.

Hall, M. C.: Cartilage changes after experimental immobilization of the knee joint of the young rat, J. Bone Joint Surg. 45-A:36-44, Jan. 1963.

Harrison, M. H. M., Schajowicz, F., and Trueta, J.: Osteoarthritis of the hip: A study of the nature and evolution of the disease, J. Bone Joint Surg. 35-B:598-626, Nov. 1953.

Lucas-Championnière, J.: Précis du traitement des fractures par le massage et la mobilisation, Paris, 1910, G. Steinheil.

McLean, F. C., and Urist, M. R.: Bone: An introduction to the physiology of skeletal tissue, Chicago, 1955, University of Chicago Press.

Menzel, A.: Ueber die Erkrankung der Gelenke bei dauernder Ruhe derselben: Eine experimentelle Studie, Arch. klin. Chir. 12:990-1009, 1871.

Müller, W.: Experimentelle Untersuchungen über die Wirkung langdauernder Immobilisierung auf die Gelenke, Z. Orthop. Chir. 44:478-488, 1924.

Peacock, E. E., Jr.: Some biochemical and biophysical aspects of joint stiffness: Role of collagen synthesis as opposed to altered molecular bonding, Ann. Surg. 164:1-12, July 1966.

Ranson, S. W., and Sams, C. F.: A study of muscle in contracture: The permanent shortening of muscles caused by tenotomy and tetanus toxin, J. Neurol. Psychopath. 8:304-320, 1923.

Salter, R. B., and Field, P.: The effects of continuous compression on living articular cartilage: An experimental investigation, J. Bone Joint Surg. 42-A:31-49, Jan. 1960.

Scaglietti, O., and Casuccio, C.: Studio sperimentale degli effetti della immobilizzazione su articolazioni normali, Chir. Organi Mov. 20:469-488, Feb. 1936.

Sokoloff, L., and Jay, G. E., Jr.: Natural history of degenerative joint disease in small laboratory animals. 4. Degenerative joint disease in the laboratory rat, Arch. Pathol. 62:140-142, July-Dec. 1956.

Solandt, D. Y., and Magladery, J. W.: A comparison of effects of upper and lower motor neurone lesions on skeletal muscle, J. Neurophysiol. 5:373-380, 1942.

Thaxter, T. H., Mann, R. A., and Anderson, C. E.: Degeneration of immobilized knee joints in rats: Histological and autoradiographic study, J. Bone Joint Surg. 47-A:567-585, 1965.

Trias, A.: Effect of persistent pressure on the articular cartilage, J. Bone Joint Surg. 43-B:376-386, May 1961.

Thomsen, P., and Luco, J. V.: Changes of weight and neuromuscular transmission in muscles of immobilized joints, J. Neurophysiol. 7:245-251, July 1944.

Tschmarke, G.: Experimentelle Untersuchungen über die Rolle des Muskeltonus in der Gelenkchirurgie 3. Mitteilung: Fixationskontrakturen und die Beeinflussung ihrer Entwicklung, Arch. klin. Chir. 164:785-797, 1931.

Fractures of the ankle joint

Ashhurst, A. P. C., and Bromer, R. S.: Classification and mechanism of fractures of the leg bones involving the ankle. Based on a study of three hundred cases from the Episcopal Hospital, Arch. Surg. 4:51-129, Jan. 1922.

Aufranc, O. E.: Trimalleolar fracture dislocation, J.A.M.A. 174:2221-2223, Dec. 1960.

Bonnin, J. G.: Injuries to the Ankle, ed. 1, New York, 1950, Grune and Stratton.

Bosworth, D. M.: Fracture-dislocation of the ankle with fixed displacement of the fibula behind the tibia, J. Bone Joint Surg. 29:130-135, Jan. 1947.

Burwell, H. N., and Charnley, A. D.: The treatment of displaced fractures at the ankle by rigid internal fixation and early joint movement, J. Bone Joint Surg. 47-B:634-660, Nov. 1965.

Childress, H. M.: Vertical transarticular-pin fixation for unstable ankle fractures, J. Bone Joint Surg. 47-A:1323-1334, Oct. 1965.

Coonrad, R. W., and Bugg, E. I.: Trapping of the posterior tibial tendon and interposition of soft tissue in severe fractures about the ankle joint, J. Bone Joint Surg. 36-A:744-750, July 1954.

Dieterle, J.: The use of Kirschner wire in maintaining reduction of fracture-dislocations of the ankle joint: A report of two cases, J. Bone Joint Surg. 17:990-995, Oct. 1935.

Fleming, J. L., and Smith, H. O.: Fracture-dislocation of the ankle with the fibula fixed behind the tibia, J. Bone Joint Surg. 36-A:556-558, June 1954.

Glick, B. W.: The ankle fracture with inferior tibiofibular joint disruption, Surg. Gynec. Obstet. 118:549-554, March 1964.

Jergesen, F.: Open reduction of fractures and dislocations of the ankle, Amer. J. Surg. 98:136-150, Aug. 1959.

Kleiger, B.: The mechanism of ankle injuries, J. Bone Joint Surg. 38-A:59-70, Jan. 1956.

Lauge-Hansen, N.: Fractures of the ankle: Analytic historic survey as the basis of new experimental, roentgenologic and clinical investigations, Arch. Surg. 56:259-317, Mar. 1948.

Lauge-Hansen, N.: Fractures of the ankle. II. Combined experimental-surgical and experimental-roentgenologic investigations, Arch. Surg. 60:957-985, 1950.

Lauge-Hansen, N.: Fractures of the ankle. IV. Clinical use of genetic roentgen diagnosis and genetic reduction, Arch. Surg. 64:488-500, Apr. 1952.

Lauge-Hansen, N.: Fractures of the ankle. III. Genetic roentgenologic diagnosis of fracture of the ankle, Amer. J. Roentgen. Radium Ther. Nucl. Med. 71:456-471, Mar. 1954.

Mayer, V., and Pohlidal, S.: Ankle mortise injuries, Surg. Gynec. Obstet. 96:99-101, Jan. 1953.

Meyers, M. H.: Fracture about the ankle joint with fixed displacement of the proximal fragment of the fibula behind the tibia, J. Bone Joint Surg. 39-A:441-444, Apr. 1957.

Portis, R. B., and Mendelsohn, H. A.: Conservative management of fractures of the ankle involving the medial malleolus, J.A.M.A. 151:102-105, Jan. 1953.

Zuelzer, W. A.: Use of hookplate for fixation of ununited medial tibial malleolus, J.A.M.A. 167:828-831, June 1958.

Fractures of the talus

Anderson, H. G.: The medical and surgical aspects of aviation, London, 1919, Hodder and Co.

Boyd, H. B., and Knight, R. A.: Fractures of the astragalus, South. Med. J. 35:160-167, Feb. 1942.

Coltart, W. D.: Aviator's astragalus, J. Bone Joint Surg. 34-B:545-566, Nov. 1952.

Davidson, A. M., Steele, H. D., MacKenzie, D. A., and Penny, J. A.: A review of twenty-one cases of transchondral fracture of the talus, J. Trauma 7:378-415, May 1967.

Dunn, A. R., Jacobs, B., and Campbell, R. D.: Fractures of the talus, J. Trauma 6:443-467, 1966.

Haliburton, R. A., Sullivan, C. R., Kelly, P. J., and Peterson, L. F. A.: The extra-osseous and intra-osseus blood supply of the talus, J. Bone Joint Surg. 40-A:1115-1120, Oct. 1958.

Hawkins, L. H.: Fractures of the neck of the talus, J. Bone Joint Surg. 52-A:991-1002, July 1970.

Kelly, P. J., and Sullivan, C. R.: Blood supply of the talus, Clin. Orthop. 30:37-43, 1964.

Kenwright, J., and Taylor, R. M. A.: Major injuries of the talus, J. Bone Joint Surg. 52-B:36-48, Feb. 1970.

McKeever, F. M.: Treatment of complications of fractures and dislocations of the talus, Clin. Orthop. 30:45-52, 1963.

Mindell, E. R., Cisek, E. E., Kartalian, G., and Dziob, J. M.: Late results of injuries to the talus: Analysis of forty cases, J. Bone Joint Surg. 45-A:221-245, Mar. 1963.

Mulfinger, G. L., and Trueta, J.: The blood supply of the talus, J. Bone Joint Surg. 52B:160-167, 1970.

Pennal, G. F.: Fractures of the talus, Clin. Orthop. 30:53-63, 1963.

Ray, A.: Fractures de l'astragale (à propos de 34

observations), Rev. Chir. Orthop. **53**:279-294, Apr.-May 1967.

Sneed, W. L.: The astragalus: A case of dislocation, excision and replacement. An attempt to demonstrate the circulation in this bone, J. Bone Joint Surg. **7**:384-399, Apr. 1925.

Taylor, R. G.: Immobilization of unstable fracture dislocations by the use of Kirschner wires, Proc. Roy. Soc. Med. **55**:499-501, June 1962.

Watson-Jones, R.: Fractures and joint injuries, ed. 4, vol. 2, Baltimore, 1955, The Williams & Wilkins Co.

Wildenauer, E. Die Blutversorgung des Talus, Z. Anat. Entwicklungsgesch. **115**:32-36, 1950.

Fractures of the calcaneus

Barnard, L., and Odegard, J. K.: Conservative approach in the treatment of fractures of the calcaneus, J. Bone Joint Surg. **52-A**:1689, Dec. 1970.

Bertelsen, A., and Hasner, E.: Primary results of treatment of fracture of the os calcis by "foot-free walking bandage" and early movement, Acta Orthop. Scand. **21**:140-154, 1951.

Böhler, L.: The Treatment of Fractures. ed. 5, vol. 3, New York, 1957, Grune & Stratton, pp. 2045-2114.

Brattström, H.: Primär arthrodes vid gray calcaneusfraktur, Nord. Med. **50**:1510-1511, 1953.

Carothers, R. G., and Lyons, J. F.: Early mobilization in treatment of os calcis fractures, Amer. J. Surg. **83**:279-280, Mar. 1952.

Cotton, F. J., and Henderson, F. F.: Results of fracture of the os calcis, Amer. J. Orthop. Surg. **14**:290-298, 1916.

Cotton, F. J., and Wilson, L. T.: Fractures of the os calcis, Boston Med. Surg. J. **159**:559-565, July-Dec. 1908.

Dautry, P.: Sur le traitement des fractures du calcanéum, Acad. Chir. Mém. **87**:249-256, Mar. 1961.

Dragonetti, L.: A proposito del trattamento incruento delle fratture di calcagno, Arch. Ortop. **82**:381-394, 1969.

Essex-Lopresti, P.: The mechanism, reduction technique, and results in fractures of the os calcis, Brit. J. Surg. **39**:395-419, Mar. 1952.

Gallie, W. E.: Subastragalar arthrodesis in fractures of the os calcis, J. Bone Joint Surg. **25**: 731-736, Oct. 1943.

Gellman, M.: Fractures of the anterior process of the calcaneus, J. Bone Joint Surg. **33-A**:382-386, Apr. 1951.

Goff, C. W.: Fresh fracture of the os calcis, Arch. Surg. **36**:744-765, May 1938.

Gossett, J.: In Nosny, P., and others, editors: Mobilisation précoce après réduction et contention par broches des fractures du tarse postérieur, Acad. Chir. Mém. **95**:370, Apr. 1969.

Hall, M. C., and Pennal, G. F.: Primary subtalar arthrodesis in the treatment of severe fractures of the calcaneum, J. Bone Joint Surg. **42-B**:336-343, May 1960.

Harris, R. I.: Fractures of the os calcis: Treatment by early subtalar arthrodesis, Clin. Orthop. **30**: 100-110, 1963.

Hazlett, J. W.: Open reduction of fractures of the calcaneum, Canad. J. Surg. **12**:310-317, July 1969.

Hunt, D. D.: Compression fracture of the anterior articular surface of the calcaneus, J. Bone Joint Surg. **52-A**:1637-1642, Dec. 1970.

Kiaer, Sv., and Anthonsen, W.: Fracture of the calcaneus treated with arthrodesis, Acta Chir. Scand. **87** (Suppl. 76):191-213, 1942.

Lance, E. M., Carey, E. J., and Wade, P. A.: Fractures of the os calcis: Treatment by early mobilization, Clin. Orthop. **30**:76-90, 1963.

Leriche, R.: Ostéosynthèse primitive pour fracture par écrasement du calcanéum à sept fragments, Lyon Chir. **19**:559-560, 1922.

Maxfield, J. E.: Treatment of calcaneal fractures by open reduction, J. Bone Joint Surg. **45-A**: 868-871, June 1963.

Maxfield, J. E. and McDermott, F. J.: Experiences with the Palmer open reduction of fractures of the calcaneus, J. Bone Joint Surg. **37-A**: 99-106, Jan. 1955.

Moberg, E., and Erfors, C.-G.: Primär terapi vid grava intraartikulära Kalcaneusfrakturer, Nord. Med. **49**:150, 1953.

Mooney, V.: Avulsion of the epiphysis of the os calcis, J. Bone Joint Surg. **17**:1056-1057, Oct. 1935.

Morretti, O., and Piovani, C.: Trattamento ed esiti in 90 osservazioni di fratture del calcagno, Chir. Organi Mov. **56**:441-453, 1967.

Nosny, P., Bourrel, P., and Caron, J.-J.: Mobilisation précoce après réduction et contention par broches des fractures du tarse postérieur, Acad. Chir. Mém. **95**:365-370, Apr. 1969.

Palmer, I.: The mechanism and treatment of fractures of the calcaneus. Open reduction with the use of cancellous grafts, J. Bone Joint Surg. **30-A**:2-8, Jan. 1948.

Piatt, A. D.: Fracture of the promontory of the calcaneus, Radiology **67**:386-390, Sept. 1956.

Rothberg, A. S.: Avulsion fracture of the os calcis, J. Bone Joint Surg. **21**:218-220, Jan. 1939.

Rowe, C. R., Sakellarides, H. T., Freeman, P. A., and Sorbie, C.: Fractures of the os calcis: A long-term follow-up study of 146 patients, J.A.M.A. **184**:920-923, June 1963.

Thompson, K. R., and Friesen, C. M.: Treatment of comminuted fractures of the calcaneus by primary triple arthrodesis, J. Bone Joint Surg. **41-A**:1423-1436, Dec. 1959.

Vestad, E.: Fractures of the calcaneum: Open reduction and bone grafting, Acta Chir. Scand. **134**:617-625, 1968.

Warrick, C. K., and Bremner, A. E.: Fractures of the calcaneum: With an atlas illustrating the various types of fracture, J. Bone Joint Surg. 35-B:33-45, Feb. 1953.

Widén, A.: Fractures of the calcaneus: A clinical study with special reference to the technique and results of open reduction, Acta Chir. Scand. (Suppl. 108), 1954.

Wilson, P. D.: Treatment of fractures of the os calcis by arthrodesis of the subastragalar joint, J.A.M.A. 89:1676-1683, Nov. 1927.

Zagra, A., and Bellistri, D.: L'artrodesi sottoastragalica immediata nelle fratture talamiche del calcagno, Minerva Ortop. 21:574-577, 1970.

Fractures of the cuboid

Böhler, L.: The treatment of fractures, ed 5, vol. 3, New York, 1958, Grune & Stratton.

Conwell, H. E., and Reynolds, F. C.: Key and Conwell's management of fractures, dislocations, and sprains, ed. 7, St. Louis, 1961, The C. V. Mosby Co.

Hermel, M. B., and Gershon-Cohen, J.: The nutcracker fracture of the cuboid by indirect violence, Radiology 60:850-854, June 1953.

Jackson, W. S. T., and Dickson, D. D.: Fractures and dislocations: In Du Vries, H. L.: Surgery of the foot, ed. 2, St. Louis, 1965, The C. V. Mosby Co., p. 347.

Wilson, P. D.: Fractures and dislocations of the tarsal bones, South. Med. J. 26:833-845, Oct. 1933.

Fractures of the navicular

Böhler, L.: The treatment of fractures, ed. 5, vol. 3, New York, 1958, Grune & Stratton.

Conwell, H. E., and Reynolds, F. C.: Key and Conwell's management of fractures, dislocations and sprains, ed. 7, St. Louis, 1961, The C. V. Mosby Co., pp. 1110-1113.

Crossan, E. T.: Fractures of the tarsal scaphoid and of the os calcis, Surg. Clin. N. Amer. 10: 1477-1487, 1930.

Day, A. J.: The treatment of injuries to the tarsal navicular, J. Bone Joint Surg. 29:359-366, Apr. 1947.

De Palma, A. F.: The management of fractures and dislocations: An atlas, Philadelphia, 1959, W. B. Saunders Co., pp. 937-941.

Dick, I. L.: Impacted fracture-dislocation of the tarsal navicular, Proc. Roy. Soc. Med. 35:760, Oct. 1942.

Eftekhar, N. M., Lyddon, D. W., and Stevens, J.: An unusual fracture-dislocation of the tarsal navicular, J. Bone Joint Surg. 51-A:577-581, Apr. 1969.

Eichenholtz, S. N., and Levine, D. B.: Fractures of the tarsal navicular bone, Clin. Orthop. 34: 142-157, May-June 1964.

Finsterer, H.: Ueber Verletzungen im Bereiche der Fusswurzelknochen mit besonderer Berücksichtigung des Os naviculare, Beitr. klin. Chir. 59:99-173, 1908.

Heck, C. V.: Fractures of the bones of the foot (except the talus), Surg. Clin. N. Amer. 45: 103-117, Feb. 1965.

Henderson, M. S.: Fractures of the bones of the foot—except the os calcis, Surg. Gynec. Obstet. 64:454-457, 1937.

Hoffman, A.: Ueber die isolierte Fraktur des Os naviculare tarsi, Beitr. klin. Chir. 59:217-228, 1908.

Joplin, R. J.: Injuries of the foot. In Cave, E. F., editor: Fractures and other injuries, Chicago, 1958, Year Book Publishers, Inc., pp. 604-625.

Lehman, E. P., and Eskeles, I. H.: Fractures of tarsal scaphoid: With notes on the mechanism, J. Bone Joint Surg. 10:108-113, Jan. 1928.

Morrison, G. M.: Fractures of the bones of the feet, Amer. J. Surg. 38:721-726, 1937.

Penhallow, D. P.: An unusual fracture-dislocation of the tarsal scaphoid with dislocation of the cuboid, J. Bone Joint Surg., 19:517-519, Apr. 1937.

Perriard, M., Dieterlé, J., and Jeannet, E.: Les lésions traumatiques récentes comprises entre les articulations de Chopart et de Lisfranc, incluses, A. Unfallmed. Berufskr. 63:318-328, 1970.

Speed, K.: A text-book of fractures and dislocations covering their pathology, diagnosis and treatment, ed. 4, Philadelphia, 1942, Lea & Febiger, pp. 1026-1030.

Waters, C. H., Jr.: Midtarsal fractures and dislocations. In American Academy of Orthopaedic Surgeons: Instructional Course Lectures, vol. 9, Ann Arbor, 1952, J. W. Edwards.

Watson-Jones, R.: Fractures and joint injuries, ed. 4, vol 2, Baltimore, 1955, The Williams & Wilkins Co.

Wilson, P. D.: Fractures and dislocations of the tarsal bones, South. Med. J. 26:833-845, Oct. 1933.

Fatigue fractures

Morris, J. M., and Blickenstaff, L. D.: Fatigue fractures: A clinical study, Springfield, Ill., 1967, Charles C Thomas, Publisher.

Dislocations of the subtalar joint

Leitner, B.: Behandlung und Behandlungsergebnisse von 42 frischen Fällen von Luxatio pedis sub talo im Unfallkrankenhaus Wien in den Jahren 1925-1950, Ergeb. chir. Orthop. 37:501-577, 1952.

Leitner, B.: Obstacles to reduction in subtalar dislocations, J. Bone Joint Surg. 36-A:299-306, Apr. 1954.

Soustelle, J., Meyer, P., and Sauvage, Y.: Luxation sous-astragalienne fermée, Lyon Chir. **60:** 119-120, Jan. 1964.

Vogt, Von H.: Drei seltene Verrenkungsformen im Talusbereich, Schweiz. Med. Wochenschr. **89:** 1005-1008, Sept. 1959.

Dislocations of the midtarsal (Chopart's) joint

Böhler, L.: The treatment of fractures, ed. 5, vol. 3, New York, 1958, Grune & Stratton.

Boidard, C. A. L.: Contribution à l'étude des luxations astragalo-scaphoidiennes. Thesis, Bordeaux, 1939.

Conwell, H. E., and Reynolds, F. C.: Key and Conwell's management of fractures, dislocations, and sprains. ed. 7, St. Louis, 1961, The C. V. Mosby Co.

Dewar, F. P., and Evans, D. C.: Occult fracture-subluxation of the midtarsal joint, J. Bone Joint Surg. **50-B:**386-388, May 1968.

Gilland, F. A. E.: Les luxations isolées du scaphoide tarsien. Thesis, Nancy, 1936.

Watson-Jones, R.: Fractures and joint injuries, ed. 4, vol. 2, Baltimore, 1955, The Williams & Wilkins Co.

Weh, R.: Ueber die isolierte Luxation im Talonaviculargelenk. Thesis, Munchen, 1939.

Willigens, J. E. F.: Contribution à l'étude de la luxation du scaphoide tarsien. Thesis, Nancy, 1936.

Dislocations of the cuboid

Drummond, D. S., and Hastings, D. E.: Total dislocation of the cuboid bone: Report of a case, J. Bone Joint Surg. **51-B:**716-718, Nov. 1969.

Dislocations of the tarsometatarsal (Lisfranc's) joint

Aitken, A. P., and Poulson, D.: Dislocations of the tarsometatarsal joint, J. Bone Joint Surg. **45-A:**246-260, Mar. 1963.

Arenberg, A. A.: Vyvikhi v sustave lisfranka [Dislocation of Lisfranc's joint], Vestn. Khir. **102:** 126-127, June 1969.

Ballerio, A.: Un caso raro di lussazione tarso metatarsale isolata, Chir. Organi Mov. **38:**286-288, 1953.

Cherkes-Zade, D. I.: Pepelomy-vyvikhi v sustave lisfranka [Fracture-dislocation of Lisfranc's joint], Vestn. Khir. **103:**102-108, Dec. 1969.

Collett, H. S., Hood, T. K., and Andrews, R. E.: Tarsometatarsal fracture dislocations, Surg. Gynec. Obstet. **106:**623-626, May 1958.

del Sel, J. M.: The surgical treatment of tarsometatarsal fracture-dislocations, J. Bone Joint Surg. **37-B:**203-207, May 1955.

Detlefsen, M.: Die Luxation im Lisfrancschen Gelenk als typische Verletzung des Motorradfahrers, Beitr. Orthop. Traumatol. **15:**242-246, Apr. 1968.

Fitte, M., and Garacotche, I.: Luxation-fracture de l'articulation de Lisfranc, J. Chir. (Paris) **56:**367, 1940.

Geckeler, E. O.: Dislocations and fracture-dislocations of the foot: Transfixion with Kirschner wires, Surgery **25:**730-733, Jan.-June 1949.

Gissane, W.: A dangerous type of fracture of the foot, J. Bone Joint Surg. **33-B:**535-538, Nov. 1951.

Groulier, P., and Pinaud, J.-C.: Les luxations tarsométatarsiennes (A propos de dix observations), Rev. Chir. Orthop. **56:**303-324, 1970.

Huet, P., and Lecoeur, P.: Sur 4 cas de luxation tarso-métatarsienne, Acad. Chir. Mém. **72:**124-219, Mar. 1946.

Perriard, M., Deterlé, J., and Jeannet, E.: Les lésions traumatiques récentes comprises entre les articulations de Chopart et de Lisfranc, incluses, Z. Unfallmed. Berufskr. **63:**318-328, 1970.

Quénu, E., and Küss, G.: Etude sur les luxations du métatarse, Rev. Chir. **39:**1-72; 281-336; 1093-1134, Jan.-June 1909.

Taussig, G., Hautier, S., and Maschas, A.: Les fractures-luxations de l'articulation de Lisfranc, Ann. Chir. **23:**1131-1141, Oct. 1969.

Schiller, M. G., and Ray, R. D.: Isolated dislocation of the medial cuneiform bone—a rare injury of the tarsus, J. Bone Joint Surg. **52-A:** 1632-1636, Dec. 1970.

Tondeur, G.: Un cas luxation-fracture tarsométatarsienne, Acta Orthop. Belg. **27:**286-290, 1961.

7

Traumatic injuries to the soft tissues of the foot and ankle

James M. Glick

Burns, freezing, and foreign bodies

A comprehensive discussion of burns and freezing is not within the scope of this text; however, because of the high incidence of frostbite of the foot and because burns of the foot from irradiation are not uncommon, at least brief recognition of these injuries is in order.

BURNS

Burns are caused by exposure to intense heat, by contact with strong chemicals or live electricity, or by overexposure to roentgen rays or radium. Burns on the soles of the feet can occur from walking on hot objects without wearing shoes, but today this causation is unlikely. In industries that require the handling of molten materials the danger of burning a foot through a shoe is always present (Fig. 7-1). London (1953), reporting on 301 burns of the feet, found that more burns occurred as a result of domestic accidents (during cooking or washing, for example) than as a result of work accidents.

Classification. Artz and Reiss (1957) classified the depth of burns into first, second, and third degrees. This classification is oversimplified, but the changes are directly related to the amount of tissue destroyed. First-degree burns may be caused

by the sun or by a minor flash and are characterized by erythema and dryness of the skin, usually without blistering. Second-degree burns are caused by flash or hot liquid; mottled redness of the skin occurs, with blistering, moistness, or edema. Third-degree burns, caused by contact with flame or chemicals, may be identified by the charred or pearly-white appearance and dryness of the skin. Unfortunately, it is difficult to determine the depth of the burn on first examination, but this description of the appearance of the burn may be helpful.

The first-degree burn involves the outer layer of the epidermis, while in the second-degree burn, generally the whole epidermal layer is affected. London suggested the use of a sterile safety pin to test for pain sensation in the burned area. Although both first and second-degree burns are painful, the first-degree burn is hyperesthetic to pinprick, while the second-degree burn is hypesthetic. The third-degree burn acts upon the subcutaneous fat and, in its most severe form, the underlying structures such as neurovascular bundles and bone. It is relatively painless and is anesthetic to pinprick.

Other agents used to help determine the depth or degree of the burn, which make it possible for the practitioner to devise a

168

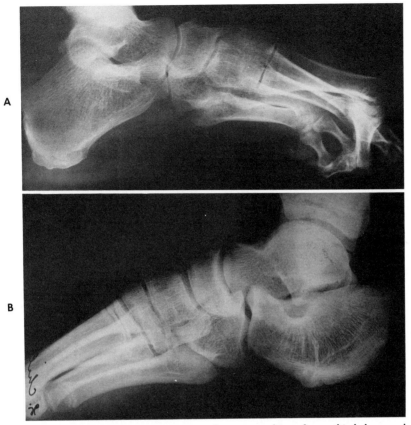

Fig. 7-1. A, Severe plantar contracture of toes resulting from third-degree burn. **B,** Destruction of calcaneal tuberosity by third-degree burn.

more complete treatment plan, are: radioactive isotopes (Bennett and Dingman, 1957) fluorescein dye injection (Meyers, 1962) and tetracycline injection and thermography (Randolph et al., 1964).

Treatment. According to London (1953) adherence to the following principles is important in order to ensure the greatest opportunity for recovery: (1) Lost skin must be replaced as soon as possible. Partly destroyed skin that may possibly regenerate must be given the best opportunity to do so, and totally destroyed skin must be replaced as soon as possible by grafting. (2) To facilitate the functional recovery of moving parts, measures should be taken to avoid infection, limit edema, and reduce pain as much as possible. (3) If necessary, reconstructive procedures may be carried out at a later time.

Artz and Reiss (1957) contend that in order to save as much of the foot as possible, it is probably better to wait to debride the eschar on the foot until it sequestrates. This treatment contrasts with that advised for burns of other parts of the body. They suggest treatment by the exposure method and emphasize that the foot should be immobilized in proper position (it should be dorsiflexed to prevent possible tendo achillis contracture).

For chemical burns, these authors recommend washing (not soaking) with water initially. If the burn is from dry lime, however, the lime should only be brushed off, as lime and water cause a chemical reaction. Attempts to neutralize the chemical agent that caused the burn are not generally recommended because some neutralizing methods have adverse effects. Baking soda for acid burns and vinegar for alkali burns are two household products that may be used without harm. Areas of the foot that have been burned by phosphorus must be protected from the air; after the burn has been washed with water, moist dressings should be applied.

Roentgen-ray burns are manifested from 6 months to a year after excessive irradiation. They are common on the plantar surface of the foot because of the extensive use of roentgen therapy for verrucae plantaris. (See intractable plantar keratosis, p. 331.) Roentgen-ray burns are resistant to all forms of therapy; however, the area should be kept clean and free from all pressures so as to stimulate healing and growth of skin. In many cases grafting of new skin is necessary.

FREEZING

Response to cold is individual and variable and therefore unpredictable. Duration and severity of exposure alter the clinical appearance. In general, the area first becomes blanched or white in response to the cold. As exposure continues, the area may become stiff and brittle. Freezing produces local sequelae similar to those of burns. Freezing injuries may be grouped as cryopathies and are classified by two principal environmental factors, wet and cold (Hermann et al., 1963). They are divided into two categories: frostbite, caused by freezing cold, and immersion foot (also known as trench foot or shelter foot), caused by a combination of wet and cold. Like burns, freezing injuries have been classified by degree of severity; unlike burns, however, the value of this classification for assessing prognosis and for planning care is limited.

Frost injuries produce pathologic changes of essentially two types: those resulting from vasomotor disturbance caused by exposure to cold, and those resulting from pathologic change caused by actual freezing of blood vessel walls or of their blood contents. If the skin has been frozen, the following effects are invariably detected: (1) local and active dilatation of the minute vessels; (2) surrounding flush caused by an arteriolar dilatation, and (3) local whealing and blistering of the skin when freezing has been extreme.

Frostbite. Frostbite represents a borderline condition between actual freezing and immersion foot (Bigelow, 1942; Brownrigg, 1943). Frostbite implies superficial freezing; however, Vinson and Schatzki (1954) observed roentgenographic changes in the bone resulting from frostbite. Edwards and Leeper (1952) analyzed seventy-one cases of frostbite of the extremities. All showed necrosis, the extent of which was in direct relation to the duration of freezing after onset of symptoms. Chronic vasospasm or hyperhidrosis, cold injury, wounds, and possibly smoking were thought to be personal contributing factors. The residual result of severe freezing may be the formidable problem of necrosis and its consequences (Lewis, 1941). Blair and associates (1957) studied 100 cases of freezing in which the persistent symptoms were cold feet, numbness, pain, hyperhidrosis, deformed nails, scarring, and mutilation of the terminal phalanges.

Treatment. Lack of understanding of the pathophysiology of frostbite makes it difficult to recommend definitive principles of care. However, two kinds of treatment are necessary: (1) the foot should be rewarmed, and (2) local care should be maintained. Contrary to the old belief that thawing should be gradual, it is now generally felt that rapid warming of the injured part is advisable. The major benefit of rapid warming is a reduction in the total time of cold exposure. The condition of treatment is explicit: The frozen part should be placed in a water bath at a temperature of between 40° C. and 42° C. (104° F. to 107° F.). Harmful effects will occur if the temperature is higher than 42° C., and maximum benefits will not be obtained if the temperature is any lower. Heavy sedation may be necessary during the rewarming period.

In the local care of the frozen foot, strict cleanliness and asepsis must be observed for the first 7 to 10 days. Either the dressing method or the exposure method may be used. The foot should be immobilized in a functional position during the acute phase, but mobilization should be started as early as possible even if the area is gangrenous. Amputation should not be rushed into; as long as there is motion, there is still a chance for revitalization of the part.

Another area of treatment exists that includes measures designed to diminish secondary vascular damage. Recently, however, the effectiveness of these methods has been challenged. Hermann and coworkers (1963) feel that sympathectomy probably is of no value, at least in the early stages of treatment. Intra-arterial vasodilation, sympathetic blocking agents (priscoline), and anticoagulants generally have not increased the good results of treatment. These measures may control pain; however, most patients require no more than the usual analgesic agents to control the pain of frostbite.

Chilblains (perniones). Repeated mild frostbite produces vasomotor instability resulting in chilblains, or perniones. The condition is characterized by recurrent attacks of hyperemia, burning, and tenderness. When the foot is affected, the symptoms generally are manifested over a bony prominence, especially the lateral side of the head of the fifth metatarsal.

Treatment is essentially mechanical and negative: the avoidance of pressure over the part by padding or shoe appliances and the avoidance of further chilling.

Immersion foot. It was not until World War II that immersion foot was given serious attention (Fausel and Hemphill, 1945). Webster and colleagues (1942) studied 142 cases of long submersion of the feet in cold water. The limbs had been immobile and constricted by boots. The result was comparable to so-called trench foot and shelter foot and to ordinary frostbite. The symptoms were increased on removal of the feet from the water. With the rapid swelling that occurred, the feet became red and hyperemic, and the temperature of the

parts became extremely elevated, although there was no sweating. The pulses in the vessels of the feet were strong. There were livid cyanosis, blebs, and extravasation of blood, with ecchymosis, vasodilation, and vascular wall impairment, especially over the medial aspects of the first metatarsophalangeal joint and the longitudinal arch. There were various degrees and patterns of anesthesia, hyperesthesia, and paresthesia.

Treatment was by dry cooling and refrigeration, effected by the application of icebags, exposure to a fan, and then slow dry cooling at room temperature while the feet were elevated. Patients were comfortable within a few hours, blebs resorbed without breaking, and the average hospitalization was about a month, although minor symptoms often persisted for up to 2 years.

Ungley (1943) suggests that massage is contraindicated and that active movements aid circulation, although walking or positions restricting circulation are dangerous. He points out that although body warmth is necessary, the extremities must be exposed to the air under dry coolness and the feet should be elevated on pillows. Bed rest and nutritional support assist the local condition. Amputation is rarely necessary.

The effects of any form of freezing are poorly understood. Experimental studies such as those of Hermann and his colleagues (1963) show that a profound reduction of blood flow occurs as a result of freezing and that ischemia occurs even though frozen tissues require less oxygen. It has also been shown that in the process of freezing the tissues become opaque; then upon thawing, small blood vessels rupture and edema occurs. Also, there is immediate intense vasoconstriction at the junction of the involved with the uninvolved tissues.

The best treatment, of course, is prophylaxis. Subsequent therapy is generally supportive. If one's feet are going to be exposed to cold, one should wear wool socks underneath a snugly fitting windproof and waterproof shoe, which will make use of

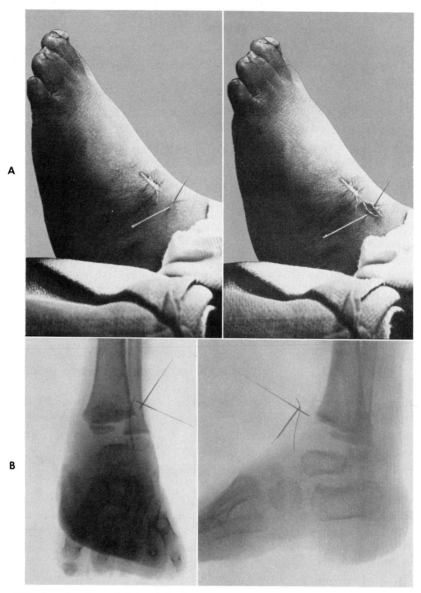

Fig. 7-2. Localization of foreign body. **A,** Two needles at right angles to each other in region of foreign body. **B,** Incision made between two needles. **C,** Biplane roentgenograms showing needles localizing foreign body.

the insulating properties of still air. Knize et al. (1969), in a study of 163 cases of frostbite, found that some tissue was lost in those victims who, in contact with metal or moisture, were exposed to temperatures of less than $-6.7°$ C. for 1 hour or more, and that a relationship existed between duration of exposure and tissue loss.

FOREIGN BODIES

Foreign bodies may produce acute symptoms or may remain asymptomatic, notwithstanding their presence in the tissues for a long time. Roentgenograms should be taken to help locate foreign bodies before any surgical attempt is made to remove them. Brown (1958) described a method

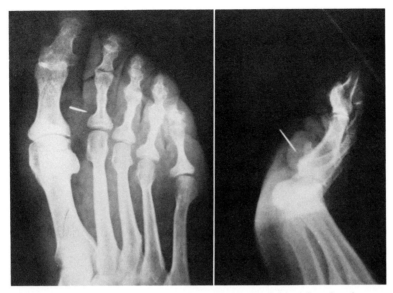

Fig. 7-3. Part of needle in foot. Acute symptoms occurred immediately after entrance.

to localize a foreign body accurately (Fig. 7-2). In this procedure two needles are inserted at right angles to each other into the area; vertical and horizontal roentgenograms are then taken. The needles may have to be replaced until their points are located in the exact region of the foreign body. With this method, tissue damage and the effects of surgery are reduced to a minimum.

Needles. Needles are the most common type of foreign body to penetrate the deep structures of the foot (Fig. 7-3). Most patients are seen soon after the accident because of disabling pain; however, asymptomatic cases are often disclosed when patients are being examined for another purpose (Fig. 7-4, A). The presence of a needle in the tissues sometimes becomes symptomatic after being dormant for years, especially if the needle is embedded in the plantar surface (Fig. 7-4, B). Long-standing needles that have not caused symptoms do not call for removal, but a needle that causes pain should be excised. Roentgenographic location of the needle in the foot should precede operation. A metal detector is helpful in locating the foreign body at operation (Moorehead, 1958). Unless the

needle is close to the surface, its removal may be difficult.

Glass. Small pieces of glass occasionally penetrate below the skin and become encapsulated (Fig. 7-5); they remain relatively superficial and are readily excised. Larger fragments may become wedged in an intermetatarsal space; when they are not removed, necrosis may result (Fig. 7-6). There are two main types of glass (Jennett and Watson, 1958). One is ordinary glass, composed of a soda lime silicate compound, from which windows, mirrors, and bottles are made. The other is lead or barium glass, which is found in the base of light bulbs, in fluoroscopic screens, and in expensive crystal glass. The former is of relatively low density and is not easily seen on roentgenogram. The latter is high-density glass and can readily be seen on roentgenogram. According to Roberts (1958), however, it should be possible to see all glass that is lodged around the foot if proper roentgenograms are taken.

Exogenous hair. Exogenous hair in the sole of the foot may become painful. While walking barefooted a person may pick up a hair which becomes embedded in the epidermis of the sole of the foot, where it re-

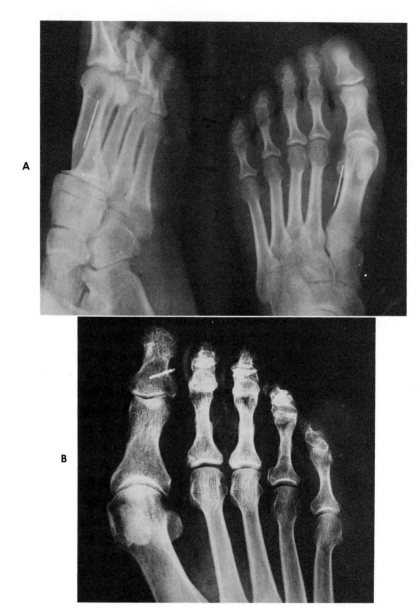

Fig. 7-4. A, Roentgenogram of foot taken for other purposes, disclosing needle. Asymptomatic. **B,** Part of needle in great toe. Foreign body dormant for long time suddenly became symptomatic.

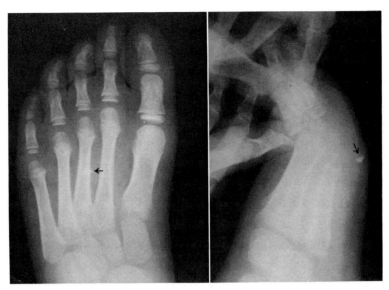

Fig. 7-5. Small piece of glass embedded in subcutaneous tissue of plantar surface. Painful.

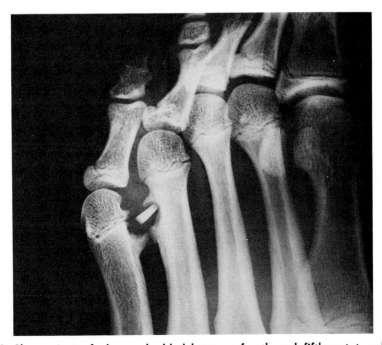

Fig. 7-6. Sharp piece of glass embedded between fourth and fifth metatarsal heads There is extensive osseous proliferation.

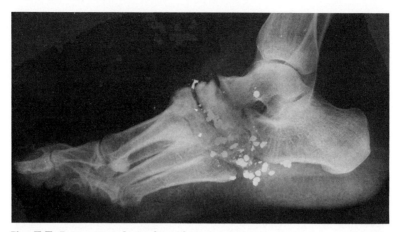

Fig. 7-7. Fragments of gunshot. There is constant pain in the tarsal joint.

mains invisible and inert. At a later date the hair may set up an acute inflammatory process. Sometimes the area must be probed under magnification until the hair is found. When the area suppurates, the hair may be exuded with the suppurative material.

Gunshot particles. Remaining particles of gunshot (Fig. 7-7) often produce delayed symptoms of varying extensiveness. Only particles that produce pain require excision. Pinpointing the site of the particles in the foot by roentgenography is always necessary preparatory to excision.

Sprains, contusions, and abrasions

A sprain is a wrenched or twisted joint. A strain is a condition of muscles, tendons, or ligaments induced by overuse or stretching in which there is no significant tear. Sudden injuries of the foot may be grouped as those that occur during violent accidents and those that occur during the normal use of the foot. Sudden injury as the result of an accident includes any degree of crushing, tearing, or breaking of one structure or of a group of structural components of the foot and ankle. Sudden injuries that take place during normal use involve the ligaments for the most part. Frequently ligaments are torn from their attachments together with a small fragment of bone. These injuries are termed sprains or chip fractures.

The foot and ankle are more subject to sprains than any other part of the body. These injuries vary from mild to severe, depending on the force involved, and may best be classified in degrees, as found in the Standard Nomenclature of Athletic Injuries (1966). A first-degree sprain is considered a mild injury, second degree a moderate one, and third degree a severe injury. The third-degree injury, therefore, is a complete rupture of the involved ligaments, tendons, or muscles. A sprain of the lateral aspect of the foot and ankle is by far the most common.

ANATOMY

The distal ends of the tibia and fibula form a mortise that maintains the trochlear surface of the talus and allows for a hinge motion in this joint. The lateral malleolus lies posterior to the medial malleolus, thereby placing the foot in slight external rotation with relation to the tibia. The articular surface of the talus is wider anteriorly, which causes some laxity of the joint when the foot is in plantar flexion. The ligaments about the ankle joint maintain the anatomic mortise. There are three groups of ligaments: (1) medial collateral (deltoid) ligaments; (2) lateral collateral ligaments; and (3) inferior tibiofibular ligaments (Fig. 7-8).

The medial collateral ligament (deltoid ligament) originates from the medial mal-

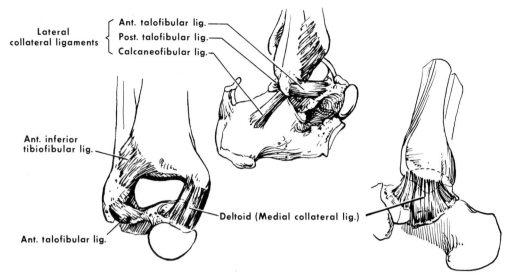

Fig. 7-8. Ligaments of foot. The three groups consist of the medial collateral (deltoid) ligaments, the lateral collateral ligaments, and the inferior tibiofibular ligaments.

leolus and extends anteriorly to attach to most of the medial aspect of the talus and the sustentaculum tali, with some filaments inserting into the navicular. The lateral collateral ligament is composed of three separate and distinct fascial bands: the posterior talofibular ligament, the anterior talofibular ligament, and the calcaneofibular ligament. These are the collateral ligaments commonly affected in an ankle sprain.

MECHANISM

Although the foot may assume varying positions of plantar flexion or dorsiflexion at the time a sprain injury is incurred, either inversion or eversion is the principal mechanism initiating the ligamentous injury. Normally, the thrust of the body weight in motion is transmitted through the leg to the talus and then through the foot to the supporting surface. When the foot is turned suddenly in extreme inversion or eversion, which may happen during walking or running, the line of force goes through the ankle laterally or medially to the body of the talus. At that moment, weight is not transferred through the foot; the line of force escapes through the side

of the ankle, thus spraining or lacerating the ligament that is not capable of absorbing the force.

Kelly (1952) is of the opinion that common ankle injuries are the result of an exaggeration of one basic foot motion, either inversion or eversion. Inversion injuries are the more common ones, however, and can generally be separated into those with only partial disruption of the lateral collateral ligament system and those with complete disruption and associated instability.

The frequent observation that a severe ankle sprain is worse than a fractured ankle may be true on occasion, if treatment is inadequate. A fracture is readily recognized; therefore, appropriate treatment is instituted at once. Sprains are often regarded lightly except in rare cases with evident ankle dislocation. Collateral ligaments may be ruptured completely in ankle sprains, and there may be associated separation of the ankle mortise. Such sprains are often reduced spontaneously and are often neglected and not treated by complete immobilization or repair of the ligaments. The resulting unstable ankle may require major surgical repair at a later date.

Injuries to lateral malleolar ligaments

Classification. There are three types of injury to the lateral malleolar ligaments: (1) sprains of the lateral collateral ligaments, (2) avulsion and momentary dislocation of the ankle joint, and (3) recurrent dislocations.

Recovery from simple, or first-degree, sprains is complete in a few weeks; nevertheless, every sprained ankle should be investigated to make certain that the sprain is actually simple. Most ankle injuries are second-degree sprains (moderate) or third-degree sprains (severe). Injury to the ligaments varies from extreme stretching of the collateral ligaments to tearing of the ligaments without complete avulsion. D'Anca (1970) has reported a case of simple rotatory dislocation of the ankle without fracture—a rare injury because of the mechanical efficiency of the mortise and the strength of the ligaments.

Symptoms. Swelling and local tenderness over the tarsal sinus, painful weight bearing, and increased discomfort on forced inversion of the foot comprise the symptoms. Edema and ecchymoses are accompanying manifestations of subdermal bleeding.

Diagnosis. First, the specific injured ligamentous structure must be sought. Usually it can be found by palpating the three segments of the lateral collateral ligament. The anterior talofibular ligament is the one most commonly injured. Whether or not the distal tibiofibular ligaments are injured should also be determined, but this is more difficult because the anterior and posterior talofibular ligaments overlie the tibiofibular ligaments. The area of swelling and discomfort helps indicate which structures are injured; also, the amount of swelling and discomfort provides a clue as to the severity of the injury. In order to make some decision about the stability of the injured ankle as compared with the ankle of the opposite side, one can stress the ankle under roentgenographic control by inverting the foot while holding it first in equinus and then in dorsiflexion. When the foot is

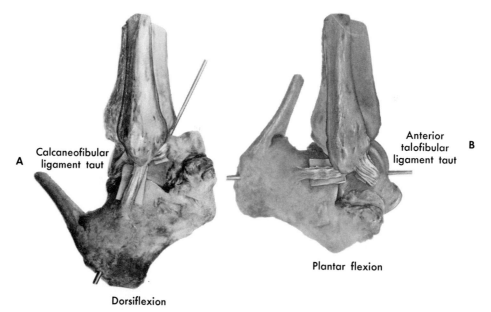

Fig. 7-9. Ligaments on lateral side of ankle joint. **A,** Dorsiflexed foot. Stability of the ankle is maintained by the calcaneofibular ligament. **B,** Plantar flexed foot. Stability of the ankle is maintained by the anterior talofibular ligament.

held in dorsiflexion, the calcaneofibular portion maintains the stability of the ankle (Fig. 7-9, *A*); when it is held in plantar flexion, the anterior talofibular portion of the lateral collateral ligament becomes the stabilizer (Fig. 7-9, *B*). It has been shown that 25 percent of normal ankles which show no talar tilt in dorsiflexion will show varying degrees (6 to 28 degrees) of talar tilt when stressed in equinus. This is apparently caused by the individual variations in the axis of the subtalar joint (the calcaneofibular ligament must be parallel to this axis in the sagittal plane) and not to the integrity of the ligaments (see Chapter 1).

Roentgenograms are helpful diagnostic tools (see Chapter 3). Lateral and anteroposterior views, as well as views of the ankle internally rotated 30 degrees, should

be taken. From these roentgenograms it is possible to see the tibiofibular syndesmosis. On occasion, one can see in the diastasis of this joint a suggestion of complete rupture of the distal tibiofibular ligaments (Fig. 7-10). Roentgenograms will not distinguish between the stable and unstable sprain injury unless stress films are taken, which may not be conclusive unless they are taken while the patient is under anesthesia (Fig. 7-11). The angle made between the dome of the talus and the articular surface of the tibia on these stress films will give the degree of the sprain (Fig. 7-12). Anderson et al. (1952) stated that a 6-degree tilt of the talus as seen in a direct anteroposterior view (with the ankle in forced inversion) indicates that the anterior talofibular ligament alone is ruptured. Anderson and Lecocq (1954) showed

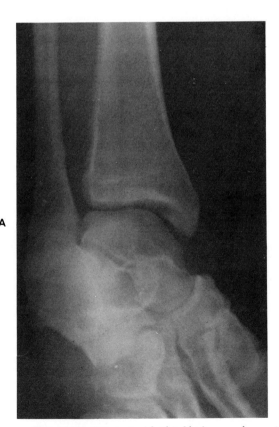

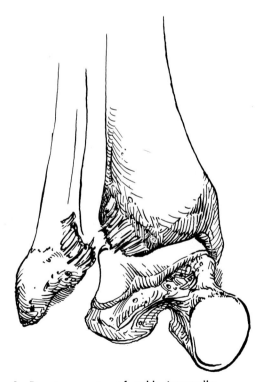

Fig. 7-10. Diastasis of tibiofibular syndesmosis. **A,** Roentgenogram of ankle internally rotated 30 degrees. **B,** Drawing showing tear of distal tibiofibular ligaments.

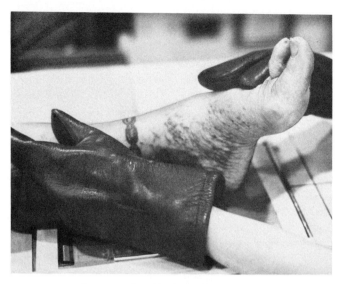

Fig. 7-11. Demonstration of tattooed ankle being stressed in inversion on cassette for roentgenogram.

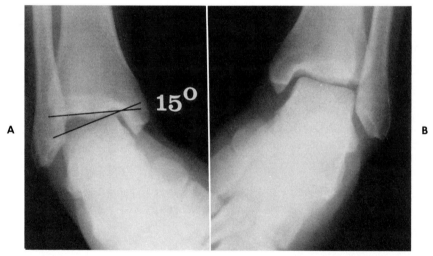

Fig. 7-12. Roentgenograms of ankle in stressed position. **A,** Fifteen degrees of talar tilt. **B,** No talar tilt.

that a 12 to 30 degree tilt meant a combined tear of the anterior talofibular and calcaneofibular ligaments.

It must be kept in mind, however, that stress roentgenograms should be taken of both ankles, since relaxation of lateral ligaments also occurs in so-called normal feet. Berridge and Bonnin (1944) found that 4 to 5 percent of the uninjured ankles they

tested showed laxity of the lateral ligaments; the laxity was usually bilateral and occurred with talar tilt of from 5 to 25 degrees. In a group of 106 football players tested at California State University, San Francisco, in the 1969 and 1970 seasons, ligamentous laxity was found in 8 percent of players with uninjured ankles, with talar tilt of from 5 to 11 degrees as seen on roent-

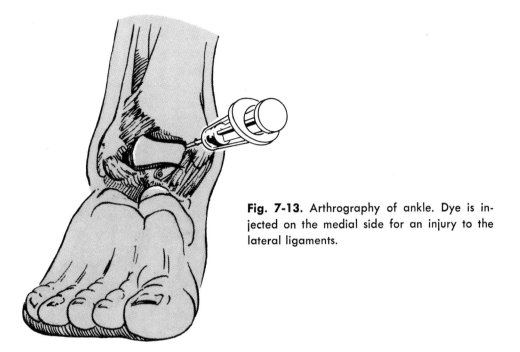

Fig. 7-13. Arthrography of ankle. Dye is injected on the medial side for an injury to the lateral ligaments.

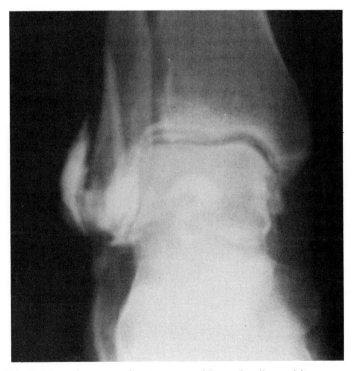

Fig. 7-14. Arthrogram showing tear of lateral collateral ligaments.

genograms. Twenty-one players actually showed a significant spread in the ankle mortises (over 5 degrees of talar tilt); however, twelve of them reported having had previous injuries. It is interesting to note that the highest percentage of ankle injuries during these two seasons occurred in the group that showed a talar tilt of 5 degrees or more (Glick, 1971).

Arthrographic studies of the ankle joint may also be made to aid diagnosis (Figs. 7-13 through 7-16). Leakage of the dye through a particular ligament or through the distal tibiofibular syndesmosis will pinpoint the structure torn. Probably the greatest benefit of this procedure is to demonstrate tears of the distal tibiofibular ligaments (Fig. 7-15). It also aids in determining whether the problem is fresh or old, especially in those patients with developmental laxity of the ligaments. Berridge and Bonnin (1944), and more recently Percy et al. (1969) and Gordon (1970), have described their methods of arthrography and their findings. Fordyce and Horn (1972) in a series of patients with recent ligamentous injuries of the ankle, correlated the findings of stress roentgenographic and arthrographic studies with

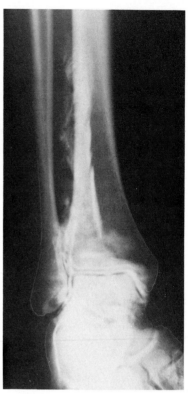

Fig. 7-15. Arthrogram showing tear of distal tibiofibular ligament. Note seepage of dye through distal tibiofibular ligament up into the interosseous membrane.

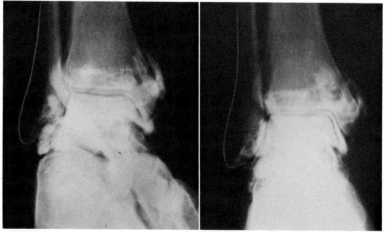

Fig. 7-16. Arthrogram showing extravasation of dye along medial malleolus. There is a tear in the deltoid ligament.

those of surgical exploration. They found that although arthrography may have been useful to demonstrate injury of the inferior tibiofibular joint and of the medial ligament, both roentgenography and arthrography were unreliable in the diagnosis of injuries to the "lateral ligament" of the ankle.

Arthrography can be performed as an office procedure. Gordon offered the following technique: The needle is inserted into the side of the ankle joint that is opposite from the side of the suspected lesion. A 1½ inch needle (22 gauge) is used. Fifty percent Hypaque, diluted with an equal amount of sterile saline to make a 25 percent solution, is injected. Five to 10 ml. of this diluted dye is then injected, depending on the amount of resistance the joint gives.

Treatment. The treatment for contusions, sprains, and strains is as follows:

Immediate treatment consists of (1) cold applications to constrict the arterial beds and reduce subdermal bleeding; (2) compression to arrest active subdermal bleeding; (3) elevation of the injured part to decrease edema; and (4) rest. Obviously, excessive manipulation of the foot aggravates a recent injury and consequently lengthens the period of disability. Cold applications begin to lose their value after 24 to 48 hours, whereas compression and elevation may be helpful for several days. Cold applications and compression are used guardedly for aged patients or patients with peripheral vascular disease.

Upon removing the compression dressing after 24 to 48 hours, assess the extent of the injury. By palpation and gentle manipulation, ascertain whether there has been a simple stretching or complete avulsion of the ligaments. When the degree of injury is uncertain, roentgenograms should be taken with the ankle stressed in eversion and inversion to rule out complete rupture of the ligaments (Fig. 7-17). It may be necessary to place the patient under anesthesia to obtain these roentgenograms. Arthrography, as described, may be of value.

In about 36 hours, if edema is minimal,

apply heat rather than cold to dilate peripheral vessels, thus speeding absorption at the site of injury.

In general, when swelling is moderate and complete rupture of the collateral ligament has been ruled out, partial immobilization with adhesive strapping or a firm ankle support, with or without the injection of procaine hydrochloride, permits healing while the patient is ambulatory. The Gibney basket-weave strapping, often used in athletic injuries, is a common method of taping the ankle. It is sometimes fortified with a heel lock. If more swelling is anticipated, the same type of ankle strapping, which leaves the ankle exposed in front, can be applied (Fig. 7-18).

Another excellent support is the Una boot type of wrap. The Gelocast bandage (Fig. 7-19) is a modification of the Una wrap, which allows for faster drying. Gelocast bandages give better support than Ace bandages, and it takes less time to apply them than it does to apply tape. Furthermore, Gelocasts are tolerated better by the patient than tape. To ensure even compression and optimal support, they should be applied from the toes to the tibial tubercle (Fig. 7-19, A); a few figure-of-eight turns should be made around the ankle (Fig. 7-19, B). These bandages can usually be left on for 5 to 7 days, maintaining the same supportive quality throughout. For participants in athletic events, however, better support is given with tape.

The sprain type of injury without complete ligamentous disruption requires only protection from additional injury and seldom requires plaster immobilization. That significant ankle instability rarely occurs as an aftermath of as common an injury as ankle sprain supports the concept that operative repair is seldom necessary.

A plaster cast will assure maximal immobilization and may be used for those patients in whom the severity of injury is in doubt or for those who cannot get along with other forms of immobilization. Some practitioners advocate immobilization with use of a short leg cast for 3 to 6 weeks in

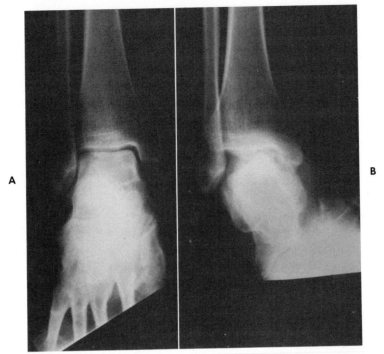

Fig. 7-17. Roentgenographic appearance of ankles with complete ruptures of lateral collateral and deltoid ligaments. **A**, No stress applied. **B**, Inversion stress applied showing rupture of lateral collateral ligaments. **C**, Eversion stress applied showing rupture of deltoid ligaments.

inversion injuries with demonstrable tilting of the talus of ±15 degrees as compared with that of the opposite side. However, the use of plaster immobilization has met with contention among those who continually treat and follow soft-tissue injuries of the ankle.

Infiltration of 5 to 10 ml. of 1 percent procaine hydrochloride has been advocated by many for sprained ankle without avulsion of the ligaments. McMaster (1943) reported 400 cases of sprained ankle in which 200 were treated by injection of procaine hydrochloride alone and 200 were treated by immobilization with adhesive strapping. He reports that treatment by injection of procaine hydrochloride alone uniformly gave the better results.

Avulsion of collateral ligaments

Avulsion of the collateral ligaments is the most severe of all injuries to the lateral side

of the ankle. In most instances the collateral ligaments are completely torn so that complete lateral instability of the ankle results. Leonard (1949), who experimented with seven cases of preserved ankle and studied fifty-one cases of sprained ankles, concluded that the most important component of the collateral group in avulsion is the anterior talofibular ligament. In all probability the calcaneofibular ligament is equally important (Fig. 7-20).

Treatment. Anderson and Lecocq (1954) showed that ankle instability is greatest when either the calcaneofibular or posterior tibiofibular ligament is torn together with the anterior talofibular ligament. They stated that although a tear of the anterior tibiofibular ligament is a severe injury, it may be treated conservatively; but combined tears should be treated surgically. Percy et al. (1969) believed that stress roentgenograms are unreliable and that an

C

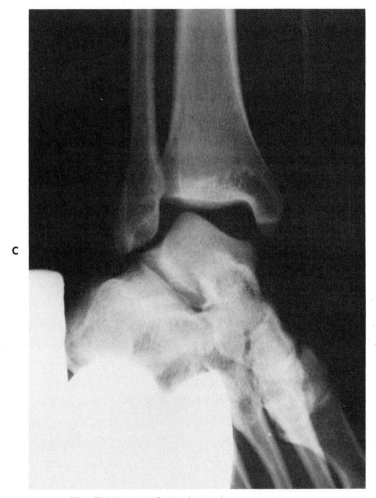

Fig. 7-17, cont'd. For legend see opposite page.

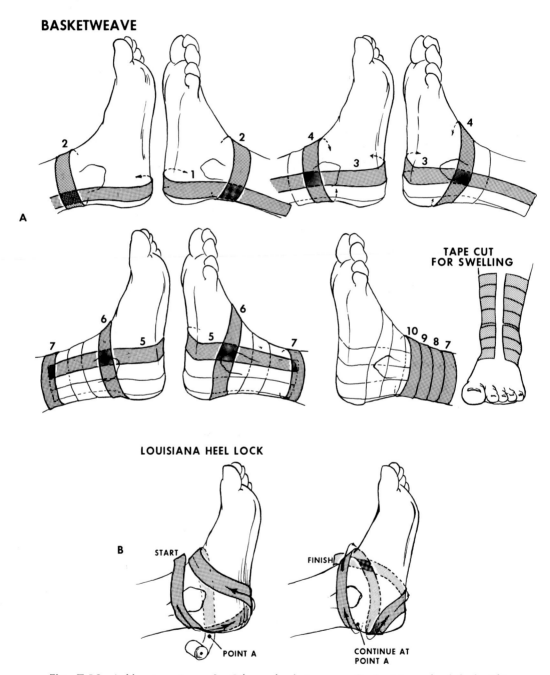

Fig. 7-18. Ankle strappings. **A,** Gibney basket-weave. **B,** Louisiana heel lock. This strapping can be applied in conjunction with the basket weave.

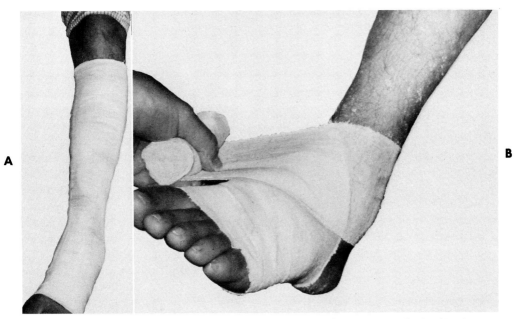

Fig. 7-19. Gelocast bandage. **A,** Completed application from toes to tibial tubercle. **B,** Figure-of-eight wrap around ankle.

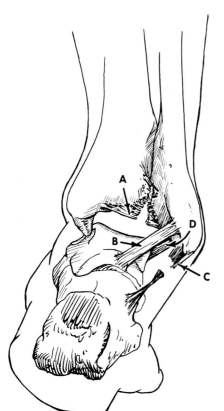

Fig. 7-20. Collateral ligaments. **A,** Torn posterior tibiofibular ligament. **B,** Posterior talofibular ligament. **C,** Torn calcaneofibular ligament. **D,** Anterior talofibular ligament.

arthrogram is of more value in determining the extent of the injury. Certainly there is a great deal of controversy—both about which methods provide the earliest and most accurate assessment of the injury and about the methods of proper treatment. So much divergent thought on the treatment of this injury indicates that results of any form of therapy have so far been imperfect. Initial therapy as previously described has proved sound; further treatment, however, seems to vary with the whim of the physician.

Freeman (1965) divided patients with lateral ligament avulsions into groups of three, with each group receiving a different type of treatment. The first group of patients were walking as soon as they were comfortable enough to do so. The second group of patients had their injured ligaments immobilized in plaster casts for 6 weeks. The third group had operative repair, with subsequent immobilization of the injured ankle for 6 weeks. The findings showed that maximum ankle stability was gained only by the patients in the third group who had been treated operatively. However, only 25 percent of these patients had symptom-free ankles after 1 year, whereas in the first group 58 percent were symptom-free after 1 year. Fifty-three percent of patients in the second group whose injured ligaments were only immobilized had symptom-free ankles after 1 year. Further evaluation of this study revealed that those who were treated without surgery showed no more than 8 degrees of instability on stress roentgenograms. Those who were walking early were disabled an average of 12 weeks; those whose injured ligaments were immobilized for 6 weeks were disabled for 22 weeks; and those who had an operative repair followed by plaster casts were disabled for 26 weeks.

In another study Freeman (1965) noted that the pathologic process which is usually responsible for functional instability of the ankle after a ligament injury is unknown. However, he and his co-workers postulated that this functional instability, which is commonly known as giving-way, is caused by a proprioceptive deficit. They therefore suggested a course of coordination exercises for all types of ankle sprain. This treatment plan is designed to control swelling and to facilitate recovery of a full range of motion and muscle strength. In the group they treated in this fashion, only 7 percent complained of giving-way, whereas 40 percent reported complaints of giving-way after other forms of treatment. In conclusion, the authors suggest that the patient perform controlled tilting exercises of the ankle as soon as he is able to stand. At first the patient stands on a board that is balanced (like a seesaw) on a stable object and tilts the board from side to side. After he has mastered this exercise, he performs another series of tilting exercises on the board, which is now placed across a spherical object (Fig. 7-21).

Despite Freeman's most interesting studies, many still claim that primary operative repair of ligaments yields the best result with the least disability. Anderson and Lecocq (1954), reporting on twenty-seven cases of repair of the collateral fibular ligaments, observed that many so-called minor ankle sprains are actually complete ruptures of these ligaments and that early surgical repair is paramount. Gillespie and Boucher (1971), in a study in which the Watson-Jones technique was used to repair lateral instability of the ankle in twenty patients, showed 80 percent excellent or good and 20 percent fair or poor results. They also stated that the presence of arthritic changes in the ankle preoperatively may contraindicate this procedure. Percy et al. (1969) felt that minor sprain should be treated by early mobilization, partial tear by immobilization, and complete tear by surgical repair. They also felt that the degree of sprain could be diagnosed properly only with the aid of an arthrogram.

Isolated posttraumatic lesions of the anterior tibiofibular ligament and of the anterior talofibular portion of the lateral collateral ligament are rare and difficult to diagnose. Disruption of the anterior talo-

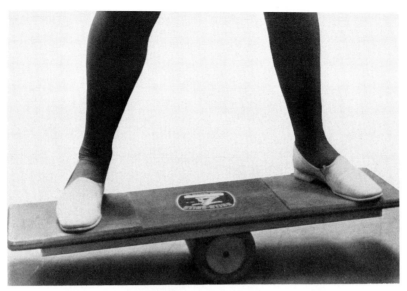

Fig. 7-21. Tilt board.

fibular ligament as described by Landeros et al. (1968) and by Anderson et al. (1952) may be more common than is generally recognized. This disruption can be demonstrated by the response of anterior subluxation of the talus to passive manipulation of the foot, the same kind of manipulation being used in this instance as is used when the attempt is made to produce the anterior drawer sign at the knee (Fig. 7-22).

Injuries to the medial malleolar ligaments

The discussion thus far has been entirely about lateral collateral ligament sprain, which is indeed appropriate since it is the most common type of ankle sprain. Injuries to the medial collateral or deltoid ligament do not occur often; when they do, they are generally caused by sudden eversion of the foot, which subjects the deltoid ligament to an extreme abduction stress. Rupture of the medial collateral ligament is a rare entity as an isolated lesion but is a common accompaniment of the bimalleolar type of fracture-dislocation of the ankle. When rupture of the deltoid ligament occurs, the ligament is usually stripped from the surface of the medial malleolus.

Conservative treatment. Treatment is selected according to the degree of injury. In simple sprains, when the deltoid ligament has not been torn, partial immobilization with adhesive or application of an ankle support for 3 weeks is sufficient for recovery. All cases of avulsion of the deltoid ligament should be considered serious, requiring complete immobilization by a plaster cast. The shape and form of this ligament allow for maintenance of apposition of the torn ends; therefore, operative repair is seldom necessary. Bonnin (1965), in an editorial, stated that rupture of this ligament "can safely be left to itself in most cases."* Dziob (1956) suggested that in the treatment of medial avulsion of the ankle, when the tilt of the talus in inversion under stress roentgenography is less than 15 degrees, plaster immobilization of the foot and leg for 6 to 8 weeks is adequate; however, when it is greater than 15 degrees, the torn ligaments must be sutured. (For surgical treatment, see Chapter 19.)

---

*Bonnin, J. G.: Injury to the ligaments of the ankle (Editorials and Annotations), J. Bone & Joint Surg. **47-B**:609-611, Nov. 1965.

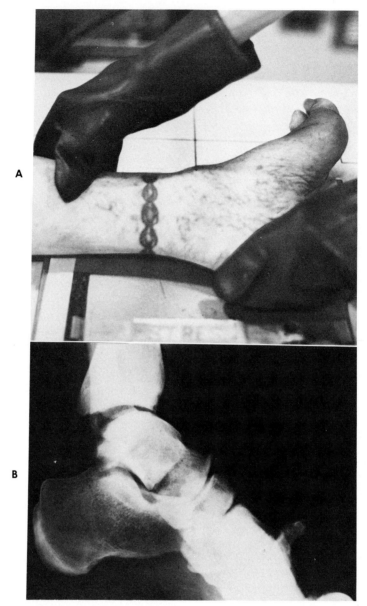

Fig. 7-22. Disruption of anterior talofibular ligament. **A,** Anterior stress on tattooed ankle. **B,** Roentgenogram demonstrating anterior instability of ankle. Note anterior subluxation of the talus.

Recurrent sprained ankles

Recurrent dislocation of the ankle, weak ankles, and chronic sprains are terms loosely applied to injured ankle ligaments. Recurrent episodes of overstretching and spraining of ankle ligaments ultimately leave them completely stretched or torn.

The condition may be caused by sudden avulsion of the collateral ligaments with spontaneous reduction of the talus dislocation, which, if not properly treated, results in an unstable ankle. A sprained ankle may and often does lead to permanent disability (Bonnin, 1944). In a report of fifty-seven cases of injury to the ankle without bony changes, Hughes (1942) recorded some lateral tilting of the ankle in about half the cases when roentgenograms were made with the ankle held in forced inversion. Bosien and his co-workers (1955) followed 133 cases of ankle sprain for an average of 27 months. Among their patients 36 percent had had previous injury to the same ankle and 33 percent had had continuous residual ankle symptoms.

Repeated twisting or giving-way of the ankle is typical, especially when the patient walks on irregular ground or wears heels worn down on the outer posterior surface. Among women, recurrent ankle sprain often results from previous injuries to the ankle coupled with the wearing of high-heeled shoes.

Supportive treatment. A good supportive shoe in addition to an elastic ankle support in some cases stabilizes the ankle sufficiently to prevent further sprains. Some patients may be helped by a short leg brace with a T-strap to prevent inversion. If this supportive treatment does not alleviate the problem, a reconstruction procedure that includes the implantation of new tissue will be necessary. (For surgical treatment, see Chapter 19.)

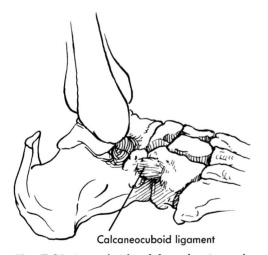

Fig. 7-23. Lateral side of foot showing calcaneocuboid ligaments.

Calcaneocuboid ligament

Forefoot sprain or sprain of the calcaneocuboid joint

This injury is a type of inversion sprain that involves a portion of the ligaments overlying the calcaneocuboid joint (Fig. 7-23). It causes immediate severe disability with pain, swelling, and tenderness that is localized to the region of this joint. Restriction of weight bearing for 48 hours usually brings enough relief to the injured patient so that he can begin to walk; thereafter, progressive healing continues to occur. On resumption of weight bearing, an Ace bandage wrap, tape strapping, or Gelocast should be worn. Any of these will provide sufficient support to the injured part and can probably be removed within a week.

Sprains of first metatarsophalangeal joint and of plantar fascia

First metatarsophalangeal joint. The first metatarsophalangeal joint is sometimes sprained by stubbing the toe or by extreme dorsiflexion. Swelling over the joint and pain on motion are symptomatic. Such sprains are for the most part simple sprains and respond to partial immobilization with adhesive tape and the wearing of a shoe with a rigid sole.

Plantar fascia. The plantar fascia may be sprained by jumping, especially from heights. The sprain may be anywhere along the length of the fascia but is seen most often at its origin. Sprains of the plantar fascia respond to strapping and the wearing of a shoe with a rigid shank and a longitudinal arch support.

Contusions and abrasions

Treatment. These injuries are best treated with ice, local compression, elevation, and protective padding when the patient begins to ambulate.

Athletic injuries
DIFFERENTIATION

Athletic injuries in many aspects are different from the usual injuries one sees in clinical practice; thus their treatment deserves special consideration. The patient is young and active, and the purpose of medical attention is not only to treat the injury so that it heals properly, but also to treat it in such a way that the patient can return to competition as quickly as possible. The injured athlete when unable to play is, in fact, no longer an athlete. Fractures, dislocations, and other major injuries constitute only a small percentage of sport injuries. Surprisingly, they present no significant problem because their diagnosis and treatment have been discussed in the literature from time immemorial. The time of disability from these injuries can be specifically measured; usually the athlete who has suffered a major injury cannot be expected to return within the same competitive season.

The greatest majority of athletic injuries however, are relatively minor ones such as mild sprains, strains, or contusions. While people of other occupations with mild sprains, strains, or contusions will probably be able to discharge their work and social responsibilities while they limp about, athletes find these injuries crippling. For example, a mild ankle strain may prevent a football player from cutting effectively but may be essentially asymptomatic while he is walking. Thus, even though they are less serious than fractures and dislocations, these injuries tax the acumen and judgment of the physician associated with athletic medicine.

Sites of injury. The foot and ankle are commonly traumatized during athletics; a sprained ankle is always a threat in sports such as baseball, football, and hockey. Thorndike (1962), in an anaylsis of athletic injuries on the Harvard football team for 15 years, found 585 ankle sprains and 15 fractured ankles. Glick and Katch (1970), in a study in which 120 joggers were observed over an 11-week period, reported that of the 241 injuries that occurred, there were 20 ankle sprains and 43 other problems of the foot consisting of blisters, arch strains, sore heels, heel bursitises, toenail injuries, bruises, metatarsalgias, and corns.

Preventive treatment is essential. Athletes who are exposed to violent twisting of the ankle should have their ankles strapped with adhesive tape so as to limit inversion and eversion. A nonelastic ankle support may also be worn during games. This applies especially to athletes who have had recurrent ankle sprains. For protection of the forefoot, shoes should have rigid or metal toe boxing and firm soles.

Treatment. Treatment for specific injuries is discussed under appropriate headings elsewhere in this book. Most soft-tissue injuries of the foot and ankle should initially be treated with the application of ice and a compression bandage; the foot should be elevated and weight bearing should be restricted. Following this treatment, graduated rehabilitative measures should be commenced under close supervision of the physician. Jogging can usually be started as soon as the athlete is comfortable enough to walk without a limp. Jogging should then progress to running and then to running in circles or tight figure-of-eights before the athlete is allowed to participate in a particular sport. If in the progression of these activities swelling of the part or increased pain occurs, progress should be terminated and the athlete should return to one of the former events mentioned. Hirata (1968) stressed the advantages of performing these rehabilitative measures right on the playing field during practice session. He also emphasized the importance of frequent examination for signs of increased swelling and pain.

Raising or lowering the heel counters of the shoe is effective in treating heel bursitis. Achilles tendinitis is best treated by elevating the heel with a ¼ to ½ inch pad. Either wearing thicker socks or placing petroleum jelly on top of and between toes seems to yield the best results for the athlete with toe blisters. Dancers frequently wrap tape around their blistered toes and do not remove the tape until it falls off by itself. For the athlete who has a contused foot, taping the protective pad over the outside of the shoe is the easiest method of application. Sprains of the first metatarsophalangeal joint will probably incapacitate the athlete for 3 weeks. He may be able to walk without pain in 1 week, but when he starts to run, more stress will be placed on this joint, so that the condition is reactivated. Therefore, if the athlete with a sprain of the first metatarsophalangeal joint is allowed to return to competition too early, a longer period of disability will probably ensue.

Traumatic injuries to the tendons of the foot and ankle

In general, traumatic rupture of the tendons about the foot and ankle is rare except for that of the tendo achillis. Traumatic tenosynovitis and peritendinitis occur more often but are usually more difficult to treat. Tenosynovitis is inflammation of a tendon sheath; peritendinitis is inflammation of a tendon that possesses no sheath. All of the tendons across the foot and ankle have sheaths except the tendo achillis.

TRAUMATIC TENOSYNOVITIS OR PERITENDINITIS

Process, symptoms, treatment. Lipscomb (1950) states that the tendons of human beings will not tolerate over 1,500 to 2,000 manipulations per hour. Acceleration of the speed of physical work, prolonged exertion, or extraordinary activity (for example, the sudden playing of three sets of tennis by a person who is usually sedentary) may cause the trauma that initiates this condition. Lipscomb also showed that the pathologic process of tenosynovitis and peritendinitis is one of either acute inflammation or chronic fibrosis. The symptom is predominantly neuritic pain; the signs are localized heat, redness, and tenderness or pain when the specific tendon is moved.

These conditions may be acute or chronic. If the patient is seen early enough, treatment should include the application of ice, elevation of the foot, and rest. After

the first 24 to 48 hours, diathermic or infrared heat may be applied. Rest, frequently best accomplished by plaster immobilization, is the most effective form of treatment. In mild cases adhesive strappings or Gelocast wraps suffice. Local steroid injections will frequently relieve acute symptoms in a short period of time, but should not be expected to heal the lesion more quickly. Repeated steroid injections, in fact, should be performed cautiously, as they may weaken the tendon and produce spontaneous rupture.

Severe cases and cases of repeated traumatic tenosynovitis or peritendinitis may produce a great deal of scarification and may freeze the tendon so that it requires extensive repair, including the formation of a new gliding mechanism. This chronic condition may present a formidable problem. Therefore, in the more severe cases of tenosynovitis, surgical excision of the inflamed tissues in which the tendon glides may be the most conservative form of treatment.

Those injuries caused by improper footwear generally involve the extensor hallucis longus tendon or the tendo achillis. The extensor hallucis longus tendon is most prominent over the dorsum of the forefoot. This is why it is often impinged upon by the margins of the vamps of pumps. Sometimes a protective fibroma of the skin and subcutaneous tissue forms just behind the first metatarsal head, which may cause recurrent infection and formation of a draining sinus in its center. The entire mass of scar must be excised and at times the gliding mechanism must be repaired.

A comparable condition is observed just above the insertion of the tendo achillis, a condition that also results from friction and pressure—in this instance of the shoe counter. This condition is commonly known as pump bump because it is frequently seen in women who wear high-heeled shoes (Fig. 7-24). Moreover, the fad of laceless shoes and loafers (shoes that must fit closely in the area of the long axis of the foot) has caused an alarming increase of

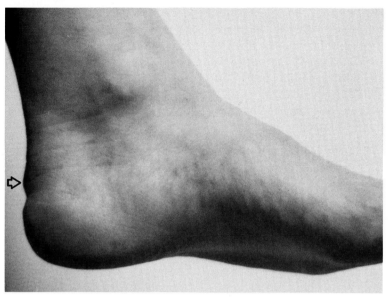

Fig. 7-24. "Pump bump."

pump bumps. Although it is anatomically related to the apophysis of the calcaneus, a pump bump is a reactive membranous bone formation that becomes an exostosis (see Chapter 13). A common anatomic variation of the calcaneus is a tuberous prominence; perhaps this variation of the normal heel predisposes to the formation of such exostoses.

A locally inflamed heel at the posterior superior surface of the calcaneus lateral or medial to the tendo achillis is a symptom of pump bump. The presence of the disorder, which occurs predominantly in adolescent and young adult females, is confirmed roentgenographically. It is best to treat it conservatively. The wearing of sandals or larger, laced shoes has been effective in promoting quiescence. At times an adventitial bursa may develop over the exostosis, which will respond to local anti-inflammatory treatment. In very select cases, excision may be considered if symptoms persist. Brahms (1967) pointed out that if the mass occurs in the midline it is apt to be a rheumatoid nodule instead of a pump bump, which usually occurs laterally. Keck and Kelly (1965) reported on

a series of eighteen patients operated upon for symptomatic bursitis of the posterior part of the heel. They found that the posterior superior border of the calcaneus was prominent in patients with this condition. Two surgical procedures were used. The first involved resection of the superior prominence of the calcaneal tuberosity with removal of the bursa, and the second consisted of a cuneiform osteotomy of the calcaneus with removal of a dorsally based wedge (see Chapter 19). Better results were achieved from the first operation, but a true statistical analysis could not be made because too few of the second operation were performed. Dickinson et al. (1966) had good results from excision of the posterior superior prominence of the calcaneus in twenty-one patients. They stressed, however, that only a small number of patients with this condition required surgical treatment; most had few or no symptoms, and those with symptoms were relieved by conservative measures.

Hemorrhagic tenosynovitis. Hemorrhagic tenosynovitis is an uncommon complication of an injury to a tendon. A direct blow to the tendon or an excessive strain of the tendon may break the endothelial lining of the tendon sheath, causing hemorrhage into the sheath, from which the blood cannot escape and therefore clots. The blood clots assume the character of a foreign body, thereby becoming an irritant and often producing muscle spasm. This accounts for the continuous pain, even when the limb is at rest. The irritation tends to induce an increase in the production of synovial fluid in the sheath, causing fluctuation over the area.

Acute pain and swelling over the injured tendon begin from 24 to 48 hours after trauma. Pain becomes worse and cannot be relieved; rest or change in position of the limb does not modify the symptoms. The area over the tendon is swollen, fluctuant, and tender to touch. The condition is differentiated from a pyogenic tenosynovitis by its rapid onset of symptoms after injury, the absence of signs of infection, and persistent, acute pain over the injured tendon, which are incompatible with simple injuries to a tendon.

Exquisite pain and fluctuation pinpoint the site of the hematoma, which must be excised through an incision in the tendon sheath. Only rarely is the clot absorbed without excision.

INJURIES TO SPECIFIC TENDONS

Lapidus and Seidenstein (1950) have reported three cases of chronic nonspecific tenosynovitis. Two involved the tibialis posterior tendon and one involved the flexor hallucis longus tendon. In all cases pain was intermittent. In the case involving the flexor hallucis longus the condition had remained unrecognized for several months. In the cases involving the tibialis posterior recognition did not occur until after 1 and 3 years, respectively. Treatment consisted of opening the tendon sheath to evacuate excess fluid and excising the thickened portion of the sheath.

In a study of tendon problems of the foot done at the Mayo Clinic, Lipscomb (1950) found that tenosynovitis of the anterior tibial tendon occurred in 24 percent,

peritendinitis of the tendo achillis in 20 percent, and tenosynovitis of the posterior tibial and peroneal tendons in 16 percent of cases. Tenosynovitis of the anterior tibial tendon was often associated with involvement of the extensor digitorum communis tendon and was frequently caused by irritation from shoes or boots. Although it was sometimes necessary to excise the synovial sheath in front of the ankle, for the most part tenosynovitis of these tendons responded to conservative treatment. Peritendinitis of the tendo achillis was more difficult to treat. Because this condition was usually caused by irritation of the shoe counter or by unusually prolonged ambulation, the most successful treatment consisted of removal of the shoe counter, followed by heel elevation and rest. Tenosynovitis of the posterior tibial tendon and tenosynovitis of the peroneal tendon were often associated with static deformities of the foot. One case was reported in which the posterior tibial and flexor digitorum communis tendons occupied the same tendon sheath. For the treatment of this condition Lipscomb suggested shoe correction, contrast baths, foot exercise, and roentgen therapy.

Ghormley and Spear (1953) reviewed twenty-one cases of tenosynovitis of the tibialis posterior diagnosed and treated at the Mayo Clinic between 1935 and 1951. Eleven of these cases were the result of anomalies of the tibialis posterior with accessory tendons, which were excised at the time of operation. The remaining ten cases were treated conservatively with roentgen therapy and strapping.

Williams (1963) reported on fifty-two patients with chronic tenosynovitis of the tibialis posterior tendon. The changes were regarded as nonspecific, with the exception of one case that showed associated manifestations of rheumatoid arthritis. Twelve patients in whom conservative treatment had failed were treated by surgical release of the tendon sheath, with complete relief resulting in eleven patients.

Cohen and Reid (1935) reported seven

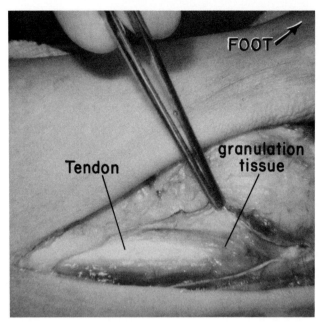

Fig. 7-25. Tenosynovitis of peroneal tendon below edge of lateral malleolus. Note granulation tissue overlying tendon. Retinaculum has already been cut.

cases of tenosynovitis crepitans associated with oxaluria. Parvin and Ford (1956) reported two cases of stenosing tenosynovitis of the common peroneal tendon sheath, and Gunn (1959) reported a similar case. Pain in the area behind the lateral malleolus was produced by forced inversion as well as eversion of the foot. Tenderness and swelling overlying the peroneal tendons were relieved by surgical release of the thickened inferior retinaculum below the edge of the lateral malleolus (Fig. 7-25).

Compression of the posterior tibial nerve at the level of the medial malleolus (tarsal tunnel syndrome) should be considered in painful conditions of the foot. This problem is discussed in Chapter 14.

TRAUMATIC SUBCUTANEOUS RUPTURE OF TENDONS

In a review of twenty patients with traumatic subcutaneous ruptures of tendons, Griffiths (1965) found most of the ruptures to be associated with open wounds. In his experience the extensor hallucis longus re-paired itself spontaneously. In one adult patient who had late repair of the posterior tibial tendon and in one who had late repair of the anterior tibial tendon, Griffiths found no functional impairment. He observed that after successful and early repair, complete functional recovery can generally be expected in adults. However, because of the plastic nature of the foot during childhood, late repair of these tendons causes deformity in children.

The two most commonly reported tendon ruptures of the foot are those of the tibialis anterior tendon and the tendo achillis.

Rupture of the anterior tibial tendon

Els (1910) was one of the first to report a rupture of the tibialis anterior tendon. Burman (1934) was first to report such a case in America. Lapidus (1941) reported two cases. Mensor and Ordway (1953) reported two cases and reviewed the published reports, of which only ten had appeared up to that time. Lipscomb and Kelly (1955) reported twelve cases of injuries to

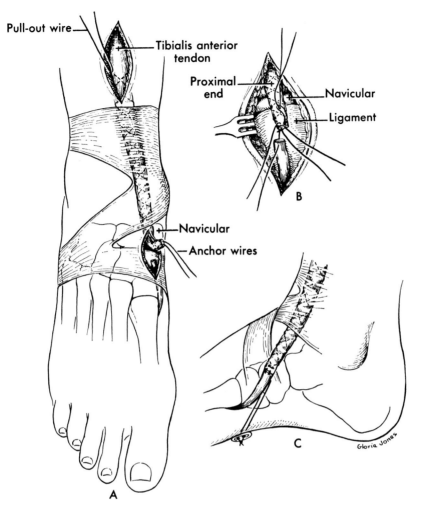

Fig. 7-26. Repair of ruptured tibialis anterior tendon. **A,** Incision over tibialis anterior tendon just above transverse crural ligament. Second incision over the insertion of the tibialis anterior. Tibialis anterior tendon pulled out through the first incision. Stainless steel wire threaded through the tendon from above downward. At the proximal end a pullout wire is looped under a threaded wire and the tendon is guided through its original channel. **B,** Fragmented ends sutured to each other. **C,** Both ends of stainless steel wire passed through plantar surface by means of Keith needle and tied to button.

the extensor tendons of the foot treated at the Mayo Clinic between 1938 and 1952; in nine of the cases the tibialis anterior tendon was involved.

Trauma causing avulsion may be powerful or mild. Usually it is caused by a fall or twisting of the ankle, especially when extreme plantar flexion is exerted. Sometimes the same area has been previously injured, probably with residual fraying of the

terminal end of the tendon, predisposing it to complete rupture.

Symptoms of a ruptured tibialis anterior tendon are sudden sharp pain and swelling over the first cuneiform, accompanied by an inability to coordinate normal foot motion. Dorsiflexion of the foot may be difficult, and there may be a tendency to stub the toes. A few days after injury, extensive ecchymosis may occur over the insertion of the tendon. On palpation, a rupture defect is observed in the tendon channel at the terminal end of the tibialis anterior. When edema subsides, the defect may become visible. The terminal end of the ruptured tendon feels like a bulbous mass.

Recommended treatment. To repair a ruptured tibialis anterior tendon, the following steps are performed:

1. Make an incision over the tibialis anterior tendon just above the transverse crural ligament.
2. Make a second incision over the insertion of the tibialis anterior tendon.
3. Pull out the tibialis anterior tendon through the first incision and thread a stainless steel wire through the tendon from above downward. At the proximal end of the threaded wire, loop a pullout wire.
4. Replace the wired tendon into its original tunnel.
5. Suture the frayed ends of the tendon to each other and to the periosteum and cortex of the first cuneiform.
6. Pass the stainless steel wires through the plantar skin surface by means of Keith needles and tie them to a button (Fig. 7-26). Bunnell (1964) may be credited with being the first to use the button innovation. Apply a boot cast for 6 weeks. After its removal cut the threaded wire at the bottom; the pullout wire permits extraction of the threaded wire.

Rupture of the tendo achillis

Fresh rupture of the calcaneal tendon is most often seen in men in their fifth decade. In a review of fifty-six cases Hooker (1963) noted the incidence of this entity in men with sedentary occupations who indulged occasionally in strenuous sports. The acute tendon rupture occurred significantly more often in the left leg than in the right leg. Histologic degeneration was evident in only some cases. Hooker's suggestion was that there were three main causes of rupture: (1) sudden extra strain on a taut tendon; (2) sudden passive stretching of a relaxed tendon into dorsiflexion; and (3) a direct blow over a taut tendon. Since pain is not always a constant factor, rupture is often unnoticed. There may or may not be a palpable gap and obvious impairment of plantar flexion in acute tendon rupture (Fig. 7-27).

Avulsion of the tendo achillis is seen frequently, even in the young. This is because of the unfavorable leverage of a long forefoot and a short posterior lever (Milgram, 1953). Rupture of the tendo achillis at its musculotendinous junction is seen more often in young persons, with the tendon fibers usually torn into irregular longitudinal strips near this junction.

Many surgical methods have been recorded for repair of this tendon. None have given perfect results; even after solid repair, residual weakness remains and adhesions often occur. Lea and Smith (1968) reported satisfactory results in eight cases treated nonsurgically. Their method of treatment consisted of a walking boot cast with the foot in gravity equinus position (without plantar flexion force) for 8 weeks, then crutches and a 2.5-cm. elevated heel for 4 weeks.

Rupture of the peroneus longus tendon

Traumatic subcutaneous rupture of the peroneus longus tendon is a rare condition caused by a sharp inversion force to the foot and ankle while the muscle is contracted. This injury may mimic an injury to the lateral collateral ligament of the ankle; the tenderness and swelling is at the same location, in the area of the lateral malleolus.

Griffiths (1965) reported four cases of nonspontaneous rupture of the peroneal tendon, which were all caused by lacerations. Three of the four ruptures occurred in children, and only one of these ruptures was repaired immediately. The two that were repaired late yielded unsatisfactory results consisting of supination deformities of the foot and failure of the first metatarsal to reach the ground during standing.

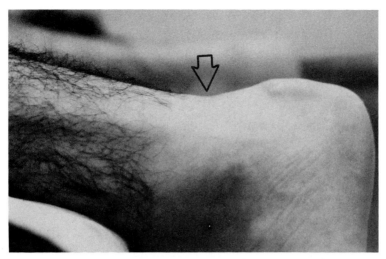

Fig. 7-27. Rupture of tendo achillis of left ankle showing palpable gap.

The adult had an immediate repair with satisfactory results. In the same article Griffiths reported a case of spontaneous rupture of the tibialis posterior tendon in an adult, which healed satisfactorily although it was never repaired.

In order to avoid a deformed foot it is mandatory that immediate repair be performed on children with rupture of the peroneus longus tendon. Since there are so few reports on the results of these ruptures, it is suggested that the condition in adults be repaired reasonably soon after the diagnosis has been made. It may be supposed that if a negative result were to occur in an adult from not repairing this tendon, it would be poor biomechanics of the foot caused by an inability to place the first metatarsal firmly on the ground just before push-off. This malfunction, in turn, would place added pressures upon the lateral portions of the foot, which could result in metatarsalgia or plantar callosities of the lateral metatarsals or both.

TENDON LUXATION

Tendon luxation is a slipping of a tendon from its natural groove. It is usually associated with congenital malformations and deformities; however, it may result from injury, arthritis, or malunited fractures. The most symptomatic tendon luxation of the foot is that of the peroneus longus.

Luxation of the peroneus longus tendon is caused by a poorly formed groove on the posterior surface of the lateral malleolus that permits the tendon of the peroneus longus to slip over it. It is characterized by recurrent episodes of sudden slipping of the peroneus longus tendon during walking. This slipping often makes the patient fall, because the peroneus longus goes immediately into spasm, thereby abducting and plantar flexing the foot. The condition can usually be reduced manually, but the attacks tend to recur with increasing frequency, because the lateral fibulocalcaneal ligament is stretched farther with each episode.

Treatment. At first occurrence the deformity is reduced and the foot immobilized for 5 to 8 weeks in a plaster cast. There are often no recurrences. If there are recurrences, surgical intervention is indicated.

Miscellaneous soft-tissue injuries of the foot

The purpose of this section is to discuss those soft-tissue injuries of the foot that have not been classified under previous headings and to investigate those condi-

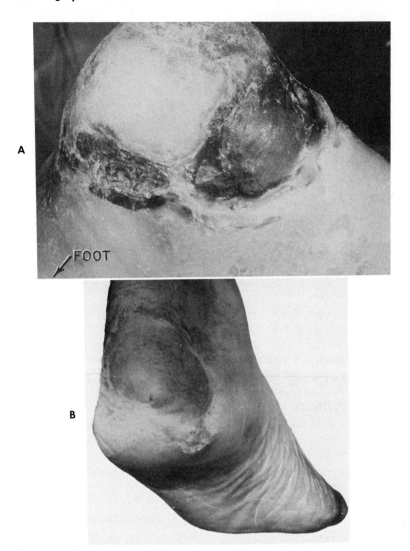

Fig. 7-28. A, Crush injury of heel showing full-thickness skin loss. **B,** Result of full-thickness, cross-leg, pedicle skin graft.

tions that are not a direct response to trauma but that may be associated with or be a sequela of trauma.

CRUSH INJURIES TO THE FOOT

A patient may complain of foot pain following an accident in which a heavy object landed on his foot, although there is no outward evidence of injury and roentgenograms show no fracture. In this case, a soft compression bandage should be applied and the foot should be elevated. Skin sloughing is to be expected (Fig. 7-28).

TRAUMATIC ULCERS

Traumatic ulcers may occur as a result of various types of sudden injury such as chemical, thermal, or mechanical injury. In the early stages they may be treated conservatively; however, for those that are accompanied by extensive skin damage and for those that become intractable, the grafting of skin on the area usually provides acceptable results. Murray and Goldwyn (1966) treated fifteen patients with intractable plantar ulcers by means of split grafts and pedicle flaps. In thirteen of the patients

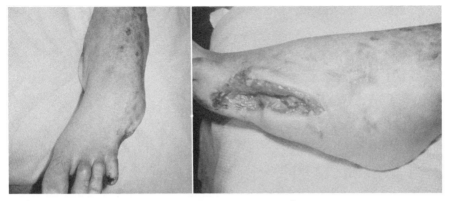

Fig. 7-29. Volkmann's ischemic contracture of foot resulting from injury to knee. The blood supply to the foot was compromised. Removal of a toe was necessary because of gangrene. Note deformity.

the results of these procedures were completely successful.

Traumatic ulcers are usually caused by excessive pressure on a weight-bearing area (see p. 340).

VOLKMANN'S ISCHEMIC CONTRACTURE

Contracture of one muscle or a group of muscles as a result of the replacement of the muscle cells by connective tissue is caused by an interference with the blood supply to the muscle involved. The condition is known as Volkmann's ischemic contracture (Fig. 7-29). A tourniquet or cast, especially over the arm, may cause the contracture by injury to a major artery. Trauma may be directly to the artery supplying the muscle or to a distal portion of the vessel, resulting in reflex vasospasm along its course through the leg. The foot is affected only indirectly.

Seddon (1966) found this condition to be more common in adults than in children. Monk (1966) reported a case of Volkmann's ischemic contracture of the lower extremity that resulted from a contusion to the calf muscles. He postulated that the contusion led to edema and decreased venous return, which ultimately led to a lack of blood supply to the muscles of the leg. The peripheral pulses in the foot remained, which demonstrated that the presence of

these pulses does not contraindicate appropriate treatment.

In the early stage the loss of blood supply produces necrosis (muscle sequestrum) in the body of the muscle. In time, fibrous connective tissue replaces dead muscle fibers. The fibrous connective tissue contracts and shortens, thereby producing a deformity of the limb.

This serious condition occurs frequently enough after injuries to the lower extremity to warrant a more determined effort to prevent it. Early signs of tenseness of the thigh or more commonly of the calf and anterior compartment, along with equinus of the foot and pain on attempted dorsiflexion of the foot, should alert the examiner to the possibility of impending ischemia. At this point all pressure should be released. Excision of the deep fascia and possibly evacuation of a hematoma beneath the muscle may save the threatened underlying structures. If the femoral or popliteal artery is injured, exploration and repair should be performed immediately.

Treatment for an already contracted lower extremity is simple because there is so little to be done. It is primarily directed toward overcoming the deformity, for it is unlikely that the muscle fibers can be revived. Treatment consists of prolonged stretching, tendon lengthening or sectioning of the contracted muscle. Amputation may be necessary.

REFERENCES

Anderson, K. J., and Lecocq, J. F.: Operative treatment of injury to the fibular collateral ligament of the ankle, J. Bone Joint Surg., **36-A:** 825-832, July 1954.

Anderson, K. J., Lecocq, J. F., and Lecocq, E. A.: Recurrent anterior subluxation of the ankle joint: A report of two cases and an experimental study, J. Bone Joint Surg. 34-A:853-860, Oct. 1952.

Artz, C. P., and Reiss, E.: The treatment of burns, Philadelphia, 1957, W. B. Saunders Co.

Bennett, J. E., and Dingman, R. O.: Evaluation of burn depth by the use of radioactive isotopes—an experimental study, Plast. Reconstr. Surg. 20:261-272, 1957.

Berridge, F. R., and Bonnin, J. G.: The radiographic examination of the ankle joint including arthrography, Surg. Gynec. Obstet. 79:383-389, Oct. 1944.

Bigelow, W. G.: The modern conception and treatment of frostbite, Canad. Med. Assoc. J. 47:529-534, Dec. 1942.

Blair, J. R., Schatzki, R., and Orr, K. D.: Sequelae to cold injury in one hundred patients, J.A.M.A. 163:1203-1208, Apr. 1957.

Bonnin, J.: The hypermobile ankle, Proc. Roy. Soc. Med. 37:282-286, Apr. 1944.

Bosien, W. R., Staples, O. S., and Russell, S. W.: Residual disability following acute ankle sprains, J. Bone Joint Surg. 37-A:1237-1243, Dec. 1955.

Brahms, M. A.: Common foot problems, J. Bone Joint Surg. 49-A:1653-1664, Dec. 1967.

Brown, J. R.: Localization of foreign bodies, Ohio Med. J. 54:908-909, 1958.

Brownrigg, G. M.: Frostbite in shipwrecked mariners, Amer. J. Surg. 59:232-247, Feb. 1943.

Bunnell's surgery of the hand, ed. 4, (revised by Joseph H. Boyes), Philadelphia, 1964, J. B. Lippincott Co.

Burman, M. S.: Subcutaneous rupture of the tendon of the tibialis anticus, Ann. Surg. 100:368-372, 1934.

Cohen, H., and Reid, J. B.: Tenosynovitis crepitans associated with oxaluria, Liverpool Med. Chir. J. 43:193-199, 1935.

D'Anca, A. F.: Lateral rotatory dislocation of the ankle without fracture, J. Bone Joint Surg. **52-A:** 1643-1646, Dec. 1970.

Dickinson, P. H., Coutts, M. B., Woodward, E. P., and Handler, D.: Tendo achillis bursitis, J. Bone Joint Surg. 48-A:77-81, Jan. 1966.

Dziob, J. M.: Ligamentous injuries about the ankle joint, Amer. J. Surg. 91:692-698, Apr. 1956.

Edwards, E. A., and Leeper, R. W.: Frostbite: An analysis of seventy-one cases, J.A.M.A. **149:** 1199-1205, July 1952.

Els, H.: Uber eine Abrissfraktur des Tibialis-anticus-Ansatzes, Dtsch. Z. Chir. 106:610-613, 1910.

Fausel, E. G., and Hemphill, J. A.: Study of the late symptoms of cases of immersion foot, Surg., Gynec. Obstet. 81:500-503, 1945.

Fordyce, A. J. W., and Horn, C. V.: Arthrography in recent injuries of the ligaments of the ankle, J. Bone Joint Surg. 54-B:116-121, Feb. 1972.

Freeman, M. A. R.: Instability of the foot after injuries to the lateral ligament of the ankle, J. Bone Joint Surg. 47-B:669-677, Nov. 1965.

Freeman, M. A. R.: Treatment of ruptures of the lateral ligament of the ankle, J. Bone Joint Surg. **47-B:**661-668, Nov. 1965.

Ghormley, R. K., and Spear, I. M.: Anomalies of the posterior tibial tendon: A cause of persistent pain about ankle, Arch. Surg. (Chicago) 66: 512-516, Apr. 1953.

Gillespie, H., and Boucher, P.: Watson-Jones repair of lateral instability of the ankle, J. Bone Joint Surg. 53-A:920-924, July 1971.

Glick, J. M.: A study of ligamentous looseness and its relation to injury, Proc. LeRoy Abbott Orthop. Soc. 1:34-39, May 1971.

Glick, J. M., and Katch, L.: Musculoskeletal injuries in jogging, Arch. Phys. Med. 51:123-126, Mar. 1970.

Gordon, R. B.: Arthrography of the ankle joint, J. Bone Joint Surg. 52-A:1623-1631, Dec. 1970.

Griffiths, J. C.: Tendon injuries around the ankle, J. Bone Joint Surg. 47-B:686-689, Nov. 1965.

Gunn, D. R.: Stenosing tenosynovitis of the common peroneal tendon sheath, Brit. Med. J. 1: 691-692, Mar. 1959.

Hermann, G., Schechter, D. C., Owens, J. C., and Starzl, T. E.: The problem of frostbite in civilian medical practice, Surg. Clin. N. Amer. 43: 519-536, Apr. 1963.

Hirata, I.: The doctor and the athlete, Philadelphia, 1968, J. B. Lippincott Co.

Hooker, C. H.: Rupture of the tendo calcaneus, J. Bone Joint Surg. 45-B:360-363, May 1963.

Hughes, J. R.: Sprains and subluxations of ankle-joint, Proc. Roy Soc. Med. 35:765-766, Oct. 1942.

Jennett, W. B., and Watson, J. A.: The radio-opacity of glass foreign bodies, with report of a case of injury of the cauda equina by fragments of glass, Brit. J. Surg. 46:244-246, 1958.

Keck, S. W., and Kelly, P. J.: Bursitis of the posterior part of the heel, J. Bone Joint Surg. 47-A: 267-273, Mar. 1965.

Kelly, R. P.: Ankle injuries, Kentucky Med. J. **50:** 281-288, July 1952.

Knize, D. M., Weatherley-White, R. C. A., Paton, B. C., and Owens, J. C.: Prognostic factors in the management of frostbite, J. Trauma 9:749-759, Sept. 1969.

Landeros, O., Frost, H. M., and Higgins, C. C.: Post-traumatic anterior ankle instability, Clin. Orthop. 56:169-178, Jan.-Feb. 1968.

Lapidus, P. W.: Indirect subcutaneous rupture of the anterior tibial tendon: Report of two cases, Bull. N. Y. Hosp. Joint Dis. 2:119-127, July 1941.

Lapidus, P. W., and Seidenstein, H.: Chronic non-specific tenosynovitis with effusion about the ankle, J. Bone Joint Surg. 32-A:175-179, Jan. 1950.

Lea, R. B., and Smith, L.: Ruptures of the Achilles tendon: Nonsurgical treatment, Clin. Orthop. 60:115-118, 1968.

Leonard, M. H.: Injuries of the lateral ligaments of the ankle: A clinical and experimental study, J. Bone Joint Surg. 31-A:373-377, Apr. 1949.

Lewis, T.: Observations on some normal and injurious effects of cold upon the skin and underlying tissues: Frostbite, Brit. Med. J. 2:869-871, Dec. 1941.

Lipscomb, P. R.: Nonsuppurative tenosynovitis and paratendinitis. In American Academy of Orthopaedic Surgeons: Instructional Course Lectures, vol. 7, 1950, pp. 254-261.

Lipscomb, P. R., and Kelly, P. J.: Injuries of the extensor tendons in the distal part of the leg and in the ankle, J. Bone Joint Surg. 37-A:1206-1213, Dec. 1955.

London, P. S.: The burnt foot, Brit. J. Surg. 40:293-304, Jan. 1953.

McMaster, P. E.: Treatment of ankle sprain: Observations in more than five hundred cases, J.A.M.A. 122:659-660, July 1943.

Mensor, M. C., and Ordway, G. L.: Traumatic subcutaneous rupture of the tibialis anterior tendon, J. Bone Joint Surg. 35-A:675-680, Oct. 1953.

Meyers, M. B.: Prediction of skin sloughs at the time of operation with the use of fluorescein dye, Surgery 51:158-162, Feb. 1962.

Milgram, J. E.: Muscle ruptures and avulsions, with particular reference to the lower extremities. In American Academy of Orthopaedic Surgeons: Instructional Course Lectures, vol.

10, Ann Arbor, 1953, J. W. Edwards, pp. 233-243.

Monk, C. J. E.: Traumatic ischaemia of the calf, J. Bone Joint Surg. 48-B:150-152, Feb. 1966.

Moorhead, J. J.: Locating and removing foreign bodies, Amer. J. Surg. 95:108-124, Jan. 1958.

Murray, J. E., and Goldwyn, R. M.: Definitive treatment of intractable plantar ulcers, J.A.M.A. 196:311-314, Apr. 1966.

Parvin, R. W., and Ford, L. T.: Stenosing tenosynovitis of the common peroneal tendon sheath, J. Bone Joint Surg. 38-A:1352-1357, Dec. 1956.

Percy, E. C., Hill, R. O., and Callaghan, J. E.: The "sprained" ankle, J. Trauma, 9:972-985, Dec. 1969.

Randolph, J. G., Leape, L. L., and Gross, R. E.: The early surgical treatment of burns. I. Experimental studies utilizing intravenous vital dye for determining the degree of injury, Surgery 56:193-201, July 1964.

Roberts, W. C.: Radiographic characteristics of glass, Arch. Ind. Health 18:470-472, 1958.

Seddon, H. J.: Volkmann's ischaemia in the lower limb, J. Bone Joint Surg. 48-B:627-636, Nov. 1966.

Standard nomenclature of athletic injuries. Prepared by the Subcommittee on Classification of Sports Injuries, American Medical Association, Committee on the Medical Aspects of Sports. Chicago, 1966, American Medical Association, pp. 99-101.

Thorndike, A.: Athletic injuries: Prevention, diagnosis, and treatment, Philadelphia, 1962, Lea & Febiger.

Ungley, C. C.: Treatment of immersion foot by dry cooling, Lancet 1:681-682, May 1943.

Vinson, H. A., and Schatzki, R.: Roentgenologic bone changes encountered in frostbite, Korea 1950-51, Radiology 63:685-694, Nov. 1954.

Webster, D. R., Woolhouse, F. M., and Johnston, J. L.: Immersion foot, J. Bone Joint Surg. 24:785-794, Oct. 1942.

Williams, R.: Chronic non-specific tendovaginitis of tibialis posterior, J. Bone Joint Surg. 45-B:542-545, Aug. 1963.

8

Acquired nontraumatic deformities of the foot

Henri L. DuVries

The foot, more than any other skeletal unit, is subject to static deformities. Its weight-transmitting and propulsive functions are restricted daily by nonyielding foot covering. Anatomic variation in the shape and stability of the joint surfaces may predispose, resist, or modify the deforming force of such footwear.

Modern civilization disregards the physiology of the foot. Fashion and eye appeal rather than function determine shoe design, especially in its forepart, where most disabilities and deformities of the foot occur. It is probably because the styles of women's footwear are more extreme than those of men that 80 percent of all forefoot problems occur in women. Men also are guilty of wearing ill-fitting shoes (Fig. 8-1), but do so to a lesser degree.

The restrictive force of poorly fitting shoes produces little deformity on the tarsus because the tarsus is made up of short heavy bones, and normal movement in the tarsal joints is limited inasmuch as the articular surfaces of the tarsal joints are comparatively flat. However, the phalanges and metatarsals are long thin bones with a normally wide range of joint motion. Restrictive force on these bones may produce most of the static deformities of the forefoot, such as most first metatarsophalangeal joint deformities, including hammertoe, tailor's bunion, overlapping toes, and many

other conditions that are deviations from the normal.

The human foot is uniquely specialized. The metatarsals and toes allow man to stand erect. The versatility of the forefoot permits him to retain his upright stance and gives him grace in walking, dancing, and athletics.

A well-developed, strong foot withstands surprising abuse; morbid changes take place only when maltreatment becomes excessive. An underdeveloped and frail foot may fail under ordinary stress and strain.

INCIDENCE AND CAUSE OF FOOT DISORDERS

Between 40 and 50 percent of civilized society has, or will have, some foot disorder. Of all disorders of the foot, 90 percent occur in the forefoot and are essentially induced by ill-fitting shoes. The forefoot is a modified square (Fig. 8-2, *A*). We have been endeavoring to educate people to this fact for many years. The forepart of a shoe, however, is generally triangular instead of conforming to the shape of the foot (Fig. 8-2, *B*). Obviously a square cannot be forced into a triangle, yet history tells us that for many thousand of years man has been forcing his foot into triangular-shaped coverings. Ordinarily shoes are without elasticity. Living tissue, however, yields to unrelenting restriction and pres-

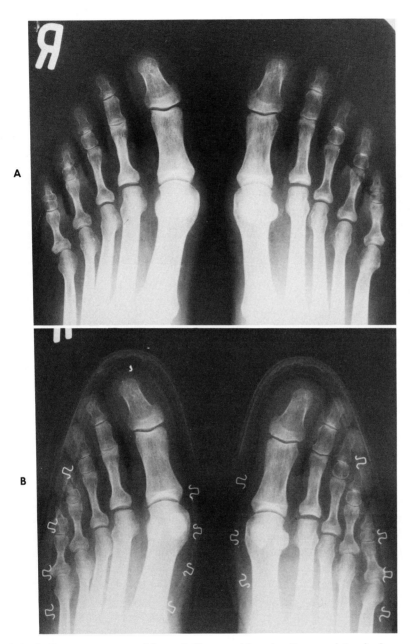

Fig. 8-1. A, Roentgenogram of feet of 42-year-old male. He complained of vague pain in the forefoot. (As a rule the forefeet are modified squares; these are more oblique than usual.) **B,** Same feet in shoes.

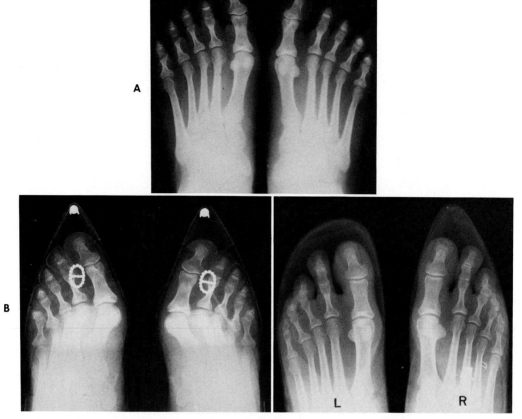

Fig. 8-2. A, Roentgenogram of average normal feet of young woman during weight bearing. **B,** Same feet in shoes during weight bearing. Note that she is developing hallux valgus. **C,** Feet in different types of shoes. Left shoe permits freedom of forefoot function. Right shoe restricts function of the four lesser toes as each step is taken.

sure, even though it is mild. The foot accommodates itself gradually to the shape of the shoe, and deformities result in accordance with Wolff's law, which maintains that "primary changes in form and function are followed by determinable changes in the outer shape and the inner architecture of the involved bone."[*]

DEFORMITIES OF THE FIRST METATARSOPHALANGEAL JOINT

The most frequent severely disabling affliction of the forefoot involves the first metatarsophalangeal joint. Anatomically this joint is the most complex part of the forefoot (Fig. 8-3); it is composed of relatively large bones with powerful intrinsic muscles inserted into the base of the proximal phalanx. It also is influenced in its function by the extensor and flexor hallucis longus, the tibialis anterior, and the peroneus longus. It plays a major role in the transmission of body weight in locomotion. General diseases, such as gout, rheumatoid arthritis, and neuropathies of the foot, have a predilection for this joint.

Bunions

According to the twenty-fourth edition of *Dorland's Illustrated Medical Dictionary*

---

[*]Weinmann, J. P., and Sicher, H.: Bone and bones: Fundamentals of bone biology, ed. 2, St. Louis, 1955, The C. V. Mosby Co., p. 174.

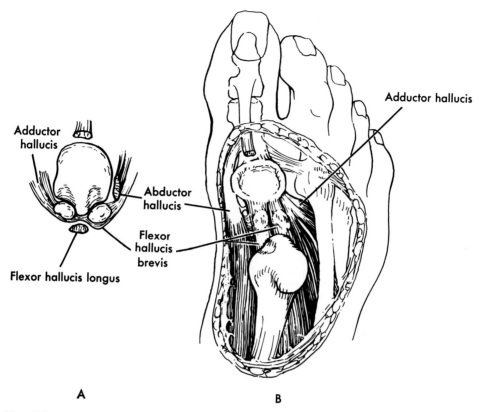

Adductor hallucis

Adductor hallucis

Abductor hallucis

Flexor hallucis brevis

Flexor hallucis longus

A

B

Fig. 8-3. A, Cross section through metatarsophalangeal joint demonstrating relation of sesamoids and tendons to first metatarsal head. **B,** Dorsal view of first metatarsophalangeal joint with toes in plantar flexion.

the term "bunion," derived from the Latin *bunio* meaning "turnip," has been confusingly misapplied to disorders of the first metatarsophalangeal joint. The term is often loosely used to connote any enlargement or deformity of this joint and has included such diverse conditions as ganglion, a congenitally wide head of the first metatarsal, hallux valgus, hallux rigidus, proliferation of the dorsum of the first metatarsophalangeal joint (dorsal bunion), and proliferative change secondary to arthritides. Hallux valgus, which is itself a symptom complex, is the most common and most disabling group of deformities included under the heading "bunion." When applied to the fifth metatarsal head (bunionette, or tailor's bunion), bunion has been misapplied to connote lateral bending of the head, congenitally wide head, and

chronic thickening of soft structures over the head. As a corollary, "bunionectomy" is an equally unscientific term.

The numerous disorders in this category will be considered separately.

Cogenitally wide first metatarsal head. A congenitally wide first metatarsal head (Fig. 8-4) often becomes a pressure area on the medial side of the great toe joint. Whether or not it is associated with hallux valgus, it may become a problem. The medial side becomes the most prominent point on the inner surface of the foot, creating a fulcrum for pressure by footwear and resulting in a chronic inflammatory process of the synovial structures over the area. The inflammation produces a further thickening of the synovia and enlargement of the prominence.

Symptoms. The symptoms of a congen-

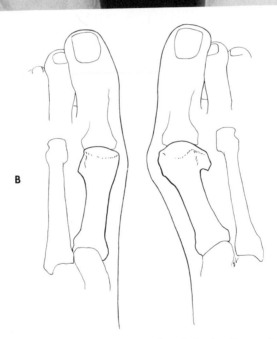

Fig. 8-4. *Left,* Normally shaped metatarsal head. *Right,* Congenitally wide metatarsal head in foot of same person.

itally wide first metatarsal head are chronic pain and swelling over the medial side. A shoe cut out over this area gives relief, but treatment requires amputation of the tibial condylar process of the first metatarsal head (Fig. 8-5). Occasionally, an enlargement of the tibial side of the first metatarsal head (bunion) forms because of the congenitally wide head, with little or no hallux valgus. Such cases require surgical correction.

Technique for reduction. The technique for reduction is as follows:

1. Make a semilunar incision with its vertex extending dorsally from the middle of the tibial side of the first

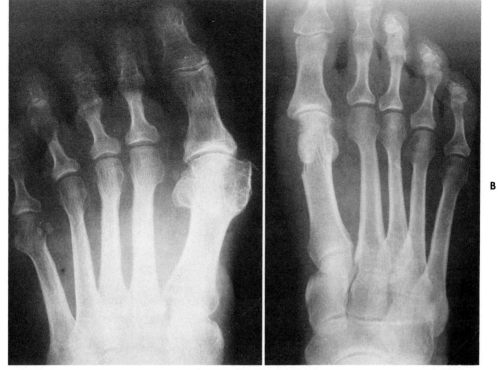

Fig. 8-5. A, Congenitally wide first metatarsal head showing some osteophytic change as result of pressure. **B,** Postoperative roentgenogram of condylectomy for wide first metatarsal head.

proximal phalanx to a point about 3 cm. proximal to the head on the tibial side of the first metatarsal.

2. Dissect and free the skin flap formed to expose the tibial side of the great toe joint.

3. Excise all excess hypertrophied or adventitious bursal tissue.

4. Make a longitudinal incision in the mediodorsal aspect of the joint capsule, dissecting it from the head of the first metatarsal.

5. Retract the capsule with the skin flap, exposing the tibial condyle of the first metatarsal head.

6. Sever the metatarsophalangeal interarticular ligament and deliver the metatarsal head dorsomedially from the wound with a periosteal or Chandler elevator.

7. The condylar ridge on the articular surface of the metatarsal head is an ideal landmark for removal of the tibial condylar process. Use a straight nasal saw or osteotome. Then round the sharp margins with a Joseph nasal rasp.

8. Make certain that the insertion of the abductor hallucis tendon is intact. If it is not, repair it; otherwise, the patient will develop a postoperative hallux valgus.

9. Suture the capsule and skin in layers, and apply a compression bandage.

Ambulation may begin in 24 hours. Full use of the joint is usually possible in 3 to 4 weeks. Complications and disability are minimal.

Hallux valgus. Lateral deviation of the great toe, with medial prominence of the head of the first metatarsal, is technically classified as hallux valgus. The deformity is actually a static partial dislocation or subluxation of the first metatarsophalangeal joint that occurs with or without an accompanying painful soft-tissue reaction over the medial prominence (bunion). It is one of the most common complaints of persons who wear shoes. In addition to the obvious outward deviation of the great toe, concomitant skeletal abnormalities are present. The hallux valgus is accompanied by rotation of the phalanges around their longitudinal axes; roentgenographic studies reveal additional abnormalities. There is always a varus deformity and a longitudinal rotation of the first metatarsal. A variable amount of periosteal reaction on the medial side of the head of the metatarsal is usually present.

With increasing angulation of the metatarsophalangeal joint, two displacements of the sesamoids occur. These displacements can be better comprehended if one considers the sesamoids to be more related anatomically and functionally to the proximal phalanx than to the head of the first metatarsal. The head of the first metatarsal, with increasing valgus, progressively moves medially off the sesamoids, which retain their essential relationship with the proximal phalanx. With this concept in mind, the proximal displacement of the fibular sesamoid and the distal displacement of the tibial sesamoid, which are often seen in standard roentgenographic views of the foot, are easily understood. Furthermore, as the ligamentous structures in which the sesamoids are embedded become bow-stringed across the joint, the sesamoids are displaced laterally. Thus, the fibular sesamoid appears to be located in the metatarsal interspace as a result of two factors: longitudinal rotation of the ray and actual lateral displacement.

Etiology. Since hallux valgus occurs almost exclusively in people who wear shoes, all investigators agree that the shoe must be an important etiologic factor. It is in-

teresting to note, however, that even among unshod people, hallux valgus, although infrequent, has been reported to occur.[*]

While it appears that the shoe may be an essential element in the causation of hallux valgus, the fact remains that many individuals who wear modern footwear do not develop this deformity. There must be predisposing factors that make some feet more vulnerable to the effects of footwear and cause some unshod feet to exhibit a tendency toward the development of hallux valgus. Rare cases of hallux valgus seen in children (juvenile type) may also be explained by these predisposing factors.

While there is no doubt that the various skeletal abnormalities mentioned above are all present in the full-blown case of hallux valgus, various authors have seized upon single aspects of the deformity and have cited them as major etiologic factors. These may be summarized under separate headings.

SHOES. That modern footwear is the principal contributor to the development of hallux valgus appears to be a certainty. A study of shoe-wearing and non–shoe-wearing individuals of the same genetic background by Lam Sim-Fook and Hodgson (1958) revealed that 33 percent of the shod individuals demonstrated some degree of hallux valgus as compared with 1.9 percent among the unshod. All studies that provide statistical data on the frequency of hallux valgus among shoe-wearing populations report that it is more frequent in females than in males. Wilkins (1941), in a study of feet with reference to schoolchildren, reported a proportion of 2 to 1 in the general population. Those reporting from surveys made among male and female recruits (Marwil and Brantingham, 1943; Hewitt et al., 1953) place the proportion at approximately 3 to 1, while authors whose statistics were obtained from clinical practice report the proportion to be 15 to 1 (Creer, 1938; Hardy

[*]See Engle and Morton, 1931; Wells, 1931; Barnicot and Hardy, 1955; Lam Sim-Fook and Hodgson, 1958; Shine, 1965; and Maclennan, 1966.

and Clapham, 1951). Certainly the shoes worn by females are less physiologic than those worn by males, and shoes of any type are prone to lead to hallux valgus in susceptible individuals (Figs. 8-1 and 8-2).

PES PLANUS. The tendency for the pronated foot to develop a hallux valgus has been noted by several observers.* Hohmann (1925) was the most definite; he asserted that hallux valgus is always combined with pes valgus and that pes valgus is always the causative factor in hallux valgus.

In general, the role played by pronation of the foot in the life history of hallux valgus has received little attention in the world literature, yet the effect of pronation as a possible initiating factor is readily demonstrated in any normal foot, as depicted in Figs. 8-6 to 8-10.

In Fig. 8-6 a pendulum has been glued to the nail of the big toe. As the foot is

*See Ewald, 1912; Mayo, 1920; Stein, 1938; Galland and Jordan, 1938; Rogers and Joplin, 1947; Joplin, 1950; and Craigmile, 1953.

pronated the rotation of the first ray around its longitudinal axis is clearly shown. In Fig. 8-7 a skeletal model has been photographed. Note that with longitudinal rotation of the first metatarsal the fibular sesamoid becomes visible on the lateral side of the first metatarsal head. In Fig. 8-8 a dorsoventral weight-bearing roentgenogram is shown of the same foot as in Fig. 8-6. Note that in the pronated position the sesamoids appear to have been displaced laterally. The fibular sesamoid is now visible in the interval between the first and second metatarsals, as one would anticipate from viewing the skeletal model in Fig. 8-7. That this appearance is due solely to the longitudinal rotation of the first metatarsal and not to an actual lateral displacement is revealed in tangential roentgenograms of the foot, in which it is seen that the sesamoids remain in a normal relationship to their facets located on the plantar surface of the metatarsal head (Fig. 8-9). In Fig 8-10 the distribution of weight bearing through the sole of the foot is demonstrated by the barograph. Note that in the pronated foot the area of weight bearing transmitted through

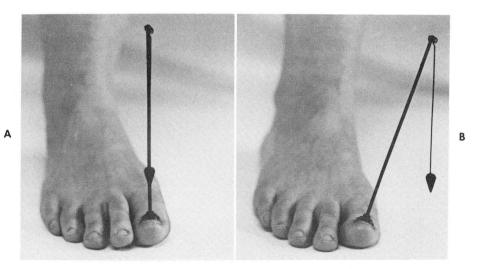

Fig. 8-6. Demonstration of longitudinal rotation of first ray with supination and pronation of foot. A pendulum is glued to the nail of the great toe. **A,** Foot supinated. **B,** Foot pronated.

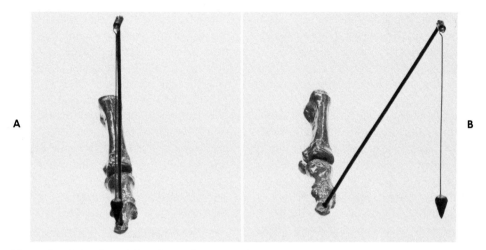

Fig. 8-7. Skeletal model with pendulum. With rotation of the first ray the lateral articular surfaces of the metatarsal head and fibular sesamoid, which cannot be seen in **A,** become clearly visible on the lateral side when the ray is rotated.

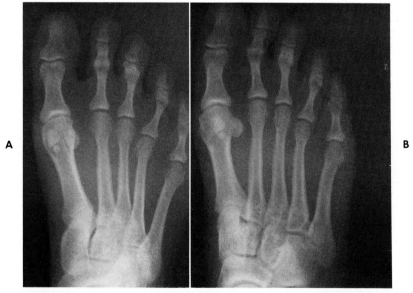

Fig. 8-8. Standard dorsoventral roentgenograms of foot shown in Fig. 8-6 during weight bearing. **A,** Foot supinated. **B,** Foot pronated. Note the apparent lateral displacement of the sesamoids.

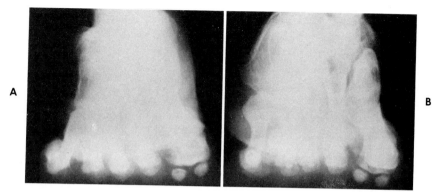

Fig. 8-9. Tangential views showing sesamoids of same foot during weight bearing. **A,** Foot supinated. **B,** Foot pronated. The degree of longitudinal rotation of the metatarsal is clearly demonstrated by the position of the sesamoids, which still retain a normal relationship to their facets on the underside of the metatarsal head.

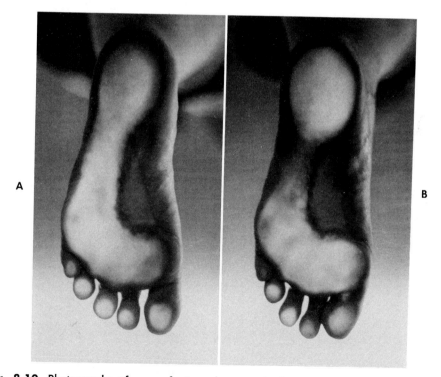

Fig. 8-10. Photographs of same foot on barograph during weight bearing. **A,** Foot supinated. **B,** Foot pronated. Note that the pressure area on the great toe has moved medially and has produced a mild hallux valgus.

the big toe has been displaced medially and a degree of hallux valgus has been created.

Pronation of the foot imposes a longitudinal rotation on the first ray (metatarsal and phalanges). This rotation places the axis of the metatarsophalangeal joint in an oblique plane relative to the floor. In this position it appears to be less able to withstand the deforming pressures exerted upon it either by the shoe or by weight bearing. Unfortunately there are no data available on the relationship between the degree of pes planus and the degree of hallux valgus in the small percentage of unshod individuals who develop this condition. Furthermore, those authors who have noted a relationship between pes planus and hallux valgus in shod individuals have presented no quantitative data.

METATARSUS VARUS. The concomitant occurrence of hallux valgus and metatarsus varus has been noted by almost all clinicians. In a careful statistical study of patients with hallux valgus, Hardy and Clapham (1951) found that of all the possible correlations between various measurements on the foot, the correlation between the degree of hallux valgus and the size of the intermetatarsal angle was by far the "most striking" (coefficient, 0.71). This study confirmed that hallux valgus and metatarsus varus go together. The question is still unanswered as to which one is the cause and which the result. Ewald (1912), while emphasizing the relationship, stated categorically that the "primary source" of hallux valgus was metatarsus varus of the first metatarsal. Truslow (1925) claims to have presented a new name, "metatarsus primus varus," for a congenital abnormality which, if present, inevitably results in hallux valgus when the individual is forced to wear shoes. However, the studies of Hardy and Clapham (1951) and Craigmile (1953) on schoolchildren seem to indicate that the metatarsus varus is secondary to the hallux valgus. In either case, any surgeon who is considering an operative correction of this deformity should be aware of the close relationship between the degree of metatarsus varus and hallux valgus.

LENGTH OF FIRST METATARSAL. Based upon minimal anthropometric data and unsubstantiated by mathematical analysis, both a short first metatarsal (Morton, 1935) and a long first metatarsal (Mayo, 1908, 1920) have been proposed as essential factors in the development of hallux valgus (Fig.

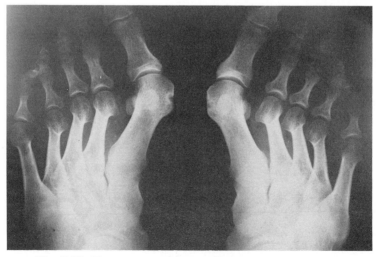

Fig. 8-11. First metatarsal longer than second metatarsal.

8-11). It appears to me that the relationship between metatarsal length and the development of hallux valgus is fortuitous and is not a direct etiologic factor.

ANATOMIC AND PHYSIOLOGIC VARIATIONS IN MUSCLES. There appears to be no question that in the presence of the typical skeletal deformities seen in the case of marked hallux valgus, an alteration in the action of the intrinsic and extrinsic muscles is acting upon the components of the first ray. It seems reasonable to believe that these al-

terations in muscular action may expedite an increasing deformity. However, whether anatomic variations in the muscles or abnormalities in their function are basic etiologic factors remains unproved. Only Kaplan (1955) has described a constant anatomic variation occurring in routinely dissected cadaver feet. In those laboratory specimens that demonstrated a definite hallux valgus, he reported that the tendon of the tibialis posterior muscle was "thicker" than in normal feet and possessed an ex-

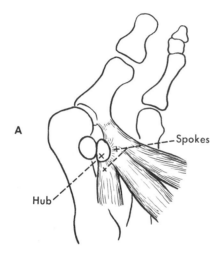

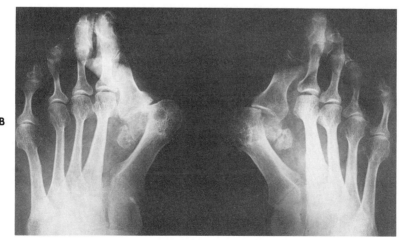

Fig. 8-12. A, Pulling off the proximal phalanx from first metatarsal head by conjoined tendon of adductor hallucis and fibular portion of flexor hallucis brevis tendon. **B,** Roentgenogram of actual case. The adductor hallicus has pulled the proximal phalanx off the first metatarsal head.

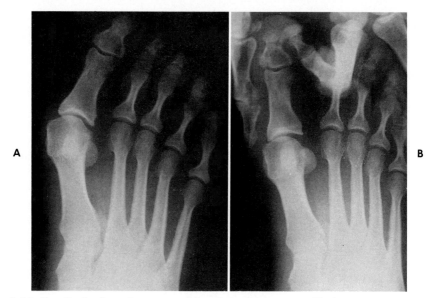

Fig. 8-13. Peculiarly shaped metatarsal head. It slopes on its fibular aspect to produce congenital hallux valgus. **A,** Normal articulation of joint. **B,** Hallux held in straight line by assistant. Note the gap in the articular surface at the fibular side of this joint.

tension of its insertion into the lateral head of the flexor hallucis brevis. This condition was not present in feet without hallux valgus.

The evidence to date is too meager to evaluate the role of the muscles alone in the production of hallux valgus. One has the intuitive feeling that the muscular variations are only one component among several which make some feet more prone than others to develop hallux valgus. However, when the deformity begins and progresses, the conjoined tendon around the fibular sesamoid becomes an important element in producing the deformity (Fig. 8-12).

MISCELLANEOUS FACTORS. Several additional factors have been suggested that may contribute to or resist the development of hallux valgus. These consist of roentgenographic variations in the appearance of the first metatarsophalangeal and first metatarsocuneiform articulations in dorsoventral views of the foot (Figs. 8-13 to 8-16). These differences may or may not be real, since the rotation of the first ray may produce apparent anatomic variations that are

caused by the projection of the articulation onto the single dorsoventral plane. Some variations in the shape of the first metatarsal head and the angle of articulation of the first metatarsal–medial cuneiform joint that may contribute to or resist deformity of the first metatarsophalangeal joint are seen in Figs. 8-15 and 8-17.

Amputation of the second toe will usually be followed by hallux valgus (Fig. 8-18).

Flaccid ligaments and poor musculature have been cited as causative factors of hallux valgus. It appears more likely that flaccidity is not the direct etiologic factor, but that the flaccid effect is produced by a generalized weak foot.

Regardless of the initiating factors of hallux valgus, the pathologic anatomy in a full-blown case is clear. The concomitant valgus position of the phalanges and the varus displacement of the first metatarsal are obvious in the two cases of hallux valgus shown in Fig. 8-19. This combination results in a lateral luxation of the metatarsophalangeal articulation. The medial half

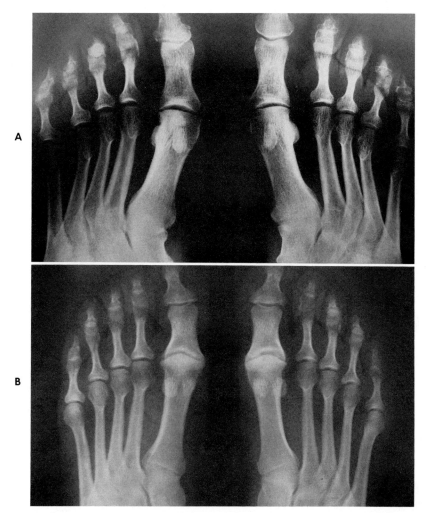

Fig. 8-14. A, Flat type of metatarsal head. This type resists hallux valgus deformity. **B,** Peculiarly shaped metatarsal heads. This type resists movement of the great toe into valgus.

of the metatarsal head becomes unduly prominent and is subject to externally applied pressure.

A massive adventitious bursa over the deformity, as shown in Fig. 8-19, *B,* is rare, although ganglionic cysts occasionally do accompany hallux valgus (Fig. 8-19, *A*). Such cysts may also occur in this area in the absence of hallux valgus.

The degree of longitudinal rotation of the metatarsal is indicated by the appearance of the lateral edge of the articular surface of the metatarsal head in the dorsoventral

roentgenographic projection and is also shown by the apparent lateral displacement of the sesamoids. Fig. 8-20 shows the relationship of the sesamoids under the first metatarsal head in a normal foot and in a foot with hallux valgus. Besides the abnormalities seen in Fig. 8-19, a lateral migration of the long flexor and extensor tendons, contractures of the adductor hallucis, and an altered direction of pull of the flexor hallucis brevis and the abductor hallucis occur as depicted in Fig. 8-21.

Over 100 surgical procedures for the

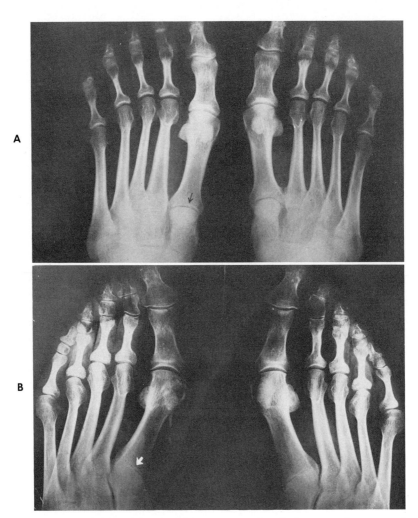

Fig. 8-15. A, Articulation of base of first metatarsal with first cuneiform at right angle, resisting hallux valgus. **B,** Articulation of base of first metatarsal with first cuneiform at obtuse angle, permitting hallux valgus.

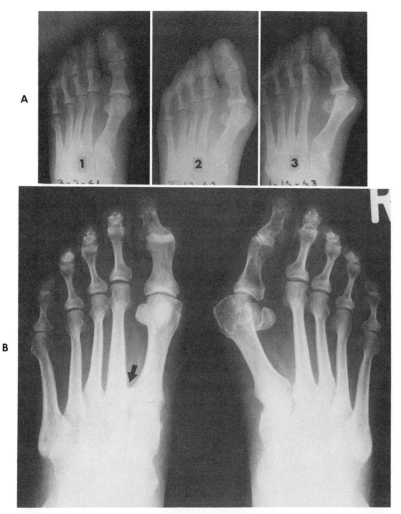

Fig. 8-16. A, Rapidly developing hallux valgus in foot of 55-year-old woman. *1,* Roentgenograms taken to explain pain at base of first metatarsal. No tenable diagnosis was made. *2,* Roentgenogram 1 year later. Hallux valgus with moderate articular changes in the first metatarsocuneiform joint is shown. *3,* Roentgenogram 1 year after this. Increase in hallux valgus and definite osteoarthritic change in the first metatarsocuneiform joint had occurred. **B,** *Left,* Congenital synostosis at bases of first and second metatarsals preventing hallux valgus. *Right,* Absence of congenital anomaly permitting hallux valgus deformity.

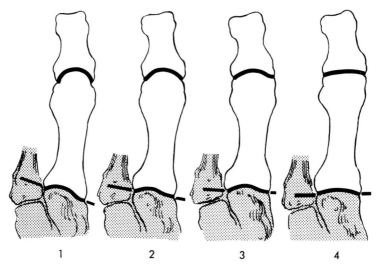

Fig. 8-17. Variations in shape of first metatarsal head and angle of articulation of first metatarsal–medial cuneiform joint of right foot. These may contribute to or resist deformity of the first metatarsophalangeal joint.

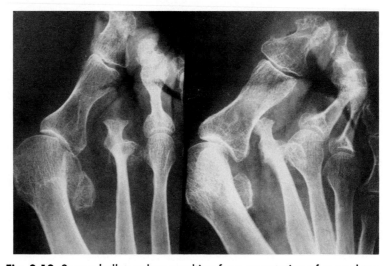

Fig. 8-18. Severe hallux valgus resulting from amputation of second toe.

treatment of hallux valgus have been described in the world literature. These vary from simple bunionectomies with capsular plication to more extensive operations such as tendon sectioning or transfers, resections of bony components, arthrodeses of joints (particularly the first metatarsocuneiform joint), and osteotomies of the first metatarsal. Before the surgeon chooses a definitive

surgical procedure, he should examine the entire foot carefully, paying particular attention to the foot during weight bearing. The presence of pes valgus as it contributes to the rotation of the first ray in producing apparent displacement of the sesamoids (shown on the dorsoventral roentgenogram) should be evaluated. The degree of metatarsus varus should be considered, along

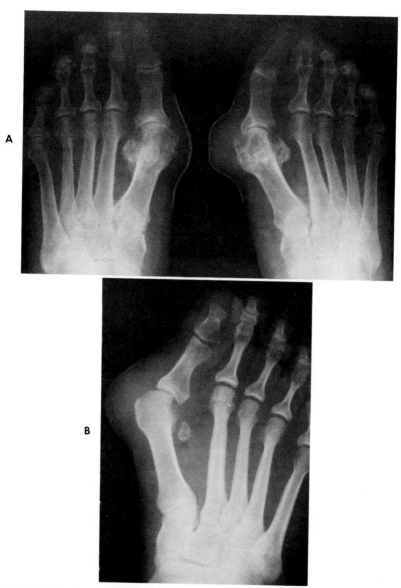

Fig. 8-19. A, Moderate, fully developed hallux valgus with ganglionic cyst, showing various skeletal abnormalities. **B,** Fully developed hallux valgus with massive adventitious bursa formation.

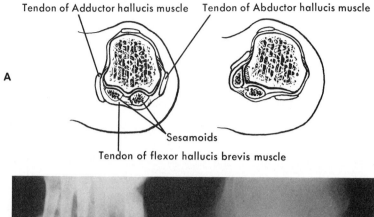

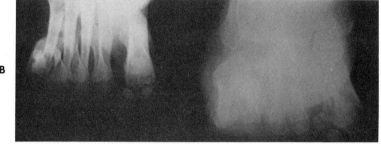

Fig. 8-20. **A,** Cross section of first metatarsal head and sesamoids. *Left,* Normal relationship between the metatarsal head and the sesamoids and tendons coursing in area. *Right,* Hallux valgus. Note distortion of all structures around the metatarsal head. **B,** Roentgenograms of sesamoids. *Left,* Normal position. *Right,* Sesamoids in hallux valgus. Note that fibular sesamoid is in the metatarsal interspace.

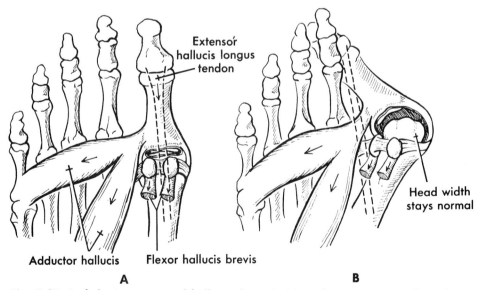

Fig. 8-21. Pathologic anatomy of hallux valgus. **A,** Normal anatomic ensemble of first metatarsophalangeal joint. **B,** Hallux valgus with distortion of all anatomic structures around first metatarsophalangeal joint.

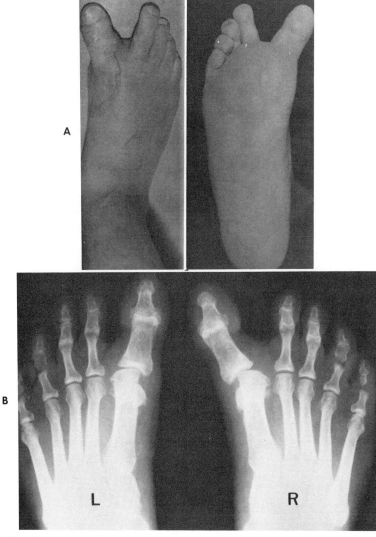

Fig. 8-22. A, Postoperative hallux varus caused by excessive shortening of abductor hallucis tendon. **B,** Bilateral postoperative hallux varus. A McBride procedure had been performed.

with any concomitant deformities that involve the structures of the forefoot. If the surgeon neglects to evaluate the entire foot properly, both he and the patient may be disappointed in the results of surgical procedures. (For procedures, see Chapter 20.)

Hallux varus. When the great toe is held or fixed in a tibialward position, the deformity is called hallux varus. The defect may be congenital (see Chapter 4) or postoperative.

Postoperative hallux varus. Occasionally, after hallux valgus reduction has been carried out hallux varus occurs as a postoperative deformity. Two surgical errors may cause the condition: excessive shortening of the capsule and tendon of the abductor hallucis on the tibial side of the great toe joint and excessive medialward angulation in subcapital amputation of the first metatarsal. It is most often a result of the McBride procedure, but hallux varus may ensue

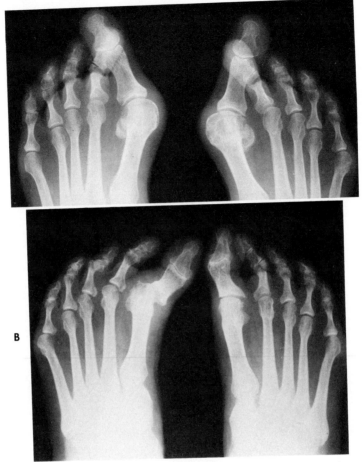

Fig. 8-23. A, Preoperative roentgenograms of hallux varus and overlapping second toes. **B,** Roentgenograms of same feet 2 years postoperatively. Keller procedure was performed.

after other procedures as well (Figs. 8-22 and 8-23).

Postoperative hallux varus in most cases is caused by an aspect of the operative procedure. Either the soft tissues on the tibial side of the first metatarsophalangeal joint are shortened too much or those on the fibular side are completely sectioned and improperly repaired.

Poor postoperative care after hallux valgus reduction may be another cause of hallux varus (see p. 527, Chapter 20).

TREATMENT OF POSTOPERATIVE TYPES. If hallux varus is caused by a severe shortening of the tibial capsule and tendon of the abductor hallucis, the capsule and tendon may be lengthened and freed by vertical sectioning of the base of the proximal phalanx on the tibial side. From this vertical incision two proximal linear incisions about 2 cm. long are made, one on the dorsal edge and one on the plantar edge of the incision. The capsule and the abductor hallucis tendon are then freed within this U-shaped incision, thus allowing the hallux to sustain a neutral position. Through a second incision over the distal end of the first metatarsal interspace the capsular structures at the base of the first proximal phalanx are sutured to the capsular structures of the second metatarsophalangeal joint. When the deformity is caused by an angulation of the

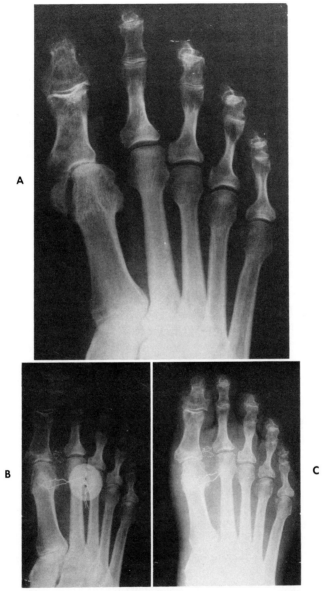

Fig. 8-24. A, Postoperative hallux varus. On weight bearing the hallux is in extreme varus. Note the tibial sesamoid lying vertically on the tibial side of the first metatarsal head. **B,** Sesamoid held in normal position by wire threaded through body and anchored to button on dorsum of foot. **C,** Sesamoid in position and hallux varus corrected 2 years postoperatively.

head of the first metatarsal, an arthroplasty must be performed and the articular surface of the metatarsal head must be rounded to form a ball-and-socket joint with the base of the proximal phalanx. Often the extensor hallucis longus is contracted and requires lengthening.

In some cases, hallux varus as an aftermath of the McBride procedure is accompanied by severe dorsal contracture of the great toe at the metatarsophalangeal joint and a severely hammered interphalangeal joint. In such cases a Jones tendon transfer (p. 535) may result in reduction of the deformity.

Each instance of hallux varus that occurs after the Keller or Mayo procedures (see Chapter 20), after excision of the first metatarsal head, or after osteotomies of the shafts of the first metatarsal or proximal phalanx must be considered an individual problem. The surgeon must study the mechanics of each particular case to determine which corrective procedure to employ, since no standardized procedure exists to correct all of them. In my experience correction of the deformity in many of these cases has been impossible.

Occasionally, in postoperative hallux varus the tibial sesamoid rotates and lies vertically on the tibial side of the first metatarsal head (Fig. 8-24, A), thereby fixing the deformity. In such cases the sesamoid tends to lock the deformity, and excision of this sesamoid can result in a hallux extensus (p. 234). The sesamoid can be replaced under the first metatarsal head by the following procedure:

1. Drill a vertical hole through the body of the sesamoid.
2. Free all adhesions holding the sesamoid in its abnormal position.
3. Loop a wire through the hole and the normal plantar aspect of the sesamoid.
4. Thread both ends of wire into a ligature carrier.
5. Pass the ligature carrier under the first and second metatarsal heads and curve them into the space between the second and third metatarsal heads to penetrate through the skin on the dorsum of the foot.
6. Retrieve both ends of the wire and remove the needle.
7. Fasten wires to a button on the dorsum of the second and third metatarsal heads, using moderate tension (Fig. 8-24, B).
8. In about 8 weeks remove the terminal ends of the wire and the button. The sesamoid will usually remain in its normal position (Fig. 8-24, C).

Hallux rigidus (hallux limitus). Hallux rigidus, or hallux limitus, is second to hallux valgus in order of prevalence among disabling deformities of the great toe joint. Indeed, it may be more disabling than hallux valgus, because in hallux valgus the patient is distressed mainly by the inability to obtain shoes to accommodate the deformity. In hallux rigidus the patient cannot obtain relief even when he does not wear shoes, because the great toe is locked in a neutral or plantar-flexed position. Dorsiflexion of the great toe is painful, yet, this movement is essential in every normal step. The degree of disability is in direct relation to the degree and extent of the deformity. The great toe is either fixed or limited in its normal motion of dorsiflexion, because of a new growth of bone around the articular surface of the head of the first metatarsal mainly on its dorsal aspect (Fig. 8-25). In most cases the discrepancy is caused by an extensive proliferation of bone around the dorsum and sides of the head of the first metatarsal, forming a collarlike mass (Fig. 8-26), which does not involve the plantar surface of the head of the first metatarsal. Often the base of the proximal phalanx is similarly affected. In advanced cases the entire hallux is fixed in a plantar attitude, which forces the patient to walk on the outer border of the foot, thereby inverting the ankle and frequently producing secondary changes in the soft tissue and the bone of the whole foot.

Types. Miller and Arendt (1940) are of the opinion that hallux rigidus is related to a congenital proximal displacement of the

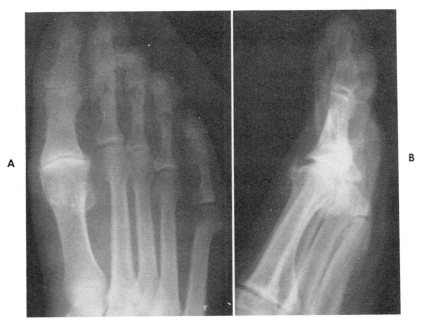

Fig. 8-25. Classic case of hallux rigidus. Note the osseous changes on the dorsum of the first metatarsal head, which project both distally and proximally. The usual projection is proximal. (See Fig. 8-32, A.)

sesamoid. Bingold and Collins (1950) studied thirty-three cases roentgenographically and histologically. When they had examined the bone and joint specimens in twelve of their cases, they concluded that there was little to differentiate between them and to classify them as to type. Mau (1928) believed that an inefficient foot, such as pes valgus or pes valgoplanus, is the forerunner of hallux rigidus.

For convenience, hallux rigidus may be divided into three types: (1) congenital (see Chapter 4); (2) acquired, as a result of traumatic arthritis; and (3) acquired, secondary to one of the general arthritides.

ACQUIRED. The acquired type is more common than the congenital. It is essentially a traumatic osteoarthritis caused by prolonged injury to the great toe joint as a result of a combination of any of the following factors: (1) a congenitally flat head of the first metatarsal (Figs. 8-27 and 8-28, 2); (2) unusually strong ligamentous tissues surrounding the joint; (3) extraordinary occupational weight bearing on the

great toe joint; or (4) repeated use of the great toe as a striking or anchor point. The normal great toe joint has a moderate ball-and-socket articulation, and the periarticular structures have normal resistance to external pressure. Abnormal variations of these structures are influenced adversely by short and pointed-toe shoes. Short shoes produce hallux valgus in the degree of accentuated ball-and-socket relationship of the joint surface and the amount of fragility or elasticity of the periarticular structures. Conversely, the flatter the articular surface of this joint (Fig. 8-28, 2) and the more resistant the periarticular structures, the more the pressure of the tibial side and the back of the shoes tends to cause low-grade traumatic arthritis, resulting in proliferative changes of the articular surface, and, eventually, hallux rigidus.

ACQUIRED SECONDARY TO ONE OF THE GENERAL ARTHRITIDES. Gout or rheumatoid arthritis is a likely cause of hallux rigidus. In gout the great toe joint is often the only joint of the foot involved, whereas in rheu-

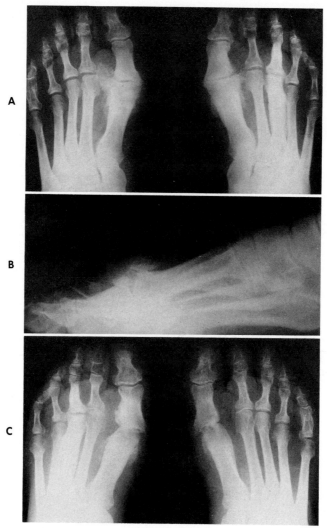

Fig. 8-26. A, Extreme case of hallux rigidus with local traumatic arthritis and violent reaction to persistent injury. Third metatarsal and proximal phalanx on the right side also show reaction to prolonged trauma. **B,** Note extensive new growth of bone on dorsum of first metatarsophalangeal joint. **C,** Roentgenograms of feet of same patient after correction by cheilectomy.

matoid arthritis other joints of the foot are also affected. Complete ankylosis of the joint may be consequent to infection after surgical correction for hallux valgus.

Treatment. Treatment for congenital cases differs because the deformity varies. The faulty articular surface of the joint must be carefully evaluated in each case and an arthroplasty performed so that a nearly normal ball-and-socket articular re-lation can be established between the base of the proximal phalanx and the head of the first metatarsal.

When the condition is acquired, Harrison and Harvey (1963) and Moynihan (1967) advise arthrodesis of the first metatarsophalangeal joint. Kessel and Bonney (1958) recommended a wedge osteotomy on the dorsum of the base of the proximal phalanx. Many surgeons prefer a Keller procedure

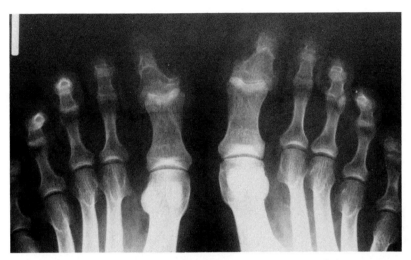

Fig. 8-27. Congenitally flat metatarsal heads of both feet.

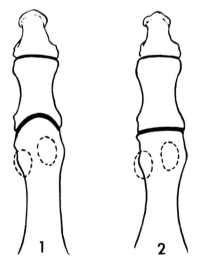

Fig. 8-28. Extreme variations in shape of first metatarsal head. *1,* Oval metatarsal head. The medial side of the shoe will force the hallux into a valgus position, producing a hallux valgus. *2,* Flat metatarsal head. The pressure of the side of the shoe cannot push the hallux into valgus but will cause constant trauma to the articular surface of the base of the proximal phalanx and to the head of the first metatarsal. Ultimately a traumatic osteoarthritis will occur, resulting in hallux rigidus.

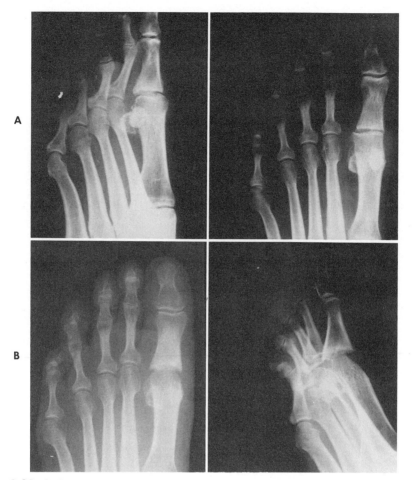

Fig. 8-29. A, Roentgenograms of postoperative hallux rigidus caused by flattened head of first metatarsal. **B,** Roentgenograms taken after remodeling of first metatarsal head.

for hallux rigidus. Gudas (1971) suggests an arthroplasty of the head of the first metatarsal and base of the proximal phalanx for hallux rigidus.

RECOMMENDED PROCEDURE FOR ACQUIRED HALLUX RIGIDUS. False ankylosis results when subcapital amputation of the first metatarsal is carried out without rounding the amputated surface (Fig. 8-29). Remodeling the metatarsal head usually will correct the disability.

Over a 30-year period the following cheilectomy procedure has given me excellent results in over 400 cases of traumatic osteoarthritis, the condition which is by far the most common.

1. Make a longitudinal incision imme-
diately over the first metatarsophalangeal joint on either side of the extensor hallucis longus tendon, extending it from the middle of the proximal phalanx to a point about the middle of the shaft of the first metatarsal.

2. Retract the skin and extensor hallucis longus tendon.

3. Incise the joint capsule longitudinally and free it from the bone lipping to which it is usually attached; retract the margins.

4. Deliver the head of the first metatarsal dorsally. Plantar flexion of the great toe at this stage aids delivery (Fig. 8-30, *1*).

5. Remove excess growth of bone on the

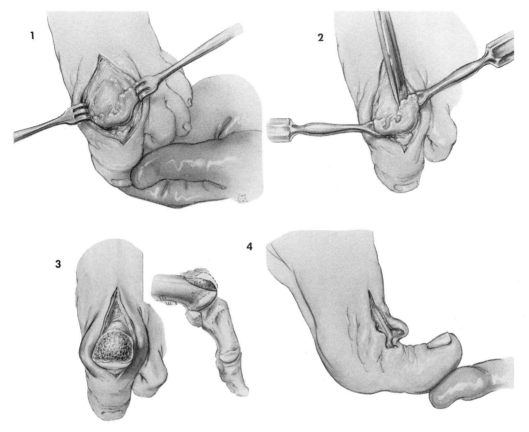

Fig. 8-30. Dorsal delivery of head of first metatarsal. *1,* Exposure of first metatarsal head with hallux plantar flexed, showing proliferated bony change. *2,* Removal of excess bone with osteotome. *3,* Smoothing and rounding of raw bone surface. *4,* Dorsiflexion of hallux in normal excursion.

dorsum and sides of the head. The bone is often granitelike in consistency. Include some of the normal bone of the head on removal so as to form an accentuated rounded surface but never a pointed surface (Fig. 8-30, *2*).

6. Smooth the surface with a rasp. If the base of the proximal phalanx is also exostotic, remove excess bone and smooth (Fig. 8-30, *3*).

7. Instill about 10 mg. of hydrocortisone acetate into the joint space to inhibit formation of extensive scar tissue in the capsule.

8. Suture the capsule with fine chromic catgut; close the skin as usual. Apply a compression bandage while the great toe is overcorrected in a dorsiflexed position.

9. Institute a gentle motion of the great toe joint on the third or fourth postoperative day to be increased in vigor and extent daily for 3 months to prevent formation of adhesions in the periarticular structures. The patient can usually be ambulatory the second or third day in a laced oxford shoe. The part of the shoe that covers the great toe and first metatarsophalangeal joint must be cut out (see Fig. 20-20).

In most cases the patient will be free from pain and have satisfactory motion in

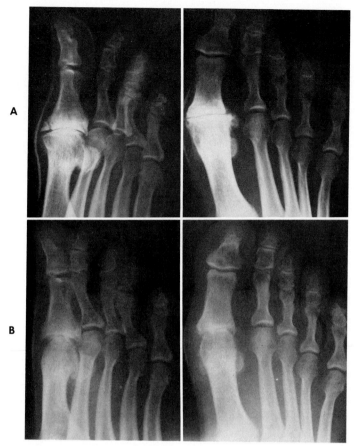

Fig. 8-31. A, Preoperative roentgenograms of right foot of 52-year-old male with hallux rigidus. **B,** Postoperative roentgenograms of same foot. A cheilectomy was performed.

the great toe joint in about 2 months (Figs. 8-31 and 8-32). Sometimes adhesions form and there is residual limitation of motion after complete healing. The adhesions are readily broken under light general anesthesia.

Hallux flexus (dorsal bunion). Most cases of hallux flexus are the result of hallux rigidus because the proliferation on the dorsum of the head of the first metatarsal is so extensive that it holds the hallux in a constant plantar-flexed position (Fig. 8-33). Only in rare cases (rare because the action of each step normally forces a dorsiflexion of the great toe) is the plantar flexion of the great toe held by unusually powerful flexor muscles or paralysis of the extensors (Fig. 8-34).

Lapidus (1940) classified the different types of hallux flexus or dorsal bunion into four groups: (1) cases secondary to hallux rigidus; (2) cases caused by a paralytic deformity of the foot, both flaccid and spastic; (3) cases associated with congenital clubfeet; and (4) cases associated with severe congenital talipes planovalgus; Lapidus attributed this type to compensation for a short tendo achillis.

Surgical approach to treatment should be based on an evaluation of the pathologic-anatomic problem in each case. In those cases in which the periarticular structures, including the tendons, are involved, it is sufficient to lengthen tendons that are shortened and shorten those that are lengthened. In those cases in which bony prolif-

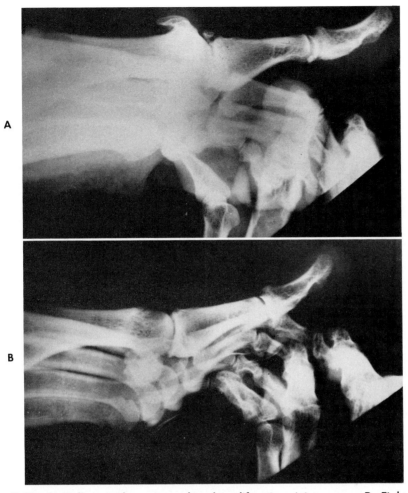

Fig. 8-32. A, Hallux rigidus; severe dorsal proliferation; joint mouse. **B,** Eight months postoperatively.

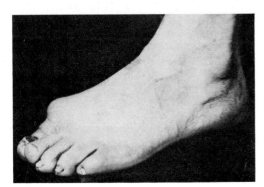

Fig. 8-33. Hallux flexus resulting from severe hallux rigidus.

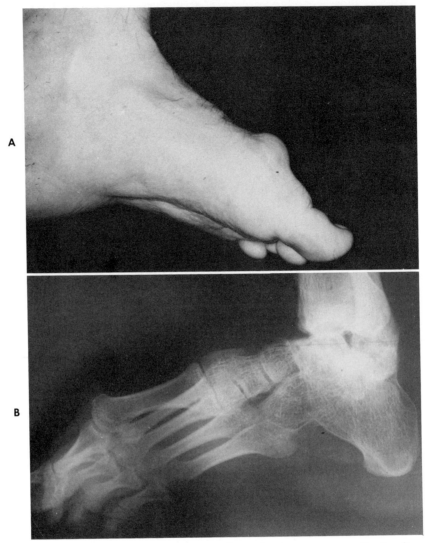

Fig. 8-34. A, Hallux flexus caused by paralysis of extensors as result of poliomyelitis. **B,** Roentgenograms of same foot and postoperative result of triple arthrodesis.

eration (hallux rigidus) limits dorsiflexion of the great toe, a cheilectomy of the first metatarsophalangeal joint must be performed.

When dorsal bunion is part of congenital talipes planovalgus, Lapidus advised transference of the terminal end of the tibialis anterior tendon into the insertion of the tibialis posterior and the tendon of the flexor hallucis longus into the dorsum of the first metatarsal, just behind its head (Fig. 8-35).

Hallux extensus. Normally the flexor hal-lucis brevis is an important opponent of the extensor hallucis longus. When this opposing structure is destroyed or severed, the extensor hallucis longus contracts, causing hallux extensus (Fig. 8-36). This often happens in cases in which the flexor tendons (especially the flexor hallucis brevis) have been sectioned, or both sesamoids have been removed, or the insertion of the flexor hallucis brevis has been destroyed. It also occurs after the base of the proximal phalanx has been amputated (e.g., in the rou-

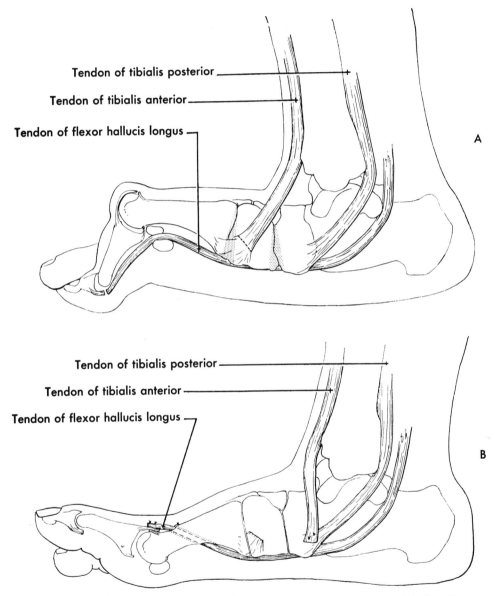

Tendon of tibialis posterior

Tendon of tibialis anterior

Tendon of flexor hallucis longus

A

Tendon of tibialis posterior

Tendon of tibialis anterior

Tendon of flexor hallucis longus

B

Fig. 8-35. A, Schematic drawing of pathologic-anatomic appearance of hallux flexus, according to Lapidus. **B,** Lapidus' technique for reduction of hallux flexus. Flexor hallucis longus is threaded, from the plantar surface to the dorsum, through a drill hole in the shaft of the first metatarsal and sutured on the dorsum of the bone of the first proximal phalanx. Terminal end of the tibialis anterior tendon is sutured into the insertion of the tibialis posterior.

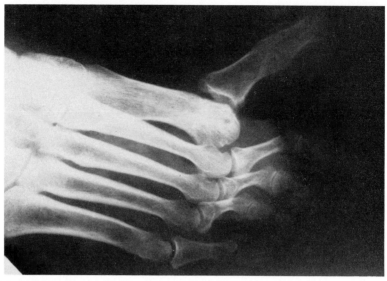

Fig. 8-36. Hallux extensus after excision of both sesamoids with arthrodesis of interphalangeal joint of hallux. Jones' tendon transfer reduced the deformity.

tine Keller procedure). The great toe becomes dorsiflexed and its interphalangeal joint becomes hammered.

In treatment, whenever possible, attempts should be made to suture the flexor hallucis brevis through a medioplantar incision; however, this is seldom possible. Lengthening of the extensor hallucis longus will usually permit the deformity to be reduced. However, when the interphalangeal joint is hammered, it must be reduced at the same time.

Tailor's bunion (bunionette). The term "tailor's bunion" is applied to any enlargement of the fibular side of the fifth metatarsophalangeal joint. In past times, tailors would sit with their legs crossed as they sewed clothes by hand, thereby placing abnormal pressure on the fifth metatarsal head and often causing painful symptoms. Hence the name "tailor's bunion." The enlargement may be the result of one or a combination of three conditions: (1) hypertrophy of the soft tissue overlying the fifth metatarsophalangeal joint; (2) a congenitally wide dumbbell-shaped fifth metatarsal head; or (3) a lateral bending of the fifth metatarsal head (Fig. 8-37).

Etiology. Hypertrophy of the soft tissue covering the fifth metatarsophalangeal joint is usually caused by either a wide metatarsal head or a lateral bending of this head; however, it is present occasionally even when the head of the fifth metatarsal is normal. In such instances the condition results from wearing tight shoes that press against the fibular side of the fifth metatarsal head. The congenitally wide metatarsal head is a constantly pressured area even though correctly fitted shoes are worn.

Lateral bending of the fifth metatarsal head is the most common cause of tailor's bunion. The fifth metatarsal is normally thin at the neck; it responds readily to pressure, especially during adolescence. The wearing of short shoes exerts constant pressure against the fifth toe, which in turn is exerted against the head of the fifth metatarsal; thus, the head tends to bend gradually lateralward on its neck.

Symptoms. In tailor's bunion the head of the fifth metatarsal is the most prominent point on the fibular side of the foot; consequently, it is subject to the greatest pressure. The area is painful, swollen, and tender and usually is covered by extensive

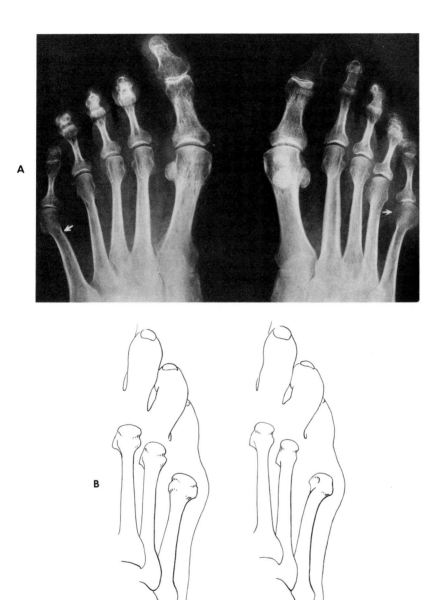

Fig. 8-37. A, Tailor's bunion. Roentgenogram illustrates two types of bone variation in the same person. *Left,* Lateral bending at the neck of the fifth metatarsal. *Right,* Wide fifth metatarsal head. **B,** Schematic drawing of case shown in **A**. *Left,* Wide head. *Right,* Lateral bending of the head.

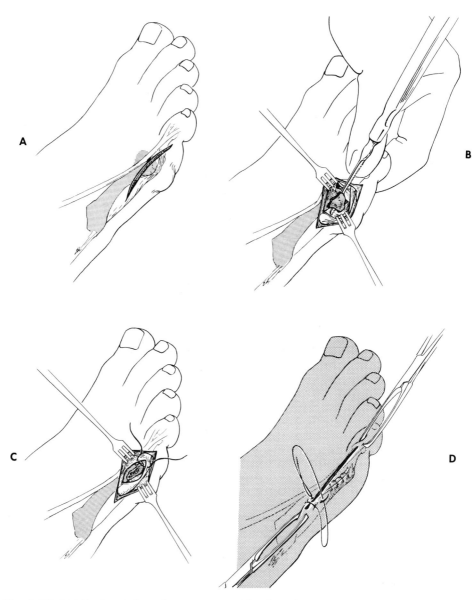

Fig. 8-38. DuVries' technique for correction of tailor's bunion. **A,** Somewhat semielliptical incision over dorsum of fifth metatarsophalangeal joint. **B,** Skin, capsule, and tendon of abductor digiti quinti retracted. Fibular condyle of fifth metatarsal head is amputated with a nasal saw. **C,** Capsule and tendon of abductor digiti quinti sutured. **D,** Skin closed.

keratosis that may have a deep-seated nucleus under which there may be a degenerative sinus into the joint. This area is a common site of chilblains

Treatment. In moderate cases shielding with pads and carefully fitting shoes allevi-

ate symptoms. In protracted cases operative correction is indicated. The recommended surgical technique follows:

1. Make a longitudinal incision over the dorsolateral border of the fifth metatarsophalangeal joint, extending it

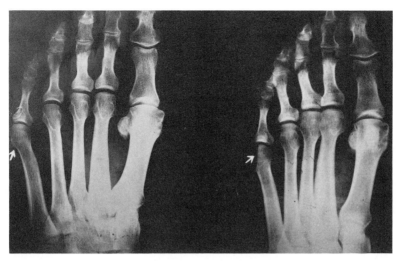

Fig. 8-39. Tailor's bunion. *Left,* Preoperative lateral bending of the fifth metatarsal head. *Right,* Same foot postoperatively.

proximally from the middle of the proximal phalanx to the juncture of the middle and distal thirds of the fifth metatarsal (Fig. 8-38, *A*).

2. Retract the skin and subcutaneous tissue to expose the joint capsule.
3. Incise the capsule longitudinally.
4. Denude the fibular border of the capsule, including the tendon of the abductor digiti quinti, from the head of the fifth metatarsal. When retracted with the skin, the fibular condyle of the head will be exposed.
5. Amputate this condylar process longitudinally by means of a nasal saw, beginning at the neck of the bone (Fig. 8-38, *B*), and round the cut surface with a nasal file. Excessive thickening of the soft tissues overlying the condyle is caused by either fibrotic infiltration or adventitious bursae which, when present, should be excised.
6. Close the capsule and skin in layers (Fig. 8-38, *C* and *D*), making certain to incorporate the tendon of the abductor digiti quinti in the capsule closure; otherwise the fifth metatarsophalangeal joint may become dislo-

cated. Figs. 8-39 and 8-40 show the end result of the operation.

Occasionally, a complication may occur after such surgery because of failure to suture the capsule and tendon of the abductor digiti quinti or because an excess amount of the fifth metatarsal head is removed or both. This results in an imbalance of the head and in dislocation of the joint (Fig. 8-41). Correction can be accomplished by remodeling the fifth metatarsal head and repairing the capsule and tendon of the abductor digiti quinti tendon on the fibular side of the fifth metatarsophalangeal joint.

DISLOCATIONS OF THE SECOND METATARSOPHALANGEAL JOINT

Dorsal dislocation of the base of the second proximal phalanx (Fig. 8-42, *A*) is common (Branch, 1937). It is the most frequent static complete dislocation in the forefoot (DuVries, 1956). Single dislocations of the other metatarsophalangeal joints are rare (Fig. 8-42, *B*). Partial or complete dislocation of all the lesser metatarsophalangeal joints is usual in talipes equinus and pes cavus, or clawfoot.

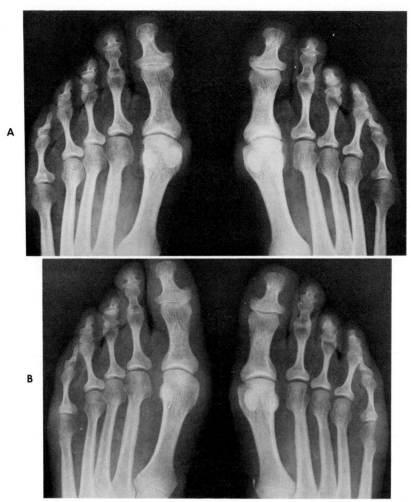

Fig. 8-40. A, Tailor's bunion caused by wide fifth metatarsal head. **B,** Postoperative roentgenogram.

Etiology. The second toe is normally the longest of the five. Because the normal position of the toes is in mild dorsiflexion, backward pressure of the short shoe is exerted mostly against the second toe, and the proximal phalanx is forced to glide over the dorsum of the head of the second metatarsal. This movement is related to the anatomic structure of the proximal phalanx, since it is the only one that has two dorsal interossei tendons inserted in its base.

Symptoms. In most cases of second metatarsophalangeal dislocations, a disabling, intractable keratosis (tyloma) is present under the second metatarsal head. The base of the proximal phalanx rests directly over the head of the metatarsal, thereby causing the shoe top to accentuate the body weight on the plantar condylar surface of the second metatarsal head. On palpation of the second metatarsophalangeal joint, the base of the proximal phalanx can be felt as it lies on the dorsum of the head of the second metatarsal. This deformity is often accompanied by hallux valgus (Fig. 8-43, A), but it may occur in a foot that has a comparatively normal first metatarsophalangeal joint.

Treatment. Open reduction of the dislocation corrects most cases and improves the

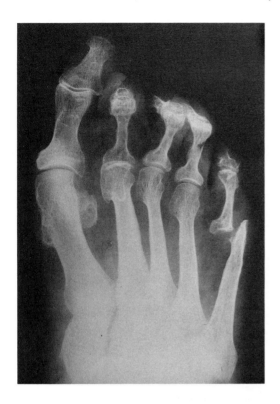

Fig. 8-41. Result of failure to suture capsule and tendon of abductor digiti minimi and excessive removal of head of fifth metatarsal.

remainder (Fig. 8-43, B). The recommended surgical technique is as follows:

1. Make a longitudinal incision immediately over the dislocation, extending distally from the midshaft of the metatarsal and curving into the first toe web as it passes over the dislocation.
2. Retract the skin and extensor tendon. In some cases this tendon has to be severed because of severe contracture.
3. Open the capsule longitudinally. Section all adhesions on both sides of the joint.
4. Reduce the dislocation and hold it in place.
5. Suture the dorsal capsule and fascia remnants with fine chromic gut while the toe is held in reduction until the reduction maintains itself.
6. Occasionally, the dorsal surface of the second metatarsal head will be found

worn and flattened, which precludes maintaining the reduced dislocation in such cases. An arthroplasty of this metatarsal head must be done.

HAMMERTOE, MALLET TOE, AND CLAWTOE

A standard interpretation of these terms is as follows:

"Hammertoe" and "mallet toe" are essentially acquired partial or complete dislocations of the proximal interphalangeal joints. Hammertoe is common and may occur in more than one toe (Figs. 8-44 and 8-45). The dislocation is usually a dorsal one, but sometimes it may be plantarward. In the lesser toes the proximal joint is frequently involved; the distal joint is involved only ocasionally, and then it is often called "mallet toe." In the fifth toe both the proximal and distal joints are usually affected, so that the toe becomes semicircular. At times a single toe may be congenitally hammered.

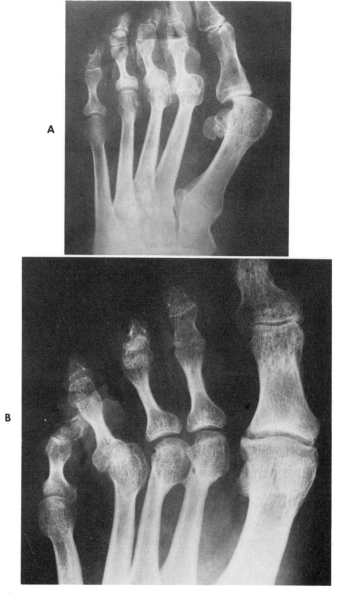

Fig. 8-42. A, Complete static dislocation of second metatarsophalangeal joint and partial dislocation of third metatarsophalangeal joint. **B,** Complete static dislocation of fourth metatarsophalangeal joint.

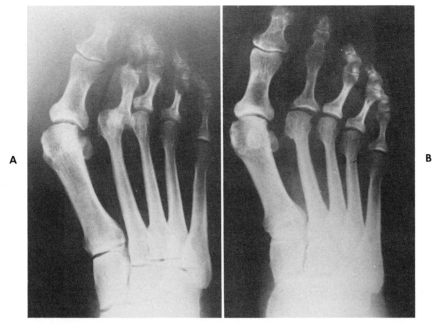

Fig. 8-43. A, Complete static dislocation of second metatarsophalangeal joint. **B,** Two years postoperatively.

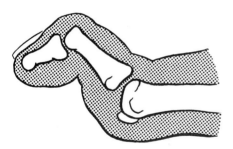

Fig. 8-44. Hammered great toe. Note articulation of the distal phalanx with the plantar surface of the head of the proximal phalanx.

When it is, the condition is usually bilateral and ordinarily is in the second toe or in the hallux (see Chapter 4).

The term "clawtoe" (Fig. 8-46) is sometimes used interchangeably with "hammertoe" (Young, 1938; Taylor, 1940). However, the term is best applied to a group of deformities that involve all the toes. Usually associated with clawfoot (pes cavus), it may be secondary to paralytic talipes equinus or rheumatoid arthritis.

Originally the hammered toe was described by Blum (1883) as a deformity of the digit simulating the configuration of a swan's neck, in which the metatarsophalangeal joint is dorsiflexed, the proximal interphalangeal joint is plantar flexed to a right angle, and the distal interphalangeal joint is slightly hyperextended. Clawtoes involve all the toes; the deformity is characterized by plantar flexion of both interphalangeal joints and dorsiflexed contracture of all the metatarsophalangeal joints. Kelikian (1965) states it is "perhaps safe to say that clawtoes constitute a multiple, exaggerated form of hammertoe."*

The frequency of hammertoe and clawtoe varies among different populations; however, hammertoe and mallet toe are common in shoe-wearing people. In reports dealing with deformities of the forefoot in natives who wear no shoes, the deformity

---

*Kelikian, H.: Hallux valgus, allied deformities of the forefoot and metatarsalgia, Philadelphia, 1965, W. B. Saunders Co., p. 305.

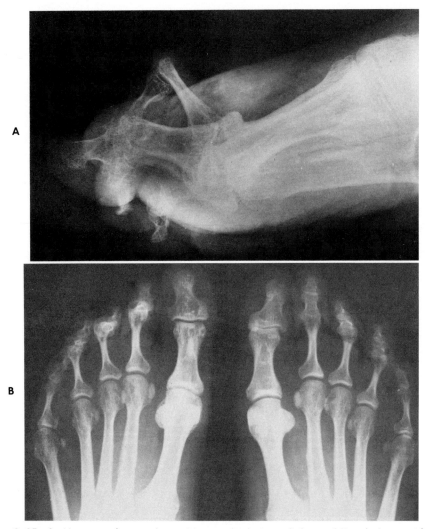

Fig. 8-45. A, Hammered second toe. Note articulation of the middle phalanx with the plantar surface of the head of the proximal phalanx. **B,** Right foot: hammered third and fourth toes. Second toe is normal. Left foot: hammered second, third, and fourth toes.

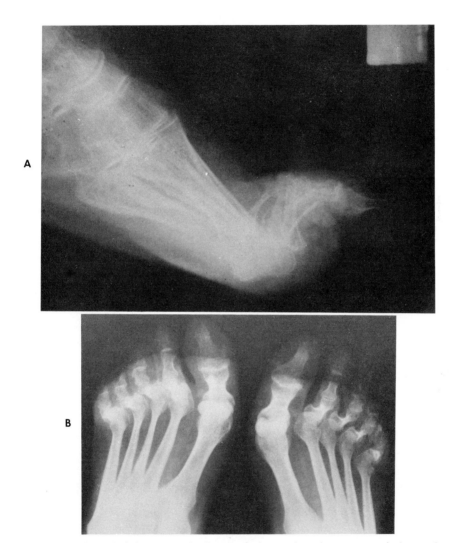

Fig. 8-46. A, Dorsal dislocation of all interphalangeal and metatarsophalangeal joints in clawtoes. **B,** Clawing of all toes.

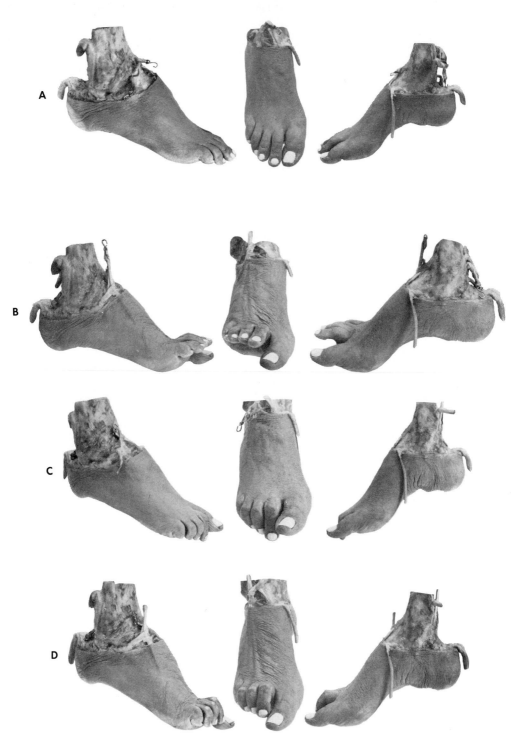

Fig. 8-47. Action of muscles in clawtoes. **A,** Fresh cadaver foot at rest. **B,** Tension on extensor digitorum longus alone. Note extension of the metatarsophalangeal joints and minimal extension of the interphalangeal joints. **C,** Tension on flexor digitorum longus alone. Note that maximal flexion occurs in the interphalangeal joints. **D,** Tension applied simultaneously to extensor digitorum longus and flexor digitorum longus. Note the resulting clawtoe deformities in all but the great toe.

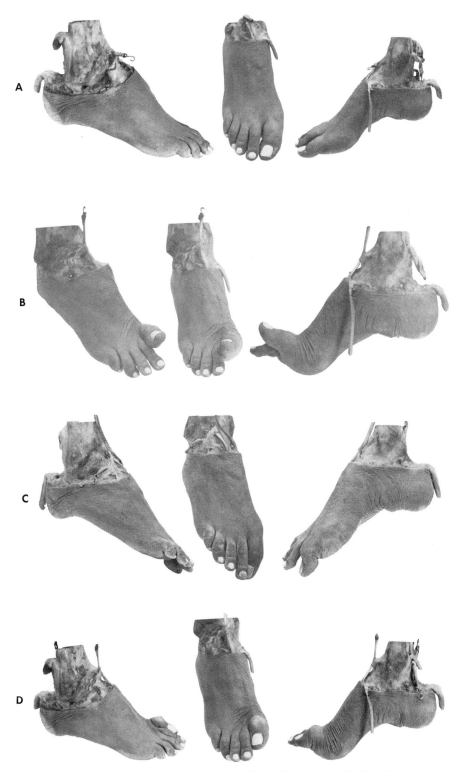

Fig. 8-48. Action of muscles in clawtoes. **A,** Cadaver foot at rest. **B,** Tension on extensor hallucis longus alone. Note the extension of the metatarsophalangeal and interphalangeal joints. **C,** Tension on the flexor hallucis longus alone. Note maximal flexion in the interphalangeal joint. **D,** Simultaneous tension on extensor hallucis longus and flexor hallucis longus, with resulting hammertoe deformity.

is hardly mentioned (Wells, 1931; Engle and Morton, 1931; James, 1939; Barnicot and Hardy, 1955). Only Lam Sim-Fook and Hodgson (1958) report an incidence of 4.7 percent of these deformities among unshod Chinese.

Hammertoe is rare in infants (Higgs, 1931). In surveys made of wartime male recruits (Hewitt et al., 1953), women reserves (Marwil and Brantingham, 1943), and industrial workers (Creer, 1938), the incidence of hammertoe and clawtoe varies from 2 to 20 percent. All studies indicate that these deformities develop slowly and insidiously; their incidence increases almost linearly with increasing age.

Etiology. The generally accepted predisposing factor to hammertoe or clawtoe is loss of function of the intrinsic muscles of the foot. There is no question that simultaneous contracture of the long flexors and extensors of the toes, without the modifying action of the intrinsic muscles of the foot, causes the typical deformities seen in these conditions. This was pointed out by Duchenne in 1867. Figs. 8-47, *D*, and 8-48, *D*, clearly demonstrate the action of the long flexors and extensors in a fresh cadaver foot in the production of the hammertoe and clawtoe deformity.

Ellis (1889) and Jones (1944) pointed out that comparing the action of the muscles of the digits of the hand to that of those of the foot was fallacious. The hand is a prehensile organ and the muscles act upon the digits from a fixed proximal segment, while the reverse is true of the foot. In orthograde progression, the forefoot is fixed by the superincumbent body, and the muscles are acting upon the moving proximal segments. The precise effect of such a reversal of the action of muscles has not been adequately investigated. Levick (1921, 1932) stimulated the intrinsic muscles of the foot electrically during weight bearing upon the forefoot. He noted, "The simultaneous action of all four dorsal interossei, with the toes fixed, is to bunch up all the metatarsal bones in such a way as to raise the transverse arch."[*] Furthermore, the mechanics of the action of the interossei and lumbricales upon the phalanges may be different in the hand and foot; rarely are the metacarpophalangeal joints of the hand in hyperextension, but in the shod foot the metatarsophalangeal joints are usually in a variable state of hyperextension because of the presence of heels on the shoes. That intrinsic muscles, particularly the interossei and lumbricales, may play a role in the development of hammertoe is supported by clinical reports of the appearance of such deformities in some neurologic diseases; but hammertoe is also seen in Sudeck's atrophy, rheumatoid arthritis, and immersion foot (Kelikian, 1965). To confuse the issue further, Taylor (1951), in a series of sixty-eight cases operated upon for hammertoe, found no evidence of abnormality in the intrinsic muscles by gross inspection, stimulation, or microscopic examination of biopsy material.

[*]Proc. Anat. Soc. Great Britain Ireland, J. Anat. **67**:196, Feb. 1932.

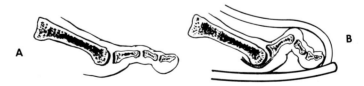

Fig. 8-49. A, Phalanx extended to its normal length. **B,** Buckling of phalanx caused by restriction of end of shoe. Interphalangeal joints and metatarsophalangeal joints become partially dislocated and, over time, the dislocation may become fixed.

Shoes play the most important role in the direct cause of hammertoe and mallet toe. As has been stated, for centuries man has chosen usually to cover the forepart of his foot (a modified square) with a shoe whose forepart is triangular in varying degrees (Fig. 8-2, *B* and *C*) or too short (Fig. 8-49). This fact unquestionably explains why acquired hammertoe and mallet toe are among the most common deformities of the forefoot in shoe-wearing societies. Shoes in general are restrictive to the normal movements of the joints and impede the normal action of the intrinsic muscles of the foot. Lam Sim-Fook and Hodgson (1958) have clearly shown that a definite inverse relationship exists between mobility and the presence of deformities of the forefoot.

It must be kept in mind that anatomic predisposing factors vary extensively, so that a large number of shod people do escape these and other deformities of the forefoot.

Pathogenesis. The clinical condition of hammertoe is readily recognized and the pathology is apparent. There is a partial or total dorsal dislocation of the proximal phalanx on the head of the metatarsal and a right-angle flexion of the proximal interphalangeal joint, with a corn overlying this joint. In addition, callosities are present under the metatarsal heads. If the distal phalanx is also flexed, a callus on the tip of the toe is present and the toenail is deformed.

Treatment. Treatment depends upon several factors. In the young individual whose deformity is not fixed, conservative measures may be employed, including avoidance of wearing footwear with a triangular forepart. Toes are manipulated by the patient or the parent to maintain mobility, metatarsal bars or anterior heels may be placed on the shoes, and strapping of the toes may be attempted. The use of conservative methods in the older individual with varying degrees of fixed deformity has been generally disappointing. The surgical procedures suggested in the literature are many and have been based largely upon the individual surgeon's concept of the etiology of the condition. These procedures may be divided into three major categories: soft-tissue releases, tendon transfers, and skeletal procedures.

Soft-tissue releases, including tenotomies. These procedures are directed toward correction of the deformity by sectioning the restrictive soft tissues and weakening the presumed deforming forces of the long flexors and extensors of the toes by elongation.

Tendon transfers. Based upon the concept that an imbalance exists between the intrinsic muscles (particularly the interossei and lumbricales) and the long flexors and extensors of the toes, various transfers have been proposed and carried out. The intent of performing these procedures is to decrease the presumed inadequacy of the intrinsic muscles.

Skeletal procedures. Many corrective procedures have been reported. They vary extensively, depending on which deformity is present and where it occurs. Some surgeons perform arthrodeses of one or more of the phalangeal joints; some excise the involved phalanx or amputate the adjacent metatarsal head.

For hammertoe and mallet toe in which the lesser toes are involved, I have found excision of the head of the proximal phalanx (in hammertoe) or excision of the head of the middle phalanx (in mallet toe) to be successful, whereas for hammered great toe or clawtoes, the procedure that is indicated varies extensively (see Chapter 20).

MORTON'S SYNDROME

A short first metatarsal, a hypermobile first metatarsal segment, and a posterior displacement of the sesamoids comprise the syndrome described by Morton (1935). This is not to be confused with Morton's neuralgia. The syndrome results in hypertrophy of the second metatarsal, tenderness at the base of the second metatarsal, and callosities under the heads of the second and third metatarsals. Morton observed that a high percentage of weak feet and of those with metatarsalgia is directly related to the syndrome. He thought that the hypermobility of the first metatarsal bones was caused by their shortness, which permits abnormally free motion in the joint between the first cuneiform and navicular bones and between the first and middle cuneiforms. The resulting instability is reflected in malfunction of the metatarsal and of the longitudinal arch of the foot.

Harris and Beath (1949) took issue with Morton's interpretation; nevertheless, in 1952 Morton again supported and enlarged his theory. Statistical studies by Hawkes (1914), among others, regarding the relative length of the metatarsals, demonstrated that in about 80 percent of human feet the first metatarsal is shorter than the second. This is in agreement with Jones (1944), who states: "The only alternative is to assume that there is such a thing as ideal foot function and that this function could presumably be carried out by an ideal but not by the normal foot"*

ACQUIRED NONTRAUMATIC DISORDERS OF THE CALCANEUS
Haglund's disease (prominent posterior superior tuberosity of the calcaneus) and related conditions

Haglund (1928) appears to have been the first to call attention to the possible relationship between the shape of the calcaneus and the appearance of pump bumps, tendo achillis bursitis, retrocalcaneal bursitis, and small spurs at the attachment of the tendo achillis. Saxl (1929) emphasized that if the upper surface of the tuberosity of the calcaneus was too prominent, the soft tissues were compressed between the counter of the shoe and the underlying bone, thus producing the variety of conditions mentioned above. Both surgeons recommended that the upper posterior lip of the calcaneus be surgically re-

---
*Jones, F. W.: Structure and function as seen in the foot, Baltimore, 1944, The Williams & Wilkins Co.

moved if chronic irritation persisted in spite of shoe modifications (Fig. 8-50).

Anatomically, the posterior superior tuberosity of the calcaneus may be variously shaped (Fig. 8-51). Occasionally, this part is markedly prominent (Figs. 8-51, A, and 12-26), and when it is it usually results in symptoms of constant pain during the wearing of shoes. Hohmann (1948) referred to such a prominence as Haglund's disease.

A congenital anomaly of the posterior tuberosity of the calcaneus (Fig. 8-52) can lead to painful symptoms from the pressure of shoes. At times a tendo achillis bursitis is produced, which may result in a subdermal enlargement immediately above the tendo achillis insertion. The condition is caused by prolonged pressure from the upper margin of the shoe counter. Any extraordinary shape or a prominent posterosuperior border of the calcaneus (see Fig. 12-26) is usually the predisposing cause.

Fowler and Philip (1945) called attention to the association of such a prominence with bursitis above the tendo achillis. They related not only the shape of the tuberosity to the development of these painful lesions, but also considered the significance of the angle made between the posterior surface and the plantar surface of the calcaneus (Fig. 8-53) as seen on the lateral roentgenogram. The normal range of the angle is between 44 and 69 degrees. If this angle is too great (above 75 degrees), abnormal pressures are likely to occur.

While Keck and Kelly (1965) expressed concern as to the possibility of measuring this angle accurately, they stated that their cases demonstrated angles between 70 and 80 degrees. From their series of twenty-six heels that were symptomatic just above the tendo achillis insertion, they concluded that an abnormally large protuberance of the posterosuperior tuberosity of the calcaneus was a basic cause in these cases of tendo achillis and retrocalcaneal bursitis. The vertical contour of the shoe counter is almost always semielliptical; therefore, when the posterosuperior margin of the

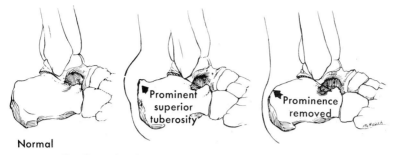

Normal

Fig. 8-50. Normally shaped calcaneus; prominent superior tuberosity; removal of posterior lip of calcaneus in Haglund's disease.

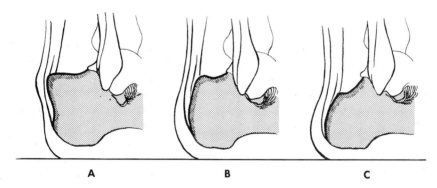

A   B   C

Fig. 8-51. Variations in shape of superior tuberosity of calcaneus. **A,** Hyperconvex (so-called Haglund's disease). **B,** Normal. **C,** Hypoconvex.

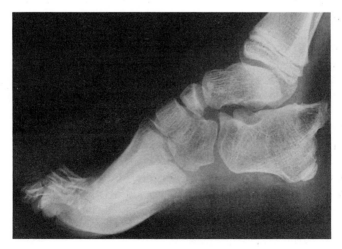

Fig. 8-52. Congenital anomaly of posterior tuberosity of calcaneus. Painful from the pressure of shoes.

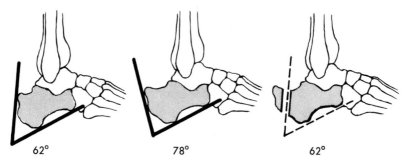

Fig. 8-53. Variation in angles of posterosuperior tuberosity of calcaneus (observations of Fowler and Philip). *Left,* Normal. *Center,* Prominence predisposing to tendo achillis bursitis. *Right,* Prominence excised. (After Keck, S. W., and Kelly, P. J.: J. Bone Joint Surg. **47-A:**267-273, Mar. 1965.)

heel bone is prominent, the upper margin of the counter constantly irritates the soft tissues over the prominence, producing hypertrophic changes. The condition usually becomes symptomatic in adolescence, before massive hypertrophy of the soft tissues develops.

For surgical treatment of these conditions, see Chapter 19.

Calcaneal spurs of the plantar tuberosity

A heel spur is an osteophytic outgrowth just anterior to the plantar tuberosity of the calcaneus, extending along its entire width for about 2 to 2.5 cm. The apex of the spur is embedded in the plantar fascia, directly anterior to its origin. The condition may exist without symptoms, or it may become painful, even disabling. Calcaneal spurs are of three types:

1. Those that are large but symptomless, because the angle of growth is such that the spur does not become a weight-bearing point, or those in which the inflammatory changes have been arrested, so that the condition is disclosed only incidentally during roentgenographic examination of the foot for some other purpose.
2. Those that are large and painful on weight bearing, because the pitch of the calcaneus has been altered by a

depression of the longitudinal arch, the spur thus becoming a weight-bearing point.
3. Those having only a rudimentary proliferation and an irregular, jagged outline accompanied by an area of decreased density around the origin of the plantar fascia, indicating a subacute inflammatory process (Fig. 8-54). All calcaneal spurs undoubtedly begin as the third type; only a few become symptomatic at that stage, because only in those few are the etiologic factors acute.

Etiology. Before the availability of roentgenograms, reports of painful heels had appeared sporadically in the medical literature, but it was difficult to determine the cause of the pain until roentgenograms demonstrated an exostosis located at the calcaneal attachment of the plantar fascia. It is not clear why at that time clinicians assumed an infectious agent rather than a mechanical factor to be the cause, but in any event Baer (1906) declared that "it seems fairly certain that we must consider the gonococcus to be the etiological factor in a great number of cases."[*] He based this statement on his experience with six patients who had painful calcaneal spurs, all

---
[*]Baer, W. S.: Gonorrheal exostosis of the os calcis, Surg. Gynec. Obstet. **2:**172, Feb. 1906.

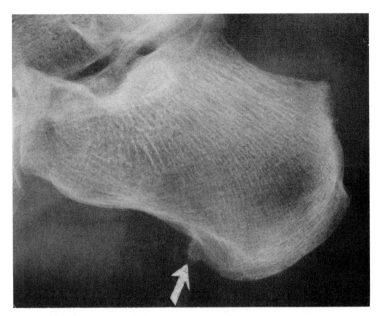

Fig. 8-54. Heel spur undergoing subacute inflammation.

of whom had a history of gonorrhea. In one, a positive culture of gonococcus was obtained, and in two others cocci were demonstrated in the microscopic sections of the excised bone. Baer's statement was accepted as truth for the next quarter of a century. As late as 1932 Liberson wrote: "The painful heel of gonorrhea is due to both bony exostosis and the soft tissue infiltration over it."[*] Later writers suggested infectious diseases and trauma as causes of spur formation. Blokhin and Vinogradova (1937) reported thirty-three cases in which arteriosclerosis, gonorrhea, and syphilis were not at all causative. The spur resulted from functional overuse or an abnormality of the bones of the foot, or both circumstances. Davis and Blair (1950) reported fifteen cases of calcaneal spurs associated with Strümpell-Marie disease. The hereditary factor has been suggested by Gould (1942), who reported exostosis of the heel in the father of six children; the third child, a son, had a spur. That son had four children, of whom the second child, a boy, had

a heel spur. Gould suggested that the abnormality passed down through the male side.

It is now generally accepted that spurs in the area of the attachment of the plantar fascia are caused by the development of abnormal tensions in the plantar aponeurosis. They are usually associated with some degree of pronation of the foot.

Anatomically, the plantar aponeurosis arises from the tuberosity of the calcaneus, passes forward, divides into five bands, and inserts into the plantar pad. The pad is firmly fixed to the base of each proximal phalanx and is continuous with its periosteum. The following chain of events occurs: During normal gait, as the body passes forward the toes are dorsiflexed and the proximal phalanx pulls the attached plantar aponeurosis over the metatarsal heads. This action produces the maximum stress on the site of origin of the plantar fascia. A weak foot and overweight aggravate the excess strain, and over time excess strain produces proliferative bone changes at the origin of the fascia, ultimately forming the spur.

Hicks (1954) compared the action of the

[*]Liberson, F.: Deep x-ray therapy in the treatment of "painful heel," J. Urol. **28**:115, July 1932.

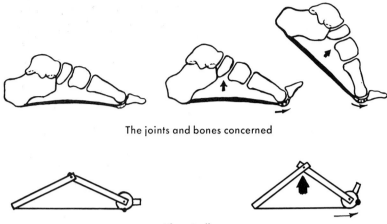

The joints and bones concerned

The windlass

Fig. 8-55. Windlass mechanism of aponeurosis and metatarsal heads: schematic illustration.

plantar aponeurosis and the metatarsal heads to a windlass mechanism (Figs. 8-55 and 1-7), with the plantar aponeurosis functioning as the cable and each metatarsal head as a drum.

Diagnosis. The principal symptom is severe pain aggravated by weight bearing, becoming progressively worse and often incapacitating, in the entire plantar surface of the heel. On palpation the entire plantar surface of the heel is tender, but the point of maximum tenderness is elicited just anterior to the calcaneal tuberosity. This tender region may be pinpointed on a roentgenogram immediately under the spur.

In the early stages fibrositis of low chronicity, with or without pain, anterior to the calcaneal tuberosity represents the pathologic change. Continuation of the process leads to osteophytic changes and bone deposits on the sulcus, just anterior to the tuberosity. The accumulation of new bone is self-limiting, the final spur varies greatly in size and shape, but mostly it has a triangular bar shape. Occasionally, an unusually shaped spur that is painful is encountered (Fig. 8-56) which requires special evaluation.

In rare instances symptoms are caused by osteolytic changes in the plantar tuberosity itself (Fig. 8-57). These symptoms can become very disabling and each case must

be given careful study. Conservative measures, such as mechanical appliances for weight distribution, are used in the treatment of this disorder. In intractable cases the entire plantar tuberosity must be flattened surgically.

The usual roentgenographic mediolateral view of the spur is two dimensional; it appears pointed like a tack, but actually extends over the entire width of the tuberosity.

Treatment. The asymptomatic type need not be treated. Since spurs are caused by mechanical factors, most symptomatic spurs will respond to those mechanical measures that reduce the tensile forces acting on the plantar aponeurosis. Reduction of these forces is readily accomplished by wedges, inserts, and other appliances that invert the heel within the shoe. Proper footwear, correction of any static foot disability, and increased rest of the foot are helpful measures. A thick, sponge-rubber heel appliance with a transverse sulcus to accommodate the spur is often used. Proper measurements should be taken to ensure that the sulcus is actually placed under the painful area. Application of dry heat daily for a few months can also help relieve the symptoms. Injection of procaine hydrochloride, alcohol, sclerosing agents, or hydrocortisone acetate has been tried, but the

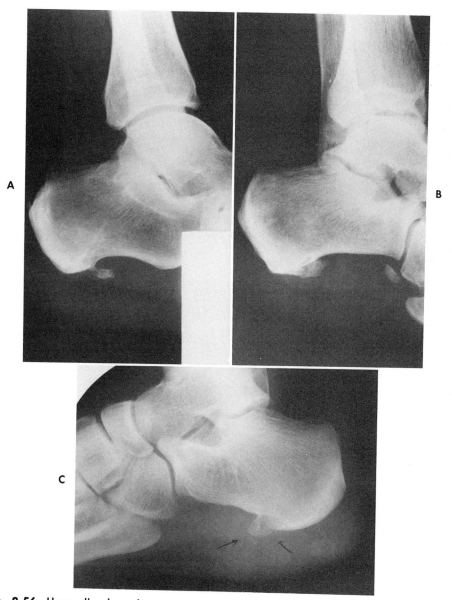

Fig. 8-56. Unusually shaped spurs requiring special evaluation. **A** and **B,** Unusually painful spurs. **C,** Osseous cyst at origin of plantar fascia.

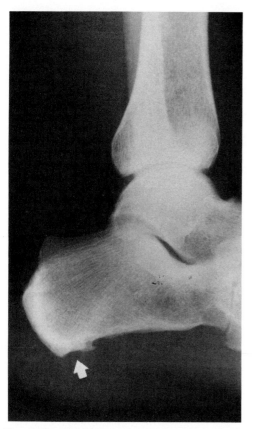

Fig. 8-57. Roentgenogram of painful heel that was caused by osteolytic changes of unknown etiology in plantar tuberosity of calcaneus. The spur was asymptomatic.

Calcaneal spurs and osteosclerosis of the posterior tuberosity

Occasionally, the surgeon encounters an abnormal insertion of the tendo achillis that is probably caused by an inward angulation of the lower half of the posterior tuberosity. This angulation causes the tendo achillis to begin its insertion at an abnormally low point; it creates an unusually deep retrocalcaneal bursa as well. Abnormal traction on the lower half of the posterior tuberosity produces a reactive osteosclerosis and the formation of a spur (Fig. 8-58). The hard leather counters of shoes undoubtedly aggravate these conditions and cause them to become painful. Occasionally, a sharp spur forms in the middle of the posterior tuberosity of the calcaneus (Fig. 8-59).

Only in rare instances are surgical procedures indicated. Usually if the patient avoids wearing shoes with hard and rigid counters (that part of the shoe that covers the posterior tuberosity must be made of soft leather), the symptoms will dissipate.

FLATFOOT (PES PLANUS)

Flatfoot, weak foot, or fallen arches, as the disorder is variously called, is difficult to classify. There is no known standard by which the longitudinal arch may be considered flat, normal, or high. Some primitive peoples in Africa and Australia are all flatfooted. When they have painful feet, however, it is only as a result of injuries; whereas in our modern society, many people with so-called normal arches have painful longitudinal arches on weight bearing.

Many people with flatfoot can walk as comfortably and as easily as others who have so-called normal arches, yet for some reason a myth exists that people with flatfoot will have difficulty with their feet. During World War II, thousands of men were rejected from the Army because they had asymptomatic flatfoot. Athletes with flatfoot (some long-distance runners particularly) are not impeded by the condition.

therapeutic effcacy is doubtful, because none of the published studies reviewed reports the use of a control group.

Surgical excision of the spur has been reported for cases in which intractable pain is unrelieved by conservative treatment. However, since the presence of the spur is simply the visual evidence of abnormal forces in the plantar aponeurosis, it is not surprising that mere resection of the spur does not always result in a cure. Reviews of reported cases indicate that not more than 50 percent of patients get prompt and permanent relief from surgical procedures (Steindler and Smith, 1938; Chang and Miltner, 1934). For procedures, see Chapter 19.

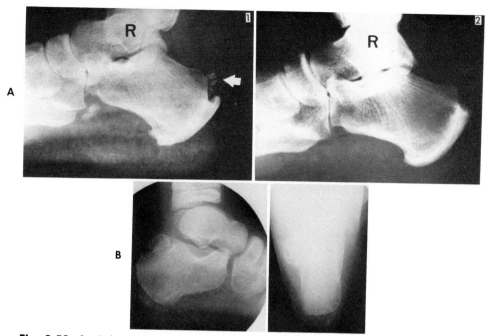

Fig. 8-58. A, Calcaneal spurs and osteosclerosis of posterior tuberosity caused by abnormal insertion of tendo achillis. Note the presence of osteophytes in retrocalcaneal bursa in 1. **B,** Osteoma at posterior tuberosity and in retrocalcaneal space in foot of 8-year-old boy.

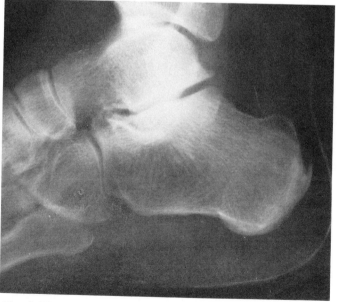

Fig. 8-59. Spur in middle of posterior tuberosity of calcaneus.

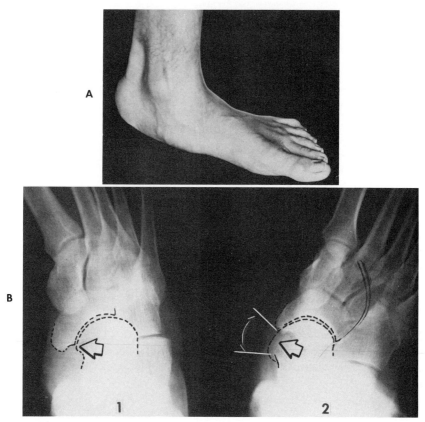

Fig. 8-60. A, Flatfoot and eversion and abduction of forefoot. **B,** Roentgenograms of flatfoot in 43-year-old male. *1,* Foot held in adduction. *2,* Same foot held in extreme abduction. Note extreme excursion of the navicular over the head of the talus.

With few exceptions, black people have flatfoot at an early age but later usually develop strong "normal" arches. Perhaps one out of a thousand people with flatfoot will have pain from the condition because of congenital or acquired abnormalities (DuVries, 1967).

Symptomatic flexible flatfoot

Harris and Beath (1948) attributed the weak, flat foot to deficiencies in the structure of the talus and calcaneus. Conversely, strong and well-shaped feet are attributed to the result of tarsal bones so shaped and so integrated into one another that they cannot shift when weight is imposed on them. In symptomatic flatfoot not involving osseous anomalies, the condition is often related to weak posterior tibial muscle function, which permits an abnormal excursion of the talonavicular joint (Fig. 8-60, *B*).

Recently, surgeons have become aware that rupture of the tendon of the posterior tibialis muscle is an etiologic factor in pes planus. These ruptures have occurred in middle-aged individuals who have had one or more injections of a corticoid preparation into the sheath of the tendon to relieve local discomfort or to alleviate an obvious synovitis. Subsequently, a rupture of the tendon has occurred, with prompt development of a markedly pronated foot. When the patient attempts to rise on his toes, he has difficulty doing so on the involved side; the heel fails to invert and

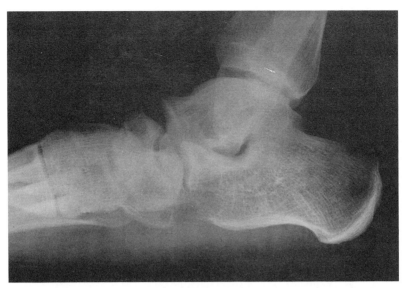

Fig. 8-61. Planovalgus caused by congenital talonavicular anomaly.

the longitudinal arch fails to rise during this maneuver. Rupture of the posterior tibial tendon should be suspected in any case in which a unilateral pes planus suddenly appears.

Use of arch supports, wedges, and heel cups has proved unsuccessful in providing relief from the symptoms of foot strain in these patients. Prompt repair of the tendon is indicated in early cases. Subtalar arthrodesis or transfer of the peroneus longus tendon to replace the posterior tibial function may be required in older patients. To date, the surgical results of these procedures have not been evaluated adequately.

The symptomatic weak foot may be flat or may have a high longitudinal arch, especially at rest. The flat foot usually has a degree of abduction of the forefoot (Figs. 8-60 and 8-61) and eversion of the ankle. The tendo achillis may be shortened and pulled at an angle instead of following a plumb line (Fig. 8-62). Pain is usually chronic but may be acute. The long, narrow, flaccid foot with a so-called normal arch is likely to become symptomatic.

Only the flatfoot that is symptomatic needs medical attention (Fig. 8-63). Cor-

rective shoes, the wedging of the shoe, the use of inlays of leather or of metal or plastic materials, or the use of both wedging and inlays is recommended. In acute cases, adhesive strapping to hold the foot in adduction and inversion usually gives immediate relief.

A few cases may become intractable. If appliances do not give relief, stabilization of the tarsus is the only resort (see Chapter 19).

Peroneal spastic flatfoot (spastic pes planus)

Spastic flatfoot has posed many questions since Jones (1916) called attention to the prevalence and disabling effect of the disorder. The term is loosely applied to a group of conditions arising from different causes. Usually it begins during adolescence and is characterized by severe pes planus, an abduction of the forefoot, and an eversion of the ankle, caused by constant spasm of the peroneal muscles.

Two distinct types of the condition are recognized: the rigid and the flexible. Under anesthesia, the spasticity of the flexible type disappears and the foot can be placed in a normal position, whereas the rigid type

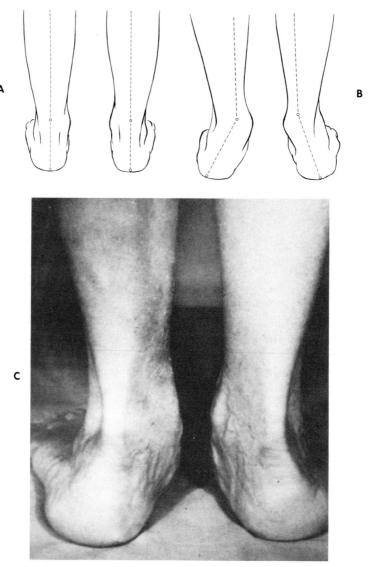

Fig. 8-62. A, Tendo achillis in vertical line. **B,** Everted foot. The tendo achillis lies medially behind the medial malleolus. **C,** Photograph of patient with everted foot. Tendo achillis lies medially behind the medial malleolus. (**C,** Courtesy Dr. Milton Lewis.)

remains fixed. Harris and Beath (1948) reported that among 3,600 candidates for Army enlistment, 74 cases (2 percent) of the rigid type and 217 cases (6 percent) of the flexible type were observed.

Etiology. The cause of spastic flatfoot is not entirely understood, probably because the condition is a symptom complex rather than a disease entity. Many factors are pre-

disposing. They may be present singly or in combination, but the same predisposing factors may be present without producing the syndrome.

The flaccid type is undoubtedly caused by excessive stress on the foot as a result of overweight and of poorly fitting shoes during adolescence. As nature attempts to force the foot to rest, as happens in frac-

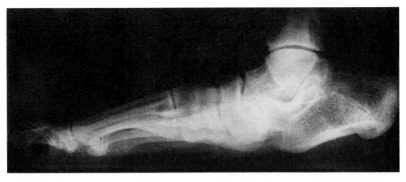

Fig. 8-63. Symptomatic severe flatfoot (rocker-bottom foot). It required major stabilization.

tures or chronic joint disease, a compensatory reflex spasm of the peroneal muscles takes place.

The rigid type is often the end result of long duration in cases of the flexible type; sometimes it is caused by a congenital tarsal anomaly (see p. 105). Harris and Beath thought that the rigid type was always caused by an anomalous talocalcaneal bridge or by a calcaneonavicular bar. Webster and Roberts (1951) supported this theory. Either or both anomalies may be present.

Kidner (1929) believed that a number of these spastic flatfoot cases are related to the presence of an accessory navicular or prehallux. Because the posterior tibial tendon is usually attached to the prehallux, its normal support of the longitudinal arch is lost. It is true, as Kidner says, that a prehallux is sometimes the cause, not because the support of the tibialis posterior is lost, but rather because irritation from the movement of the prehallux against the body of the navicular occurs. A reflex peroneal spasm is produced in an attempt to avoid irritation of the head of the talus (see Fig. 6-29). Lapidus (1946) regarded spastic flatfoot as the result of a lesion of the interosseous talocalcaneal ligament in the subtalar joint. In my experience, the majority of cases of peroneal spastic flatfoot have been related to tarsal coalition, especially to calcaneonavicular bar. The calcaneonavicular bar is usually completely

osseous (synostosis, Fig. 8-64); occasionally the bar has a cartilaginous bridge (synchondrosis, Fig. 8-65), and both conditions predispose to spastic flatfoot.

Sometimes spastic flatfoot has occurred as the aftermath of trauma to the neck of the navicular (see Fig. 6-29). Congenital anomalies of the talonavicular joint (Fig. 8-61) have also been other predisposing factors. If anomalies of the tarsus are not present, one should suspect arthritic changes in the subtalar joint as initiating factors. These changes may be traumatic, degenerative, or rheumatoid.

The peroneus longus and brevis are the muscles in spasm, but there is evidence that the peroneus brevis is more productive of deformity. Merryweather (1955), in his study of sixty cases of spastic flatfoot, observed tarsal anomalies in only 40 percent. Fifty-two out of the sixty were treated successfully by conservative measures, such as immobilization with overcorrection, which was suited equally to those with or without anomalies.

Many cases occur in short, squatty, overweight adolescents who have endocrine deficiency bordering on cretinism. With glandular therapy and proper footwear and shoe wedging, many respond and become asymptomatic. However, there is usually a relationship between this malady and tarsal coalition.

Treatment of flatfoot. The type of flatfoot that is caused entirely by muscle

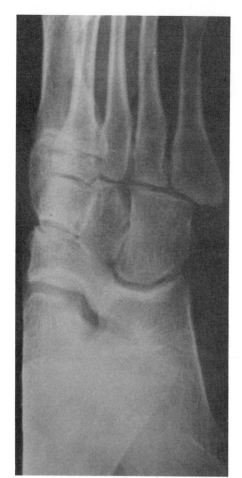

Fig. 8-64. Calcaneonavicular bar completely ossified (synostosis).

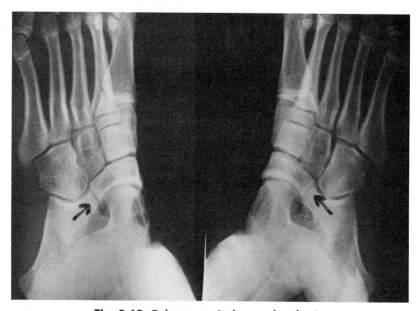

Fig. 8-65. Calcaneonavicular synchondrosis.

spasm, after anomalies such as tarsal coalition, talonavicular joint anomalies, or prehallux have been ruled out, can usually be controlled by conservative measures. To differentiate between the flexible and rigid types, it is often necessary to place the patient under general anesthesia for complete voluntary muscle relaxation. If the deformity is readily reduced under anesthesia, a plaster cast with walking caliper may be applied with the foot overcorrected. Many will remain corrected and require only corrective shoes for a time after removal of the cast. Some will require repetition of overcorrection under anesthesia and immobilization.

In a few cases, I have found that injection of 10 to 20 ml. of 1 percent procaine hydrochloride at the neck of the fibula relieved the peroneal spasm.

Recurrent cases of the flexible type of flatfoot without peroneal spasm may be corrected by Schoolfield's (1952) operation (see Fig. 19-10), which shortens and reinforces the deltoid ligament.

In selected cases in which the tibialis anterior has become paralyzed or has lost most of its power, the peroneus longus may be transferred into the insertion of the tibialis anterior or into the body of the medial cuneiform. Sectioning the peroneus brevis will further reduce the pull of the foot in abduction.

Treatment of the rigid type is difficult. Numerous stabilization procedures and wedge osteotomies have been reported. After a review of the end results of several operative procedures on 102 feet of children for the correction of flatfoot, Crego and Ford (1952) were forced to conclude that arthrodesing operation for flatfoot should never be done for cosmetic reasons only, and is justified solely for the relief of pain. Weil (1955) likewise reviewed the end result of treatment in 400 cases (561 feet) of rigid flatfoot; 189 had been treated conservatively and the remainder were treated by a variety of surgical procedures, such as tendon transference and osteotomies. In only 36 percent were results of operation satisfactory.

Hoke (1921, 1931), an early student of foot deformities, proposed the following stabilizing procedure for flatfoot: (1) lengthen the tendo achillis; (2) through an incision along the medial border of the foot, exposing the naviculocuneiform joint, denude and reflect the ligamentous covering; (3) force and maintain the foot in extreme plantar flexion while excising a rectangular block of bone from the navicular and medial cuneiform joint on the longitudinal plane; (4) remove a segment of cortical bone of equal dimension from the tibia and fit it into the rectangular slot bridging the joint (see Fig. 19-31, A).

Zadek (1935) recommended a wedge osteotomy of the talocalcaneal joint. White (1940) removed a wedge of bone from the medial side of the neck of the talus and then inserted it into an opened osteotomy on the lateral side of the neck of the calcaneus. Harris and Beath (1948) advised a subtalar and talonavicular fusion.

No single procedure can be used in all cases. Conservative measures should always be exhausted before resorting to surgical treatment of osseous disorders. Each case should be evaluated and a procedure selected that is best suited to the case.

Generally, Schoolfield's shortening and reinforcement of the deltoid ligament and Hoke's naviculocuneiform bone graft are the most useful operations for the flexible type of flatfoot, whereas triple arthrodesis must usually be resorted to for the rigid type. (For surgical procedures, see Chapter 19.)

CLAWFOOT

Clawfoot, described in detail in Chapter 5 (see pp. 103 to 105) is a deformity that is largely one of the forefoot, with typical dorsal contracture of all the toes and dislocation of the metatarsophalangeal joints. The apex of the deformity on the inner border of the foot is usually the naviculocuneiform joint.

It is ironic that all flat feet are considered to be potentially disabling, while little consideration is generally given to pes cavus (high arched) feet. As a matter of fact, most cavus feet are poorly functioning feet, whereas flat feet become symptomatic only in the presence of other abnormalities.

Clawfoot appears more often during early childhood or adolescence and occurs about as frequently in boys as in girls. No relationship to race or social status has been demonstrated. It may be associated with many known disorders or may occur independently. Saunders (1935) concluded that congenital abnormalities of the spinal cord often produce clawfoot but that unlike the congenital talipes, clawfoot of independent congenital origin as seen at birth or during infancy is rare. Kochs (1927) reported a case in which laminectomy was performed for spina bifida; spontaneous correction of the deformity of the foot ensued.

For a discussion of the symptoms of clawfoot, see Chapter 5; for treatment of the deformity, see Chapters 5 and 19.

DROPFOOT

In dropfoot the foot is in a constant equinus position and the patient is unable to dorsiflex the foot actively. There are two types of dropfoot: congenital talipes equinus, which is discussed in Chapter 5, and the more common type, paralytic dropfoot (see Fig. 19-6, A).

Symptoms of paralytic dropfoot. Although the foot is held most frequently in an equinus position in paralytic dropfoot, in some cases it is held in a varus or valgus attitude. The condition differs from congenital talipes equinus in that in typical paralytic dropfoot the foot is limp but can be dorsiflexed passively because the calf muscles are not contracted and the ligaments or bones are not fixed in this deformed state. The extent of the deformity is dependent upon such factors as the severity of the paralysis of the dorsiflexors, the strength of the antagonistic muscles, adaptive growth alterations that occur as a result of the deforming forces, and the effectiveness of the after-treatment. Sensory function is usually normal but may be diminished. The patient is unable to dorsiflex the foot, trips easily, and stumbles frequently unless the foot is kept clear of the ground.

Etiology. The condition is usually caused by paralysis of the anterior compartment of the leg muscles, often as a result of poliomyelitis and sometimes as a result of injury to the common peroneal nerve. The common peroneal nerve is superficial as it courses around the neck of the fibula; injury to the neck of the fibula, and hence to the peroneal nerve, may result in dropfoot. Many other conditions, such as intraspinal compression neuropathy, cerebral nervous system disease such as multiple sclerosis, paralysis and spasticity after a stroke, and cerebral palsy, are causes of dropfoot.

Treatment. The paralysis responsible for the dropfoot deformity may be reversible or can be permanent. Prevention of overstretching of the dorsiflexors is very important, since recovery of muscle tone and strength may not occur in the overstretched attitude. A dropfoot control brace worn continuously, or until dorsiflexion power returns, is the treatment of choice. Return of muscle power of the dorsiflexors has been observed in cases where a dropfoot control brace has been applied many months after paralysis. Operative treatment may require arthrodesing, bone blocking, and tendon transposing, or a combination of these to control dropfoot. The best results occur when foot stabilization, such as triple arthrodesis, is followed by tendon transposition to the dorsum of the foot. In some circumstances transposition of the tendon of a strong muscle that is producing a deformity may be corrected without a stabilizing bone procedure. The results are less predictable, generally, as to ultimate function of the foot. The following tendon transpositions to aid in overcoming dropfoot have been used:

1. Extensor hallucis longus tendon transposed to the neck of the first metatarsal

2. Peroneus brevis tendon transposed to the dorsum of the foot
3. Peroneus longus tendon transposed to the dorsum of the foot
4. Both peroneal tendons transposed to the dorsum of the foot
5. Posterior tibial tendon transposed through the interosseous ligament to the dorsum of the foot

Dynamic forces acting on the foot must be evaluated accurately before any attempt is made to rebalance. It is not uncommon that the foot will be deviated to a new deformity after a tendon transposition done to improve dorsiflexion. This applies especially to the immature foot, since the shape of the foot may change with growth.

Stabilization operations to control drop-foot. Many operations to eliminate or reduce the number of joints upon which the weakened muscles must act have been devised, such as triple arthrodesis, pantalar arthrodesis, ankle arthrodesis, and posterior bone block.

Triple arthrodesis is perhaps one of the more refined procedures of orthopaedic surgery. Two methods are common in current use: (1) Ryerson triple arthrodesis, and (2) Lambrinudi triple arthrodesis. If sufficient motor power to produce dorsiflexion is absent, the stabilization of the foot may be supplemented by the addition of a posterior bone block of the ankle joint. (For surgical procedures, see Chapter 19.)

REFERENCES

Barnicot, N. A., and Hardy, R. H.: The position of the hallux in West Africans, J. Anat. 89:355-361, July 1955.

Bingold, A. C., and Collins, D. H.: Hallux rigidus, J. Bone Joint Surg. 32-B:214-222, May 1950.

Blokhin, V. N., and Vinogradova, T. P.: Shpory pyatochnykh kostey [Calcaneal spurs], Ortop. Travmatol. Protez. 11:96-113, 1937.

Blum, A.: De l'orteil en marteau, Bull. Mém. Soc. Chir. Paris, 9:738-745, 1883.

Branch, H. E.: Pathological dislocation of the second toe, J. Bone Joint Surg. 19:978-984, Oct. 1937.

Craigmile, D. A.: Incidence, origin, and prevention of certain foot defects, Brit. J. Med. 4:749-752, Oct. 1953.

Creer, W. S.: The feet of the industrial worker. Clinical aspect: Relation to footwear, Lancet 2:1482-1483, Dec. 1938.

Crego, C. H., Jr., and Ford, L. T.: An end-result study of various operative procedures for correcting flat feet in children, J. Bone Joint Surg. 34-A:183-195, Jan. 1952.

Chang, C. C., and Miltner, L. J.: Periostitis of the os calcis, J. Bone Joint Surg. 16:355-364, Apr. 1934.

Davis, J. B., and Blair, H. C.: Spurs of calcaneus in Strümpell-Marie disease: Report of 15 cases, J. Bone Joint Surg. 32-A:838-840, Oct. 1950.

Duchenne, G. B.: Physiology of motion (translated and edited by E. B. Kaplan), Philadelphia, 1949, J. B. Lippincott Co. (Original French edition appeared in 1867.)

DuVries, H. L.: Dislocation of toe, J.A.M.A. 160:728, Feb. 1956.

DuVries, H. L.: Five myths about your feet, Today's Health 45:49-51, Aug. 1967.

Ellis, T. S.: The human foot: Its form and structure, functions and clothing, London, 1889, J. & A. Churchill.

Engle, E. T., and Morton, D. J.: Notes on foot disorders among natives of the Belgian Congo, J. Bone Joint Surg. 13:311-318, Apr. 1931.

Ewald, P.: Die Ätiologie des Hallux valgus, Dtsch. Z. Chir. 114:90-103, 1912.

Fowler, A., and Philip, J. F.: Abnormality of the calcaneus as a cause of painful heel, Brit. J. Surg. 32:494-498, Apr. 1945.

Galland, W. I., and Jordan, H.: Hallux valgus, Surg. Gynec. Obstet. 66:95-99, Jan.-June 1938.

Gould, E. A.: Three generations of exostoses of the heel: Inherited from father to son, J. Hered. 33:228, June 1942.

Gudas, C. J.: An etiology of hallux rigidus, J. Foot Surg. 10:113-124, 1971.

Haglund, P.: Beitrag zur Klinik der Achillessehne, Z. Orthop. Chir. 49:49-58, 1928.

Hardy, R. H., and Clapham, J. C. R.: Observations on hallux valgus, J. Bone Joint Surg. 33-B:376-391, Aug. 1951.

Harris, R. I., and Beath, T.: Etiology of peroneal spastic flat foot, J. Bone Joint Surg. 30-B:624-634, Nov. 1948.

Harris, R. I., and Beath, T.: The short first metatarsal: Its incidence and clinical significance, J. Bone Joint Surg. 31-A:553-565, July 1949.

Harrison, M. H., and Harvey, F. J.: Arthrodesis of the first metatarsophalangeal joint for hallux valgus and rigidus, J. Bone Joint Surg. 45-A:471-480, Apr. 1963.

Hawkes, O. A. M.: On the relative lengths of the first and second toes of the human foot from the point of view of occurrence, anatomy and heredity, J. Genet. 3:249-274, Apr. 1914.

Hewitt, D., Stewart, A. M., and Webb, J. W.:

The prevalence of foot defects among wartime recruits, Brit. Med. J. **2**:745-749, Oct. 1953.

Hicks, J. H.: The mechanics of the foot. II. The plantar aponeurosis and the arch, J. Anat. **88**: 25-30, 1954.

Higgs, S. L.: "Hammer-toe," Postgrad. Med. J. **6**:130-132, May 1931.

Hohmann, K. G. G.: IV. Der Hallux valgus und die übrigen Zehenverkrümmungen, Ergeb. Chir. Orthop. **18**:308-376, 1925.

Hohmann, K. G. G.: Fuss und Bein, ihre Erkrankungen und deren Behandlung, ed. 4, Munich, 1948, J. F. Bergmann, p. 299.

Hoke, M.: An operation for stabilizing paralytic feet, Amer. J. Orthop. Surg. **3**:494-505, 1921.

Hoke, M.: An operation for the correction of extremely relaxed flat feet, J. Bone Joint Surg. **13**:773-783, Oct. 1931.

James, C. S.: Footprints and feet of natives of the Soloman Islands. Lancet **2**:1390-1393, Dec. 1939.

Jones, F. W.: Structure and function as seen in the foot, Baltimore, 1944, The Williams & Wilkins Co.

Joplin, R. J.: Sling procedure for correction of splay-foot, metatarsus primus varus, and hallux valgus, J. Bone Joint Surg. **32-A**:779-785, Oct. 1950.

Kaplan, E. B.: The tibialis posterior muscle in relation to hallux valgus, Bull. Hosp. Joint Dis. **16**:88-93, Apr. 1955.

Keck, S. W., and Kelly, P. J.: Bursitis of the posterior part of the heel: Evaluation of surgical treatment of eighteen patients, J. Bone Joint Surg. **47-A**:267-273, Mar. 1965.

Kelikian, H.: Hallux valgus, allied deformities of the forefoot and metatarsalgia, Philadelphia, 1965, W. B. Saunders Co.

Kessel, L., and Bonney, G.: Hallux rigidus in the adolescent, J. Bone Joint Surg. **40-B**:668-673, Nov. 1958.

Kidner, F. C.: The prehallux (accessory scaphoid) in its relation to flat-foot, J. Bone Joint Surg. **11**:831-837, Oct. 1929.

Kochs, J.: Spontanheilung einer Fussdeformität bei Spina bifida occulta nach Laminektomie, Münch. Med. Wochenschr. **74**:1877-1879, Nov. 1927.

Lam Sim-Fook, and Hodgson, A. R.: A comparison of foot forms among the non-shoe and shoe-wearing Chinese population, J. Bone Joint Surg. **40-A**:1058-1062, Oct. 1958.

Lapidus, P. W.: "Dorsal bunion": Its mechanics and operative correction, J. Bone Joint Surg. **22**:627-637, July 1940.

Lapidus, P. W.: Spastic flat-foot, J. Bone Joint Surg. **28**:126-136, Jan. 1946.

Levick, G. M.: The action of the intrinsic muscles of the foot and their treatment by electricity, Brit. Med. J. **1**:381-382, Mar. 1921.

Levick, G. M.: On the arch-raising rôle of certain intrinsic muscles of the foot, Proc. Anat. Soc. Great Britain Ireland J. Anat. **67**:196-197, Feb. 1932.

Maclennan, R.: Prevalence of hallux valgus in a neolithic New Guinea population, Lancet **1**: 1398-1400, June 1966.

Marwil, T. B., and Brantingham, C. R.: Foot problems of women's reserve, Hosp. Corps Quart. **16**:98-100, Oct. 1943.

Mau, C.: Das Krankheitsbild des Hallux rigidus, Münch. Med. Wochenschr. **75**:1193-1196, July 1928.

Mayo, C. H.: The surgical treatment of bunion, Ann. Surg. **48**:300-302, July-Sept. 1908.

Mayo, C. H.: The surgical treatment of bunions, Minn. Med. **3**:326-331, 1920.

Merryweather, R.: Spastic valgus of foot, Proc. Roy. Soc. Med. **48**:103-106, 1955.

Miller, L. F., and Arendt, J.: Deformity of first metatarsal head due to faulty foot mechanics, J. Bone Joint Surg. **22**:349-353, Apr. 1940.

Morton, D. J.: The human foot, New York, 1935, Columbia University Press.

Morton, D. J.: Human locomotion and body form: A study of gravity and man, Baltimore, 1952, The Williams & Wilkins Co.

Moynihan, F. J.: Arthrodesis of the metatarsophalangeal joint of the great toe, J. Bone Joint Surg. **49-B**:544-551, Aug. 1967.

Rogers, W. A., and Joplin, R. J.: Hallux valgus, weak foot and the Keller operation: An endresult study, Surg. Clin. N. Amer. **27**:1295-1302, Oct. 1947.

Saunders, J. T.: Etiology and treatment of clawfoot, Arch. Surg. **30**:179-198, Feb. 1935.

Saxl, A.: Die Schuhgeschwulst der Ferse, Z. Orthop. Chir. **51**:312-320, 1929.

Schoolfield, B. L.: Operative treatment of flatfoot, Surg. Gynec. Obstet. **94**:136-140, Feb. 1952.

Shine, I. B.: Incidence of hallux valgus in a partially shoe-wearing community, Brit. Med. J. **1**:1648-1650, June 1965.

Stein, H. C.: Clinical surgery: Hallux valgus. Surg. Gynec. Obstet. **66**:889-897, Jan.-June 1938.

Steindler, A., and Smith, A. R.: Spurs of the os calcis, Surg. Gynec. Obstet. **66**:663-665, Mar. 1938.

Taylor, R. G.: An operative procedure for treatment of hammer-toe and claw-toe, J. Bone Joint Surg. **22**:608-609, July 1940.

Taylor, R. G.: The treatment of claw toes by multiple transfers of flexor into extensor tendons, J. Bone Joint Surg. **33-B**:539-542, Nov. 1951.

Truslow, W.: Metatarsus primus varus or hallux valgus? J. Bone Joint Surg. **7**:98-108, Jan. 1925.

Webster, F. S., and Roberts, W. M.: Tarsal anomalies and peroneal spastic flatfoot, J.A.M.A. **146**:1099-1104, July 1951.

Weil, F.: Über Erfahrungen an operativ behandelten kontrakten Plattfüssen, Z. Orthop. **86**:204-210, 1955.

Wells, L. H.: The foot of the South African native, Amer. J. Phys. Anthropol. **15**:185-289, Jan.-Mar. 1931.

White, J. W.: Congenital flat-foot: A new surgical approach, J. Bone Joint Surg. **22**:547-554, July 1940.

Wilkins, E. H.: Feet, with particular reference to schoolchildren, Med. Officer **66**:5, 13, 21, 29, July 1941.

Young, C. S.: An operation for correction of hammer-toe and claw-toe, J. Bone Joint Surg. **20**:715-719, July 1938.

Zadek, I.: Transverse-wedge arthrodesis for relief of pain in rigid flat-foot, J. Bone Joint Surg. **17**:453-467, Apr. 1935.

9

Neuromuscular diseases affecting the foot

Robert L. Samilson
Elmer E. Specht

Any condition affecting the innervation of the musculature of the foot and ankle, or directly affecting the muculature itself, can result in an alteration of function and lead to deformity. Similarly, conditions that affect the afferent impulses arising in the foot can produce significant disturbance. In considering these conditions one should be mindful of the functional impositions placed on the foot from deformities above. For the treatment of the deformities described in this chapter that require surgical procedures, see Chapter 19.

Upper motor neuron diseases (e.g., cerebrovascular accidents, brain tumors, tuberous sclerosis, and cerebral palsy) differ from lower motor neuron diseases (e.g., myelodysplasia, poliomyelitis, Charcot-Marie-Tooth syndrome) in the character of the neuromuscular changes that they produce. Spasticity, rigidity, ankle clonus, positive Babinski's reflex, and synchronous muscle activity are alterations imposed by upper motor neuron disease. Flaccidity, weakness, atrophy, an electrical reaction of degeneration, and deformity caused by muscle imbalance are commonly encountered in lower motor neuron disease. Reflexes are diminished or absent.

CEREBROVASCULAR ACCIDENTS

There are approximately two million stroke patients in the United States, whose care costs four billion dollars annually. One third of these patients are wage earners under age 65, made unemployable by the residua of stroke (U. S. Dept. of H. E. W., 1971). In addition, there are untold numbers of patients with head injury who manifest symptoms and signs of stroke.

Spastic hemiplegia

The most common manifestation of cerebrovascular accident is spastic hemiplegia. Sensory and motor loss are present in varying degrees; the former may seriously affect the return of motor function. In the lower extremity, spastic hip adductors, spastic quadriceps, and spastic equinovarus are commonly seen, as well as circumduction of the adducted thigh, extended knee, and equinovarus foot. Loss of reciprocal upper-limb–lower-limb swing and failure to incorporate the many rotatory displacements of the individual segments into a smoothly functioning unit are characteristics of spastic hemiplegia. Observation and analysis of the patient's gait are essential in order to provide a rational treatment program.

Treatment. Conservative splinting to avoid contracture, which appears with surprising rapidity in spastic muscle, is of benefit initially. Peripheral nerve blocks, first with a local anesthetic and then with phenol, will offer transitory relief of a non-fixed deformity (but not of a contracture) and thus may be of some use as a diagnostic measure for spastic equinovarus associated with a cerebrovascular accident. If a contracture exists, it is beneficial to lengthen the tendo achillis. Obviously the tendo achillis should be lengthened before ankle dorsiflexion is reinforced with a posterior tibial tendon transfer through the interosseous membrane to the dorsum of the midfoot. A split anterior tibial tendon transfer sometimes obviates the varus component and produces better balance in the foot, but in using such a procedure one should anticipate further weakening of ankle dorsiflexion. Finally, release of tight toe flexors may be necessary in some instances. Postoperative management should include appropriate splinting, bracing, or both (Treanor et al., 1955; Mooney et al., 1967).

CEREBRAL PALSY

No official figures are available as to the existing number of cases of cerebral palsy in the United States, but the United Cerebral Palsy Association estimates the figure at approximately 750,000 persons, with 25,000 babies born each year with cerebral palsy. In a New York State survey in 1971, six infants out of a thousand live births were found to have cerebral palsy (U. S. Dept. of H. E. W., 1971).

Increased mortality of persons with cerebral palsy has been documented by Schlesinger et al. (1959) with data from upstate New York. Cohen and Mustacchi (1966), in a survival study of a group of over a thousand individuals with cerebral palsy under the age of 21 years who resided in northern California, found an eightfold to ninefold excess over "expected mortality" in their sample of cases.

Characteristics

Spasticity is the most common finding in ambulatory patients with cerebral palsy. We have noted (1968) the following characteristics that make functional ambulation difficult:

1. Increased resistance to manipulation, hyperactive reflexes, and clonus
2. Exaggerated contraction of muscles subjected to stretch
3. Synchronous electrical activity of agonist-antagonist muscles, without regard to phase
4. Voluntary contraction that begins simultaneously in all parts of a spastic muscle, with peaks of activity that frequently occur at the same time in different parts of a muscle (voluntary contractile activity in normal muscle is asynchronous)
5. Enlarged reflexogenic area (e.g., tonic reflexes of the foot)
6. Persistent neonatal reflexes with their postural impositions (e.g., asymmetrical tonic neck reflex)
7. Failure of developmental milestones to appear in an orderly fashion
8. Slowness of voluntary movement (probably a function of 2, 3, and 4)
9. Perceptual and conceptual deficits
10. Varying degrees of sensory loss

To consider the deformities in cerebral palsy a consequence of muscle imbalance alone, without careful consideration of the above factors, is to reduce a complex subject to an absurdly simple one. The genesis of deformity in cerebral palsy is different from that of deformity in lower motor neuron disorders (e.g., poliomyelitis or myelomeningocele). To suppose that it is the same—whether for diagnosis, treatment, or both—is to assure an unsatisfactory result.

Obviously, consideration of one anatomic part (e.g., the foot) to the exclusion of others) (e.g., the ankle, leg, knee, hip, pelvis, spine, and upper limb) is another source of error that the practitioner may make in his clinical judgment of cerebral palsy. One of the most common questions asked about the orthopaedic management of the spastic child who walks with flexed hip, flexed knee, and equinus foot is "Where do I start?" The answer is not difficult. Begin by examining the child; the examination, if detailed enough, will indicate what to do or not to do first. It would be an error, for example, for the surgeon to perform a hamstring transfer (Eggers procedure) without first releasing a hip-flexion contracture of 30 degrees or more. Similarly, equinus may resolve following a hamstring transfer. One should predict this outcome by preoperative cylinder cast or by a simple electromyographic test as follows: With an electrode over the triceps surae, the child stands in the crouched equinus position as the examiner rapidly extends the child's hip and knee, while constantly recording. If the potentials in the triceps surae fall to zero when the hip and knee are extended and remain at zero throughout the hip and knee extension activity, it is probable that hamstring transfer will correct the equinus. In such a circumstance, injudicious lengthening of the triceps surae may result in a calcaneus deformity (Samilson, in press).

Equinus deformity. Equinus is a common deformity in cerebral palsy that may at first be due to spasticity alone, but eventually permanent contracture results which requires surgical correction (Baker and Hill, 1964). Conservative management of incipient equinus includes light and comfortable splints at night and proper heel-cord stretching exercises during the day. (In these exercises it is important to lock the subtalar joint in inversion before dorsiflexing the ankle in order to avoid producing a rocker-bottom foot.) In cases in which the deformity has been corrected surgically, the same conservative measures should be adopted as part of postoperative management.

When the clinician examines the child who has an equinus deformity, he should attempt to determine whether any function exists in the tibialis anterior muscle. Tibialis anterior activity may become apparent in the "dorsiflexion confusion test," in which the child sits on the edge of a table and flexes his hip against the resistance of the examiner's hand (Fig. 9-1). It is also important for the examiner to determine which muscles (the tibialis posterior, the peroneals, or the toe flexors) contribute to the

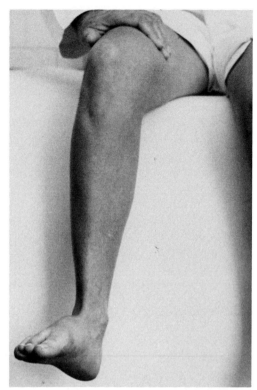

Fig. 9-1. Dorsiflexion "confusion" test. The patient flexes the hip against resistance of the examiner's hand. In so doing, tibialis anterior function may become apparent.

equinus. The tibialis posterior muscle is usually a stance-phase muscle (see Chapter 1), but when it is overactive in cerebral palsy it stands out like a band on the medial aspect of the ankle during swing phase. The peroneals, when overactive, frequently cause an elevation of the lateral border of the foot. When the toe flexors are tight, the toes claw.

In children with hemiplegia it is unwise to correct all the equinus on the hemiplegic side because some equinus is necessary to compensate for the shortening of the entire leg, a condition that often coexists.

For contracture of the triceps surae selective heel-cord lengthening is effective. It is rarely necessary to perform a capsulotomy of the ankle joint posteriorly. If the gastrocnemius is tight but the soleus is not, length-

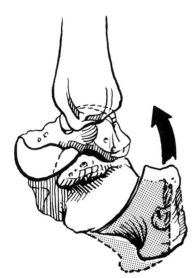

Fig. 9-2. Crescentic osteotomy of calcaneus for calcaneocavus deformity. The posterior fragment is moved upward.

ening or dividing the aponeurosis of the gastrocnemius (Strayer, Vulpius, Baker procedures) is effective. Occasionally, lengthening of the toe flexors is required if these muscles contribute to the equinus, and sometimes tibialis posterior lengthening may be done if that muscle is functionally short.

Since our experience with the tibialis posterior slide in front of the medial malleolus has been disappointing, we cannot recommend it. However, in cases in which the tibialis posterior muscle does contribute to the equinovarus deformity and in which the dorsiflexors are weak and contracture of the triceps surae in absent, posterior tibial tendon transfer through the interosseous membrane of the dorsum of the foot into the middle cuneiform has proved to be helpful. Most of the time, the result of this procedure is an effective tenodesis. Neurectomies have provided inconsistent and transient results and we cannot recommend them for the correction of equinus.

Calcaneus deformity. This deformity is rarely found in cerebral palsy, but when it is present it is frequently associated with

cavus. Occasionally it occurs as a result of injudicious triceps surae lengthening. The biomechanical genesis of the deformity should be investigated whenever possible. Plantar fasciotomy may be helpful initially; crescentic osteotomy of the calcaneus, with displacement of the heel fragment upward, may be performed at a later time (Fig. 9-2). This procedure has proved to be effective if the deformity is actually calcaneocavus and not primarily midtarsal cavus. In the latter instance a midtarsal wedge resection may be indicated.

Varus and valgus deformities. These deformities may be associated with any of the disorders mentioned above (Fig. 9-3). Excessive valgus can be controlled conservatively with a "heel hugger" (UC-BL) insert (Fig. 9-4). In patients between 4 and 10 years old, excessive valgus that has not responded to conservative measures may be treated surgically by the Grice procedure. Careful follow-up to determine whether secondary changes in the ankle mortise have occurred should be part of the treatment plan; ball-and-socket ankle joints sometimes appear (Fig. 9-5).

A word of caution about possible overcorrection of the foot in Grice operations: A standing anteroposterior roentgenographic view of the ankle should be obtained preoperatively. It may show a valgus tilt of the talus in the ankle mortise (Fig. 9-6) and if the surgeon does not notice this tilt, he may overcorrect for it in the subtalar bone block and produce a varus deformity at the subtalar joint.

Triple arthrodesis may be used for the correction of excessive varus and valgus in a child 11 years of age or older for whom other treatment methods have failed. Here again, long-term follow-up of the patient to determine whether secondary ankle-joint changes have occurred should be part of the treatment program.

Some surgeons advocate osteotomy of the calcaneus (Dwyer procedure) for the correction of varus or valgus deformity. However, this procedure merely creates a cosmetic illusion of correction and we feel it

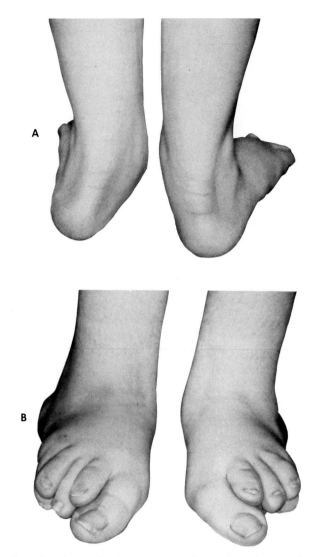

Fig. 9-3. A, Valgus feet in cerebral palsy. **B,** Hallux valgus frequently associated with valgus (pronated) feet in cerebral palsy.

should be avoided, especially if talocalcaneal relationships are altered.

Spastic abduction of the great toe (Fig. 9-7) is rarely found in patients with cerebral palsy; when it does occur, the deformity responds to abductor release (Bleck, 1967). Clawtoes may be corrected by the use of extensor tendon transfers (Hibbs procedure). Hallux flexus sometimes requires the transfer of the long toe flexors to the extensors. One should make certain that the hallux flexus is not secondary to a dorsal bunion (strong tibialis anterior, weak peroneus longus as illustrated in Fig. 9-8) or to excessive supination of the forefoot. If it is, these deformities should be corrected first.

Cold, blue feet, indicative of vasomotor dysfunction, are sometimes seen in patients with cerebral palsy. Before performing elective orthopaedic surgical procedures on such feet, the surgeon should first

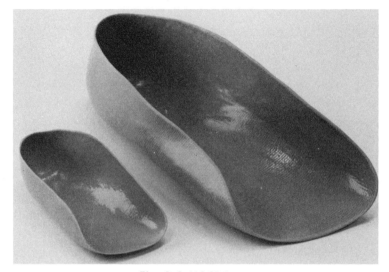

Fig. 9-4. UC-BL insert.

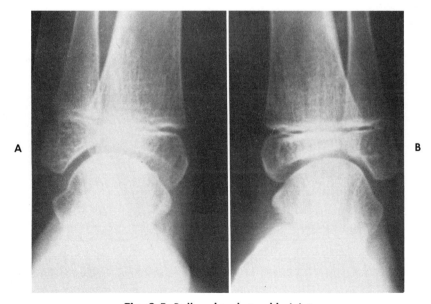

A   B

Fig. 9-5. Ball-and-socket ankle joint.

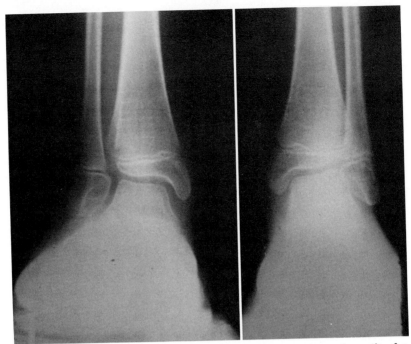

Fig. 9-6. Standing anteroposterior roentgenogram demonstrating valgus tilt of talus in ankle mortise. If this tilt is unrecognized and an attempt is made to overcorrect it in subtalar extra-articular arthrodesis (Grice), overcorrection of the hindfoot into varus will result.

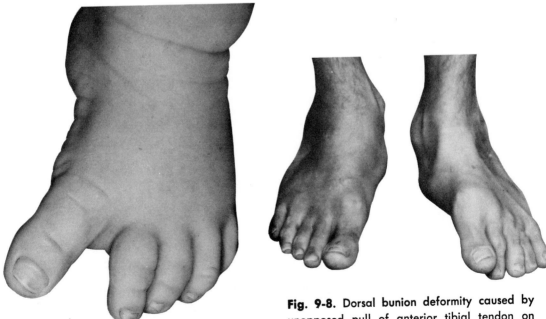

Fig. 9-7. Spastic hallux varus in cerebral palsy.

Fig. 9-8. Dorsal bunion deformity caused by unopposed pull of anterior tibial tendon on first metatarsal.

carry out a diagnostic lumbar sympathetic block, followed by lumbar sympathectomy if the block is successful.

Retention of the gains obtained as a result of surgical procedures has been discussed by Evans (1966), who advocates appropriate night splinting.

Again, it should be emphasized that long-term follow-up is a cardinal principle in the management of patients with cerebral palsy.

TUBEROUS SCLEROSIS

Tuberous sclerosis is characterized by mental retardation, adenoma sebaceum, epilepsy, and occasional orthopaedic disorders. Cystic changes in the phalanges and metatarsals and pathologic fracture occur at times, but the most common orthopaedic problem encountered in this disease is spastic equinus (Smith et al., 1969). The principles mentioned for its management in cerebral palsy apply here as well.

MULTIPLE SCLEROSIS

It is estimated that there are 500,000 patients with multiple sclerosis and related diseases in the United States, whose care costs one billion dollars annually. Multiple sclerosis is a long-term progressive disease, which usually makes itself manifest between the ages of 20 and 40 years (U. S. Dept. of H. E. W., 1971). The etiology of the disease is unknown; the condition is more common in females than in males. Widespread neurologic abnormalities may occur, and the disease is characterized by remissions and exacerbations (Gordon, 1951). In the extremities, numbness, tremor, awkward gait, and weakness may be the presenting symptoms.

Because of the unpredictable natural course of the disease, orthopaedic surgeons are loath to perform surgical procedures on these patients. Death occurs at an average of 16 to 20 years after the onset of the disease. Braces and splints are used in the conservative management of this disease. Avoidance of contracture, prevention of decubitus, and maintenance of maximal functional capacity are principles of this kind of treatment. In cases in which a true triceps surae contracture is present, heelcord lengthening may be considered.

FRIEDREICH'S ATAXIA

This condition, believed to be an inherited degenerative spinocerebellar disease, first appears in childhood or adolescence. Ataxia, loss of position sense, loss of deep tendon reflexes, nystagmus, and positive Babinski's reflexes are encountered sometimes. The progress of this disease is slow, steady, and unpredictable; its etiology is unknown.

The two most common abnormalities of the foot that occur in this disorder are first cavus deformity with clawtoes, then equinovarus deformity. Despite the unpredictable progression of this disease, surgical intervention to correct deformity is considered to be worthwhile (Makin, 1953).

Triple arthrodesis together with plantar fasciotomy can help to correct excessive cavus and to prevent metatarsalgia. Extensor tendon transfer (Hibbs procedure) to the middle cuneiform is effective for the correction of clawtoes.

CHARCOT-MARIE-TOOTH DISEASE

This condition, which may be inherited through a sex-linked recessive trait, is characterized by peroneal muscle atrophy in the legs or intrinsic atrophy in the hands or both, leading to the typical "champagne bottle" legs and "pancake" hand deformities. Varus deformity caused by peroneal muscle atrophy is sometimes seen in the feet of children with this disease. Since neurologic wasting can involve other muscles of the leg, the results of tendon transfers are unpredictable. Correction of varus by triple arthrodesis is more likely to be successful (Jacobs and Carr, 1950).

MYELODYSPLASIA

Myelodysplasia is the generic term for a number of developmental defects of the spinal cord. The condition most often affects the lower segments of the spine and

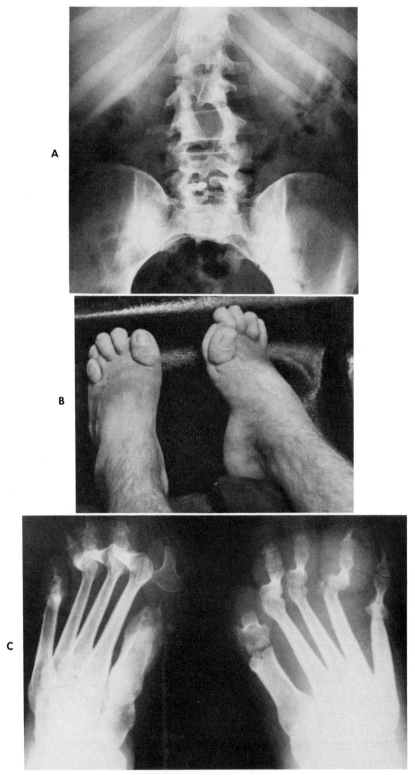

Fig. 9-9. A, Defects of lumbosacral vertebra in patient with spina bifida. **B,** Deformity of feet. **C,** Trophic destruction of first metatarsophalangeal joints.

includes both spina bifida (Figs. 9-9), with meningocele and myelomeningocele, and spina bifida occulta, as well as "lipoma" of the cord, diastematomyelia (bony, cartilaginous, or fibrous separation of the lateral halves of the cord), sacral agenesis, and tight filum terminale. These conditions may produce a congenital paraplegia caused by involvement of the spinal cord or cauda equina.

There are approximately 27,500 children with spina bifida in the United States, whose care costs fifty-five million dollars annually (U. S. Dept. of H. E. W., 1971). It is the most common cause of congenital paraplegia. Several theories of its pathogenesis exist, which pertain to the failure of the posterior neural arch to close or to remain closed. Studies have indicated an increased risk of occurrence in siblings born to parents of a child with spina bifida (Lorber, 1966); polygenetic factors of inheritance may account for this increased risk. Infants with myelodysplasia have a high incidence of hydrocephalus and the Arnold-Chiari malformation, both of which require continuous neurologic surveillance. In addition, the presence of bladder paralysis dictates the need for continuous urologic management, often with urinary diversion, as well as for pediatric and social care. Orthopaedic and rehabilitative planning must take into consideration the spine, hips, and knees, as well as the feet, but areas other than the feet are beyond the scope of this book.

Often the greatest difficulty with regard to spina bifida occulta is the recognition of the underlying process, inasmuch as the spinal defect is not clinically apparent. Neurologic signs may not appear until later in childhood, at which time progressive development of a cavus or equinovarus foot, with or without urinary incontinence, may be the initial finding. Any child in whom the onset of a progressive foot disorder is apparent deserves a careful neurologic evaluation as well as roentgenograms of the lumbar spine. It must be borne in mind, however, that many x-ray films will show minor and inconsequential failure of fusion of the posterior elements of L5 or S1, and that, conversely, a cartilaginous diastematomyelia, which may be producing cord damage, will not show on routine films of the spine.

The treatment of deformity of the foot in patients with spina bifida occulta does not differ significantly from treatment of this deformity in patients with open spinal lesions. In both instances, it is vital to recognize that the deformity is caused by a dynamic muscle imbalance, which differs from the relatively static situation one often encounters in deformities caused by old poliomyelitis. Deformity may progress slowly over a prolonged period of time because a minimal imbalance of forces may be acting on the foot during that time. To view a child with the condition as a *growing paraplegic* is useful in understanding this tendency of progression of deformity. Serial evaluations throughout childhood are essential.

Orthopaedic management of the foot (as well as the spine, hips, and legs) in myelodysplasia must always be directed toward the ultimate goals of the educability and employability of the patient. A mobile, plantigrade, balanced, shoeable foot is essential, and one of the first responsibilities of the orthopaedist in the management of this disorder is to determine the level or pattern of the remaining neurologic function and to predict the type of deformity which this pattern can be expected to produce. Thus, with a functional L4 level, the tibialis anterior muscle may be innervated, but its action may be unbalanced because of functioning plantar flexors and evertors. A varus force may be produced; but more importantly, a progressive and severe calcaneus deformity may develop, which can be minimized by early transfer of the tibialis anterior tendon to the heel. With a functional L5 level, a calcaneus deformity will almost certainly develop if tendon transfer is not done by the time the patient is from 1 to 2 years old, and at present no satisfactory means of managing a fully developed calcaneus deformity exists. At the S1-S2 level, ankle plantar flexors and foot evertors will be functioning, so that clawing of the toes and a planovalgus foot are more apt to develop. At the S3 level, intrinsic muscular imbalance obtains, and a cavus foot is most likely. The equinus portion of the deformity that is commonly present is a positional rather than a dynamic problem and is thus less apt to recur following tenotomy. All dynamic deformities, however, must be brought into balance by tendon transfers or releases if recurrence is to be avoided.

The two deformities of the foot in myelodysplasia that most commonly require correction are equinovarus and equinocavovarus (Carr, 1956; Hayes, Gross, and Dow, 1964; Sharrard, 1968). Opinion on the management of these deformities varies. Sharrard (1963, 1964, 1967, 1968) feels that splinting, manipulation, and serial plaster casting for these insensitive feet result in disaster. Hayes, Gross, and Dow (1964), Tzimas (1966), and Walker (1971), on the other hand, believe that such measures are useful, although all of these authors warn against the injudicious use of plaster on feet in which sensation is lacking, and all resort to the use of surgical procedures if they are necessary in order to achieve correction. Sharrard and Grosfield (1968) have reported their results of the management of 241 feet with various deformities. They found soft-tissue releases and tendon transfers to be most effective. For equinovarus deformity they advised medial and posterior releases, and their rate of success in this group was 22 percent. Usually, the tendo achillis, both long toe flexors, both tibial tendons, and the medial ligaments of both the ankle and the subtalar joints will require division. An unopposed anterior tibial tendon should be transferred to the lateral side of the foot if no tendency to calcaneus deformity is present; if it is, the tendon should be transferred posteriorly. For simple equinus contracture, subcutaneous tendo achillis tenotomy and toe flexor tenotomy often will suffice.

Talectomy may also be of value in the management of rigid feet in which equinovarus deformity cannot be controlled and the potential for walking is limited. Menelaus (1971) reported on his use of this procedure in fourteen feet with equinovarus deformity due to spina bifida. He believes that best results can be obtained if talectomy is performed between the ages 1 and 5 years, but that triple arthrodesis is preferable for the older child or adult.

Planovalgus and equinovalgus feet are also commonly seen in myelodysplasia, and convex pes valgus (vertical talus) has been described (Drennan and Sharrard, 1971). The Grice subtalar arthrodesis is useful in the correction of planovalgus deformity.

Paralytic vertical talus is a difficult deformity to manage. Dorsolateral release with open reduction is indicated, along with such tendon transfers as are necessary to bring the musculature of the foot into balance.

The fully developed calcaneus and calcaneovarus deformities which the clinician occasionally encounters are among the most difficult to manage. In cases in which an unbalanced overpull of the peroneus tertius, the tibialis anterior, or both cause an elevation of the arch, both tendons should be transferred through the interosseous membrane to the heel at the midline of the foot. These tendons are usually not sufficiently strong to act as plantar flexors or to cause equinus deformity, but in the event that equinus ensues, the deformity is easily held in a dropfoot brace, whereas a calcaneus deformity cannot be held in any brace. These transfers should be done when the child is about 1 year old.

In order to salvage some feet, triple arthrodesis may be necessary, but the performance of this procedure should not be undertaken lightly. In their series of forty-five triple arthrodesis operations, Hayes, Gross, and Dow (1964) found that eight feet required procedures for revision, and bone nonunion occurred in thirteen feet.

It should be borne in mind also that in the past, at least, osteomyelitis in the insensitive foot often required amputation in order to control the infection. Pantalar arthrodesis should be avoided; unwanted ankle motion can be controlled by the placement of appropriate anterior and posterior stops on short leg braces. Neuropathic arthropathy may occur after attempted arthrodesis of joints, especially the ankle joint; furthermore, even if fusion is accomplished, there is no virtue in a completely rigid ankle and hindfoot.

Finally, it must be stressed that nonplantigrade feet, particularly those that have been immobilized under plaster, but also those that have been supported by braces for prolonged periods of time, are vulnerable to trophic ulceration. Casts, if they are used at all, must be well padded and bivalved; removable splints are preferable. Skin should be inspected for rubor at pressure points at least twice daily. It is better to maintain a surgically induced correction by passive movement of the involved joint than by the use of plaster.

POLIOMYELITIS

Once the scourge of millions of children who became orthopaedic patients, poliomyelitis is now relatively rare in the United States because of the efficacy of a well-directed immunization program. The disease, which affects the anterior horn cells of the ventral cord, results in deformity caused by muscle imbalance, which, if left untreated, leads to contracture.

Much of what was learned from experience with patients with poliomyelitis has been applied to those with myelodysplasia, often successfully. However, when the same application is made to patients with cerebral palsy, the results are often disastrous.

Some principles that are essential to the success of surgical procedures performed on postpoliomyelitic patients must be reiterated:

1. Fixed deformities must always be corrected (contractures must be released) *before* tendons are transferred.
2. The function of every tendon that is

to be transferred should be evaluated. It is foolhardy to use a thin muscle with short excursion to do the work of a thick muscle with long excursion.
3. A weak muscle always becomes weaker when it is transferred.
4. Whenever possible, transplant tendon to bone rather than to tendon.
5. A transferred tendon should have as straight a direction of pull as possible in its new position.
6. Proper tension of a transferred tendon is essential. One that is too tight produces reverse deformity or, at best, tenodesis; one that is too loose is an ineffectual motor.

The balance between the plantar flexors (triceps surae, tibialis posterior, peroneals, toe flexors) and the dorsiflexors (tibialis anterior, peroneus tertius, toe extensors) determines whether calcaneus or equinus deformity will occur. Weak calf muscles produce calcaneus; strong calf muscles and weak dorsiflexors produce equinus (Abbott, 1951). Similarly, invertor (tibialis anterior and tibialis posterior) weakness results in valgus, while evertor (peroneal) weakness results in varus deformity. Cavus, planus, dorsal bunion, clawtoes, and hallux flexus are all caused by the unbalanced action of muscles upon the foot. Any combination of the above deformities may be seen, and the correction of them depends upon an accurate analysis of the problem.

In the surgical treatment of paralytic feet, tendon transfer by itself often cannot provide stability. Correction of deformity by stabilization (arthrodesis of unstable joints), with subsequent tendon transfer, is an effective method of achieving balance in the foot. Thus, triple arthrodesis is the most common surgical operation to correct lateral instability (Hallock, 1951).

In performing tendon transfers in and about the foot and ankle, one should try to preserve a set of invertor-evertor muscles. If paralysis prevents the retention of at least one set of these muscles, then triple arthrodesis is a necessity. Unopposed pull of the tibialis anterior on the first metatarsal, together with a weak peroneus longus, will result in a dorsal bunion.

For the treatment of calcaneocavus deformity caused by weakness of the triceps surae, the peroneals and the tibialis posterior may be transferred to the calcaneus. Stabilization of the foot by triple arthrodesis will frequently be necessary. If the dorsiflexors are weak, the transplantation of a strong posterior tibial tendon through the interosseous membrane to the dorsum of the midfoot is often successful. In our experience the use of the extensor hallucis longus by itself as a dorsiflexor of the ankle has been a mistake and should be discouraged. Furthermore, we have found that transplantation of the peroneals, except to the calcaneus in the calcaneocavus foot, produces poor results, although others have transplanted the peroneals to the dorsum as dorsiflexors.

Protection of the transferred tendons postoperatively and instructions to the patient about how to make active use of the transfers should be included in the treatment plan.

Problems of inequality of leg length may be dealt with according to established principles (Green, 1951; Anderson, 1963; see also Bibliography, Chapter 2).

CHILDHOOD MYOPATHIES (MUSCULAR DYSTROPHY)

There are approximately 200,000 patients with muscular dystrophy in the United States whose care costs four hundred million dollars annually (U. S. Dept. of H. E. W., 1971). A detailed classification of the myopathies is not within the scope of this chapter, but essentially there are three main types: (1) the Duchenne, or pseudohypertrophic type, which is inherited through an X-linked recessive trait and most often affects young males; (2) the limb-girdle type, which begins in adolescence or early adult life and involves the pelvic musculature, the shoulder-girdle musculature, or both; and (3) the facioscapulohumeral type, which is the most benign of all the myopathies and may begin at any age.

Procedures that are of value in the diagnosis of the myopathies are (1) manual muscle examination, (2) the use of serum enzymes (adolase and creatine phosphokinase), (3) electromyographic examination, and (4) muscle biopsy.

Spencer and Vignos (1962) have indicated that when the patient is no longer able to stand for at least 2 hours daily or to walk independently, and when the strength of the quadriceps is fair to minus, he should begin to wear braces. Because of the presence of contractures, however, braces cannot always be fitted. Their preferred method of treatment is to cut tight illiotibial bands, carry out a closed tendo achillis tenotomy, and transfer the posterior tibial tendon through the interosseous membrane to the dorsum of the foot to prevent the redevelopment of equinus. Patients use walking casts for 3 or 4 weeks, after which they wear long leg braces.

REFERENCES

Abbott, L. C.: The orthopedic care in anterior poliomyelitis, J. Pediat. 39:663-671, July-Dec. 1951.

Alter, M.: Anencephalus, hydrocephalus, and spina bifida, Arch. Neurol. 7:411-422, Nov. 1962.

Anderson, M., and Messner, M. B.: Growth and predictions of growth in the lower extremities, J. Bone Joint Surg. 45-A:1-14, Jan. 1963.

Baker, L. D., and Hill, L. M.: Foot alignment in the cerebral palsy patient, J. Bone Joint Surg. 46-A:1-15, Jan. 1964.

Bleck, E. E.: Spastic abductor hallucis, Dev. Med. Child Neurol. 9:602-608, Oct. 1967.

Carr, T. L.: The orthopaedic aspects of one hundred cases of spina bifida, Postgrad. Med. J. 32:201-210, Apr. 1956.

Cohen, P., and Mustacchi, P.: Survival in cerebral palsy, J.A.M.A. 195:642-644, Feb. 1966.

Drennan, J. C., and Sharrard, W. J. W.: The pathological anatomy of convex pes valgus, J. Bone Joint Surg. 53-B:455-461, Aug. 1971.

Evans, E. B.: The status of surgery of the lower extremities in cerebral palsy, Clin. Orthop. 47:127-139, July-Aug. 1966.

Gordon, E.: Multiple sclerosis: Application of rehabilitation techniques, New York, 1951, National Multiple Sclerosis Society.

Green, W. T., and Anderson, M. S.: Discrepancy

in length of the lower extremities. In American Academy of Orthopaedic Surgeons: Instructional Course Lectures, vol. 8, Ann Arbor, 1951, J. W. Edwards, pp. 294-305.

Hallock, H.: The surgical treatment of poliomyelitis, Surg. Clin. N. Amer. 31:397-415, 1951.

Hayes, J. T., and Gross, H. A.: Orthopedic implications of myelodysplasia, J.A.M.A. 184:762-767, June 1963.

Hayes, J. T., Gross, H. P., and Dow, S.: Surgery for paralytic defects secondary to myelomeningocele and myelodysplasia, J. Bone Joint Surg. 46-A:1577-1597, Oct. 1964.

Jacobs, J. E., and Carr, C. R.: Progressive muscular atrophy of the peroneal type (Charcot-Marie-Tooth disease): Orthopaedic management and end-result study, J. Bone Joint Surg. 32-A:27-38, Jan. 1950.

Lorber, J.: Incidence and epidemiology of myelomeningocele, Clin. Orthop. 45:81-83, Mar.-Apr. 1966.

Makin, M.: The surgical management of Friedreich's ataxia, J. Bone Joint Surg. 35-A:425-436, Apr. 1953.

Menelaus, M. B.: Talectomy for equinovarus deformity in arthrogryposis and spina bifida, J. Bone Joint Surg. 53-B:468-473, Aug. 1971.

Mooney, V., Perry, J., and Nickel, V. L.: Surgical and non-surgical orthopaedic care of stroke, J. Bone Joint Surg. 49-A:989-1000, July 1967.

Neurological and sensory disabilities: Estimated numbers and cost, U. S. Dept. of Health, Education and Welfare, Public Health Service, National Institutes of Health, Public Health Service Publication No. 1427, revised 1971.

Samilson, R. L., editor: Orthopaedic aspects of cerebral palsy, Philadelphia, J. B. Lippincott Co. (In press.)

Schlesinger, E. R., Allaway, N. C., and Peltin, S.: Survivorship in cerebral palsy, Amer. J. Public Health 44:1124-1133, Sept. 1954.

Sharrard, W. J. W.: The mechanism of paralytic deformity in spina bifida, Dev. Med. Child Neurol. 4:310-313, June 1962.

Sharrard, W. J. W.: Spina bifida, Physiotherapy 50:44-49, Feb. 1964.

Sharrard, W. J. W.: Paralytic deformity in the lower limb, J. Bone Joint Surg. 49-B:731-747, Nov. 1967.

Sharrard, W. J. W., and Grosfield, I.: The management of deformity and paralysis of the foot in myelomeningocele, J. Bone Joint Surg. 50-B:456-465, Aug. 1968.

Smith, T. K., Gregersen, G. G., and Samilson, R. L.: Orthopaedic problems associated with tuberous sclerosis, J. Bone Joint Surg. 51-A:97-102, Jan. 1969.

Spencer, G. E., and Vignos, P. J., Jr.: Bracing for ambulation in childhood progressive muscular dystrophy, J. Bone Joint Surg. 44-A:234-242, Mar. 1962.

Treanor, W.: The hemiplegic posture and its correction, Clin. Orthop. 63:113-131, Mar.-Apr. 1969.

Tzimas, N. A.: Orthopaedic care of the child with spina bifida. In Swinyard, C. A., editor: Comprehensive care of the child with spina bifida manifesta, New York, 1966, Institute of Rehabilitation Medicine, New York University Medical Center, pp. 45-65.

Walker, G.: The early management of varus feet in myelomeningocele, J. Bone Joint Surg. 53-B:462-467, Aug. 1971.

10

Vascular and metabolic disorders affecting the foot

William R. Murray
Verne T. Inman

METABOLIC DISORDERS AFFECTING THE FOOT
Rheumatoid arthritis

Rheumatoid arthritis is a systemic disease of unknown etiology that affects connective tissue. Joint inflammation is its dominant clinical feature. The disease, which affects women three times as frequently as men, is said to occur in 2 to 3 percent of people over 55 years of age. No clear-cut racial or occupational predisposition is evident. There are geographic aggregations of people with rheumatoid arthritis, but it is unclear whether these clusters of rheumatoids appear because of genetic or environmental influences.

In most patients the course of the disease is variable. It assumes a chronic form, which leads to progressive joint destruction and disability. Even though all joints may be involved, the small joints of the hands and feet are most frequently affected. Careful questioning of patients reveals that rheumatoid arthritis begins as frequently in the feet as in the hands (17 percent in each instance).

A diagnosis of rheumatoid arthritis is based on clinical, laboratory, and roentgenographic findings. For a list of eleven diagnostic criteria for rheumatoid arthritis, the reader is referred to the primer published by The Arthritis Foundation (1964).

Even though all the joints of the foot and ankle may be and frequently are involved in the rheumatoid process, involvement of the metatarsophalangeal, interphalangeal, ankle, and subtalar joints produces the greatest degree of disability. Swelling of the joints precedes (but often shortly) the joint destruction and deformity that ensue (Figs. 10-1 to 10-3). Initially one sees swelling with tenderness, increased skin temperature, and erythema over the involved joint; finally, the characteristic deformities appear. End-stage deformities seen in the forefoot are (1) hallux valgus; (2) marked claw and hammertoe deformities caused by hyperextension of the metatarsophalangeal joints and flexion of the interphalangeal joints; (3) loss of the plantar fat pad; (4) plantar callosities under the heads of the metatarsals; (5) dorsal callosities over the interphalangeal joints caused by shoe pressure; and (6) terminal callosities at the tips of the phalanges caused by direct pressure secondary to the flexed position. Hyperextension of the proximal phalanges pulls the plantar fat pads under the metatarsal heads forward where they are no longer in a position to be effective. This situation, combined with the effect of the windlass action of the plantar fascia described by Hicks (see Chapter 1), leaves the metatarsal heads palpable directly beneath the skin.

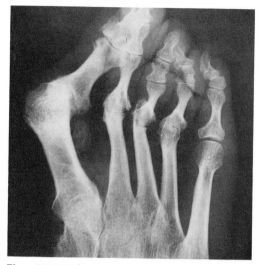

Fig. 10-1. Rheumatoid arthritis of first four metatarsophalangeal joints. Note atrophic changes of the articular surfaces of these joints.

With the involvement of the hindfoot (subtalar and ankle joints, as well as possible rupture of the posterior tibial tendon), progressive valgus deformity occurs along with loss of the longitudinal arch. Eventually the patient seems to be walking on the tuberosity of the navicular with a deformed rocker-bottom flatfoot. Occasionally varus deformity occurs but with less frequency.

Treatment. An appreciation of the clinical course of the disease is essential for the proper planning of a treatment program (Fig. 10-4). Treatment is directed toward (1) relief of pain, (2) prevention of deformity, (3) correction of deformity, (4) restoration of function, and (5) preservation of function.

Medical management (stages I to IV). Medical management must be continued throughout all four stages of the disease and may be the only treatment necessary throughout the early phases of the process (stage I). It should include rest, drug therapy, local steroids, and orthopaedic appliances.

REST. Both general and articular rest should be included, and the latter is

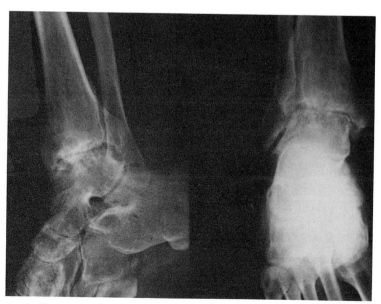

Fig. 10-2. Rheumatoid arthritis of tarsus and ankle joints.

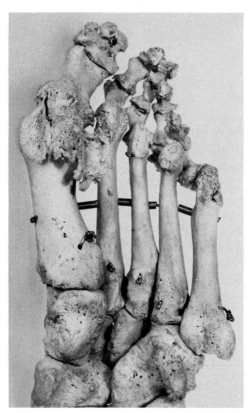

Fig. 10-3. Rheumatoid arthritis in skeletal specimen.

achieved through the use of perfectly fitted splints. A proper balance of rest and exercise must be maintained in order to prevent loss of joint motion and to preserve muscle power. Depending on the activity of the disease, the splints may be left on from 8 to 18 hours but should be removed at least once (and preferably several times) a day for passive, active-assistive, and active exercises.

DRUG THERAPY. The agents used are those that reduce inflammation or relieve pain. Aspirin is prescribed as the first line of defense and may be the only drug needed. The minimal maintenance dose in adults is twelve (300 mg.) tablets daily; an average adult dose is fourteen to eighteen tablets, and many adults easily tolerate from twenty to twenty-four tablets daily. Other drugs such as phenylbutazone, the corticosteroids, antimalarials, and gold salts may also have their place in the treatment of rheumatoid arthritis in specific patients, but a discussion of these drugs is not within the scope of this chapter.

LOCAL STEROIDS. Injections of local steroids are of greatest use in the ankle and

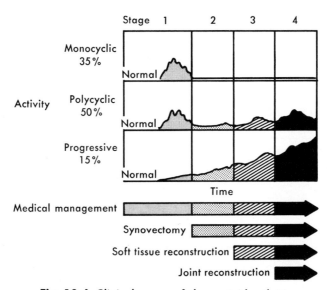

Fig. 10-4. Clinical course of rheumatoid arthritis.

subtalar joints, and injection into the swollen interphalangeal joints may also be performed. The dosage varies, but a practical amount for the ankle or subtalar joint is 20 mg. of triamcinolone acetonide, with 10 mg. for the metatarsophalangeal and interphalangeal joints. These injections should not be given in excess of once every 2 weeks for three injections during the acute phase and once every 2 months for a maximum of six injections thereafter.

ORTHOPAEDIC APPLIANCES. Besides resting splints and braces, dynamic appliances and those that are designed to permit more comfortable function are necessary as the disease process progresses. In the hindfoot progressive involvement of the subtalar joint often occurs, producing pain with inversion-eversion stresses. Before a fixed deformity is present, fitting with the UC-BL insert (see Fig. 9-4) may suffice to relieve pain that arises from the transverse tarsal and subtalar joints, as well as pain from the plantar fascia. However, if the deformity is advanced or if the tuberosity of the navicular is prominent or the posterior tibial tendon is ruptured, the insert will not suffice. The patient must then be fitted with a short leg double upright brace with a free ankle. Relief of forefoot pain caused by plantar and dorsal callosities requires proper shoe fitting and adjustment. Frequently a metatarsal bar or pad will suffice to reduce excess plantar pressures; if not, it may be necessary to fit the patient with a molded "space" shoe.

Surgical treatment (Stages II-IV). Although medical management continues during stages II to IV of the disease, surgical procedures are indicated in these later stages.

STAGE II. In this stage there is early involvement without fixed deformity and with minimal erosive change as seen on roentgenogram. Synovectomy as a prophylactic and therapeutic measure may be employed. This procedure is indicated if there has been unremitting synovitis in spite of adequate nonsurgical measures for a period of not less than 6 months and if the patient

has had the disease for not less than 1 year. The ankle, metatarsophalangeal, and interphalangeal joints lend themselves to synovectomy.

STAGE III. At this later stage of involvement, soft-tissue deformity has occurred, but there has been no significant erosive change. Under these circumstances, synovectomy, plus repair, transfer, or release of tendons is indicated, as well as capsulotomy.

STAGE IV. At this late stage of involvement, deformity and articular destruction have occurred. Stage IV requires reconstructive surgical procedures such as arthroplasties or arthrodeses. A general rule in the surgical treatment of rheumatoid arthritis is that arthrodesis is seldom indicated. However, under some circumstances an exception is made to this rule with regard to the foot.

Hindfoot and ankle deformity. Usually rheumatoid involvement of the hindfoot is clinically most apparent as an affection of the subtalar joint; the ankle joint is frequently spared. If significant involvement of the subtalar joint has failed to respond to nonsurgical measures (including inserts or short leg braces) and if the talotibial joint is only minimally involved, triple arthrodesis is indicated. However, if the ankle joint is involved—that is to say, if the patient has "pantalar arthritis" or if the patient has the dry, stiff type of rheumatoid arthritis—triple arthrodesis will place intolerable stresses on joints proximal and distal to the site of fusion. In a patient with "pantalar arthritis" a talectomy is most apt to result in optimal rehabilitation.

Forefoot deformity. The typical forefoot deformities are hallux valgus, hyperextension of the metatarsophalangeal joints, and flexion of the interphalangeal joints of the lesser toes. Loss of the effectiveness of the plantar fat pad causes painful plantar callosities to develop under the metatarsal heads, and with flexion of the interphalangeal joints dorsal callosities form because of shoe pressure. When conservative treatment has failed, surgical treatment must be directed toward reestablishment of the

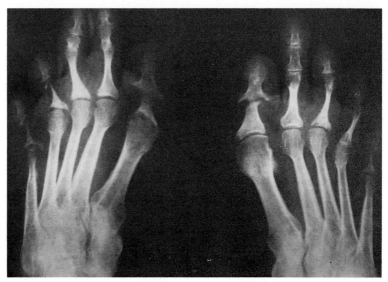

Fig. 10-5. Psoriatic arthritis of both feet. Note extensive destruction of some of the proximal phalanges.

alignment of the metatarsals and phalanges, restoration of adequate padding on the plantar surface of the foot, and correction of the deformed position of the interphalangeal joints.

For surgical procedures to correct deformities of the foot in rheumatoid arthritis, see Chapter 19.

Limited surgical procedures. Excision of rheumatoid nodules, which may be necessary to permit adequate function or shoe fitting, is definitely indicated when the nodules interfere with function. However, one must realize that there is a recurrence rate of approximately 20 percent. Occasionally a limited procedure such as the correction of a flexion deformity of the proximal interphalangeal joint is necessary. In most instances, this correction can be made with a modified DuVries type of procedure. Sometimes it may be necessary to reset the distal half of the proximal phalanx in order to correct the flexion contracture.

Psoriatic arthritis

Psoriatic arthritis is a form of arthritis occasionally observed in cases of longstanding psoriasis in which there are episodes of acute exacerbation of joint symptoms. The joints of the feet are often involved (Fig. 10-5). The changes may vary from an inflammation of the synovia to complete atrophic destruction of the joint and adjacent bone. It has been suggested that this phase of psoriasis is closely related to rheumatoid arthritis.

Gout

Gout has been known since antiquity and is recognized as a perversion of purine metabolism. It occurs more frequently in males than in females, and a definite family history exists in relation to the disease. It is basically a medical problem; therapy has been improving with greater knowledge of the chemistry of purines and with the advent of better uricosuric agents. However, a short discussion of gout is appropriate in a surgical text on the foot for two reasons, the first of which is a historical one. Manifestations of this disease occurred so frequently in the foot that it was called "podagra," a name derived from the Greek meaning a "foot seizure" (*pod,* foot, *agra,* seizure). Approximately 50 percent of initial attacks involve the great toe and 90 per-

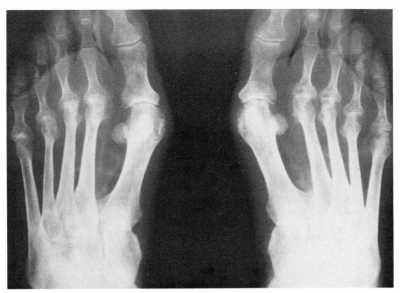

Fig. 10-6. Gouty arthritis in 65-year-old woman who has long history of high blood levels of uric acid and tophi in other parts of her body.

cent of gouty patients will experience one or more attacks of acute gout in their great toes during their lifetime (Stanbury et al., 1972). The acute attack usually begins to abate in from 1 to 2 weeks. While its mode of action is not clearly understood, colchicine remains an effective drug and the response to its administration constitutes an important diagnostic test.

The second reason for discussing gout is that during the past two decades surgical intervention is becoming more frequent. Prior to the excellent article by Linton and Talbott (1943), only a few sporadic reports appeared in the literature. These authors pointed out that it is not the acute gouty episodes that are surgical problems; it is rather the chronic tophaceous deposits that begin insidiously and progress not only to involve soft tissue but to invade and destroy joints and bone (Fig. 10-6). This occurs in approximately 10 percent of patients with gout.

Categories of tophaceous gout. For convenience, tophaceous gout may be divided into three categories: (1) deposits that occur superficially in bursae and in subcutaneous tissues and that may be unsightly

and painful to pressure; (2) deposits below the deep fascia that may encircle and invade tendons (nerves and blood vessels are not attacked but may be surrounded by the deposit); and (3) deposits that arise in joints and lead to cartilage destruction and bony absorption, which may extend superficially to involve adjacent tendons, bursae, subcutaneous tissues, and skin, and may break down to form sinuses.

Tophi in soft tissues tend to have a thin fibrous capsule-like shape. The capsule is not a membrane but is apparently formed as the extending tophus causes compression of the surrounding tissue. Such deposits can be removed by extracapsular excision. If a bursa is involved, the bursal sac should be removed completely.

In deeper tissue, deposits must be removed piecemeal with a curet. If the deposits are old they are dry and chalky. Our experience has been that the use of irrigation with buffered solutions is of no avail. Incomplete removal of all tophaceous material is usual, but this is rarely followed by return of the deforming overgrowth, and the wounds usually will heal (Woughter, 1959). In an excellent review, Kurtz (1965) emphasizes the following points: Amputation is rarely indicated. In cases of draining sinuses over tophi, local curettement of as much as possible of the deposit, followed by the application of wet dressings, will usually result in healing. Should the skin slough and a surgical wound exude urates, treatment with wet dressings and antibiotics will result in healing with surprisingly little scarring.

Balasubramaniam and Silva (1971) reported a case in which large tophaceous deposits on the dorsum of both feet involving the tarsal bones were excised and bone grafting was carried out.

It should be remembered that an acute attack of gout may follow any surgical procedure. The attack may occur at any time from 24 hours to 1 week after the operation has been performed.

Indications for surgical procedures. Surgical procedures are indicated for the treatment of tophaceous gout in the presence of (1) large tophi that are cosmetically unacceptable or interfere with the wearing of shoes; (2) tophi that are painful because of pressure; (3) extensive deposits that interfere with movement of the toes and are likely to destroy joints; and (4) discharging sinuses caused by tophaceous deposits. Surgical procedures are also indicated to decompress tophi that appear to be in danger of breakdown or are pressing on nerves.

Bursitis from gout. An acute attack of bursitis is frequently characterized by an acute periarthritis of the great toe joint, often referred to as gouty bursitis. It has a sudden onset; the great toe joint is extremely swollen and excruciatingly painful. The attack is self-limiting but recurs at intervals.

Bed rest for 3 to 7 days, hot compresses over the involved joint, and the use of colchicine, aspirin, butazolidin, cortisone, or injection of a hydrocortisone of any combination comprise the treatment. This therapy shortens the course of the acute stage. To prevent acute episodes the patient should have the regular supervision of an internist.

VASCULAR DISORDERS AFFECTING THE FOOT
Diabetes

The relationship between diabetes and some neurovascular disabilities of the lower extremity is still not crystal clear. The subject continues to be surrounded with conjecture and assumptions (Oakley et al., 1968). Peripheral arterial disease is similar in character in diabetics and nondiabetics; the differences are quantitative rather than qualitative. All studies appear to support the contention that diabetics develop peripheral vascular disease more often than do nondiabetics. Furthermore, diabetics seem to develop arteriosclerotic manifestations in the arterial system below the knee and to manifest peripheral neuropathy with greater frequency.

Diabetic neuropathy. The neuropathic phase of diabetes is a specific degeneration closely resembling the neuropathic changes of latent syphilis, and, like diabetic gangrene, it has a predilection for the foot. The severity of diabetes does not appear to be directly associated with trophic changes; however, most cases reported have been those of long-standing diabetes. Changes are essentially caused by destruction of the posterior horns of the spinal cord. The most drastic results of the trophic changes are complete collapse and distortion of the tarsometatarsal articulation.

Although first described by Marchal de Calvi as far back as 1864, few early publications appeared on the subject of diabetic neuropathy. Later reports indicate that the syndrome is not uncommon.*

Etiology. The cause of diabetic neuropathy remains unknown. At one time vitamin B_1 (thiamine) deficiency was proposed as a probable cause of diabetic neuropathy (Rudy, 1945). However, subsequent studies have shown that the response to treatment

---

*See Rundles, 1945 (125 new cases); Bailey and Root, 1947; Parsons and Norton, 1951; Sheppe, 1953; Antes et al. 1954; Martin, 1954; Lippman and Grow, 1955; Bolen, 1956; and Goodman et al. 1953.

with thiamine has been far from clear-cut.

The vascular theory of the etiology of neuropathy began with the report of Woltman and Wilder (1929) of ischemic nerve lesions in ten cases. From their evidence it has often been supposed that disease of small arteries is sufficient cause for all neuropathy. Jordan (1936) thought that about one-third of his cases were associated with arteriosclerosis. However, many investigators have been skeptical of ischemia as the cause of more than a small number of cases. Hutchinson and Liversedge (1956) reported that the findings of neuropathies in severe peripheral vascular disease are different from those in diabetes. In the arteriosclerotic case the neuropathic symptoms are overshadowed by those of ischemia. Recently the vascular theory has revived with the notion that neuropathy is related to a specific capillary angiopathy (Seitz, 1956). Fagerberg (1957) found lesions of the intraneural arterioles to be closely associated with the incidence of neuropathy.

Some investigators adhere to the view that neuropathy is essentially the result of a metabolic disturbance associated with uncontrolled diabetes. The view of Malins (1968), supported by the study of Mayne (1964), is that there are two types of neuropathy in diabetes. The common form is almost asymptomatic, occurs in old age in both diabetics and nondiabetics but begins at an earlier age in the diabetic. The acute neuropathy is less common, and Malins believes that this type of neuropathy begins when the diabetes is uncontrolled and that the symptoms may continue long after control has been established.

Symptoms. There are no specific manifestations of diabetic neuropathy that do not also appear in other forms of neuropathy. Its incidence is rare in persons under the age of 20 years, and it increases with the duration of the diabetes. Interestingly, the findings are confined to the lower limb and are usually distal, symmetrical, and sensory. Absent or diminished tendon reflexes are the most characteristic findings. The ankle jerk is mainly affected and is ab-

sent four times as frequently as the knee jerk. Diminution or loss of vibratory sense in the area of the foot and ankle is the next most common finding. In more advanced cases diminished appreciation to light touch and to thermal and painful stimuli may occur. In severe cases deep pain sensibility is lost and the individual may experience spontaneous pain, which may be described as burning, aching, or gnawing. The sensation of coldness or burning of the feet may simulate that produced by ischemia. In the latter condition, cooling may be effective in alleviating the symptoms but it is apt to be less so in neuropathy. Hyperesthesia may make contact with clothing and bed covers unbearable.

The onset is gradual, although development of osteolytic changes in the bone may be rapid, the foot becoming deformed in a comparatively short time. The remnants of the metatarsals are displaced laterally (Figs. 10-7 to 10-10). The foot is greatly misshapen and distorted, and there are both osteolytic and osteophytic changes. Often deposition of new bone is an accompaniment, as in Charcot's joint. Relative or complete absence of pain during the process of bone degeneration is typical; but the patient notices that his foot is becoming unstable and its shape is changing rapidly.

Pathogenesis. Most changes in the foot are of Charcot's type of destruction at the tarsometatarsal articulation. The articular surfaces are destroyed at the same time that hypertrophic changes take place. Often loose bodies are formed. Relaxation or destruction of the ligaments results in distortion of the joints from the weight of the body.

Treatment. Control of diabetes is accepted as the one effective form of treatment for neuropathy. No quick treatment is available beyond medication for relief of pain; improvement is slow and somewhat uncertain. Full courses of vitamin B_{12}, liver extracts derived from pregnant mammals, and adenosine triphosphate with

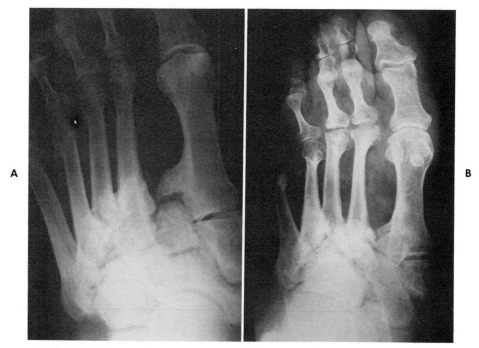

Fig. 10-7. A, Diabetic neuropathy, with complete collapse of tarsometatarsal articulations. **B,** Diabetic neuropathy of tarsometatarsal articulations. There was a previous episode of diabetic gangrene of the fifth toe. (**B,** Courtesy Dr. C. W. Grinstead.)

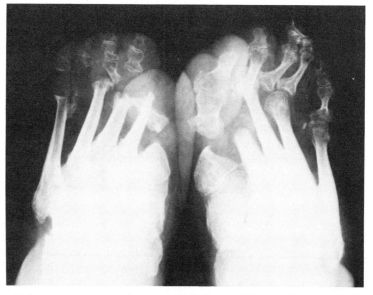

Fig. 10-8. Diabetic neuropathy of metatarsophalangeal joints. (Courtesy Dr. D. Dickson.)

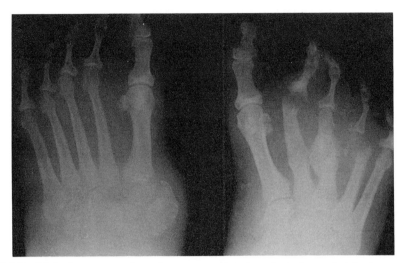

Fig. 10-9. Diabetic neuropathy of tarsometatarsal articulations of left foot and of metatarsophalangeal joints of right foot.

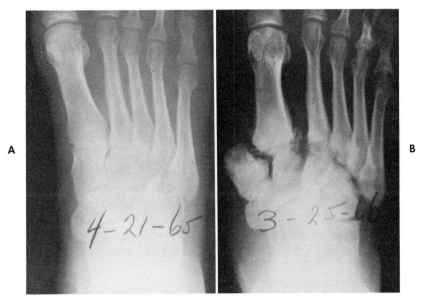

Fig. 10-10. Right foot of 48-year-old diabetic woman. Diabetic neuropathy developed in less than 1 year.

thiamine or pantothenic acid (Shuman and Gilpin, 1954) failed to improve a group of diabetic neuropathic patients.

Lesions of the feet are the most frequent complications of diabetes. These lesions are usually complex in nature and should not be considered purely as manifestations of vascular disease. While ischemia is the most important factor in ulceration and gangrene, neuropathy contributes to the loss of sensation, trophic defects in the skeletal system, and impaired function of the foot. Hyperglycemia in poorly controlled diabetes encourages the development and spread of infection. Only occasionally does one of these three factors appear in a pure form; usually combinations are encountered and it is difficult to assess the degree to which each is contributing to the clinical picture.

Only recent changes are to some extent reversible. In advanced cases destruction is so extensive that surgical intervention is of little benefit. Stability can be improved by use of metal inlays, pads, high shoes, or leg braces. In many instances amputation is advisable because of the likelihood of diabetic ulcers leading to gangrene.

Diabetic gangrene. There are two types of diabetic gangrene. The first occurs in diabetic patients with advanced arteriosclerosis. When gangrene sets in, the course is similar to that seen in all occlusive vascular disease. It is rarely reversible and represents a terminal stage.

Under these conditions all local measures should be taken, and the patient's peripheral arterial system should be evaluated thoroughly. If the lesion is in the major arterial system supplying the leg and is occlusive but appears amenable to surgical procedures, the possibility of performing reconstructive arterial surgical procedures should be considered, together with local treatment. In addition, if an arterial reconstructive procedure is successful, the eventual outcome will be enhanced should amputation become necessary, and benefit will accrue both in the choice of amputation level and the healing of the amputation stump (de Takats, 1959).

The second type of diabetic gangrene may occur in a warm foot with circulation not seriously impaired and little if any arteriosclerosis. In such a foot it may even be possible to obtain a pulse. Usually this type is encountered in uncontrolled diabetes but may occur even when diabetes has been controlled. However, the condition is reversible, as seen in the thirty cases of DuVries. When such a foot, sometimes called diabetic foot, is threatened by gangrene, treatment by conservative methods is often successful, and amputation may be avoided. Amputation is most often needed if there is intractable pain or extensive tissue destruction. When these indications exist and amputation seems to be justified, the medical status of the patient should be evaluated to determine whether sympathectomy concomitant with amputation is advisable. In the presence of trophic changes sympathectomy is not indicated (Classen, 1964). It must be borne in mind that the amputation of part of one foot demands increased strain on the other foot. Excessive strain on the stable foot can result in a similar complication of the vessels, and complete or partial loss of a diseased foot greatly increases chance of injury in the remaining foot. Every factor should be evaluated carefully before resorting to amputation.

Treatment. The diabetic patient with gangrene of the foot (Fig. 10-11) must rest. The control of diabetes is in the province of the internist. When gangrene is limited to a toe or toes, conservative management should be exhausted in every case. When the gangrene of the foot progresses rapidly and the local and systemic symptoms do not respond to conservative measures and become alarming, then amputation is imperative.

Lowrie and associates (1955) suggested the following general criteria for differentiating between terminal and nonterminal diabetic gangrene:

> . . . if the skin of the foot is warm, elastic, of normal thickness, with some subcutaneous fat, and if pulsations can be felt in the dorsalis pedis and the posterior tibial arteries, it can be assumed that the body of the foot

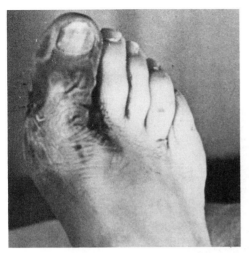

Fig. 10-11. Diabetic gangrene.

has a supply of blood, and healing could be expected without loss of the foot.

If the skin of the foot is thin, tightly applied to the tendons with absence of subcutaneous fatty tissue, colder than the other foot, and arterial pulsations are absent, it can be assumed that there has been gradual arterial occlusion above the ankle. . . .*

The foot should be left exposed to air and protected by a foot cradle; the sides of the cradle should be padded to prevent further injury. The position of the foot should be changed frequently to prevent the development of pressure sores. Since the heel is the commonest area of pressure gangrene, a doughnut pad applied around the heel, held on by gauze around the foot and ankle, is a helpful measure.

Because of impaired circulation that accompanies infection, antibiotic therapy must be instituted immediately. The antibiotic dosage should be large, and the antibiotic used should be one to which the sensitivity of the organism involved has been previously ascertained. By this means an effective concentration in the affected area may be assured. Vasodilators such as Priscoline or Roniacol may be of value. A sali-

cylate combined with a barbiturate may be prescribed for the relief of pain.

Dry gangrene ordinarily is painless and spreads slowly. There is always the possibility that dry gangrene will be self-limiting and end in spontaneous amputation of the dead part, thus arresting the progress of the disease. It is advantageous, therefore, to keep dry gangrene as dry as possible. Moist gangrene is painful and spreads rapidly. Fairbairn and co-workers (1972) pointed out that diabetic lesions are likely to be moist and infected; therefore, attempts at drying up the moist gangrene should be made as early as possible.

Ulcers caused by vascular deficiency

Diabetic ulcer. Ulcer of the foot is a common complication of diabetes. The ulcer appears on the plantar surface, especially under a weight-bearing pivot. The plantar surface of the metatarsal heads, usually the middle three, is a likely area. The ulcer is chronic and has a small orifice that exudes a seropurulent material. The ulcer may penetrate the fascial layers. The orifice is surrounded by a thick, brawny, white callus (Fig. 10-12). On removal of the callus the surface is seen to be covered with granulation tissue.

First in importance in treatment is control of the underlying diabetes. Cleanliness is imperative. The brawny tissue surrounding the ulcer must be removed. All secondary infections should receive careful attention. The application of 5 percent silver nitrate to the granulation tissue, repeated about twice a week, destroys the granulation tissue and permits healing by third intention. All pressure should be removed from the area by means of padding or a sponge-rubber shoe. Local applications on large dressings, using a hydrophilic ointment containing water-soluble derivatives of chlorophyll (chloresium), as described by Cady and Morgan (1948), are worth trying. Cady and Morgan sought a healing preparation that would be applicable to all types of ulcers and effect early healing.

Necrotic ulcer. A necrotic ulcer is a slough of devitalized tissue such as occurs

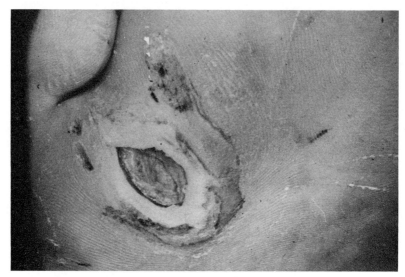

Fig. 10-12. Diabetic ulcer under fourth metatarsal head.

in diabetes, Buerger's disease, arteriosclerosis, and other vascular deficiencies. The ulceration is often invaded by low-grade pathogens that cause the type of chronically sloughing, draining ulcer that forms on a weight-bearing surface.

Treatment should be initiated by an attempt to control or ameliorate any underlying disease that could contribute to the formation of the ulcer. The ulcerous area should be relieved of as much pressure as possible. If the ulcer is on the plantar surface of the foot, weight bearing must be held to a minimum and heavy padding or any appliance to protect the area should be used during weight bearing. Frequent debridement is essential, as is scrupulous cleanliness of the ulcerous area.

Varicose ulcer (indolent ulcer). Congestive ulcers are caused by a circulatory deficiency resulting in reduced tissue vitality. Any interference in the blood supply to the foot ultimately may produce an ulcer, especially if the area is subjected to secondary irritating factors. Varicose ulcer is the commonest congestive ulcer of the ankle. It is sometimes called indolent ulcer. It is a phlegmonous destruction of tissue caused by prolonged venous congestion or stagnated venous blood. Such ulcers are sec-

ondary to long-standing varicose veins. They occur just above the medial malleolus (Fig. 10-13), rarely over other surfaces of the foot or ankle. Usually they lie over a varix and are surrounded by varying degrees of pigmentation. Because of prolonged and progressive deterioration of all the surrounding soft tissue, varicose ulcers are resistant to treatment. They may hemorrhage spontaneously.

The primary objective in the treatment of varicose ulcers is occlusion of the varices proximal to and under the ulcer. This may be accomplished by one of the following procedures, utilizing any combination of appropriate steps.

A sponge-rubber compression bandage, sometimes called venous heart, may be used. A nonirritating medication, such as a dye or an antibiotic ointment, is applied, and the lesion is covered with sterile gauze. A sponge-rubber pad about 1.3 cm. thick is placed over the gauze, covering the entire ulcer and extending about 3 cm. proximally to the ulcer; then an elastic bandage is wrapped around the foot and leg.

A second method of treatment is to eliminate the varices that caused the ulcer by sclerosing, ligating, or stripping the varicosed vein. Supportive measures, such as

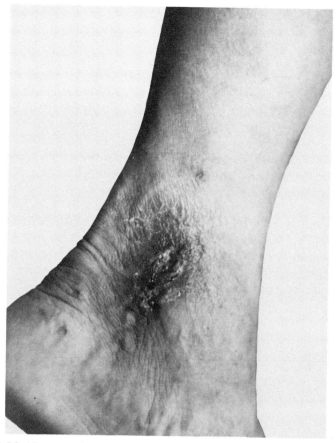

Fig. 10-13. Varicose ulcer over medial malleolus. (Courtesy Dr. Ned Pickett.)

wearing elastic stockings or bandages, should be used after the ulcer has healed to prevent recurrence. A finely powdered, specially treated sterile gelatin (Gelfoam), which possesses tissue stimulating and hemostatic properties, has been used in the treatment of chronic recalcitrant stasis of leg ulcers.

Lucca (1956) reported on 100 cases of leg ulcers, of which 75 were the chronic varicose type. Results in his series were better when sympathectomy was performed before skin graft or when skin graft was not performed at all. He recommended a one-stage operation for extirpation and skin grafting. He reported 7 percent recurrence after the skin grafting in patients with other complications.

Peripheral vascular disease

Peripheral vascular disease is a general term that encompasses all diseases of the blood vessels and lymphatics except those of the heart. The circulation to the lower extremity may be modified by many conditions. These may be local pathologic processes specifically involving the vessels or functional responses to such factors as ingestion of food and alcohol, smoking of tobacco, exercise, temperature, and emotions. (The phenomenon of "cold feet" has a real physiologic basis, since anxiety or fear causes a drop in peripheral skin temperature.)

The literature dealing with the various conditions that may alter peripheral blood flow is enormous, and even a cursory survey in such a text as this would be inadequate and inappropriate. For more detailed information the reader should refer to one of several standard reference books.

When the circulation to the lower extremity is markedly impaired, dire consequences result that can hardly be overlooked by the examining surgeon. However, in incipient vascular disease it may prove difficult to distinguish between symptoms caused by orthopaedic conditions and those arising from impaired circulation. Paresthesias, numbness, nocturnal ache, cramps, and pain on activity can result from circulatory disturbances in the leg and foot. The possibility of impaired circulation should always be considered in the differential diagnosis of foot strain, tarsal tunnel syndrome, perineural fibroma, plantar fasciitis, spurs, the effects of tight shoes, and osteoporosis.

Symptoms. Abnormalities in the peripheral circulation should be suspected if the patient complains of one or more of the following symptoms: (1) pain that appears in the leg or the foot after exercise and is promptly relieved on cessation of activity (pain due to vascular insufficiency is related to muscular activity and not to mechanical factors); (2) rest pain, relieved by foot-down position and made worse by heating; (3) swelling about the legs, ankles, and feet; (4) excessively cold or excessively warm extremities; (5) abnormal sweating or dryness of skin; and (6) numbness, paresthesias, or muscular weakness.

If none of the foregoing complaints are elicited, a rapid examination can confirm the impression that no vascular impairment is present. However, if the history is suggestive, a more detailed examination is indicated. The examination is usually simple and can be carried out quickly. With the patient standing, the surgeon should look for swelling, ulcers, varices, scleroderma, and thrombophlebitis. He should note the color and temperature of the skin. The amount of dryness or wetness of the skin should be estimated, since it is indicative of vasomotor activity. The significance of

temperature and tint of skin has been outlined by Lewis (1936) as follows: (1) warm, pale skin through which the blood flows quickly for many minutes; (2) warm, deeply colored, red skin that has been irritated or inflamed, or in which arterial vasodilation has recently occurred; (3) warm, deeply colored, cyanosed skin that has been made warm by external heating and has an imperfect supply of blood; (4) cold, pale, cyanosed skin to which the blood flow is slow or absent; (5) cold, deeply colored, cyanosed skin in which circulation is very slow; and (6) cold, deeply colored, red skin in which the damaged minute vessels dilate if the skin is cold enough, making it bright red. (Immersion of a hand in ice water produces these changes, for example.)

The most informative procedure to determine the adequacy of the blood supply to the lower extremity has been described by Gilfillan (1958). The patient is placed supine on the examining table, his leg elevated so that the foot is at least 60 cm. above the level of the chest. Gravity will thereby assist in the drainage of blood from the extremity. Stroking the foot and leg toward the body will facilitate the emptying of blood from the venous channels. With the patient's leg elevated, the clinician may note the degree of blanching of the skin. In severe arterial obstruction, the skin may appear white and waxy. Blotchy color changes may be caused by anatomic vasoconstriction or small-vessel obstruction resulting from microemboli. If caused by vasoconstriction the skin will be moist; is caused by small-vessel obstruction the skin will be dry. After a few minutes of elevation of the leg, the patient should be asked to quickly sit up and let the leg hang over the edge of the table. If the arterial supply is adequate, pinking of the skin will be noted within 10 to 15 seconds. If the return of color requires a minute or more to occur, circulation is inadequate.

It is now incumbent on the surgeon to investigate further in the hope of determining the etiologic basis of the impaired

Table 1. Criteria for differential diagnosis of some vascular diseases affecting the foot

Differential factors	Organic vascular diseases		Functional disorders		
	Thromboangiitis obliterans (Buerger's)	Arteriosclerosis obliterans	Raynaud's disease	Acrocyanosis	Erythromelalgia
Age at onset (years)	Below 40	Over 40	Below 40	Below 40 (20-30)	Below 40
Sex incidence	Rare In females	More frequent in males (11:1)	70% females	90% females	70% females
Skin color	Normal to cyanotic	Normal to cyanotic, or marked pallor	Pale to waxy	Persistent cyanosis	Red to cyanotic
Skin color on elevation of leg	Blanching, usually restricted to digits	Pale to waxy (entire foot)	No change	Cyanosis may decrease slightly	No change
Skin color on dependency of leg	May be normal to red to cyanotic in digits	Slow return to red or to cyanosis (30 sec. +)	No change	No change	No change
Pain					
Spontaneous	Aching and gnawing (present at rest)	Moderate to severe aching (present at rest, often nocturnally)	Rare	Rare	Continuous and burning
On elevation of leg	May increase	May increase	No change	No change	May decrease
On dependency of leg	May decrease	May decrease	No change	No change	May increase
On cooling of leg	May decrease	May decrease	Increases	Increases	Decreases
On warming of leg	Increases	Increases	Relieves discomfort	Little or no change	Increases
Intermittent claudication	Common	Usual	Absent	Absent	Absent
Diabetes mellitus	Absent	Present in 20%	Absent	Absent	Absent
Superficial thrombophlebitis	Frequent	May occur	Absent	Absent	Absent
Trophic changes	Frequent	Frequent	Only tips of digits	Absent	Absent
Skin temperature	Low	Low	Low	Low	High (above 32° C.)
Pulses	Usually present	Absent or impaired	Good	Good	Usually bounding
Bruits (aortic, iliac, femoral)	Absent	Present in 85%	Absent	Absent	Absent

circulation. Palpation of pulses and auscultation over major arteries for the presence of bruits may assist in determining the highest level of vascular occlusion.

Finally, arteriographic studies may be necessary to evaluate the condition fully.

Intermittent vasoconstriction, such as occurs in Raynaud's disease, can stop blood flow more effectively if the size of the lumen of the small vessels has been encroached upon by a disease process. Embolism to the microcirculation from large-vessel thrombi (aortic, iliac, femoral, or popliteal aneurysm) is probably responsible for a good deal of the small-vessel disease of feet in older persons. The common forms of small-vessel disease (thromboangiitis obliterans, lupus, and other forms of inflammatory arteritis) are not as common in the feet as in the hands.

It should be noted that many of the symptoms and signs are shared by several vascular diseases. For the surgeon who may not be an expert in the field of peripheral vascular disease, the accompanying table of signs and symptoms may be of assistance in arriving at a tentative diagnosis.

REFERENCES
Rheumatoid arthritis

American Rheumatism Association: Primer on the rheumatic diseases, New York, 1964, The Arthritis Foundation.

Gout

Balasubramaniam, P., and Silva, J. F.: Tophectomy and bone-grafting for extensive tophi of the feet, J. Bone Joint Surg. 53-A:133-136, Jan. 1971.

Kurtz, J. F.: Surgery of tophaceous gout in the lower extremity, Surg. Clin. N. Amer. 45:217-229, Feb. 1965.

Linton, R. R., and Talbott, J. H.: The surgical treatment of tophaceous gout, Ann. Surg. 117:161-182, Feb. 1943.

Stanbury, J. B., Wyngaarden, J. B., and Fredrickson, D. S., editors: The metabolic basis of inherited disease, ed. 3, New York, 1972, McGraw-Hill Book Co.

Woughter, H. W.: Surgery of tophaceous gout: A case report, J. Bone Joint Surg. 41-A:116-122, Jan. 1959.

Diabetes

Antes, E. H.: Charcot joint in diabetes mellitus, J.A.M.A. 156:602-603, Oct. 1954.

Bailey, C. C., and Root, H. F.: Neuropathic foot lesions in diabetes mellitus, N. Eng. J. Med. 236:397-401, Mar. 1947.

Bolen, J. G.: Diabetic Charcot joints, Radiology 67:95-98, July 1956.

Fagerberg, S.-E.: Studies on the pathogenesis of diabetic neuropathy. IV. Angiopathia diabetica vasae nervorum, Acta Med. Scand. 159:59-62, Oct. 1957.

Goodman, J. I., Baumoel, S., Frankel, L., Marcus, L. J., and Wasserman, S.: The diabetic neuropathies, Springfield, Ill., 1953, Charles C Thomas, Publisher.

Hutchinson, E. C., and Liversedge, L. A.: Neuropathy in peripheral vascular disease: Its bearing on diabetic neuropathy, Quart. J. Med. 25:267-274, Apr. 1956.

Jordan, W. R.: Neuritic manifestations in diabetes mellitus, Arch. Intern. Med. 57:307-366, Feb. 1936.

Lippman, E. M., and Grow, J. L.: Neurogenic arthropathy associated with diabetes mellitus, J. Bone Joint Surg. 37-A:971-977, Oct. 1955.

Malins, J.: Clinical diabetes mellitus, London, 1968, Eyre & Spottiswoode.

Marchal de Calvi, C. J.: Recherches sur les accidents diabétiques, et essai d'une théorie générale du diabète, Paris, 1864, P. Asselin.

Martin, M. M.: Neuropathic lesions of the feet in diabetes mellitus, Proc. Roy. Soc. Med. 47:139-140, 1954.

Mayne, N. M.: Diabetic neuropathy: A clinical study, M.D. Thesis, Univ. of Birmingham, 1964.

Oakley, W. G., Pyke, D. A., and Taylor, K. W.: Clinical diabetes and its biochemical basis, Oxford, 1968, Blackwell Scientific Publications.

Parsons, H., and Norton, W. S.: The management of diabetic neuropathic joints, New Eng. J. Med. 244:935-938, June 1951.

Rudy, A.: Diabetic neuropathy, New Eng. J. Med. 233:684-689, Dec. 1945.

Rundles, R. W.: Diabetic neuropathy: General review with report of 125 cases, Medicine 24:111-160, May 1945.

Seitz, D.: Zur Klinik und Pathogenese der Polyneuritis diabetica, Dtsch. Z. Nervenheilkd. 175:15-37, 1956.

Sheppe, W. M.: Neuropathic (Charcot) joints occurring in diabetes mellitus, Ann. Intern. Med. 39:625-629, July-Dec. 1953.

Shuman, C. R., and Gilpin, S. F.: Diabetic neuropathy: Controlled therapeutic trials, Amer. J. Med. Sci. 227:612-617, June 1954.

Woltman, H. W., and Wilder, R. M.: Diabetes mellitus: Pathologic changes in the spinal cord and peripheral nerves, Arch. Intern. Med. 44:576-603, Oct. 1929.

Diabetic gangrene

Classen, J. N.: Neurotrophic arthropathy with ulceration, Ann. Surg. 159:891-894, June 1964.

de Takats, G.: Vascular surgery, Philadelphia, 1959, W. B. Saunders Co.

Fairbairn, J. F., II, Juergens, J. L., and Spittell, J. A.: Allen-Barker-Hines' peripheral vascular diseases, ed. 4, Philadelphia, 1972, W. B. Saunders Co., p. 189.

Ulcers caused by vascular deficiency

Cady, J. B., and Morgan, W. S.: Treatment of chronic ulcers with chlorophyll, Amer. J. Surg. 75:562-569, Apr. 1948.

Lucca, D.: Management of leg ulcers, J. Int. Colloq. Surg. 25:718-726, June 1956.

Peripheral vascular disease

Fairbairn, J. F., II, Juergens, J. L., and Spittell, J. A.: Allen-Barker-Hines' peripheral vascular diseases, ed. 4, Philadelphia, 1972, W. B. Saunders Co.

Gilfillan, R. S.: A test for evaluating pedal gangrenous lesions: Observations of elevation reactive hyperemia as a gauge of blood supply, Calif. Med. 88:364-368, May 1968.

Lewis, T.: Vascular disorders of the limbs: Described for practitioners and students, London, 1946, Macmillan & Co., Ltd.

11

Infectious disorders and noninfectious inflammatory diseases of the foot

Stanford F. Pollock
James M. Morris

INFECTIOUS DISORDERS AFFECTING THE FOOT

Although several of the infectious conditions considered in this chapter are relatively uncommon in the United States, many of them are endemic to locales that are easily accessible by air travel. Sporadic cases may be seen all over the world.

Bailey (1957) has discussed the subject of infections of the foot, particularly in terms of specific areas of the foot: infected adventitious bursae associated with a corn; infected bursae over a hallux valgus; infections of the terminal pulp space; suppurative tenosynovitis; infections of the interdigital subcutaneous spaces, of the heel space, the web spaces, the deep fascial spaces of the sole; infections of the central, medial, and lateral plantar spaces; and infections of the dorsal subcutaneous and the dorsal subaponeurotic spaces. He also includes a brief description of infected blisters and of paronychia in the lateral region of the nail, which is especially common in the great toe as a complication of an ingrown nail.

Tuberculosis

Osseous tuberculosis of the foot. The bones of the foot are seldom sites of tuberculous lesions, but in establishing a diag-

nosis the possibility of tuberculous lesions must not be overlooked (Fig. 11-1). Since the advent of antimicrobial agents, especially isonicotinic acid hydrazide, tuberculosis of the bone has decreased in severity. It may be difficult to diagnose because it often simulates other diseases of bone.

Tuberculosis of bone and joints is a slow, unrelenting, destructive manifestation of a systemic disease induced by the tubercle bacillus. Since the lesion is always secondary to a tuberculous focus elsewhere in the body, this focus should be located.

Tuberculosis of the bones of the foot may occur at any age. As a rule, the chronic infection is fairly widespread, although isolated foci may be found, particularly in the calcaneus and talus.

According to Miltner and Fang (1936), the most important weight-bearing bones are affected in cases of multiple infection. The order of incidence, from highest to lowest, is as follows: calcaneus, talus, first metatarsal, navicular, and first and second cuneiform bones.

Complete excision or curettage of a localized tuberculous focus and adequate antibacterial therapy have been consistently successful. If a bone or bones can be removed in entirety without producing excessive deformity and disability, exci-

299

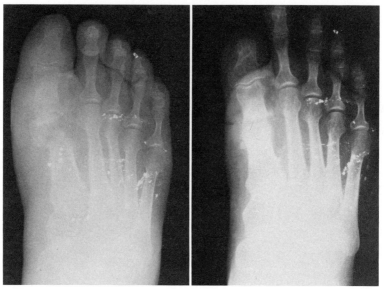

Fig. 11-1. Roentgenograms showing tuberculosis of first metatarsal. Buckshot wounds antedated the onset of this involvement. Infection was proved by biopsy and guinea pig inoculation. (Courtesy Dr. D. D. Dickson.)

sion may be possible (Mukopadhaya and Mishra, 1957). Instillation of streptomycin and other antimicrobial agents (e.g., iso-nicotinic acid hydrazide, para-aminosalicylic acid) through a drainage tube has also been of value; these drugs probably should be administered exclusively by this local route. In cases in which the state of generalized illness requires the use of triple systemic therapy, an exception may be made to this statement. Such drugs as vio-mycin sulfate and cycloserine may be considered in particularly resistant infections. Recently ethambutol, rifampin, and cap-reomycin have been used in the treatment of pulmonary tuberculosis. The efficacy of these drugs in treating osseous lesions has not been clearly established in the literature.

In general, tuberculosis should be suspected in the presence of an unrelenting, prolonged, chronic destructive process in the bone with recurring acute exacerbations. Skin tests for tuberculosis should be performed, since this disease is apt to be present in such cases. Reeves (1958) presents a thorough discussion of differential diagnosis of tuberculosis of the talus in a case in which the clinical diagnostic impressions included arthritis, degenerative disease, and granulomatous proliferation. Reeves emphasizes a sign that is almost pathognomonic: roentgenographic evidence of partial sclerotic reaction, indicating unsuccessful healing, the fragmented talus being more severely diseased in one part than another. Reeves also calls attention to the need for follow-up roentgenograms, because the first ones may show no abnormality.

Syphilis

Syphilitic neuropathy. Until the advent of antibiotics, latent syphilis was the most common destroyer of the joints of the body (Figs. 11-2 and 11-3). Although the late manifestations of syphilis have now become rare, it must be remembered that the venereal disease rate for both syphilis and gonorrhea has continually increased throughout the world. Charcot's joint was frequently encountered as a result of syphilis, but its predilection was for the knee rather than the foot, although the ankle was often

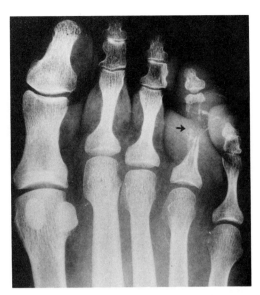

Fig. 11-2. Necrosis of fourth digit in latent syphilis.

affected and other joints were not unaffected. Antibiotics and antianemia therapy have greatly diminished the incidence of arthropathies caused by syphilis and anemia.

Coccidioidal infection

Coccidioides immitis. *Coccidioides immitis,* a specific fungus, gains entrance through the respiratory tract or skin and is disseminated through the blood or lymph channels or is spread by direct extension. Spores settle in cancellous bone and bone lesions form. The resulting infection is usually chronic and shows clinical and roentgenographic changes similar to those in chronic osteomyelitis.

McMaster and Gilfillan (1939) reported twenty-four cases of coccidioidal osteomyelitis with multiple foci involving various parts of the body, including the foot. The average age of their patients, who were predominantly men, was 32 years. Thirteen

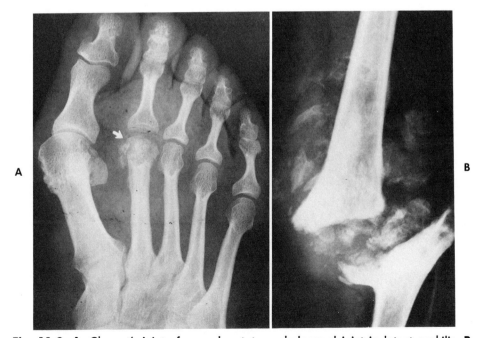

Fig. 11-3. A, Charcot's joint of second metatarsophalangeal joint in latent syphilis. **B,** Knee joint in same case. Bizarre destruction and new bone formation.

of the patients died; all were proved to have had an associated active pulmonary involvement.

Grebe (1954) reported a case of monostotic coccidioidal infection in which the bone lesion occurred in the left calcaneus. Evidence of disease or injury had not been observed. There was no response to wide excision of the bone lesion, but rapid healing was accomplished by treatment with 2-hydroxystilbamidine diisethionate.

More recently, the use of amphotericin B as described by Winn (1955, 1963) has produced encouraging results in cases which might previously have been fatal. Amphotericin B has been particularly useful in preventing massive dissemination of the disease in patients who undergo surgical procedures for coccidioidal lesions. A fall in the coccidioidal complement fixation titer indicates successful treatment and may occur after surgical removal of the infected tissue. Although treatment with amphotericin B has effectively reduced the toxicity of the disease, it should also be noted that amphotericin B is an extremely toxic drug and that *Coccidioides immitis* is among the most resistant of fungal infections to it.

Mycetoma (Madura foot)

Mycetoma is a chronic granulomatous disease (Fig. 11-4) found mainly in tropical countries, especially in some districts of India. It is caused by a fungus belonging to the genus *Nocardia* or *Madurella*. The disease begins as a granuloma, generally subcutaneous in location (Fig. 11-5). The deep structures are involved only late in the course of the disease (Oyston, 1961). New tumors form while old ones soften, and the foot increases enormously in size, becoming deformed. Franz and Albertini (1954) found extensive osteoporosis of the tarsal bones in one of their patients. Primary mycetoma of bone is a more uncommon condition. According to Majid and colleagues (1964), all primary intraosseous infections that have been studied mycologically are caused by *Madurella mycetoma*.

A similar condition indigenous to the United States is caused by *Actinomyces bovis*, a gram-positive, non–acid-fast, nonmotile filamentous organism related to true bacteria but resembling fungi.

The characteristic lesion in this condition is a firm, relatively nontender abscess with

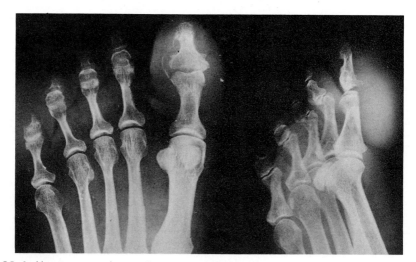

Fig. 11-4. Massive granuloma of great toe. Result of a mycotic infection acquired in a tropical country.

central necrosis that may drain to the surface. Consequently, the sinus tract produced has little tendency to heal spontaneously.

Mycologic identification of the organisms and appropriate antimicrobial sensitivity studies are important, since treatment may depend to some degree on the use of antimicrobial agents. Actinomyces may be sensitive to penicillin, tetracycline, erythromycin, and chloramphenicol, whereas nocardial species show only moderate sensi-

tivities to penicillin, sulfonamides, and sulfones. Mycetomas caused by *Madurella* types of organisms are fairly resistant to antimicrobial therapy, although Neuhauser (1955) reported promising therapeutic results with diaminodiphenylsulfone. In spite of the encouraging results of antimicrobial treatment, surgery is usually necessary. In all these conditions superficial lesions excised in the early stages result fairly often in cure. In advanced cases amputation above the diseased area may be necessary.

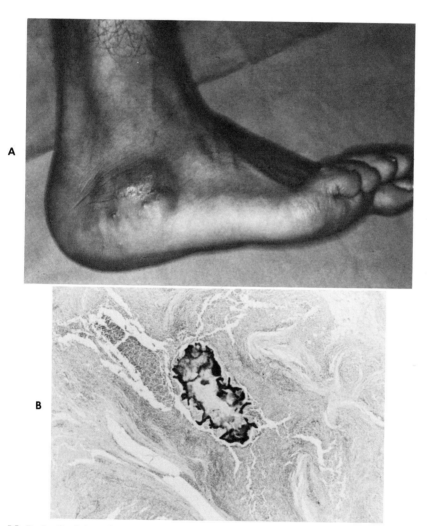

Fig. 11-5. A, Draining sinus tracts on lateral side of heel. Biopsy of the extensive nodular lesion of the soft tissues revealed *Nocardia*. **B,** *Nocardia* colony with chronic inflammation showing sulfur granule of lesion in **A.**

Leprosy (Hansen's disease)

Leprosy is a specific chronic disease of man. It is believed to be caused by *Mycobacterium leprae,* although until recently cultivation of the organism and the production of subsequent disease in inoculated animals could not be accomplished. A recent successful effort to cultivate the organism and produce the disease in the armadillo opens avenues for research in this area that have hitherto been impossible.

The mode of transmission of leprosy is unknown, but direct and prolonged contact appears to be necessary. Once in the body, the bacilli are probably spread through the lymphatics and the bloodstream. Localization occurs in the skin, nerves, or both, but in advanced cases bacilli are found in all parts of the body with the exception of smooth muscle.

Types of lesions. There are three types of lesions in leprosy—lepromatous, tuberculoid, and intermediate.

Lepromatous. These lesions are characterized by the formation of lepromas, nodules that are made up of large macrophages which contain numerous bacilli and fat droplets.

Tuberculoid. Areas of asymmetric lesions form tubercles containing epithelial cells, giant cells, lymphocytes, and plasma cells, with few or no bacilli present. These nodules may affect the skin and nerves.

Intermediate. These lesions contain a few bacilli and produce a slight cellular reaction that is limited to the perivascular and perineural areas. The diagnosis is established when acid-fast bacilli are found in scrapings of the nasal mucosa and in the tissue fluid expressed from superficial incisions of the skin in some areas.

Effects of leprosy upon the feet. The foot may be affected in several ways: (1) Leprous lesions may develop in the feet directly; (2) lepromatous involvement of the peripheral nerves may result in anesthetic feet; and (3) involvement of the peroneal nerve may result in dropfoot.

Harris and Brand (1966) indicated two distinct methods of destruction of the foot once pain sensibility is lost. The first is slow erosion and shortening associated with perforating ulcers under the distal weightbearing end of the foot. The second is a proximal disintegration of the tarsus in which mechanical forces often determine the onset and progress of the condition. The treatment of such feet is as follows:

1. The patient must be educated to use the feet only for gentle walking.
2. Immobilization of the feet in plaster or complete bed rest is necessary for the treatment of ulcers.
3. One should be alert to signs of tarsal disintegration. The earliest signs may be local warmth, swelling, or both. When these signs occur, gait analysis should be carried out and suitable shoe adjustment should be made until the patient can walk a limited distance without developing tarsal heat at points of stress.
4. When definite bone damage is seen, full immobilization is imperative.
5. In cases in which joints are disintegrating, surgical fusion should be performed without delay.

Warren (1971), in a study of tarsal bone disintegration in over 1,500 leprosy patients treated at the Hong Kong Leprosarium during a 12-year period, found that early detection and treatment by immobilization permitted healing with minimal deformity or disability, and that feet with advanced lesions could be similarly treated, without the need for amputation.

Involvement of the common peroneal nerve frequently results in dropfoot. Carayon and colleagues (1967) described promising results in the correction of this deformity with a dual transfer of the posterior tibial and flexor digitorum longus tendons.

Although the sulfones appear to be helpful in the medical management of bacterial infection, surgical procedures continue to play an important role in the treatment of neurogenic manifestations of this disease.

Pyogenic infections

Superficial pyogenic infections are often induced or are aggravated by footwear. The distal portion or segment of the toe is susceptible to a felon similar to that which occurs in the finger. The troublesome, ubiquitous tinea pedis organisms may combine with other bacterial organisms to infect the foot by means of neglected minor scratches, irritations caused by friction, or injury from such instruments as scissors. In the presence of such infection, continued wearing of shoes and weight bearing may lead to extension of the infection into the fascial planes, tendon sheaths, or lymphatic channels. Pyogenic organisms may invade any part of the foot through an abrasion in the skin surface. The abrasion may be microscopic, and the patient may be completely unaware of its presence.

Cellulitis. Cellulitis may result from the entrance of pyogenic bacteria to the tissues underlying the epidermis. The most commonly encountered organism is *Staphylococcus* and the most common sites of entry of the organism are the numerous hair follicles. Continued irritation such as that caused by the eyelets of the shoe over the dorsum of the first metatarsocuneiform joint, generally the highest point on the dorsum of the midfoot, may aggravate the condition.

Cellulitis is best treated by complete bed rest, elevation of the foot, continual hot compresses, and appropriate systemic antibiotics. If pus is allowed to accumulate in a localized area, adequate drainage is mandatory.

Lymphangitis. Lymphangitis is generally caused by staphylococcal or streptococcal organisms that penetrate small wounds or abrasions. The onset of symptoms of lymphangitis is sudden; a history of injury or abrasion may or may not be present. Pain and tenderness are experienced over a local point; chills often occur, followed by a rapidly rising temperature. Within 12 to 24 hours, bright red streaks may appear along the course of the lymphatic channels; inflammation and edema surround the streaks. The lymph glands proximal to the focus of infection become swollen, painful, and inflamed. Symptoms of general toxicity may be severe, out of all proportion to the appearance of the local lesion. In a few cases, organization of pus takes place at the focus of infection. Occasionally the infection spreads rapidly despite treatment until general septicemia develops. Koch (1934) has contributed a long study of the disease as it applies to the hand.

Treatment. Patients with lymphangitis should be hospitalized and kept at complete bed rest. The leg should be elevated, and moist hot compresses should be applied to the entire foot and leg continuously. High blood levels of appropriate antibiotics should be maintained. Close attention should be paid to such complications of toxemia as dehydration and electrolyte imbalance. Incision and drainage is rarely indicated; it may even be harmful (Kanavel, 1939; Koch, 1929). Even if there is evidence of partial organization, it is better to err on the conservative side by not incising. The only indication for incision and drainage is the presence of localized loculated areas of material. That condition is manifested by the presence of a blister or fluctuant mass directly under the skin, which ordinarily occurs at the focal point of infection but occasionally appears along the course of the lymphatic channels or in the area of the regional lymph nodes.

Felon. A felon, or whitlow, is a septic infection of the pulp space of the distal phalanx of the finger or toe (Fig. 11-6). Purulent material collects in the pulp space and may develop considerable pressure, causing accompanying severe throbbing pain. The pressure may cause decrease or obliteration of the blood supply to bone, which results in necrosis and sequestration. Osteomyelitis of the distal phalanx and the interphalangeal joint is a common complication of a felon (Fig. 11-7).

The distal segment of the toe becomes indurated, swollen, and throbbing 24 to 48 hours following the onset of infection. Pain may be severe, with sleep impossible. The

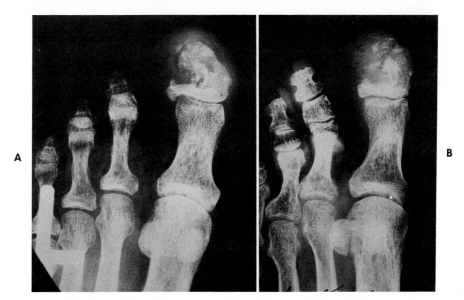

Fig. 11-6. Felon of great toe with involvement of distal phalanx.

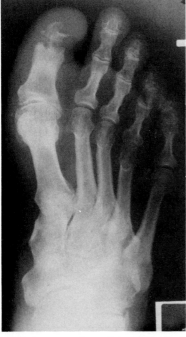

Fig. 11-7. Osteomyelitis of first distal phalanx and of heads of proximal phalanges after injury.

discrepancy between objective observations and the severity of the pain is characteristic of a felon. After several days the pain diminishes as necrosis of bone progresses. Roentgenographic examination at the time may disclose early osteomyelitis of the distal phalanx.

Treatment. Local and systemic measures, which include bed rest, elevation of the foot, and warm compresses should be instituted immediately. Appropriate systemic antibiotics, which tend to localize the infectious process, should also be started immediately.

Except during the early stages in the development of a felon, incision and drainage is mandatory under general anesthesia or adequate regional block. The pulp space should be opened widely by a semicircular (fishmouth) incision extending from one side of the toe to the other and encircling the distal half of the distal phalanx. Secondary vertical incisions may be made into the pulp space to facilitate drainage. If sequestrae are present they may be removed. In most cases the process subsides in 2 to 3 weeks and the bone regenerates. If the bone of the distal phalanx has sequestered completely, it is occasionally advisable to leave the sequestrum in position in the hope that it will serve as a scaffold for the new bone formation and thereby conserve the contour of the toe. In most cases, however, it is recommended that the entire sequestered bone be removed.

On occasion, the infection may progress so rapidly and with such local destruction of bone and tissues that amputation of the distal phalanx or of the entire digit is necessary. This destructive process is generally seen in diabetes or peripheral small-vessel disease. In cases in which amputation is necessary, the skin flaps should be left open for free drainage and subsequent secondary closure.

Infectious tenosynovitis. *Bacterial tenosynovitis* is an inflammation of tendon sheaths, which may be suppurative or non-suppurative. It is always caused by invasion of the bacteria into the involved tendon sheaths. The course of the disease depends largely on the virulence of the invading oragnism and the extent of invasion of the tendon sheaths.

Acute infectious tenosynovitis (Christie, 1956) is caused by a spread of infection from adjacent tissues from direct inoculation by accidental laceration or by contamination from an incision made because of a subcutaneous infection. The laceration or puncture may be microscopic. Occasionally the infection may spread to other parts of the body.

The invader in most cases is one of the common pyogenic organisms, although infections from other more unusual organisms have been reported.

Diagnosis is based on the classic signs of inflammation along the course of the tendon. The inflammation produces extreme pain, which is especially severe at the insertion of the tendon (even though the active infection may be distant from it) because the infected tendon is immobilized. Any tendon or its sheath may be involved, but the extensor tendons of the foot are most commonly affected. Sliding of the tendon or tendons is a complication that may lead to extreme contracture.

Treatment consists of complete bed rest and prompt administration of appropriate antibiotics. Continuous, hot, moist compresses should be applied, and when fluctuation gives evidence of the organization or localization of purulent material, surgical drainage should be carried out promptly. The local injection of antibiotics into the tendon sheath may occasionally reduce the necessity for incision and drainage but should not be relied upon to the exclusion of surgical drainage.

Chronic infectious tenosynovitis is caused by a specific disease, such as syphilis or tuberculosis. It may be the only manifestation of active tuberculosis. Chronic infectious tenosynovitis is rare, but when it occurs it involves the sheaths of the extensors and peroneal tendons around the ankle joint.

Treatment consists of immobilization of the affected tendons and general treatment of the underlying systemic disease. Surgical repair of the gliding mechanism may be necessary when injury to the tendon and its sheath is severe.

Bursitis. Infectious bursitis includes acute septic bursitis and retrocalcaneal bursitis.

Acute septic bursitis. Inflammation of an adventitial bursa may be caused by the invasion of pyogenic organisms. It is often accompanied by pus formation and is usually the result of a wound such as a small abrasion or laceration in the vicinity of the bursa. It may also occur subsequent to a simple acute or traumatic bursitis as a result of the implantation of organisms from the circulatory system during a period of transient bacteremia.

Treatment consists of complete rest, hot compresses, appropriate antibiotics, and incision and drainage if localization or loculization has occurred. After the acute stage subsides, the patient may be ambulatory, provided pressure has been completely removed from the affected area.

Retrocalcaneal bursitis. Retrocalcaneal bursitis is an inflammation of the only consistent anatomic bursa of the foot. This bursa is situated between the posterosupe-

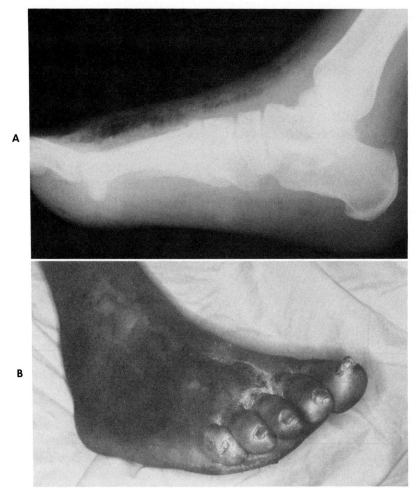

Fig. 11-8. Gas gangrene of foot. **A,** Lateral x-ray film of foot showing gas formation in subcutaneous tissue on dorsum of foot as a result of clostridial cellulitis. **B,** Clostridial cellulitis of dorsum of foot. Note the fluctuant swelling of subcutaneous tissue. **C,** View of dorsum of foot at time of wide incision and drainage, with excision of necrotic tissue.

rior surface of the calcaneus and the tendo achillis. The condition is usually acute but may be chronic and may or may not suppurate.

ETIOLOGY. Tension from a tight heel cord, friction, and pressure from the shoe counter, with ensuing secondary infection, are ordinarily the causative factors. Infection may be metastatic. Because the bursa is enclosed in a limited area, the infected area is under pressure. The symptoms of swelling and inflammation above the posterosuperior portion of the calcaneus, pain, and tenderness to touch may be acute. Dorsiflexion of the foot increases the pain.

TREATMENT. In the acute stage, treatment is the same as that for acute cellulitis: complete rest, hot packs, and antibiotics. If the infection becomes organized, drainage should be instituted. In chronic or recurrent cases the heel cords must be stretched or lengthened and the bursa may need to be excised; however, such excision is at times followed by lengthy and painful convalescence because· of the difficulty of occluding dead space left by removal of the

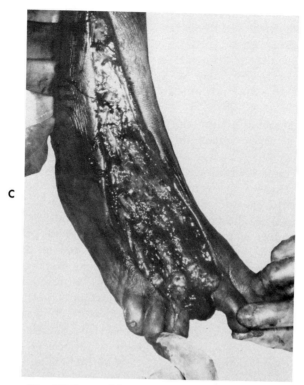

C

Fig. 11-8, cont'd. For legend see opposite page.

bursa. (For surgical procedure, see Chapter 19.)

Gas gangrene. The term "gas gangrene" refers to a group of pure or mixed clostridial infections. Most cases (90 percent) occur because of infection caused by *Clostridium perfringens*. Infection occurs when devitalized tissue is present, especially devitalized muscle, as a result of crushing or severe soft-tissue trauma. The severity of the infection ranges from cellulitis of a localized area of tissue necrosis to so-called clostridial cellulitis (known as gas abscess or anaerobic cellulitis), which is an infection of the subcutaneous tissues rendered susceptible by ischemia or crush injury. In this case muscle is generally not affected, and the symptoms are much less severe than in the so-called full-blown form of gas gangrene caused by myonecrosis, in which there is infection of the dead or damaged muscle tissue. In the case of involvement of muscle, the progress of the disease may be extremely rapid, with severe systemic effects caused by the production of toxins by the infecting organism. In the foot clostridial cellulitis is more commonly encountered because, compared with the leg or thigh, the foot has relatively little muscle tissue (Fig. 11-8).

Diagnosis. The possibility of a clostridial infection should be considered whenever there is a crush injury with devitalized tissue of even a small amount. This is especially true if there has been the possibility of contamination by foreign body, soil, or feces. The diagnosis is made essentially by physical examination. The characteristic picture of gas gangrene is tissue edema, necrosis, discoloration, characteristic autopsy room odor, brown exudate, and crepitation due to gas formation in the soft tissues. Care should be taken, however, not to assume that any infection associated with gas formation is clostridial; many other organisms can produce gas, or air can be trapped in the soft tissues as a result of open injury. Diagnosis is confirmed by the findings of characteristic gram-positive bacilli on gram stain of exudate or debrided soft tissue. Cultures are rarely of value in making the diagnosis because of the prolonged delay.

Treatment. Gas gangrene is almost always preventable. The most important single aspect in the prevention of gas gangrene is thorough, adequate debridement of all dead avascular tissue. The wound must be debrided back to bleeding tissue and, in the case of muscle, to the point at which the muscle contracts when gently pinched. Prophylactic use of antibiotics is of some value; generally, penicillin in very high intravenous doses is the drug of choice. It must be pointed out, however, that no antibiotic can prevent gas gangrene in the absence of thorough surgical debridement.

The use of polyvalent gas gangrene antitoxin is controversial; probably it should not be used prophylactically. Its value in treatment remains questionable. Also used in treatment is hyperbaric oxygen (3 atmospheres), which is probably a helpful adjunct. However, it should not be considered as a substitute for adequate, thorough surgical treatment. Despite adequate local debridement and the use of antibiotics and hyperbaric oxygen, it is occasionally impossible to control the infection without amputating the involved limb.

NONINFECTIOUS INFLAMMATORY DISEASES

Plantar fasciitis

The classic symptom of plantar fasciitis is severe pain that is aggravated by weight bearing and becomes progressively severe and often incapacitating. On palpation the entire plantar surface is tender, but the point of maximal tenderness is elicited just anterior to the calcaneal tuberosity. Presumably in the early stages, fibrositis—with or without pain anterior to the calcaneal tuberosity—represents the pathologic change.

The etiology of the fibrositis is unknown. It is probably related to degenerative and inflammatory changes in other fibrous structures such as the rotator cuff of the shoulder or the medial collateral ligament of the knee. These changes are aggravated by mechanical factors in the susceptible foot (see p. 253), and ultimately a calcaneal spur may form. It must be emphasized that the spur is a reaction to the inflammation and degeneration of the plantar fascia. It is not the spur per se but rather the process within the origin of the plantar fascia that causes the painful symptoms. The spur may be present with or without any painful symptoms; conversely, severe and incapacitating pain may be present without evidence of spur formation.

Treatment. The treatment of plantar fasciitis, with or without spur formation, ranges from simple modification of footwear to the use of surgical procedures in cases of intractable incapacitating pain.

The simplest form of treatment is the use of a felt heel pad with a cutout in the area of maximal tenderness, combined generally with a short course of anti-inflammatory agents such as phenylbutazone or oxyphenbutazone. In those cases that fail to respond to these measures, considerable success has been obtained by the use of appliances such as a UC-BL insert, a heel cup, or a medial felt wedge, which places the heel in a varus position and thus relaxes the tension in the plantar fascia. Occasionally, injection of lidocaine and steroid locally in the area of origin of the plantar fascia is successful. Rarely is surgical release of the plantar fascia from the calcaneus indicated, with or without excision of the accompanying spur. (For surgical treatment of calcaneal spurs, see Chapter 19.)

Bursitis

The term "bursitis" as applied to conditions in the foot is often misleading. It implies an inflammation of an anatomic bursa. However, the retrocalcaneal bursa is the only constant anatomic bursal sac in the foot. In most people a rudimentary bursa remains on the tibial side of the great toe joint. It contains little or no synovial bursal fluid except when diseased, at which time it forms a ganglion—a pathologic, not an anatomic, entity.

Synovial structures are characteristically lined with endothelial cells and include such tissues as tendon sheaths, joint capsules, pleura, and the peritoneum as well as anatomic bursae. To describe painful areas of the foot as bursitis when these areas do not have anatomic bursae is erroneous. The tissues referred to in this way are usually joint capsules or formations of adventitious bursae or ganglia. By way of analogy, myositis is always understood to mean an inflammation of a muscle, a muscle present in everyone, and no one would apply the term to tissues in which there are no muscles. Bursitis, however, is a term which has been carelessly applied to areas that have no anatomic bursae, although synovial membranes may be present.

Lieberman (1936) described enlarged intermetatarsophalangeal bursae, but apparently he meant ganglia. The term "bursitis" is often applied to inflammation in various parts of the foot, especially to joints and tendons, where indeed there is synovial tissue but normally no anatomic bursae. Pathologic or adventitious bursae likewise form in the foot, mostly under the great toe joint, over the fifth metatarsophalangeal joint, over tendon sheaths, and under hard corns. Normal bursae are monolocular, whereas pathologic or adventitious bursae are usually multilocular. As applied to the foot, therefore, one should refrain from using the loose term bursitis, which may mean an inflammation of (1) an anatomic bursa, (2) a joint capsule or tendon sheath, (3) an adventitious bursa, or (4) a ganglion.

Acute simple bursitis. An inflammation of the synovial lining of an adventitious bursa that is without suppuration, and is caused by irritation or injury to a bursa, joint capsule, or tendon sheath, most frequently occurs over the medial side of the great toe joint, the fifth metatarsophalangeal joint, the tendo achillis insertion, or the dorsum of the first metatarsal cuneiform. It is induced by ill-fitting shoes.

Removal of all irritation and protection of the area by padding gives relief in mild cases. In severe cases injection of a hydrocortisone preparation and partial or complete immobilization may be necessary.

Chronic serous bursitis (hygroma). The onset of chronic serous bursitis, sometimes referred to as a hygroma, may follow an attack of acute bursitis. Continuation of the causative factors, such as prolonged friction and pressure, leads to the chronic condition. The synovium of the adventitious bursa becomes thickened and distended. The bursa is generally multiloculated, and a variable amount of fluid is present within the bursal tissue. Occasionally a sinus forms leading to the skin surface, into the joint, or into a cavity formed by the breakdown of subdermal tissues. Chronic serous bursitis most frequently affects the tibial side of the great toe joint; a sinus may develop which penetrates into the joint or along the shaft of the metatarsal (see Fig. 12-7). The condition also occurs over the phalangeal joints of the lesser toes, where the hygroma may or may not be under a hard corn. When a hygroma forms over the tendo achillis just above its insertion, a sinus may drain or communicate from the bursal sac to the skin surface. Occasionally, a hygroma may develop into a fibrotic mass.

Hygromas should be removed surgically by excising hypertrophied and distended synovium, including all sinus tracts leading from the bursa. Whenever possible, the entire mass, including the skin and all surrounding tissue, should be excised, after which appropriate skin closure is carried out. All necrotic bone should be curetted from under the bursa. Great caution should be exercised in the removal of these chronic lesions in cases of arteriosclerosis, diabetes, and peripheral nerve disease because of the possibility of delayed wound healing.

Adventitious bursae under the first metatarsal head. An adventitious bursa under

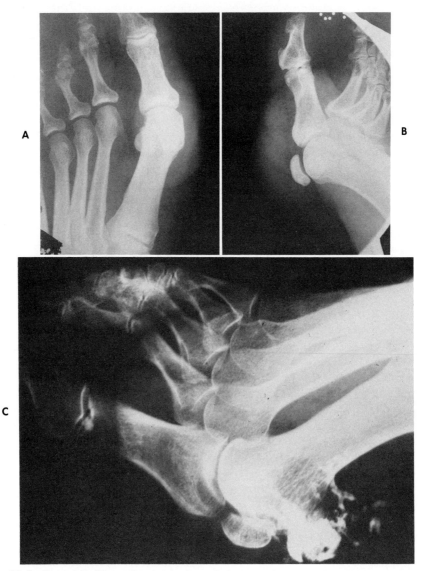

Fig. 11-9. A and **B,** Dorsoplantar and medial view of large adventitious bursa under first metatarsophalangeal joint. **C,** Contrast dye injected in adventitious bursa under first metatarsophalangeal joint. (**C,** Courtesy Dr. Helen Numbers.)

the first metatarsal head is an accumulation of lobular, multiloculated bursal tissue under the great toe joint. The accumulation may reach massive size (Fig. 11-9). It is observed most frequently in girls during adolescence or in early adult life. It is caused by a chain of conditions, such as hypermobile sesamoids, sesamoids that articulate immediately under the great toe joint space, and bifurcated tibial sesamoids, especially if the tibial bone is distorted or abnormal in size. These factors, in combination with the wearing of high-heeled shoes before the sesamoids have completely ossified, and excessive dancing and pivoting on the first metatarsophalangeal joint cause the defensive formation of a bursa. On palpation the mass feels like a large bulbous structure under the skin, which is freely movable and compressible.

Treatment by recommended surgical technique. Excision of the mass is indicated. If the tibial sesamoid is dislocated, hypertrophied, or anomalously shaped, it should be excised in addition to the bursal mass.

An incision is made following the curve of the medial plantar border of the great toe joint. The skin margins are retracted and a plantar flap is freed from the entire plantar surface of the great toe joint. This is retracted as high as possible. The bulbous mass is exposed, dissected, and excised. If, on palpation of the tibial sesamoid, sharp points are felt or if the shape of the plantar surface is anomalous, the tibial sesamoid is excised. A horizontal incision is made in the tibial side of the metatarsophalangeal capsule at the juncture of the superior surface of the tibial sesamoid with the inferior surface of the head of the first metatarsal. The medial margin of the sesamoid is grasped and freed from its entire attachment with a scalpel, and the bone is completely enucleated. The capsule is closed with interrupted catgut sutures, and the skin is closed in the usual manner. A compression bandage is applied and ambulation is started in 48 hours.

Postoperative pain is generally mild; the sutures are removed 9 to 11 days later. A dressing that will partly immobilize the great toe joint should be maintained for 4 weeks, at which time full weight bearing may be resumed.

Adventitious bursae under other weight-bearing surfaces. A comparable adventitious bursa sometimes forms as a protection against excessive pressure under any other weight-bearing surface, such as the plantar surface of the lesser metatarsal heads or the tuberosity of the calcaneus. Malformation, deformities, or anomalies of those bones induce formation of adventitious bursae. Such bursae vary from small to large proportions, depending on the cause. The plantar surface of the fifth metatarsal is the next most likely area where they may form (Fig. 11-10). Excision of the bursa, correction of the causative bone de-

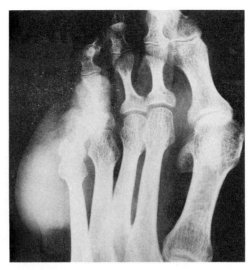

Fig. 11-10. Large adventitious bursa under fifth metatarsophalangeal joint.

formity, and prevention of excessive pressure under the area through proper weight distribution resolve the problem.

Adventitious bursae under a corn are multilobular masses filled with a synovial-like fluid, frequently encountered under helomas. They are formed as a protection against pressure on a bony prominence; however, they increase that irritation inasmuch as the original cause of the pressure persists. Usual sites are on the fifth toe or over a hammered toe of any of the three middle toes. On the fifth toe, they may be excised through a dorsal longitudinal incision at the same time that the offending condyle is excised. (See heloma on fifth toe operation, p. 319). Over a hammered toe the skin and the bursa may be excised through a transverse elliptical incision. (See fifth toe hammertoe operation, p. 540.)

Ossification of tendons

Ossification of the tendo achillis. Ossification of the tendo achillis is a distinct, although rare, clinical entity. Höring (1908) and Jacobsthal (1909) were among the early writers to call attention to this condition. Ghormley (1938) reviewed the published reports of twenty-one cases, of which sixteen occured in males. In eighteen

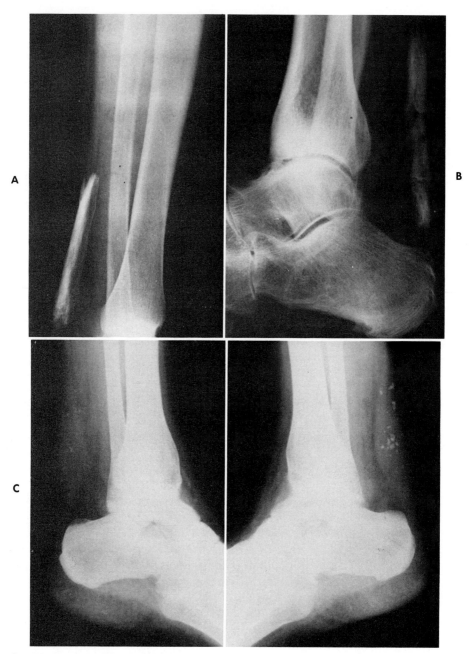

Fig. 11-11. A and **B,** Ossification of tendo achillis resulting from Z-plasty lengthening. **C,** Bilateral fibromatosis with ossification of tendo achillis.

instances the ossification developed free in the tendon, and in three it was an outgrowth of the posterior tuberosity of the calcaneus. In many of the patients there had been a history of previous trauma.

The cause of the condition is obscure; many suggestions have been offered, such as causation by (1) myositis ossificans, (2) a neoplasm, or (3) an accessory sesamoid. None of these conjectures explains why ossification occurs mostly in this tendon of the foot, the tendo achillis. Extensive ossification of the body of the tendon (Fig. 11-11) is uncommon and occasionally is accompanied by fibrosis of the tendon (Fig. 11-12), but ossification at the insertion of the tendon is common (Fig. 11-13). The only consistent symptom is limitation of motion of the ankle, the degree of limitation depending on the extent of ossification.

Asymptomatic cases need not be treated. If pain ensues and motion is greatly lim-

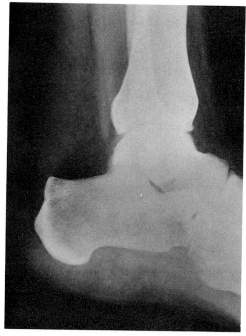

Fig. 11-12. Extensive fibrosis of tendo achillis.

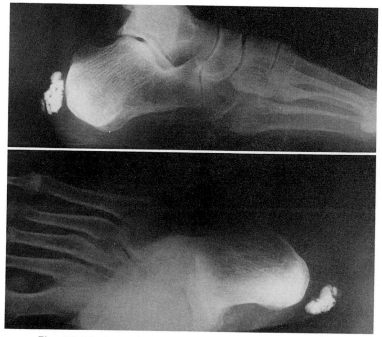

Fig. 11-13. Osteochondroma at insertion of tendo achillis.

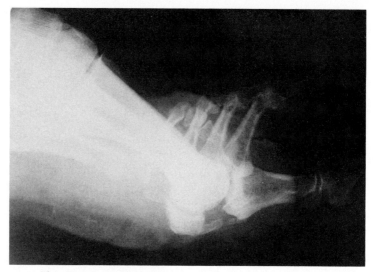

Fig. 11-14. Ossification of flexor hallucis brevis tendon.

ited, then the entire mass should be excised. When the entire tendo achillis must be removed, the terminal end of the triceps surae can be sutured to the peroneus longus and the terminal end of the peroneus longus tendon transferred into the insertion of the tendo achillis.

Ossification of tendons other than the tendo achillis. Any tendon in the foot may undergo ossification but seldom does. The rare case does not become symptomatic except when the site is under a weight-bearing area or the tendon glides around an angle; then weight bearing or movement of the part becomes painful. The diagnosis is made by pinpointing the painful area and confirming ossification of the tendon at that location in the roentgenogram. At times, however, ossification may be overshadowed by adjacent bone. In one such case, ossification of the fibular half of the flexor hallucis brevis tendon caused persistent pain in the first metatarsophalangeal joint for a period of 3 years. The patient had to walk on the outer border of the foot. The pathologic condition was not disclosed in repeated roentgenograms until one of a series of medioplantar views showed the flexor hallucis brevis tendon ossified from the fibular sesamoid to its insertion (Fig. 11-14). Excision of the fibular sesamoid

and the ossified area effected symptomatic cure.

REFERENCES

Altemeier, W. A., and Fullen, W. D.: Prevention and treatment of gas gangrene, J.A.M.A. **217:** 806-813, Aug. 1971.

Bailey, H.: Infections of the foot, J. Int. Colloq. Surg. **27:**475-482, Apr. 1957.

Carayon, A., Bourrel, P., Bourges, M., and Touzé, M.: Dual transfer of the posterior tibial and flexor digitorum longus tendons for drop foot: Report of thirty-one cases, J. Bone Joint Surg. **49-A:**144-148, Jan. 1967.

Christie, B. G. B.: The diagnosis and treatment of tenosynovitis, Brit. J. Clin. Pract. **10:**677-680, Oct. 1956.

DeHaven, K. E., and Evarts, C. M.: The continuing problem of gas gangrene: A review and report of illustrative cases, J. Trauma **11:**983-991, Dec. 1971.

Franz, A., and Albertini, B.: Sul micetoma primitivo del piede: Piede di Madura, Chir. Organi Mov. **40:**412-430, 1954. (Abstracted in Int. Abstr, Surg. **102:**196, Feb. 1956.)

Ghormley, J. W.: Ossification of the tendo achillis, J. Bone Joint Surg. **20:**153-160, Jan. 1938.

Grebe, A. A.: Monostotic coccidioidal infection: Report of a case successfully treated with 2-hydroxystilbamidine, J. Bone Joint Surg. **36-A:** 859-862, July 1954.

Harris, J. R., and Brand, P. W.: Patterns of disintegration of the tarsus in the anaesthetic foot, J. Bone Joint Surg. **48-B:**4-16, Feb. 1966.

Höring, F.: Ueber tendinitis ossificans traumatica, Münch. Med. Wochenschr. **55:**674-675, Mar. 1908.

Jacobsthal, H.: Ueber Fersenchmerzen: ein Beitrag zur Pathologie des Calcaneus und der Achillessehne, Arch. klin. Chir. **88**:146-190, 1909.

Kanavel, A. B.: Infections of the hand, ed. 7, Philadelphia, 1939, Lea & Febiger.

Koch, S. L.: Felons, acute lymphangitis and tendon sheath infections: Differential diagnosis and treatment, J.A.M.A. **92**:1171-1173, Apr. 1929.

Koch, S. L.: Acute rapidly spreading infections following trivial injuries of the hand, Surg. Gynec. Obstet. **59**:277-308, Sept. 1934.

McMaster, P. E., and Gilfillan, C.: Coccidioidal osteomyelitis, J.A.M.A. **112**:1233-1237, Apr. 1939.

Majid, M. A., Mathias, P. F., Seth, H. N., and Thirumalachar, M. J.: Primary mycetoma of the patella, J. Bone Joint Surg. **46-A**:1283-1286, Sept. 1964.

Miltner, L. J., and Fang, H. C.: Prognosis and treatment of tuberculosis of the bones of the foot, J. Bone Joint Surg. **18**:287-296, Apr. 1936.

Mukopadhaya, B., and Mishra, N. K.: Treatment of tuberculosis sinuses and abscesses of osteoarticular origin, J. Bone Joint Surg. **39-B**:326-333, May 1957.

Neuhauser, I.: Black grain maduromycosis caused by *Madurella grisea*, Arch. Dermatol. **72**:550-555, July-Dec. 1955.

Oyston, J. K.: Madura foot: A study of twenty cases, J. Bone Joint Surg. **43-B**:259-267, May 1961.

Reeves, J. D.: Differential diagnosis in case 44122: Presentation of case. New Eng. J. Med. **258**: 612-615, Jan.-Mar. 1958.

Warren, G.: Tarsal bone disintegration in leprosy, J. Bone Joint Surg. **53-B**:688-695, Nov. 1971.

Winn, W. A.: The use of amphotericin B in the treatment of coccidioidal disease, Amer. J. Med. **27**:617-635, July-Dec. 1955.

Winn, W. A.: Coccidioidomycosis and amphotericin B, Med. Clin. N. Amer. **47**:1131-1148, 1963.

12

Disorders of the skin and toenails

Henri L. DuVries

Disorders of the skin to which the foot is especially susceptible are either excrescences caused by friction and pressure over a bony prominence, which are by far the most common lesions of the foot, or diseases of the skin itself, which may be intrinsic or extrinsic and are covered in all texts on dermatology. Friction or pressure may result in hard or soft corns, calluses, keratoses, suppurating sinuses, ulcers, or fibromatoses. Keloids and hypertrophic scars are usually secondary to the healing of lacerations, burns, or surgical wounds. Some intrinsic diseases of the skin are verrucae, dermatoses (especially tinea infections), epidermal cysts, and the rare diastasis of the fifth toe known as ainhum.

The various types of solitary lesions appearing on the plantar surface of the foot are (1) common diffuse calluses; (2) small, deep-seated, circumscribed nucleated calluses; (3) solitary or multiple verrucae plantaris; (4) circumscribed fungating areas; (5) epidermal cysts; and (6) intractable plantar keratoses. These conditions are frequently misdiagnosed, and are often treated as though they were verrucae plantaris.

EXCRESCENCES CAUSED PRIMARILY BY FRICTION, PRESSURE, OR FAULTY WEIGHT BEARING

Corns and calluses are common disorders of this type. They are essentially localized keratoses caused by intermittent pressure from without and solid resistance from within; the outside pressure is produced by the shoe, which is resisted from within by the bones. For this reason, we rarely see a corn or callus over the shaft of a long bone. They occur either on the condyles of the epiphyses of long bones or on the prominent projections of short bones. A hard corn (heloma durum) forms primarily on the exposed surfaces of the toes. The tibial side of the fifth toe is by far the most common site of the hard corn; occasionally one may occur on the fibular side of the fifth metatarsal head. A soft corn (heloma molle) forms over a condyle of a phalanx between the toes. A callus (tyloma) may form over or under any bony prominence of the foot but commonly does so on the ball of the foot, on the plantar surface of the heel, or on the plantar surface of the base of the fifth metatarsal. The terms heloma and tyloma are misleading because they imply that the lesion is neoplastic, whereas the lesion may actually be a reactive proliferation of dead epithelium secondary to pressure. The findings of an extensive study of corns by Bonavilla (1968) support this hypothesis.

Corn (heloma, clavus)

A corn is an accumulation of horny layers of skin over a bony prominence.

Etiology. The outline of the bones of the

318

foot is irregular; the bones have numerous projections, especially over the condyles of the heads and bases of the metatarsals and phalanges. The shoe presses on these prominent condylar processes and the soft tissues over the prominences bear the brunt of pressure and friction exerted on the foot by ill-fitting shoes. Nature attempts to protect the irritated part by accumulating horny epithelium, but the accumulation elevates the prominence so that the shoe increases the pressure on the underlying live tissues. Excrescences and numerous other morbid changes are inevitable over such pressured areas.

That the prominences under excrescences represent proliferative changes in bone is an erroneous concept. Galland (1933) and McElvenny (1940) spoke of exostosis under corns. A study of 5,000 roentgenograms of such cases disclosed that only in rare instances are there cortical changes of bone in the condyle. In those rare instances causation of the changes was unrelated to causation of the corn.

General treatment. Palliative measures, such as reduction of the horny accumulation and then padding of the area to distribute the pressure, give relief in most cases, especially if the site of the corn is a non–weight-bearing area. Excrescences on a weight-bearing surface call for orthopaedic appliances as well as corrective shoes. Intractable conditions over a non–weight-bearing area respond to excision of the condylar prominence immediately under the excrescence (Rutledge and Green, 1957; Billig, 1956). Excrescences on a weight-bearing area usually occur under the metatarsal head and are caused by the deforming restriction of modern footwear on the forepart of the foot; they are only occasionally associated with some degree of deformity or anomaly of the involved bone. They will be discussed later in this chapter.

Corns on the lateral side of the fifth toe. These are common, because the fifth toe receives the maximal pressure of the curve of the outer border of the forepart of stan-

dard shoes. Ordinarily the head of the proximal phalanx of the fifth toe is the most prominent surface at that point, and that is why the corn is nearly always over the fibular condyle of the head of the proximal phalanx.

OPERATIVE TREATMENT. The following procedure for condylectomy of the phalanges under a corn on the fibular side of the fifth toe usually involves the head of the proximal phalanx, but it may also involve condyles of the middle phalanx:

1. With the patient under infiltration anesthesia (0.5 ml. of 1 percent procaine hydrochloride), make an incision over the dorsolateral aspect of the toe, extending it from just proximal to the nail to about the base of the proximal phalanx (Fig. 12-1, *A*). The corn itself should not be incised, because the scar would be exposed to further friction; moreover, callous tissues are devitalized and, therefore, healing is poor.
2. Retract the lateral margin of the skin and subcutaneous tissue to expose the condylar projection covered by capsule and fascia.
3. Carry the line of the skin incision into the capsule; denude the bone of the lateral margin of the capsule and retract with the skin (Fig. 12-1, *B*).
4. Excise the condyle, which has been exposed (Fig. 12-1, *C*).
5. Smooth the surface with a small rasp.
6. Close the skin and capsule with a single mattress suture (Fig. 12-1, *D*).

Postoperative pain is usually slight. Ordinarily healing is rapid, and ambulation may begin in 24 hours. The toe need never be deformed by this operation.

In cases comprising the 2 percent incidence of recurrence the head of the proximal phalanx may be amputated or the middle phalanx may be excised as an alternative procedure, depending on which structure lies under the corn. If the patient also has a soft corn in the fourth web (usually caused by pressure of the head of the proximal phalanx), amputation of

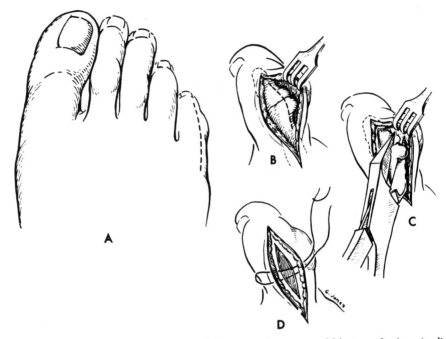

Fig. 12-1. DuVries' technique for condylectomy of corn on fifth toe. **A,** Longitudinal incision over dorsolateral aspect of fifth toe. **B,** Skin and capsule retracted. **C,** Fibular condyles of phalanges amputated. **D,** Skin and capsule closed by mattress suture.

the head should be done initially. However, a flail toe deformity does occasionally result (Fig. 12-2), sometimes making amputation of the entire toe necessary.

EXCISION OF THE HEAD OF THE FIFTH PROXIMAL PHALANX. The technique for excising the head of the fifth proximal phalanx is as follows:

1. Make an incision over the dorsum of the fifth toe, extending from the matrix to about the middle of the shaft of the proximal phalanx.
2. Retract the skin and extensor tendon.
3. Continue the original incision through the capsule and retract its margins together with the skin and the extensor tendon.
4. Flex the distal end of the toe to expose the head of the proximal phalanx. Excise it at its neck.
5. Close the skin and capsule with a single layer of sutures. Apply a compression dressing to occlude the dead space.

6. Remove the sutures on the seventh to tenth day. The corn will usually lift off in about a month.

Corn on the dorsum of the middle three toes and the great toe. These corns are for the most part secondary to hammertoe. (See p. 249.)

Soft corn in the web between the fourth and fifth toes. These are caused by long-continued compression of the skin between the head of the fifth proximal phalanx and the base of the fourth proximal phalanx (Fig. 12-3). Corns in this area are a common disability. A sinus leading into the metatarsal interspace may produce recurrent episodes of acute infection, which often complicate this lesion.

TREATMENT BY CONDYLECTOMY. Condylectomy of the tibial side of the head of the fifth proximal phalanx gives relief. The procedure is similar to that described for hard corn of the fifth toe, except that the incision is made on the dorsomedial aspect of this toe. In cases in which a corn on the

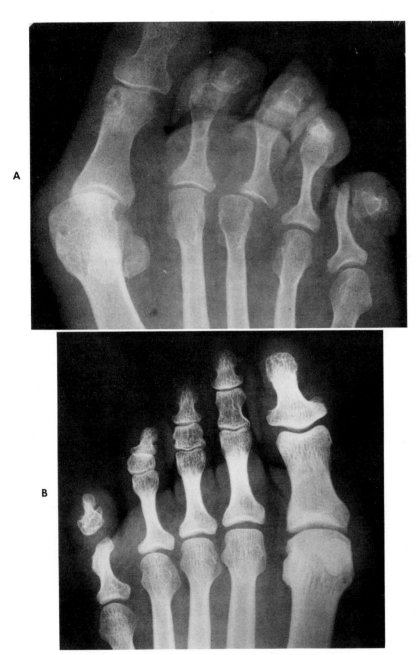

Fig. 12-2. Flail toes produced by phalangectomy.

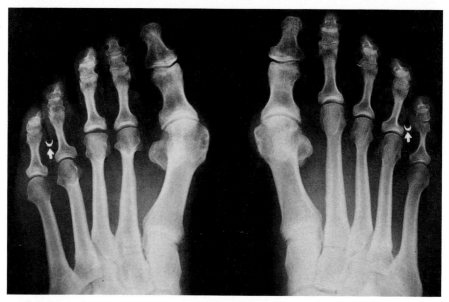

Fig. 12-3. *Right foot,* Head of fifth proximal phalanx adjacent to base of fourth proximal phalanx impinging on soft tissue in fourth web. Severe soft corn is caused. *Left foot,* Same patient; no impingement. Sharp point on the tibial side of the head of the right first metatarsal is a frequent cause of sinus formation over it. (See Fig. 12-7.)

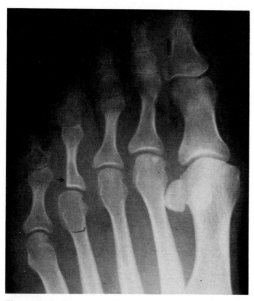

Fig. 12-4. Postoperative appearance of amputation of condyle of base of fourth proximal phalanx.

fibular side of the fifth toe is also present, excision of the head of the fifth proximal phalanx will usually dispose of both. Amputation of the condyle on the fibular side of the base of the fourth proximal phalanx also gives relief (Fig. 12-4). This more traumatic procedure is outlined here; it is only occasionally indicated.

1. Make an incision over the dorsolateral aspect of the fourth proximal phalanx, extending from the middle of the shaft of this phalanx to a point just proximal to the head of the fourth metatarsal (Fig. 12-5, *A*).
2. Open and retract the capsule of the metatarsophalangeal joint to expose the offending condyle for removal by a nasal saw (Fig. 12-5, *B*).
3. Close the skin and capsule by a single layer of sutures (Fig. 12-5, *C*).

Soft corn on the lesser toes. Soft corn on the lesser toes may form over any condylar process of the phalanges. Condylectomy immediately under the excrescence by a pro-

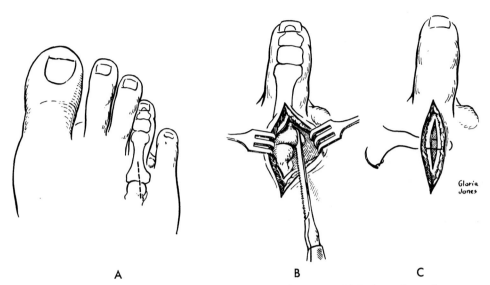

Fig. 12-5. Technique for excision of base of fourth proximal phalanx for soft corn in fourth web. **A,** Incision over dorsolateral aspect of fourth metatarsophalangeal joint. **B,** Skin and capsule retracted; fibular condyle of base of fourth proximal phalanx excised with nasal saw. **C,** Skin and capsule closed with single layer of sutures.

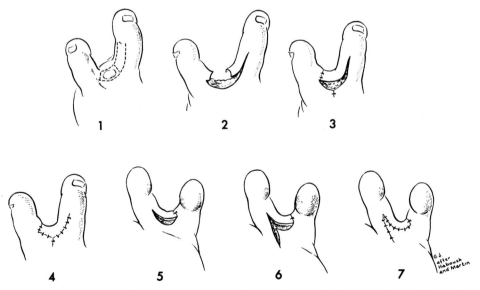

Fig. 12-6. Haboush and Martin's technique for excision of soft corn. **1,** Incisions; **2,** corn excised and flap mobilized; **3,** flap sutured and web advanced; **4,** dorsal closure; **5,** plantar aspect with remaining defect; **6,** flap made and raised; **7,** final suturing.

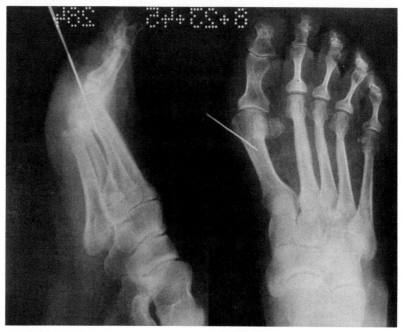

Fig. 12-7. Probe leading into sinus under corn over tibial side of first metatarsal head, coursing along head and neck of metatarsal.

cedure similar to that described for a corn of the fifth toe is effective.

Elaborate procedures have been described, but they are all mutilating and are not physiologic. Such a technique, for example, is described by Haboush and Martin (1947), who performed a skin plastic operation for soft corn in the fourth toe web (Fig. 12-6). After excision of the soft corn on the fifth toe, a skin flap is turned up on the lateral aspect of the fourth toe, based distally, and is sutured to the distal edge of the skin where the corn has been removed. The free dorsal edges of the wound on the fourth and fifth toes are then sutured together. On the sole of the foot, from the base of the fifth toe in the lateral angle of the still open plantar wound, a 2 cm. incision is made, extending proximally. The skin flap is then undermined and mobilized, thus effecting closure of the plantar defect.

Corn over the tibial side of the great toe. Corn over the tibial side of the great toe joint ordinarily is secondary to hallux valgus or to an abnormally wide first metatarsal head. Such corns often have a degenerative sinus that penetrates to an osseous projection on the tibial side of the head of the first metatarsal (Fig. 12-7).

In mild cases protective padding and proper fitting of shoes relieve the condition. In protracted cases open reduction of the hallux valgus is necessary for relief. In a few cases without valgus deformity in which the condition is caused by a congenitally wide head of the first metatarsal, a simple condylectomy on the tibial side of the first metatarsal head suffices. (See Chapter 19, hallux valgus procedures.)

Corn over the base of the fifth metatarsal. This corn is caused by an unusual prominence of this bone and is often associated with pes cavus or metatarsus adductus. In most cases, correction is possible by the use of padding to shield the part and by the wearing of shoes that do not exert pressure over the area. In cases in which this corn occurs because of a major deformity of the foot, the deformity must be corrected in order to relieve the condition. In the occasional case in which the condition is the result of an abnormally prominent bone as an entity by itself, reduction of this bony prominence is indicated.

TECHNIQUE FOR REDUCTION. The following steps accomplish reduction:

1. Make a linear incision over the dorsolateral aspect of the base of the fifth metatarsal, extending from the proximal third of the fifth metatarsal to the lateral aspect of the calcaneocuboid articulation.
2. Retract skin and incise down into the fascia.
3. Detach the base of the fifth metatarsal from the lateral margin of the fascia, which includes the insertion of the peroneus brevis tendon, taking care to preserve the peroneal tendon.
4. With an osteotome or nasal saw amputate the lateral prominence of the base of the fifth metatarsal.
5. Repair the tendon and fascia with fine chromic catgut, and close the skin in the usual manner.
6. Apply a compression bandage that may be released in 24 hours. The patient may bear weight in 48 hours, provided an oxford is worn that has been cut out over the area of operation.

Neurovascular corn. Neurovascular corn is an extremely painful lesion. It is encountered most often on the ball of the foot; it may occur on the fifth toe but rarely occurs on other parts of the foot. It is often mistaken for a wart.

This lesion is often secondary to an old, deeply nucleated corn under a metatarsal head or on the fifth toe. After paring or enucleating the corn (a considerably more painful procedure), or both, one uncovers a glossy surface, which contains fibers and small vessels. Occasionally a minute area appears at the periphery, which under magnification seems to be loosened. When this area is even lightly touched with a sharp instrument, the patient will experience violent, excruciating pain. The condition is caused by an invagination of live epithelium with nerves and blood vessels along the border of the hard, dead epithelium of a callus.

Treatment. Because neurovascular corn is usually caused by prolonged trauma from shoe pressure, the live epithelium underneath it is relatively devitalized and as a result does not respond readily to therapy.

If a localized painful area at the periphery of the corn is found, it is well to stab it and permit it to bleed (which it will do profusely). The small vessels will then collapse. To destroy the neurovascular bundle of the peripheral portion, 95 percent phenol should be applied. Destruction of the major portion of the lesion may be accomplished by repeated applications of the escharotics commonly used for the eradication of small skin growths.

First and foremost, care must be taken to avoid any additional friction and pressure over the area.

Callus (tyloma)

Calluses are large keratotic masses that form on the plantar surface of the foot and are histologically similar to corns. Except for calluses under the talonavicular joint, which may occur in severe cases of flatfoot, these masses are caused by excessive pressure imposed by restrictive footwear upon a weight-bearing surface. The metatarsal head, the heel, the plantar surface of the base of the fifth metatarsal, or the area under the phalangeal joint of the great toe are such surfaces.

Etiology. Calluses are basically caused by shoes with pointed toes, short shoes, or both, that force the toes to buckle and thus produce a hammertoe deformity (see p. 249) at the metatarsophalangeal joints. Normally, the dorsal angle of the metatarsophalangeal joint is about 160 degrees. In hammertoe the angle may be reduced to 90 degrees, at which angle the base of the proximal phalanx articulates with the dorsum of the head of the metatarsal. The pressure of the shoe on the head of the proximal phalanx is transmitted to the metatarsal head, which is depressed plantarward.

Callus under the first metatarsal head. This callus is a circumscribed keratotic area which may or may not be associated with a hammered great toe. It is formed by the bearing of weight on the pointed area of a malformed or displaced tibial sesamoid or, occasionally, a fibular sesamoid. The keratosis often resembles verruca plantaris, for which it is mistakenly treated until the keratosis breaks down and ulcerates or leaves a permanent scar.

In mild cases of callus under the first metatarsal head, proper redistribution of weight bearing by means of a shoe inlay or Thomas bar relieves the lesion. In severe cases, reduction of the hammered toe or excision of the offending sesamoid or both are necessary.

Callus under the middle three metatarsals. Callus under the middle metatarsals is secondary to a depression of the anterior arch and is often accompanied by contracted or hammered toes (clawtoes). It is most pronounced in congenital clawfoot.

Callus under the fifth metatarsal head. This callus is generally the result of faulty weight distribution of the foot, which forces the fifth metatarsal to bear an excessive amount of total body weight. Sometimes the callus is caused by an unusually pointed plantar condyle of the metatarsal head.

A metatarsal inlay or Thomas bar added to a properly fitted shoe corrects most mild cases. However, if the lesser toes are greatly contracted, a dorsal tenotomy and capsulotomy of the fifth metatarsophalangeal joint is advisable. The toes are then maintained in a normal position for about 5 weeks. If any of the toes are extremely hammered, that deformity should also be reduced. (See Chapter 19.)

Proper weight redistribution by means of an appliance and well-fitting footwear gives relief. In resistant cases either a procedure to free the skin under the metatarsal

head or a plantar condylectomy is indicated. Sometimes both procedures are necessary.

Callus on the fibular side of the fifth metatarsal head. Callus on the fibular side of the fifth metatarsal head occurs because the head of the fifth metatarsal is the most prominent point on the outer border of the forefoot. The prominence, known as tailor's bunion, results from either an extraordinarily wide fifth metatarsal head or an outward bending of that head. Constant pressure over the prominence often produces keratotic changes. The skin covering it is thin, so that pressure of the shoe keeps it constantly exsanguinated. In cold climates frequent chilling destroys the capillary beds in the skin and subcutaneous tissues, so that the condition is complicated by painful chilblains. (Treatment is discussed under "Tailor's bunion," p. 236 and "Chilblains," p. 171.)

Callus under the heel. Callus under the heel is usually the result of faulty mechanics of the foot, such as pes planus or pes cavus. In either instance the calcaneus is rotated, so that it bears more weight on one side or the other of the tuberosity. In rare instances the callosity is caused by faulty weight bearing due to an anomalous shape of the tuberosity.

In most cases of callus under the heel, correction of the mechanical fault by appliances and proper shoes eliminates the callus. In rare cases in which the condition is caused by bony projection of the tuberosity of the calcaneus, the prominent area must be reduced and the surface of the tuberosity must be leveled. The surgical approach to such a prominence can be made from either side of the calcaneus, depending on the site of the prominence.

Intractable lesions under metatarsal heads

Most cases of so-called intractable verruca plantaris under the middle three metatarsal heads are essentially a reactive callus (keratosis) resulting from bearing weight on a pointed condylar process under those metatarsal heads (DuVries, 1953, 1954, 1960). It is noteworthy that many reports on intractable verruca plantaris illustrate the lesion as being situated under the second metatarsal head (Blair et al., 1937; Anderson, 1957; Dickson, 1948; Hauser, 1957; Dingman and Grabb, 1962). In 53 years' experience in the treatment of such problems I have encountered few true warts immediately under a metatarsal head. Keratotic lesions on the plantar surface, especially those under the heads of the metatarsals or under any weight-bearing area of the foot, often become disabling. A deep-seated callus or residual scar, when located under a weight-bearing area, can make standing or walking extremely painful. Small, deep, keratotic masses are commonly found under any of the metatarsal heads, especially under the middle three, where they are most likely to become intractable. However, a comparable problem occurs under the first metatarsal head, although the anatomic factors differ. Under the fifth metatarsal head the condition only occasionally becomes intractable. The degree of disability that these growths may cause varies from constant discomfort to complete inability to bear weight on the area.

Intractable keratosis under the first metatarsal head. Although intractable keratosis under the first metatarsal head is common, in general it is not so disabling as when it occurs under the middle three metatarsals. In most instances, it occurs under the tibial sesamoid. In rare cases the fibular sesamoid is the offending ossicle (Fig. 12-8). The tibial sesamoid normally assumes most of the weight-bearing function transmitted to the head of the first metatarsal. Its articulation with the tibial facet under the head of the first metatarsal is unique. The plantar surface of the tibial sesamoid is convex. Because the sesamoids are embedded in the tendon of the flexor hallucis brevis, which inserts into the base of the proximal phalanx, any degree of hallux valgus tends to rotate both sesamoids on the long axis. The fibular sesamoid tends to rotate into the first metatarsal interspace, thereby disposing of the possibility of its becoming a weight-bearing focus; the tibial sesamoid may rotate on its side and thus become a weight-bearing pivot. Because the sesamoids are variously shaped, they may be unusually thick or pointed. A sharp ridge or point on the plantar surface of a sesamoid may cause a

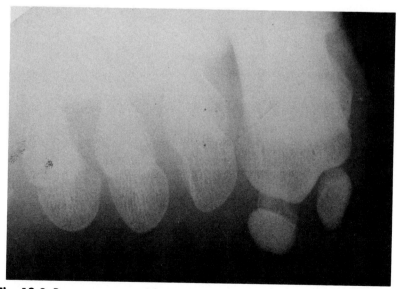

Fig. 12-8. Roentgenogram of foot with hyperkeratosis under fibular sesamoid.

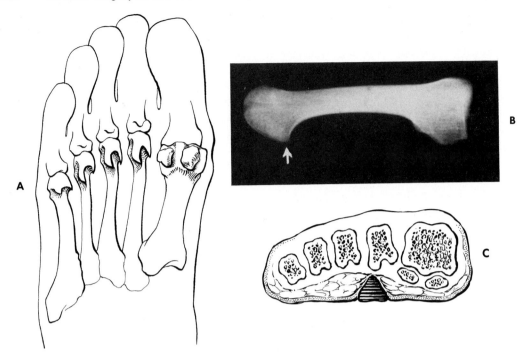

Fig. 12-9. A, Plantar view of sharp condylar process of three middle metatarsals. **B,** Side view of one metatarsal. Note the sharp condylar process. **C,** Cross section of metatarsal heads. Hyperkeratosis under the sharp condylar process of the second metatarsal head.

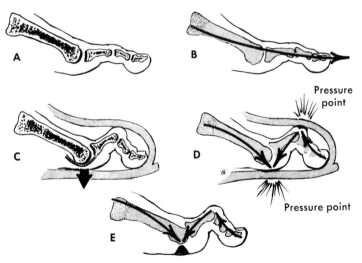

Fig. 12-10. A and **B,** Normal escape of force from body weight. **C,** Contraction of intrinsic muscles as toes strike against end of shoe. (These muscles are inserted into the bases of the proximal and middle phalanges.) **D** and **E,** Counterforce on plantar surface of the metatarsal heads with each step during walking.

deep-seated callus to form under it. That callus is also often erroneously diagnosed and treated as verruca plantaris; consequently it may also become an intractable lesion. Excision of the sesamoid usually offers relief.

Intractable keratosis under the middle three metatarsal heads. The plantar surface of the head of each of the lesser metatarsals has two condylar projections. The condylar projection on the fibular side is always the larger of the two. The condylar projections of the middle three metatarsals end in sharp points extending proximally (Fig. 12-9). The middle three metatarsals form the dome of the anterior metatarsal arch, which functions as a shock absorber and was meant to bear weight only briefly during each step. Because modern footwear buckles the metatarsophalangeal joints (Fig. 12-10), almost everyone in civilized areas has a depressed anterior arch; therefore, the plantar condyles of the metatarsals almost always bear full weight. As a result, the condylar points gouge the soft structures underneath.

The condylar projections vary in size and shape from one metatarsal to another and from one person to another. The projection may be a mere rudiment, or it may extend higher than any other weight-bearing point under all the metatarsal heads. Its surface may be as small as a pinpoint or it may be larger and ball-like in appearance. The sharper and more projecting these processes are, the more the skin and subcutaneous tissue are subject to fibrotic changes, especially if the fat pad is thin. The skin under such a condyle accumulates horny cells as a protective measure. The greater the accumulation of horny layers, the less space there is between the condylar surface and the contact area. Thus, further compression of the soft tissues covering these areas occurs, along with further displacement of the epithelium of the skin and subcutaneous tissue by fibrous connective tissue. The fibrous connective tissue that invades the stratum corneum tends to become frayed from friction and is cauli-

flower-like in appearance (Fig. 12-11). It resembles verruca plantaris (plantar wart, see p. 342) and the lesion is often mistakenly treated as such. Repeated attempts are made to destroy it, using the usual methods for destruction of verrucae, and the scar tissue increases. If the erroneous treatment is repeated, as it often is, the lesion becomes more intractable. (For a differential diagnosis of plantar warts, see p. 344.)

I made a survey of 139 cases of intractable keratosis under the lesser metatarsals and found the lesions to be distributed in the areas illustrated in Fig. 12-12.

Many patients with intractable keratosis become apprehensive of any new treatment for recurrent so-called plantar warts because of their experience with treatment by escharotics, fulguration, excision, and radiation, after which the scar and disability increased. The Montgomerys (1949) have called attention to frequent plantar radiodermatitis, which occurs because of improper diagnosis and treatment of plantar lesions.

Because of the aforementioned chain of events, drastic operations have been recommended. Dickson suggested excision of the entire metatarsal shaft, including the dorsal and plantar soft structures covering it and the toe (Fig. 12-13). Blair et al. (1937) advised excision of the growth and its surrounding skin, with subsequent pedicle grafting from a non–weight-bearing surface of the sole of the foot. Giannestras (1954) shortened the metatarsal shaft by a step-down osteotomy (Figs. 12-20 and 12-21). McKeever (1952) stated that an arthrodesis of the first metatarsophalangeal joint corrects many of the problems.

In recent years there has been a trend toward amputation of the metatarsal head over such lesions. Figs. 12-14 to 12-17 show the feet of patients who experienced greater disability after surgical operations than they did initially. Two hundred fifty such patients have come under my care during the last 15 years.

No roentgenographic method has been

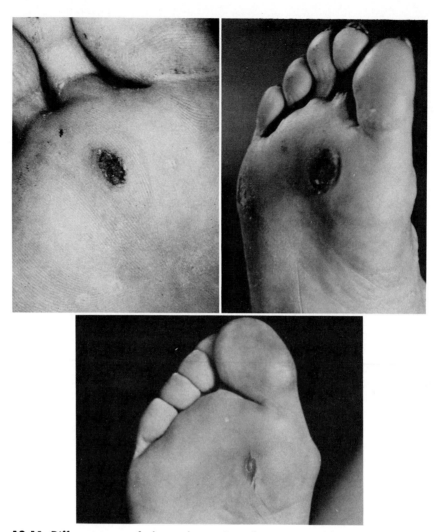

Fig. 12-11. Different types of plantar keratosis under metatarsal heads. Each resembles verruca plantaris.

Metatarsal head involved

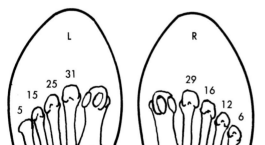

Fig. 12-12. Distribution of lesions in 139 cases of intractable plantar keratosis.

devised whereby plantar condyles can be visualized accurately. From whatever angle the roentgenogram is taken, the plantar condyles either appear distorted or are not seen at all. If the keratosis is located directly under a metatarsal head, it may be assumed that the condylar process is the causative factor. The relationship of the keratosis to the condylar processes can be positively ascertained by comparing two distances on a dorsoplantar roentgenogram of the foot—one from the keratosis to the end of the toe immediately distal to the keratosis and the other from the keratosis to the medial or lateral border of the foot. One can also effectively compare these measurements on a roentgenogram of the foot taken after a metallic substance has been painted on the keratotic area.

Keratosis under the fifth metatarsal head. Keratotic changes under the fifth metatarsal head rarely become intractable because the plantar condylar surface of the head of this bone is usually flat and broad, giving it a good weight-bearing area. When a callus does form, it is widespread and is most frequently associated with functional foot disabilities that force the patient to bear excess weight on the outer border of the foot. The callus usually disappears after the disability has been corrected. In a few instances the condylar process of the fifth metatarsal head becomes distorted or pointed. When that happens, the problem is comparable to distortion under the other metatarsal heads.

Procedures for intractable keratosis under the metatarsal heads. Plantar keratosis under the *first metatarsal head* mainly occurs under the tibial sesamoid. In 95 percent of cases, excision of this sesamoid will dissipate the lesion:

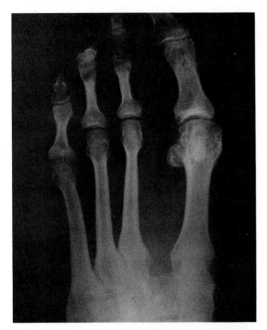

Fig. 12-13. Increased disability after Dickson's pie technique for intractable keratosis.

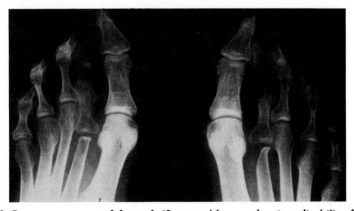

Fig. 12-14. Roentgenograms of feet of 42-year-old man showing disability from previous surgical procedures performed elsewhere.

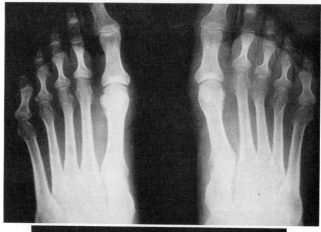

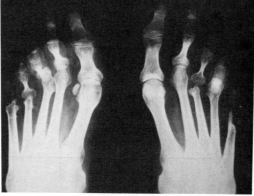

Fig. 12-15. Preoperative and postoperative roentgenograms of feet of 28-year-old woman. She had sought help elsewhere for keratosis under the metatarsal heads.

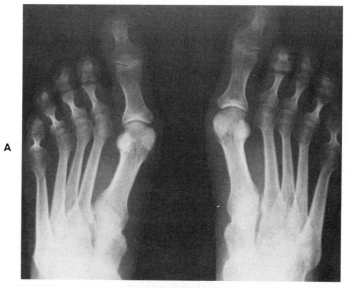

Fig. 12-16. A, Roentgenograms of feet of 51-year-old woman. She had sought my advice in 1961 for calluses under the metatarsal heads caused by moderate clawtoes. **B,** Roentgenograms taken in 1964. She then sought help for severe disability after surgical procedures had been performed elsewhere in 1963.

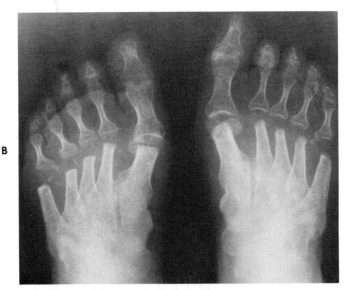

Fig. 12-16, cont'd. For legend see opposite page.

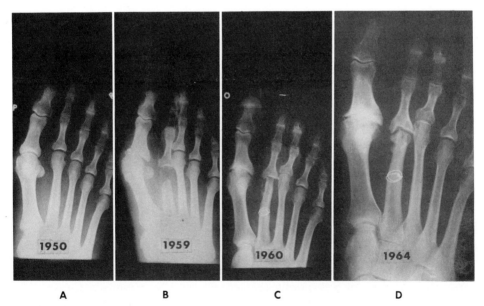

A   B   C   D

Fig. 12-17. Intractable keratosis under right second metatarsal head in foot of 30-year-old woman. **A,** 1950 preoperative roentgenogram. **B,** 1959 roentgenogram. A surgical procedure had been performed elsewhere for the same lesion 8 years previously. She now sought help because of disability, especially because the second toe was lying on the dorsum of the foot. Note that the first metatarsophalangeal joint had also been surgically treated. A fibular graft on the second metatarsal remnant was implanted, and the first metatarsophalangeal joint was repaired. **C,** Roentgenogram taken 1 year postoperatively. **D,** Roentgenogram taken 4 years postoperatively.

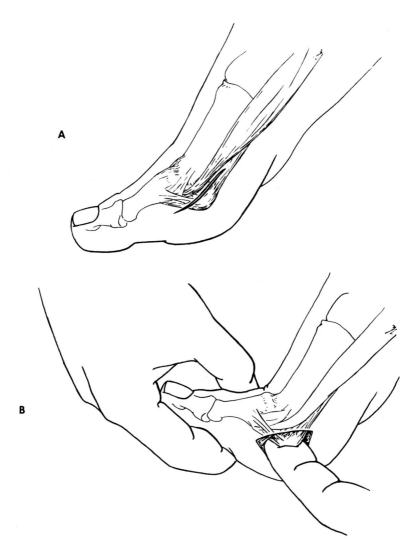

Fig. 12-18. Technique for excision of tibial sesamoid. **A,** Semielliptical incision following medioplantar border of first metatarsophalangeal joint. **B,** Retraction of skin margin and insertion of surgeon's right index finger into wound. When the great toe is dorsiflexed the sesamoid glides over the index finger, pinpointing the sesamoid. **C,** Incision into capsule along mediosuperior surface of sesamoid. **D,** Grasping of periosteum of sesamoid with Allis forceps. Sesamoid is excised by sharp dissection. **E,** Closing of capsule and fascia with interrupted catgut sutures. Skin is closed in layers as usual.

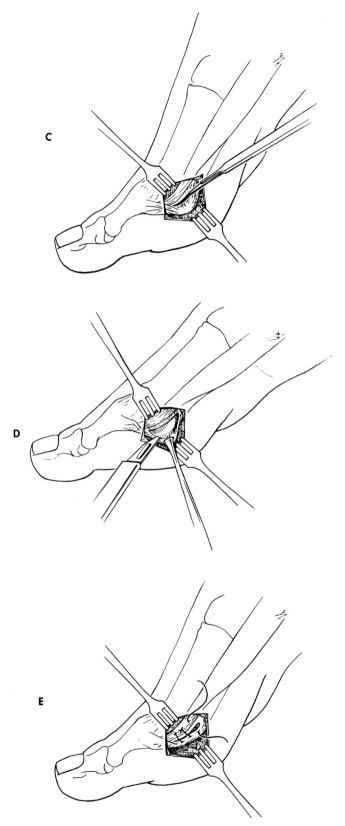

Fig. 12-18, cont'd. For legend see opposite page.

1. Under hemostasis make a semielliptical incision along the contour of the medioplantar border of the great toe joint, extending the incision from the middle third of the metatarsal to the middle of the proximal phalanx (Fig. 12-18, *A*).
2. Dissect and retract the plantar skin and subcutaneous tissue from the plantar surface of the great toe joint.
3. Place the index finger against the plantar surface of the sesamoid while the great toe is dorsiflexed. The outline of the tibial sesamoid is revealed (Fig. 12-18, *B*).
4. Make an incision about 1 cm. long over the mediosuperior surface of the sesamoid (Fig. 12-18, *C*). Grasp the plantar margin in this incision, including the superior margin of the sesamoid, with Allis forceps (Fig. 12-18, *D*).
5. Remove the sesamoid by sharp dissection, using its own outline as a guide.
6. Close the capsule and fascia with interrupted catgut sutures, and close the skin as usual (Fig. 12-18, *E*).
7. A compression bandage is applied for 24 hours. Ambulation may begin in 48 hours.

In most cases the lesion under the sesamoid will disappear in 2 to 4 months. In rare cases where the intractable lesion is under the fibular sesamoid (Fig. 12-8), relief can usually be obtained by excising this ossicle as described under reduction of hallux valgus, p. 522.

Over a 22-year period, more than 900 patients were treated with the DuVries plantar condylectomy (1953) for intractable keratosis under the lesser metatarsal heads. In 1965 the technique was modified to include an arthroplasty. A survey was made in 1971 of 100 patients on whom 142 of the latter procedures were performed. In 112 instances (79 percent) the lesions disappeared, in twenty-three (16 percent) the keratoses lessened, and in seven instances (5 percent) no improvement occurred.

For the recommended procedure for the treatment of intractable keratosis, see Fig. 12-19. The legend to the figure gives a full description of the procedure.

Giannestras (1954) recommended a step-down osteotomy for the treatment of plantar keratosis, in which the metatarsal shaft was shortened (Figs. 12-20 and 12-21). In this procedure a 2.5 cm. step cut is outlined (Fig. 12-20, *A*). Each tongue of the step cut is rongeured to produce a 1 cm. shortening of the shaft (Fig. 12-20, *B*). A drill hole is made in each remaining portion and a suture is passed through each hole and is tied, holding the two bone ends in the shortened position (Fig. 12-20, *C*).

In a small percentage of cases of intractable plantar keratosis the lesion itself must be excised, usually because the lesion is entirely composed of scar that penetrates to the transverse metatarsal ligament. This condition is invariably a result of previous treatment of the lesion as a wart by escharotics and roentgen therapy. After the keratotic area has been excised, the patient should use crutches and should not be allowed to bear weight on the area for about 6 weeks. Because the skin of the plantar surface has little elasticity, early weight bearing on the foot may separate the incisional margins and cause the formation of a new scar or a keloid. The wire two-button retention suture keeps the margins in coaptation without tension (Fig. 12-22).

Anderson (1957) performs a rotation flap graft (Fig. 12-23), in addition to plantar condylectomy, in a one-stage procedure. This might be advantageous in selected cases, but almost 5 percent of his cases were complete failures. They had received the maximum amount of irradiation elsewhere preoperatively. Poor results were in direct relation to the amount of previous therapy for plantar warts. The advantage of condylectomy as an initial approach is that, among those who have obtained only partial relief and those who have had no relief, none was worse than before the operation.

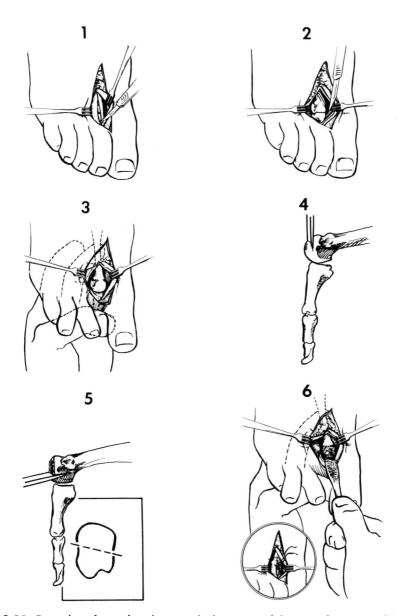

Fig. 12-19. Procedure for arthroplasty and plantar condylectomy for intractable keratosis under lesser metatarsal heads. *1,* Make incision from middle of metatarsal shaft to web. Retract skin and extensor tendon and incise capsule longitudinally. *2,* Section capsule on both sides of metatarsal head vertically. *3,* Plantar flex involved toe with thumb of left hand while applying pressure against metatarsal shaft with index finger of same hand. *4,* Remove about 2 mm. of articular surface. *5,* Remove plantar condyle with osteotome. Note angulation to facilitate removal of more of the fibular aspect. *6,* Smooth surface with nasal rasp. Close capsule and skin.

Suppurating sinuses of the foot

Suppurating sinuses of the foot are newly formed channels lined with granulation tissue. They discharge a serosanguineous material, which may become purulent from secondary infection. The sinus may form in a corn or callus over a bony prominence. Such suppurating sinuses ordinarily are chronic, but acute exacerbations are typical.

Etiology. A suppurating sinus of the foot is produced in the same way as are corns and calluses—by persistent sharp pressure over a bony prominence, which devitalizes the tissue under the excrescence and, in some cases, causes necrosis of the central portion. The presence of a debilitating disease worsens the degenerative process. Lusskin (1961) reports a case of serpentine sinus of the foot that led to a dead end; the disorder proved to be a congenital dermal defect.

Site. Suppurating sinuses of the foot oc-

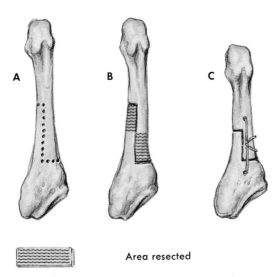

Area resected

Fig. 12-20. Giannestras' step-down osteostomy. The metatarsal is shortened in order to alleviate plantar keratosis.

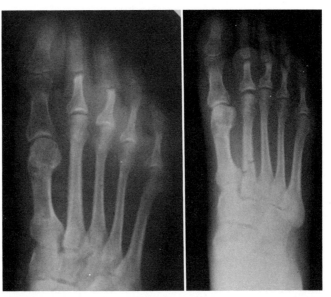

Fig. 12-21. Roentgenograms of foot of 24-year-old woman. Severe hyperkeratosis had occurred under the second metatarsal head after the first metatarsal had been shortened by osteotomy for hallux valgus elsewhere. The second metatarsal was forced to carry an abnormal part of the body weight. Giannestras' operation relieved the problem.

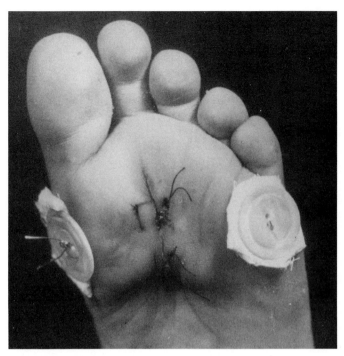

Fig. 12-22. Coaptation of skin margins after excision of plantar lesion. Margins are held by a retention wire suture deep below the incision.

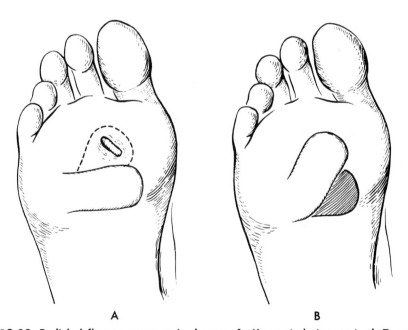

A   B

Fig. 12-23. Pedicled flap to cover excised area. **A,** Keratotic lesion excised. Transverse pedicle flap formed immediately below it. **B,** Flap graft rotated to cover excised area. (After Anderson, R.: Plast. Reconstr. Surg. **19**:384-388, May 1957.)

cur in the following areas: under a hard corn on the lesser toes; in the center of a soft corn, generally in the web between the fourth and fifth toes; and on the tibial side of the great toe joint, usually over the tibial condyle of the first metatarsal head and often associated with a hallux valgus deformity, especially if there is a sharp projection on the tibial side of the head. In rare instances, the sinus may digress along the shaft of the first metatarsal (see Fig. 12-7). On the fibular side of the fifth metatarsal head, it is often associated with tailor's bunion.

A degenerative sinus may occur under any of the metatarsal heads, especially the middle three. In the young and middle-aged they are often secondary to unusually large condylar processes on the plantar surface of the head of the metatarsals. When they are situated under the first metatarsal, they are usually caused by an uncommonly large or malshaped sesamoid. Claw-toe or clawfoot may produce such a sinus under a metatarsal head. In older persons, this type of sinus is often associated with a degenerative disease, such as diabetes. Trophic changes as a result of peripheral nerve disease also produce this kind of sinus, typically under the head of the first metatarsal. They usually retrogress and produce extensive ulceration. Under the head of the second metatarsal a degenerative sinus often results from the static dislocation of the second metatarsophalangeal joint. (See p. 239.)

Treatment. When the sinus is present over a non–weight-bearing area and is not complicated by a degenerative disease, excision of the condyle or bony prominence beneath the sinus, without excision of the necrotic tissue, disposes of the problem in most cases. Excision to eliminate the sinus itself may or may not be required.

On the plantar surface, in cases such as hammertoe or metatarsophalangeal dislocation in which debilitating disease is not a complication, healing usually takes place after open reduction of the deformity underlying the sinus or excision of the offend-

ing plantar condyle or sesamoid is performed.

Patients in whom there is an underlying degenerative disease should be treated conservatively to achieve balanced weight distribution through such mechanical measures as shoe inlays, Thomas bars, shoe wedging, and padding. Total weight bearing should be reduced as much as possible. Close cooperation with the internist to improve the general medical status is important. The sinus itself must be kept clean. Rough handling or the application of chemical irritants is likely to worsen the degenerative process. Only the most conservative surgical procedure is ever indicated, and then only in extreme cases.

Traumatic ulcer

Traumatic ulcers are usually caused by excessive pressure on a weight-bearing area over a long period of time. Degeneration of the skin surface and the underlying soft structures leads to ulceration. Traumatic ulcers most commonly occur under the metatarsal heads, but they may appear over any bony prominence (Figs. 12-24 and 12-25). They are often seen in older persons, because in these people the general tissue vitality is reduced and the irritation has been long-standing. General disease, such as diabetes and peripheral neuritis, can accelerate the process.

Such ulcers are characterized by large amounts of granulation tissue surrounding a small orifice that exudes a nonpurulent discharge; they are subject to recurrent secondary infection that may become intractable.

To treat these ulcers:
1. Excise all the surrounding overlying callus.
2. Cauterize the granulation tissue with 90 percent phenol or 10 percent silver nitrate.
3. Paint the ulcer with a dye such as carbolfuchsin or gentian violet.
4. Protect the area from further pressure by the use of padding or a foot appliance.

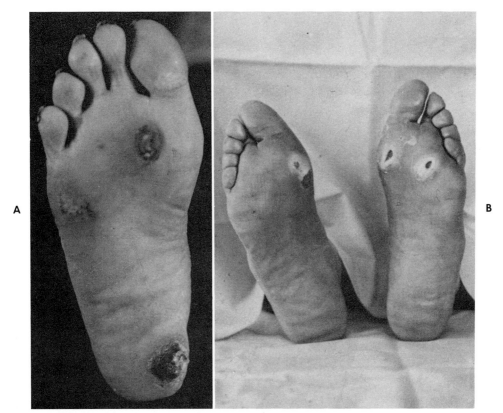

Fig. 12-24. A, Traumatic ulcers under second and fifth metatarsal heads and under heel. **B,** Traumatic (pressure) ulcers. *Right foot,* First metatarsal head. *Left foot,* First and third metatarsal heads.

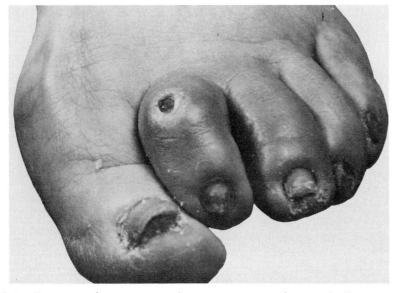

Fig. 12-25. Traumatic ulcer over second toe. Acute tinea infection of all toes. (Courtesy Dr. Ned Pickett.)

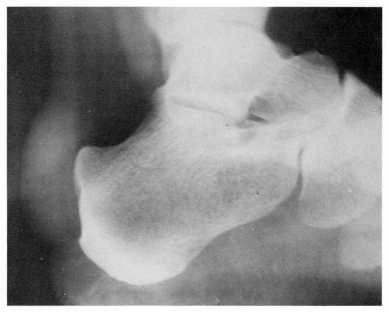

Fig. 12-26. Fibromatosis of insertion of tendo achillis. The condition is a result of a prominent posterosuperior tuberosity of the calcaneus.

Traumatic ulcers may also occur as a result of various types of injury (see Chapter 7).

Hypertrophy of the skin and soft tissues over the tendo achillis

Hypertrophy of the skin and soft tissues over the tendo achillis is an accumulation of connective tissue of the skin over the tendo achillis immediately above its insertion. The condition, often referred to as tendo achillis bursitis, develops in persons in whom the upper posterior border of the calcaneus juts out acutely posteriorly. This enlargement is sometimes referred to as Haglund's disease (see p. 250). A heel bone thus shaped makes the contour of the back of the heel a straight line (Fig. 12-26). The shoe counter is always convex; therefore, its upper margin exerts an abnormal amount of friction and pressure on this prominence. The condition is more common in women as a result of wearing pumps and high heels. The growth is solid connective tissue in which a cavity appears only if the tissue breaks down, producing a draining sinus. Occasionally an adventitious bursa forms.

The growth may be excised through an incision on either side of the tendon. Great care must be taken in dissection, since the mass is not encapsulated and the skin may be irreparably injured. The skin should be sutured subdermally to prevent dead space and consequent hematoma formation. A walking plaster cast should be applied with the foot in mild plantar flexion to avoid movement of the wounded area, which may interfere with healing. It should be borne in mind that this area is notoriously poor in healing. A window in the cast over the field of operation permits redressing. The cast is removed in about 3 weeks. Dorsiflexion is begun gradually.

DISEASES OF THE SKIN ITSELF
Verruca plantaris (papilloma wart)

Verruca plantaris does not produce the high incidence of disability erroneously attributed to it, because other lesions on the weight-bearing surfaces of the foot assume the appearance of this innocent neoplasm.

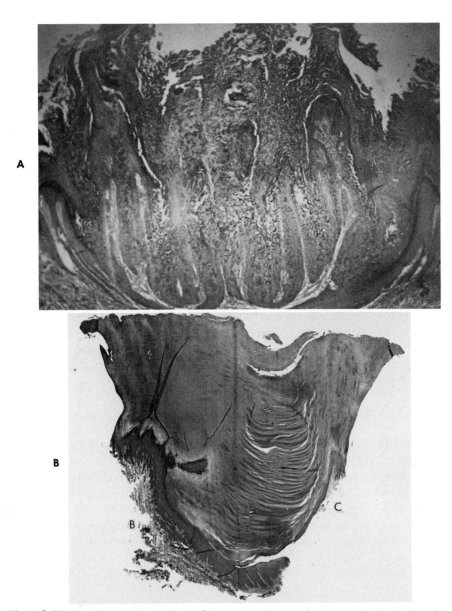

Fig. 12-27. A, Microscopic section of verrucae. Verruca here reveals typical mushrooming of the entire epidermis. Note thickening of rete pegs with some fusion at the base and degeneration at the top. **B,** Compression of subdermal living epithelium. **C,** Hyperkeratosis. Hyperkeratinization of the uppermost layers of the epidermis. Rete malpighii, flushed.

(See intractable plantar keratosis, p. 326.) The accepted method of treating warts is to destroy them by fulguration, escharotics, excision, or any other means of eradication. Lesions that are not verrucae but resemble them (pseudoverrucae), when treated in the manner listed, become intractable. Histologically verrucae plantaris are similar to verrucae vulgaris; they differ grossly in that they are embedded below the skin by the pressure of weight bearing. Microscopically they differ entirely from deep-seated keratoses (Fig. 12-27). Warts may occur anywhere on the plantar surface of the foot, but they only occasionally form under weight-bearing points of pressure, such as under the metatarsal heads or the tuberosity of the calcaneus.

Etiology. It is generally accepted that warts are caused by a filterable virus infection. They often spread from one part of the body to another. A student may acquire a wart and then many in the same classroom may exhibit the growth. Kile (1956) concluded that some strains of wart virus are more communicable than others.

Diagnosis. There are several factors to keep in mind in the differential diagnosis of plantar warts:

1. Warts on the bottom of the foot are usually more painful than those that are located elsewhere on the body because of the weight-bearing function of the foot.

2. The typical wart rarely occurs under a weight-bearing surface such as a metatarsal head, whereas a deep-seated, keratotic callus will develop under a metatarsal head because of ill-fitting footwear.

3. If the location of a wart-like lesion can be pinpointed under a metatarsal head, it is far better to assume that it is a reactive keratosis due to pressure and to treat it as such, rather than to attempt its destruction.

4. Typical verrucae are unequivocally circumscribed, are either oval or circular in outline, and are completely encapsulated. Margins are sharply de-

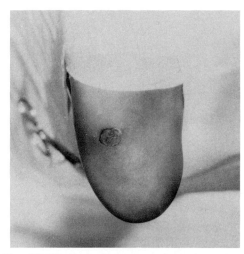

Fig. 12-28. Typical verruca plantaris on heel.

fined (Fig. 12-28); the center is spongy, pale, and furrowed.

Treatment. There are numerous methods of destroying verrucae. Many dermatologists and roentgenologists advise radiation therapy; Reeves and Jackson (1956) believe it to be the treatment of choice. An editorial in the *New England Journal of Medicine* (1953) gives an excellent summary of the treatment of patients with warts by autosuggestion. Allington (1952) also discusses psychotherapy of persons with warts, and Dunbar (1954) reviews the psychosomatic origin of warts. Montgomery (1964) classified plantar warts into (1) single, (2) mother-daughter, and (3) mosaic. He points out that the first and second are radiosensitive, whereas the third is not. Among the different methods of therapy for the first two he suggests the application of carbon-dioxide snow or liquid nitrogen.

Duthie and McCallum (1951) advise the use of Elastoplast and podophyllum resin. Ducourtioux (1950) suggests the use of electrocoagulation. Blank (1947) outlines the following procedure: (1) Reduce the overlying callus from the verruca, (2) apply a drop of 90 percent phenol, and (3) apply a drop of fuming nitric acid on top of the phenol. Ignatoff (1954) sums up the status of treatment of verrucae plantaris and suggests that once the diagnosis has been established, any of the following procedures will eradicate the growth: (1) application of caustics, (2) cauterization, (3) surgical excision, (4) radiation therapy, (5) application of solidified carbon dioxide, or (6) application of liquid nitrogen.

Allyn and Waldorf (1968) and McGee (1968) suggested treating warts with injections of smallpox vaccine; however, the Committee on Cutaneous Health and Cosmetics (1968) disapproved of the treatment.

In treating single or mother-daughter warts one must first differentiate them from the solitary, circumscribed keratotic lesion.

Brown and Fryer (1951) believe that plantar warts are the cause of most of the surgical repair of the sole of the foot.

Upon confirmed diagnosis of a plantar wart, the personal choice of procedure for eradication must be made from among those recommended. It has been our experience that radiation therapy should be reserved as a last resort because of potential radiodermatitis (Montgomery et al., 1949). Such dermatitis on the plantar surface of the foot can become an intolerable condition.

Since a small percentage of plantar warts tend to recur, regardless of the mode of eradication instituted, it is better to begin with the least disabling method of therapy (cryotherapy), and if necessary resort to fulguration by excision or radiation as a secondary procedure.

Mosaic plantar wart. Typically, the mosaic wart appears on the heel but may form on any other part of the plantar surface, including the web of the toes. These warts extend over a wide area and seem to be a coalescence of multiple small warts. They are rather superficial and relatively painless. Montgomery and Montgomery (1937) first called attention to the lesion as a distinct entity. Mosaic warts are radioresistant (Montgomery and Montgomery, 1944) and unresponsive to the usual treatment of warts. The Montgomerys (1948) reported 89.9 percent cure in 109 cases by the following recommended procedure: The area

is pared until the capillary tips are visible or bleeding. Capillary bleeding is stopped with silver nitrate solution. The wart is swabbed lightly with saturated solution of monochloroacetic acid or 20 percent silver nitrate solution. Salicylic acid plaster, shaped to the size of the warty patch, is applied. The same treatment is given to the satellites.

For hornier lesions the plaster is fortified with a thin coating of 60 percent salicylic acid ointment. For a deeper reaction a saturated solution of monochloroacetic acid instead of silver nitrate solution is rubbed in. The plaster is held in place with adhesive strapping. The area is kept dry during treatment. The lesion is pared down weekly to active warty tissue and the aforementioned steps are repeated. When the area thins, silver nitrate solution alone is used. Every vestige of wart must be removed to prevent recurrence.

When reaction to the application of monochloroacetic acid is severe, the medication is discontinued and a wet dressing is applied. The tissue is pared down to release the subwart fluid. Foam-rubber pads, placed posterior to the wart, relieve pressure.

Dermatophytosis

Dermatophytosis, or tinea infection (commonly called ringworm), is almost always present on the foot. Spores of one or more strains of trichophytes are commonly harbored between the toes and under the nails but may invade any part of the foot. The spores may lie dormant for months or years before they mature and multiply under favorable conditions, such as excessive moisture, friction, pressure, or trauma, either accidental or iatrogenic. When the disease is active, it assumes various forms and degrees, from minute fissures between the toes to a vesicular scaly dermatitis over large areas on the entire foot (Fig. 12-29), and from a low-grade inflammatory process to a violent infection, although serious illness is rare. Dermatophytosis is resistant to all forms of ther-

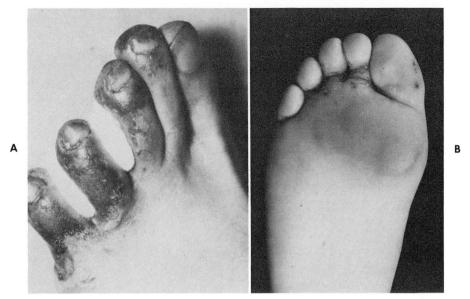

Fig. 12-29. A, Acute dermatophytosis of toes. **B,** Dermatophytosis in plantar creases of toes.

apy. Griseofulvin, taken internally for many months, has proved to be of value in many cases.

One theory in many cases of thrombophlebitis is that the causative pyogenic organism may have found entrance in a fissure caused by trichophytosis between the toes. Such a fissure may be microscopic. Retardation of the healing of a wound in the foot may be caused by the invasion of dormant fungi into the wound. According to some observers, fungi may even act to make certain organisms resistant to antibiotics.

Special precautions in cleanliness and the generous use of fungicides preoperatively and postoperatively reduce the incidence of morbidity from surgical procedures on the foot.

Dermatophytosis is generally thought to be contagious; however, Baer and his associates (1956), in an experimental attempt to infect sixty-eight subjects proved to be free of the disease, were not able to infect a single patient.

Dermatitis from shoe irritants

Niles (1938) reported two cases of severe dermatitis of both feet that were first assumed to be caused by tinea infection but later were proved conclusively to have been caused by allergens in shoe leather.

Gaul and Underwood (1949) made an exhaustive study of 160 cases of dermatitis pedis which they traced to allergens in various fabric and leather parts of shoes. The onset of dermatitis varied from a few hours to 7 months after the offending shoes had been worn. The allergens affected persons of all ages, including a 16-month-old child.

Many of the chemicals employed in processing leather or fabrics of which shoes are made may cause dermatitis, not necessarily on an allergic basis but because they are irritants. Dolce (1944), in a study of cases of shoe-leather dermatitis, found chromic acid and potassium dichromate to be the most common irritants.

Epidermal cyst (inversion cyst, epidermoid cyst)

An epidermal cyst is an encapsulated mass filled with caseous material; it is often erroneously called a sebaceous cyst or atheroma. Epidermal cysts appear on any part of the body, most often on the scalp, and occasionally on the plantar surface of

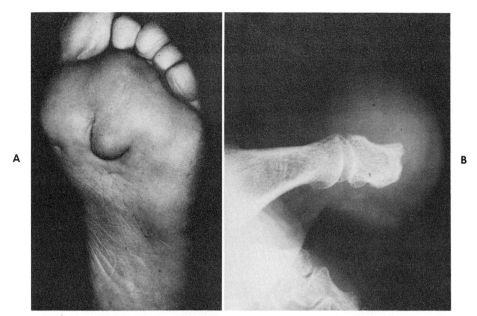

Fig. 12-30. A, Epidermal cyst on ball of foot. It became the most prominent weight-bearing area. **B,** Large epidermal cyst. Lesion formed on the dorsum of the distal phalanx after partial amputation of this bone.

the foot (Fig. 12-30, *A*). There are no sebaceous glands in the plantar surface of the foot; hence the term "sebaceous" is a misnomer, since this type of cyst cannot form there. In fact, on sectioning many so-called sebaceous cysts from other parts of the body, pathologists have found that glandular epithelium is absent and that the caseous material does not contain fat. Invagination and destruction of the epidermis are typical. Epidermal cysts on the plantar surface vary in size from 0.5 to 3 cm. They are painful only when they form on a weight-bearing surface, such as on the ball of the foot, where they do form commonly. They also form on other areas of the foot, however, even on the dorsum of a hammertoe and in old incisions (Figs. 12-30 to 12-32). They are extremely painful under a metatarsal head, as if a pebble were in the sole of the foot. The cyst sometimes degenerates, becomes infected, and produces a discharging sinus.

Epidermal cysts on the foot are often erroneously diagnosed because they are relatively uncommon and because the skin surface may appear normal. A diagnosis is made by finding, on palpation, a freely movable, circumscribed, subdermal mass of medium hardness. Occasionally, an epidermal cyst may become calcified (Fig. 12-31) and further confuse the diagnosis.

Excision of the mass is simple. When possible, the incision should be made on a non–weight-bearing surface. If the growth is immediately under a metatarsal head, the incision should be made on one side of the cyst, so that if a scar forms at the incision, it will be under the metatarsal interspace. Epidermal cysts are readily shelled out; the thick, white, glistening capsule is only loosely adherent to the surrounding tissue. After the skin incision has been made the cysts can be extruded by applying pressure on the sides of the mass.

If a large space is left by the removal of the cyst, it must be closed to prevent formation of a hematoma. This is accomplished by suturing the skin subdermally to the fascia with fine catgut before suturing the skin margins. Another method is to apply a thick plug of gauze over the su-

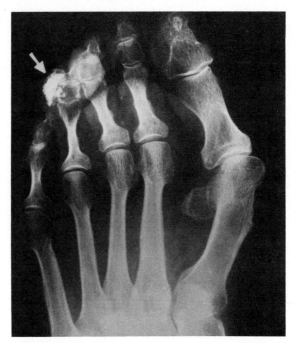

Fig. 12-31. Calcified epidermal cyst over distal end of fourth toe.

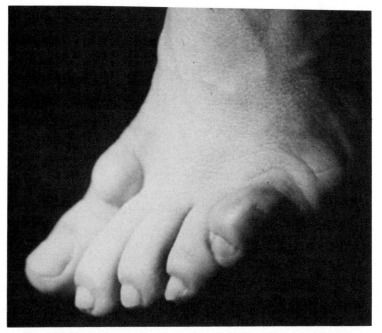

Fig. 12-32. Epidermal cyst over first metatarsophalangeal joint.

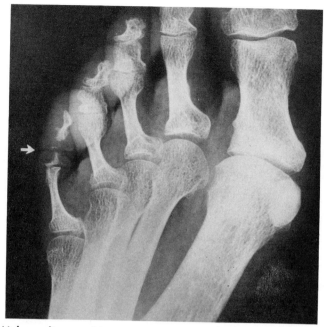

Fig. 12-33. Ainhum disease. Note constricting band and destruction of the middle phalanx.

tured incision, where it is held in compression for 24 hours. Healing is by first intention. Ambulation may begin in 24 to 48 hours.

Ainhum disease

Ainhum derives its name from an African dialect, from a word meaning compression. The disease is a diastasis (dactylolysis spontanea), usually of the fifth toe, rarely of the other toes. It is characterized by a spontaneous formation of a constricting ring near the proximal phalangeal joint, which strangulates the distal portion of the toe until it falls off. The ring appears first on the plantar surface and finally produces complete encirclement (Fig. 12-33). This is primarily a tropical disease, especially among the Negroes of Africa, but it has been observed in the southern part of the United States (Spinzig, 1939; Stack, 1950) and rarely in temperate regions. Tye (1946), Norton and associates (1957), and Auckland and associates (1957) have contributed thorough reviews of the publications on the subject. Aggarwal and Singh

(1963) report a case of a young girl in whom ainhum disease began on the left great toe and terminated in involvement of all but the second toe.

The cause is unknown. It is more common in men and is believed to be caused by local endarteritis. The disease is localized and without symptoms. The toe drops off in about 2 years. There is no known treatment.

Nevus (mole, birthmark)

Benign pigmented nevi are commonly observed in the white race. Usually little attention is paid to nevi, particularly when the sites are as inconspicuous as they are on the foot.

The nevus may or may not be elevated in the skin. It varies in color from dark brown to black, is often covered with hair, and is usually small, although sometimes it may grow to great size. Junctional nevi, so-called juvenile melanomas, are ordinarily benign. Pack and associates (1952) stated that in their experience with more than 1,220 verified cases of malignant melanoma, they never observed a single instance in which a juvenile melanoma metastasized to nodes and viscera, and they never observed a fatal outcome. These authors also found that in their series of cases, more than 17 percent of pigmented moles occurred in the lower extremities.

Nevi on the feet, especially the soles, should be watched for pressure and trauma. Notwithstanding the slight possibility that they may become malignant, there is always a chance that such a tumor was malignant at the outset. Therefore, removal is advisable, particularly when the lesion is on the sole of the foot. Despite the uneventful course of most nevi, any sudden increase in size should suggest malignancy (see malignant melanoma, p. 351). The mass should be widely excised and the regional lymphatic vessels should be dissected.

Glomus tumor

In the skin of the extremities, especially of the digits, normal areas are present wherein the blood passes directly from artery to vein without passing through capillaries. The channel through which the blood passes is surrounded by large epithelioid or glomus cells. Small nodular masses sometimes form in these areas and are exceedingly painful or produce a burning sensation. The masses, which King (1954) regards as malformations rather than as neoplasms, consist of a network of blood vessels within a capsule of typical glomus cells. The tumors occur mostly in the skin and subcutaneous tissues, but they may originate in muscles, tendons, bone (see Chapter 13), and even in deeper parts of the body. Abramson (1956) observed them in the nail beds of fingers and toes and in the palm of the hand and the sole of the foot. When located in the fingers and toes, they remain benign and do not invade other structures. They recur only when removal has been incomplete. Ottley (1942) observed that the tumor was solitary in all but thirteen instances of 173 cases. Smyth (1971) pointed out that glomus tumors often mimic other ortho-

paedic conditions and delay for long periods a diagnosis of the patient's acute pain.

A patient was observed who had violent pain on the lateral side of a lesser toe; there was no rational explanation for the pain, nor was there response to palliative therapy. When the excised subnormal tissue in the painful area was sectioned, a glomus pattern was disclosed, and excision brought complete relief. In two other cases in which a diagnosis of neurofibroma (neuroma) of the medial plantar nerve had been made, the symptoms resembled those of an exaggerated Morton's neuralgia. Histologic study showed the presence of a glomus tumor. The lesions are benign, and complete extirpation brings immediate relief.

The diagnosis is based on severe pain or agonizing throbbing in a small area of the foot where pathologic disturbance is not clinically demonstrable. Even the pressure of bedclothes can produce excruciating pain that may not be localized but may be of a neuralgic radiating type. The growth may exist for years before it is disclosed by a careful evaluation of symptoms. The definitive diagnosis may not be made until the removed specimen has been examined. Ottley (1942) reported two cases of needless amputation as a result of faulty diagnosis.

Eccrine poroma

Eccrine poroma is a benign epithelial tumor that occurs essentially on the sole of the foot and arises from the intraepidermal sweat gland ducts. It often resembles a granuloma, basal cell epithelioma, or seborrheic verruca. Pinkus, Rogin, and Goldman (1956) were probably the first to classify this lesion.

Morris, Wood, and Samitz (1968) reported two cases of eccrine poroma on the sole of the foot and gave an exhaustive list of references on the lesion.

Gibbs (1968) points to the fact that the lesion is not easily differentiated clinically, but is readily diagnosed histologically.

This neoplasm usually responds to electrodesiccation.

Carcinomas

Carcinomas rarely occur in the foot. When they do, they are usually primary, and are either squamous or basal cell carcinomas. Secondary carcinoma in the foot caused by metastasis from some other part of the body is hardly ever reported.

Epithelioma. Epitheliomas or squamous cell carcinomas of the extremities comprise about 1 percent of carcinomas in the body. An extensive study was made by Browne (1953) of reported cases as well as of a series of 511 cases at the Mayo Clinic from 1908 to 1946. Of the Mayo Clinic series, 164 epitheliomas (32 percent) occurred in the lower and 347 (68 percent) occurred in the upper extremities. In 55 cases the epitheliomas occurred in the foot itself.

Squamous cell carcinomas arising from the sites of warts and scars are reported frequently. Charache (1939) reported the distribution of carcinoma in thirty-two cases. In order of frequency, the sites were the dorsum of the hand and wrist, the leg, the arm, the forearm, the foot, the fingers, and the thighs; only rarely were they present in the toes. In four instances the growth originated in warts; in three, the growth originated in scars from burns received from 24 to 35 years earlier.

Schreiner and Wehr (1933) reported a case of squamous cell epithelioma that originated at the undersurface of the fourth toe on the site of a corn; it involved both the fourth and fifth toes and the dorsum and sole of the foot.

Epithelioma cuniculatum, a variety of squamous carcinoma peculiar to the foot, has been discussed by Aird and associates (1954). They reported the case of a 64-year-old man who had had a bulbous mass on the sole, covered with skin containing many sinuses, most of which opened at the apex of a separate bulge. Aird suggests that a low-grade, highly keratinizing, squamous carcinoma developed on the ball of the foot and that repeated pressure forced portions of the growth into the soft tissues, probably accelerating growth of the carcinoma.

Malignant melanoma. Malignant melanomas arising from nevi of the soles and palms are frequently observed (Fig. 12-

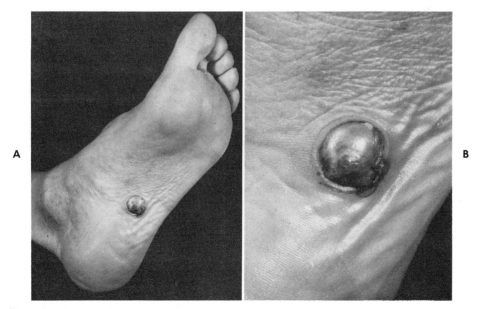

Fig. 12-34. A, Malignant melanoma on plantar surface of foot. B, Enlargement of A.

34). Allen and Spitz (1953) described the clinical and histologic features of this growth in a series of 934 cases occurring on the palms, soles, and genitalia. Two-thirds of the patients were 31 to 60 years of age. Juvenile melanoma may be confused with this malignant growth. Unless landmarks have been destroyed, differentiation between the primary and metastatic tumor is not difficult. Allen and Spitz thought that the junctional nevus rather than the intradermal nevus was the source of malignant melanomas of the skin, except for those arising from the blue nevus; however, only a small percentage of junctional nevi become malignant. The authors stated that because of the vulnerability of moles in the soles and palms, moles at these sites should be excised whenever feasible, preferably before puberty. Care must be exercised in differentiating malignant melanomas from benign juvenile melanomas that persist into adulthood.

Another series of twenty-five cases of malignant melanoma of the plantar surface of the foot was reported by Decker and Chamness (1951). Nine of their patients had noted a preexisting mole. Two of them reported having had the moles since birth, and the others reported having had them from 3 to 20 years. Six patients reported plantar injuries; three of these were reported to have occurred from nail punctures. Local therapy had been received before hospital admission in seventeen cases. In apparently no instance was a correct diagnosis made; malignancy was suggested in only five cases. Some of the malignant melanomas were shaded from brown to black; others were only slightly colored. Eight of the twenty-five malignant melanomas were not grossly pigmented; no melanin granules could be observed microscopically in six of them.

A biopsy is required for all nevi on the sole of the foot, whether pigmented or not. If the plantar lesion proves to be malignant melanoma microscopically, a radical operation is necessary. Local excision is adequate when the lesion is less than 2 cm. in diameter and does not show a tendency to deep fixation.

Pack and Adair (1939) reviewed sixty-nine reported cases of subungual melanoma and described sixteen others. Of the total, thirty-four were located in the great toes and three were located in other toes. The growth usually appears in the form of a black fungating ulcer involving the nail sulcus and matrix and elevating the nail. A black border along the edge of the nail is pathognomonic. Subungual melanomas contrast with benign forms, which do not break through the nail.

The percentage of cures for malignant subungual melanomas is higher than for malignant melanomas elsewhere, but the prognosis depends on whether or not metastasis is present. After the diagnosis has been made, amputation should be performed promptly. Pack and Adair advise amputation first and dissection of the lymph nodes 1 or 2 weeks later if gross evidence of metastatic involvement exists, and 6 weeks later if dissection is then considered to be prophylactic.

Malignant ulcer or rodent ulcer

The malignant or rodent ulcer is a slowly growing variety of basal cell carcinoma. The skin and subcutaneous tissues of the area slowly erode. The base of the area is adherent to the surrounding tissues. The ulcer resists all forms of medicinal therapy. If the diagnosis is confirmed by biopsy, wide excision of the growth is indicated. It rarely occurs on the foot.

KELOIDS AND HYPERTROPHIC SCARS
Keloids

A keloid is an idiopathic new fibrous mass of the corium raised above the skin surface anywhere on the body. It is typically regular in outline, it is often multiple, and it varies in size from a pinhead to an entity of massive proportions. Keloids are white or reddish globular masses, either round or oval. A single lesion or many, even dozens, may appear. Keloids form between the ages of 10 and 19 years. They rarely form in older persons. The tendency to keloid formation is not constant throughout life but may come and go. Dark-complexioned persons apparently are more susceptible to keloid formation.

Keloids become painful only from secondary irritation; they are otherwise symptomless. For true keloids, Kitlowski (1953) advises an erythema dose of roentgen rays, with partial excision to be performed about a month later. Strict precautions must be taken to ensure primary union, and the normal skin must not be sutured. Some patients require additional postoperative roentgen therapy. A high percentage of recurrence has been reported after excision alone with the recurrent keloid being larger than the original.

Hypertrophic scar (hyperplasia)

Hypertrophic scar is a false keloid, found only in healing wounds. It is limited to the area of injury and follows the outline of the original injury, but the growth is raised above the surface of the skin. Histologically, a hypertrophic scar cannot be differentiated from a true keloid. It is symptomless except when the tissue is irritated by friction or pressure. It can become annoying on the foot, especially when it appears on a weight-bearing surface.

The cause of the hyperplasia is not clear. A hypertrophic scar seems to be related to excessive irritation of a wound. Exposure to the radiation of an atomic explosion tends to precipitate hyperplasia. Excessive tension in a wound, burns, severe lacerations, strong chemicals, and excessive surgical handling induce hyperplasia.

A hypertrophic scar can usually be softened and reduced in size by rubbing castor oil into it for 15 minutes daily for several months. This procedure may also be used to differentiate the scar from the true keloid because this treatment has no effect on a true keloid.

Hypertrophic scars may be excised in their entirety; however, without roentgen therapy a high percentage recur. Gathings (1954) and Van den Brenk and Minty

(1960) believe that roentgen therapy is the most satisfactory method of treatment. Whitehill (1954), in a series of cases of excision of hypertrophic scar, applied a 1 to 2.5 percent hydrocortisone ointment in the lower half of the wound and, as a control, applied none in the upper half. There were no recurrences in the treated half of the wound, but there were some recurrences in the untreated half. Asboe-Hansen and associates (1956) injected hydrocortisone in fifty-six patients with false and true keloids. Their results were better in patients with the false type.

The procedure recommended here is to soften the scar and reduce its size by rubbing castor oil into it for 15 minutes daily for about a month and then to administer an erythema dose of roentgen rays. If necessary, the scar may be excised later and from 0.5 to 1 ml. 25-mg. hydrocortisone solution instilled into the wound. The skin is underscored for some distance so that there will be minimal tension on it. If possible, all suturing should be subdermal. Additional irradiation is indicated if there is any threat of recurrence.

DISEASES AND DEFORMITIES OF THE TOENAILS

Diseases of the nail may be local or constitutional affections or may be the result of congenital malformations. The nails are cutaneous appendages, which is why diseases of the skin and constitutional diseases affecting the skin often involve the nails. White and Laipply (1958) classify diseases of the nail as those caused by (1) infection, (2) psoriasis, (3) contact, (4) eczema (atopic dermatitis), (5) hypovitaminosis, (6) tumor, (7) trauma, or (8) general disease. Pardo-Castello (1960) published what is probably the most exhaustive review of diseases of the nails. His classification covers divisions according to (1) affections peculiar to the nails, (2) onychodystrophies, (3) ungual manifestations of dermatosis and of systemic disease, and (4) congenital affections of the nails.

Congenital nail deviations are errors of

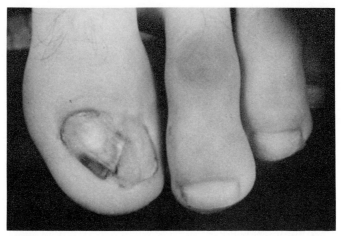

Fig. 12-35. Congenital double nail of great toe. (Courtesy Dr. C. E. Krausz.)

development that produce such anomalies of the nail as pachyonychia (hypertrophy of the nail and the nail bed), polyonychia (Fig. 12-35), and anonychia. Tauber and associates (1936) reported a case of pachyonychia congenita and reviewed the published reports of the disease. It is a rare disease involving the nails, which is accompanied by palmar and plantar keratoses, among other symptoms. Krausz (1970), in a review of 6,754 cases of disorders of the nail, reported 81 percent to be caused by local factors, such as trauma or *Candida albicans* infection.

Constitutional diseases involving the nails are in the province of the internist; skin diseases involving the nails are in the domain of the dermatologist. Only local and surgical nail problems are considered here.

Onychia

Onychia is an inflammation of the matrix, which usually extends into the nail grooves (paronychia). If the disturbance involves multiple digits, it is usually caused by systemic disease. In some instances local tinea infection may cause onychia in multiple nails. Onychia affects the great toe most frequently, where it is caused by trauma from pressure of the shoe and from superimposed secondary infection.

Treatment consists of relief of all pressure and daily application of a germicide and a fungicide dressing. In rare instances the condition may become acute, requiring antibiotic therapy, chemotherapy, or both.

Paronychia

Paronychia is an inflammation of the nail groove that commonly affects the great toe but sometimes affects the lesser toes; at times it extends to the matrix (onychia). Unlike onychia, however, paronychia is by itself rarely caused by constitutional or skin diseases. The severity of the condition varies. It may occur as a mild cellulitis, but in cases in which mechanical pressure (such as pressure from the boxing of the shoe) has crowded the tissue on the side of the nail, a severe state of suppuration may be present. Granulation tissue and extensive ulceration in the groove are characteristic. Paronychia is either accompanied by or is the forerunner of so-called ingrown nail.

Treatment consists of the following steps:
1. Relieve all pressure from shoes.
2. Excise a linear portion, about 2 mm. of the nail margin, to relieve the cutting effect on the edematous nail groove.
3. Paint the granulation tissue with 10 percent silver nitrate or 90 percent phenol.
4. Apply a fungicide dye and cover with a sterile dressing.

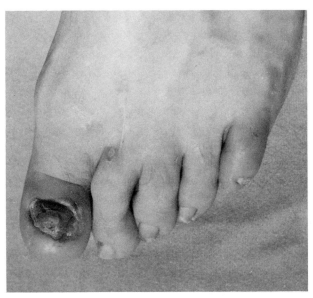

Fig. 12-36. Typical clubnail.

Onychauxis (clubnail)

The hypertrophied nail, termed onychauxis, or, popularly, clubnail, for the most part involves the great toenails, but the nails of the lesser toes may be affected (Fig. 12-36). The deformity may be caused by constitutional conditions, such as nutritional deficiencies or psoriasis. Most cases, however, are the result of local conditions: trauma to the matrix and nail bed, tinea infection, or both; indeed, tinea infection is by far the most frequent cause. In most "ringworm fungi" infections of the nail, the undersurface of the nail can become tremendously thickened from the accumulation of debris from the infection (Zaias, 1972).

The affected nail and its bed are thickened and deformed. When the disorder is caused by tinea gypsum, the surface of the nail may have white dead streaks or patches, which can be readily excised. When the undersurface of the nail contains a yellowish or brown powdery substance, destruction of the nail bed has been by tinea purpureum.

In about 10 percent of cases of clubnail, the nail bed and the dorsal distal surface of the distal phalanx undergo hypertrophic bone changes.

Two methods of treatment are available. In the first, the hypertrophied nail and bed are gradually reduced by grinding them down and then applying antifungal dressings. In the second, avulsion of the nail and repair of the bed are advised. The second method is reserved for severely deformed clubnails. The method of repair of the bed is outlined under "Incurvated nail," p. 365.

Onychogryposis (ram's horn nail, hostler's toe)

Onychogryposis is uncommon. It is known also as ram's horn nail and hostler's toe because of its occurrence in men who tended horses. The great toe alone or several toes may be affected (Fig. 12-37). The massive growth folds over the anterior surface of the toe, often terminating on the plantar surface. The condition does not appear to have any relation to tinea infection. In most cases it is the result of a congenital tendency and repeated trauma to the matrix associated with poor hygiene. For this last reason it is more likely to be

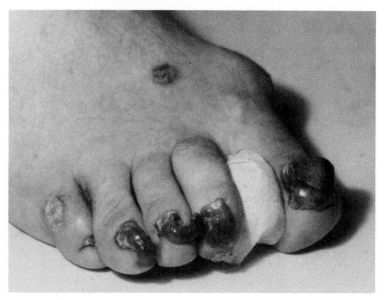

Fig. 12-37. Ram's horn nails of first four toes.

seen in derelicts than in those who are careful of cleanliness.

The entire horn up to the nail bed and to the matrix is readily removable with a pair of strong nail nippers. By frequent subsequent trimming the condition becomes asymptomatic. Treatment as outlined under onychauxis is indicated when there is pain and recurrent infection.

Onychoma: neoplasms of and around the nail

Verrucae, periungual fibromas, and subungual exostoses are common tumors about the nail. Verrucae and periungual fibromas usually appear in the nail groove but may occur in the nail bed under the nail. They respond readily to fulguration or excision. Subungual exostosis is discussed on p. 394.

Malignancy of the nail bed has been encountered, and its possibility should not be overlooked. Ashby (1956) found reports of twenty-five cases of primary carcinoma of the nail bed and added two proved cases of his own. Subungual melanoma, or melanotic whitlow, is a malignancy in the aged often unrecognized (Gibson et al., 1957), notwithstanding signs that should arouse diagnostic interest: increasing pigmenta-

tion, chronic nonhealing, painless granular excrescences, and persistent splitting of the nail. Differential diagnosis is essential. Treatment should be studied in each case with the advice of competent consultants.

Onychocryptosis (ingrown nail)

Diseases and deformities of the great toenail are one of the most common and disabling foot problems; about 5 percent are the result of general diseases, such as psoriases, endocrine disorders, or trophic changes. Intrinsic factors account for 95 percent, and of these about 15 percent are directly or indirectly related to tinea infection. The rest are the result of mechanical causes and constitute one of the most trying groups of foot problems. Unfortunately, diseases and deformities of the great toenail are generally taken lightly and are grouped under the lowly term "ingrown nail" and treated empirically. Because of the lack of differential diagnosis and the lack of understanding of the diagnosis, in numerous instances these patients are subjected to a series of unsuccessful operative procedures, which often produce more complicated problems than the original disease, including recurrence and consequent

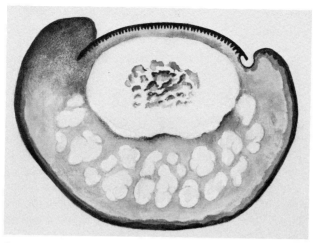

Fig. 12-38. *Left,* Hypertrophy of nail lip and occlusion of nail groove. *Right,* Normal relation of nail margin to nail groove.

iatrogenic deformity. I have seen patients who have been subjected to ten operative procedures for "ingrown nail," often with a result worse than the original complaint.

The terms "ingrown nail" and "onychocryptosis" are misleading because they imply that the side of the nail grows down into the nail groove. The unfortunate terminology has given rise to misinformation regarding this common disability, but because of its common usage, the term will be used in the following discussion.

All evidence points to the fact that the growth of nails in all vertebrates depends on the matrix, and that the width of the nail is in direct relation to the width of the matrix (Pardo-Castello, 1960; Bloom and Fawcett, 1968; Bean, 1963). There is no evidence that the matrix becomes wider in persons suffering from this malady. The old term "ingrown nail" was chosen on the assumption that ingrowth of the nail, or growing down of the nail into the nail groove, was caused by growth of the width of the convexity of the nail. Therefore, at first surgeons aimed at destroying the growth of the nail margin, but their attempts at correction failed (DuVries, 1933, 1944). Bartlett (1937) also concluded that the terms "ingrown nail" and "ingrowing nails" are misnomers. The coined term

"hypertrophy of the ungualabia" (DuVries, 1933, 1944) is more descriptive of the true pathologic condition in most cases of this sort.

Frost (1950) recognized three types of so-called ingrown nails: (1) a normal nail plate, but as a result of improper nail trimming, a fish hook or spur remains in the nail groove; (2) an inward distortion of one or both lateral margins of the nail plate (incurvated nail); (3) a normal nail plate, but the lip is hypertrophied (Fig. 12-38). Lloyd-Davies and Brill (1963) suggest that avulsion of the nail, which is commonly practiced as a treatment for ingrown nail, is probably the cause of hypertrophy of the lip distal to the nail and causes the entire nail to become embedded and clubbed (Fig. 12-39). Unlike the fingernails, if the nail of the great toe has been taken off, the new nail frequently becomes deformed as it grows out because of the upward pressure placed on it during weight bearing.

There are two distinct conditions that produce the symptoms. The first, which accounts for about 75 percent of cases, is primarily hyperplasia of the nail groove and nail lip (hypertrophy of the ungualabia). The second, which accounts for 25 percent, is essentially a deformity of the nail plate

Normal toe

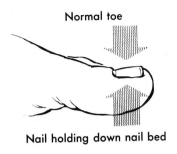

Nail holding down nail bed

After nail avulsion

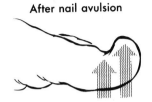

Upward pressure forces causing upward
deformation of distal nail bed

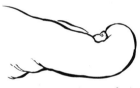

Regrowing nail approaching soft tissue wall

Fig. 12-39. Avulsion of nail as treatment for "ingrown nail" causing hypertrophy of the nail lip, resulting in embedded and clubbed nail. (After Lloyd-Davies and Brill: Br. J. Surg. **50:** 592-597, May 1963.)

itself. It is caused by a malformation of the dorsum of the distal phalanx or by hypertrophy and irregular thickening of the nail bed, often the result of tinea unguium. The normal nail plate and its bed is 2 or 3 mm. thick; its contour is determined largely by the shape of the dorsum of the distal phalanx. The shape and contour of the dorsum of this bone may vary widely because of secondary changes in the bone from irritation and pressure. Such variations often produce nail deformities, the symptoms of which are grouped and diagnosed as in-

grown nail. The most common type is an incurvation of the nail margins.

Etiology. Normally the space between the nail margin and the nail groove is about 1 mm. The groove is lined with a thin layer of epithelium and lies immediately under and on the sides of the nail margin (Fig. 12-38). This space is sufficient to protect the groove from irritation under normal conditions. The boxing of shoes, however, often exerts a downward pressure upon the nail plate or upon the nail lip on the side of the toe, and that pressure obliterates the space between the nail margin and nail groove, thus producing constant irritation to the groove. The reactive swelling in the groove creates a cycle that results in gradual hyperplasia of the groove and nail lip and ultimately in permanent hypertrophy (Fig. 12-40).

As the process continues, the nail groove is finally incised by the nail margin, often with ensuing suppuration and secondary infection. To relieve the acute symptoms a triangular section of the nail margin is excised; however, the area left by excision is the forerunner of the fishhook formation (Fig. 12-41), about which Frost (1950) speaks. Hypertrophy of the groove fills the space of the excised nail margin. As the nail continues its growth distally, it collides with the elevated nail groove, which results in recurrent episodes of infection and massive formation of granulation tissue.

Congenitally thick nail lips predispose to ingrown nail. This congenital factor explains why ingrown nails are sometimes seen in infants, or even in newborns who have thick nail lips or an absence of freedom between the nail groove and nail margin, or even both conditions. In adults the disorder is an acquired condition.

The size, shape, and contour of the nail plate and bed are usually normal. Hyperplastic changes of the nail groove and lip are accompanied by formation of granulation tissue on the lip and groove. The granulation tissue bleeds freely on slight provocation. Hypertrophy may mask a large part of the nail or even most of it.

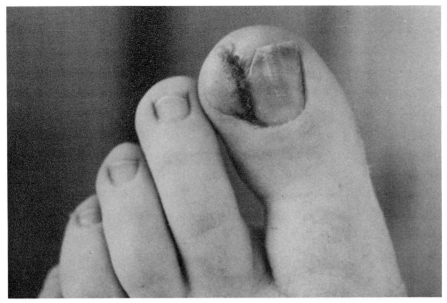

Fig. 12-40. Hypertrophy and overlapping of nail lip.

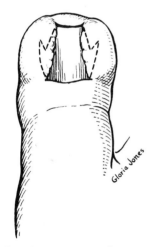

Fig. 12-41. Consequence of repeated cutting of distal end of nail margin. Note fishhook.

Correction of the hypertrophied nail lip of the great toe. The variety of procedures reported for the cure of the so-called ingrown nail indicates that none is completely satisfactory; indeed, postoperative recurrence is frequent. Keyes (1934) reviewed 110 cases in which five different procedures resulted in fifteen recurrences.

The procedures generally practiced fall into three distinct groups: (1) excision of the nail margin up to the matrix and the nail groove, as illustrated by Winograd (1929), Graham (1929), and Jansey (1955), among others (Fig. 12-42), and by Steinberg (1954), who devised a punch to simplify the procedure (Fig. 12-43); (2) avulsion of the entire nail—Frost (1958) devised an instrument (Fig. 12-44) to avulse a nail atraumatically; and (3) reduction of the hypertrophied lip, as recommended by Bartlett (1937), Ney (1923), and DuVries (1944). The first and second procedures and their varied modifications, notwithstanding their mutilating and often poor results, are more generally employed than the third procedure, probably because they are simpler to perform than plastic repair of the nail lip, just as digits are often needlessly amputated because it is easier to amputate than to repair. Polokoff (1961) reports successful treatment of hypertrophied nail lips of the great toes with the negative galvanic electrode (Fig. 12-45). Bose (1971) has reported a technique for the excision of the nail fold.

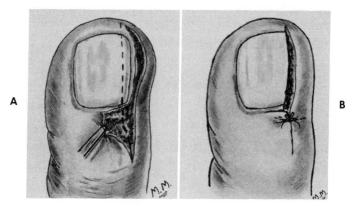

Fig. 12-42. A, Nail margin, groove, and part of nail lip excised. **B,** Eponychium sutured over matrix.

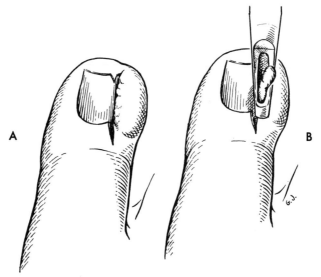

Fig. 12-43. A, Incision over nail matrix. **B,** Removal of the nail margin, groove, and part of nail lip with Steinberg's trephine.

To remove the hypertrophied nail lip, Ney (1923) devised an operation based on the flap skin graft used in plastic surgery. Two skin flaps of the entire surface on the affected side of the toe are formed; then all the subcutaneous tissue perpendicular to the nail margin is removed. The flaps are replaced and sutured into place (Fig. 12-46). This procedure is complicated, and the possibility that flaps will slough must be kept in mind.

Recommended procedure. The treatment for the different stages of hypertrophied ungualabia is as follows.

MILD CASES. Relief may be obtained by inserting a few loose strands of cotton in the nail groove to which an astringent is applied, such as 10 percent silver nitrate. Permit the nail to grow out freely over the distal end of the nail groove. The wearing of footwear that does not exert constant pressure against the great toe is required.

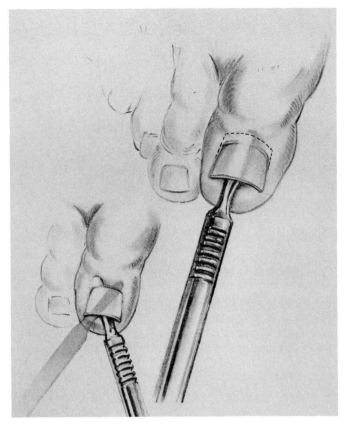

Fig. 12-44. Nail avulsed and nail plate underscored with Frost elevator.

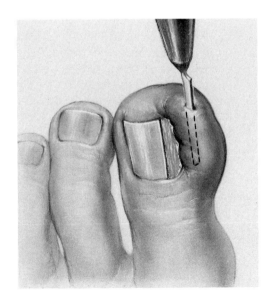

Fig. 12-45. Reduction of hypertrophied nail lip after excision of nail margin. A negative galvanic electrode is used. (After Polokoff, M.: J. Amer. Podiatry Assoc., **51:**805-808, Nov. 1961.)

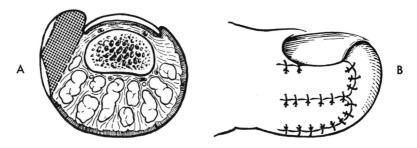

Fig. 12-46. A, Hypertrophied lip and subdermal fat excised at side of toe (shaded area). **B,** Skin on side of toe made into two flaps and sutured.

In the presence of acute cellulitis (with or without infection) the offending nail margin must be excised, a loose cotton packing is inserted into the nail groove, and an astringent is applied to the cotton pack. This procedure is repeated at frequent intervals until the nail margin becomes completely free up to the distal end of the toe.

MODERATELY SEVERE CASES. Plastic reduction of the nail lip usually corrects moderately severe cases of hypertrophied nail lip.

1. Remove a spindle-shaped section, about 3 by 1 cm. from the side of the nail lip, which is triangular on cross section (Fig. 12-47, *A* and *B*). The incisions extend from the most distal portion of the toe to about 0.5 cm. proximal to the nail fold, meeting about 2 mm. under the nail groove.
2. Excise the excess subdermal fat.
3. Coapt and suture the skin margins, drawing the nail groove downward Fig. 12-47, *C* and *D*.

The wound heals by first intention, and the procedure results in a free space between the nail groove and margin.

ADVANCED HYPERTROPHY OF THE NAIL LIP. Advanced cases are likely to be accompanied by large nail lips with excessive granulation tissue in the nail groove. The nail contour is normal, but there is a history of repeated infection of the involved nail groove. In a series of 900 cases in which the ages of the patients ranged from 2 to 80 years, the DuVries operation for reduction of hypertrophy of the ungualabia gave uniformly good results. A description of the procedure follows:

1. Make an elliptical incision, extending from 0.5 cm. proximally to the eponychium, to the distal portion of the toe from above, downward alongside the nail margin and on the side of the distal phalanx, with its base plantarward. The two incisions of the ellipse meet at the base. All the hypertrophied tissue of the nail groove and nail lip is thus excised and a skin flap is formed of the side of the nail lip (Fig. 12-48, *A* and *B*).
2. Excise all excess fat (Fig. 12-48, *C*).
3. Underscore the nail margin for a distance of about 2 mm. from its bed all the way to the matrix (Fig. 12-48, *D*).
4. Pass a suture through the dorsum of the nail and carry it under the freed portion of the nail and through the deepest portion of the wound, letting it escape through the flap.
5. Return the suture and pass it through the nail from its undersurface (Fig. 12-48, *E*).
6. When that suture has been tied, fold the skin flap under the nail margin (Fig. 12-48, *F*). Place a small bolster 0.5 cm. in diameter and 1.5 cm. long (made of gauze, Telfa, or rubber tubing), under the suture on the side of the nail lip to prevent suture strangulation.
7. Place additional sutures at the epo-

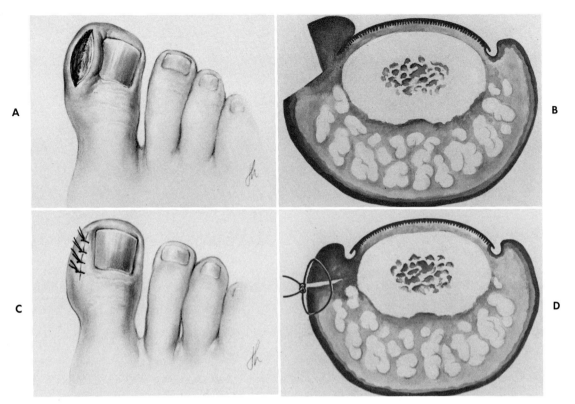

Fig. 12-47. A, Triangular section removed from side of toe. **B,** Cross section after excision. **C,** Nail lip and nail groove pulled down after suturing of nail margins. **D,** Cross section after suturing.

nychium and at the distal end of the incision if they are necessary (Fig. 12-49, *D*).

The nail margin grows freely over the new groove. Fig. 12-49, *E* shows end results.

POSTOPERATIVE CARE. Change the dressing in 24 to 48 hours. If any of the sutures are strangulating, which often occurs because of edema, they should be cut but not removed until 6 to 8 days later. Thereafter, change the dressing every 5 to 7 days until healing is complete. During that period granulation tissue may form in the wound; if it does, it should be destroyed promptly by painting it with 95 percent phenol or 20 percent silver nitrate. It may be necessary to repeat these applications a number of times until healing is assured.

The underscored nail margin will not ad-

here again but will remain detached from the bed; however, the new nail will grow normally because the matrix is not disturbed in the technique. During the growth of the new nail, the old nail margin may impinge on the lip because of residual edema secondary to the healing process. However, because its margin is not adherent, a cotton pack can be cushioned under it readily. The new nail grows out freely, does not impinge on the nail lip or groove, and results in a normal nail and lip. About 1 percent of the patients in my series failed to obtain complete relief and required secondary procedures.

Panhypertrophy of the nail lip, or embedded toenail, is usually a consequence of congenital clubbed toes or repeated complete avulsion of the nail (Figs. 12-39 and 12-50, *A*). The periungual soft tissues may

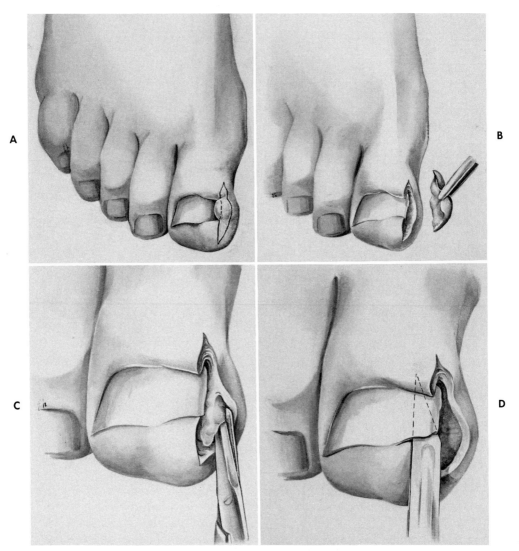

Fig. 12-48. DuVries' plastic reduction of hypertrophy of ungualabia. **A,** Linear incision along nail margin. A second semielliptical incision is made lateral to the first incision; these incisions meet at both ends. **B,** Hypertrophied lip removed. **C,** All excess fat excised. **D,** Nail margin detached from nail bed for about 2 mm. **E,** Suture carried through dorsum of nail plate, under freed nail margin, through floor of incision, and then outward through skin flap and back under freed nail margin. **F,** Automatic invagination of skin flap under nail margin by tying ends of suture. **G,** Additional sutures at eponychium and at distal end of incision.

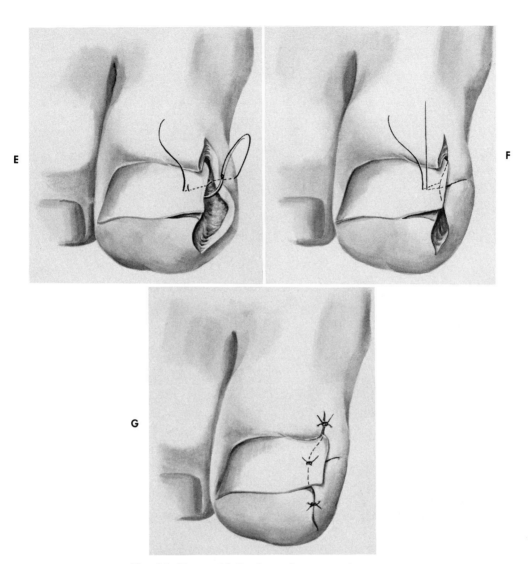

E

F

G

Fig. 12-48, cont'd. For legend see opposite page.

cover most of the nail. It may be corrected by excision of a horseshoe section of the hypertrophied lips and suturing of the skin margins (Fig. 12-50, B and C).

Incurvated nail (inverted nail; involuted nail)

Incurvated nail, also called inverted and involuted nail, is included ordinarily in the term "ingrown nail"; it comprises about 25 percent of such cases. The disorders are essentially deformities of the nail plate and

nail bed and may vary widely, from deformity of the nail margins, which curve into the side of the distal phalanx, to deformity of the entire nail plate, which, on cross section, appears horseshoe shaped (Fig. 12-51). Generally, the nail margins invert toward the sides of the distal phalanx. Because the contour of the nail depends largely on the contour of the dorsal surface of the distal phalanx, deformity of the nail often occurs secondary to an anomalous dorsal surface of that bone. It may

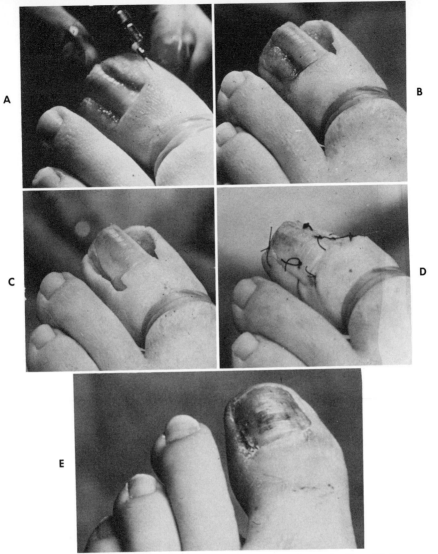

Fig. 12-49. Steps **A** to **D**, and end result, **E**. Procedure shown in Fig. 12-48 was performed on this patient.

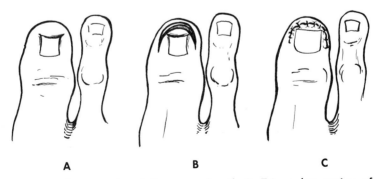

Fig. 12-50. A, Panhypertrophy of lips around nail. **B,** Triangular section of skin and subcutaneous fat excised horseshoelike around toe. **C,** Skin margins sutured.

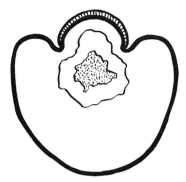

Fig. 12-51. Incurvation of nail margins.

also be caused by hypertrophy of the nail bed.

No single surgical procedure can be recommended as being applicable to all the variations of the deformity; however, the following procedures give relief in the general types as outlined:

1. When only the margin of the nail is deformed, excision of the nail margin and nail groove, including the matrix of the nail, gives relief. This can be performed by the procedures described by Winograd (Fig. 12-42) and by Steinberg (Fig. 12-43). Dyer and Cohen (1955) make use of negative galvanic current to destroy the groove and matrix after removal of the nail margin. (Regardless of the procedure chosen, it is important that the cells of the matrix under the eponychium be completely destroyed; otherwise, spicules of nail may arise from that part of the matrix and grow into the scarified nail groove.)

2. When the entire nail plate is deformed, Zadik (1950) removes the nail and makes a longitudinal incision on each side of the eponychium, thereby forming a flap of the eponychium. He excises the matrix and its bed and elevates the remaining nail bed distally; he sutures the eponychium to the proximal border of the nail bed.

3. The DuVries procedure for avulsing the nail, denuding the nail bed of hypertrophied tissue, and reducing

any dorsal deformity of the distal phalanx is as follows:

a. Underscore the plate with small Sistrunk scissors or a Frost elevator and remove it in its entirety. This leaves a smooth nail bed surface.

b. Make a U-shaped incision with its curved end directed distally, following the outline of the nail bed.

c. Denude the dorsum of the distal phalanx of the nail bed, elevating the bed from the bone.

d. Excise all hypertrophied tissue from the undersurface of the nail bed.

e. Flatten the dorsal surface of the phalanx with a rasp.

f. Remodel the distal end of the distal phalanx and the distal nail lip so that the dorsal end of the toe is flat.

g. Replace the nail bed over the phalanx.

h. Apply a compression dressing over the nail bed that is tight enough to prevent a large amount of blood from accumulating under the nail bed; otherwise, a hematoma would form and cause the bed to slough off.

Extensive surgical trauma prolongs healing. Drainage may be present for many weeks, requiring frequent dressings. Because tinea spores are often present in those regions, fungicides should be applied with each dressing. Although a rudimentary or malformed nail usually results, at least the nail is symptom-free.

4. A few extremely deformed nails resist plastic repair; hence, partial amputation of the distal phalanx must be resorted to for removal of the entire nail assembly. (For the technical steps, see Chapter 17.)

"Ingrown" nail of lesser toes

The lesser toes are subject to disease and deformity similar to that which affects the great toe but such disorders occur less frequently and rarely in severe form. When the primary problem is hypertrophy of the nail lip, the area is smaller and more manageable than in the area of the great toe. The distal phalanges of the lesser digits are small bones in comparison with the hallux; they are also comparatively more easily managed when the primary problem is one of deformity of the nail. The nail lip may be congenitally hypertrophied or become so from restriction of shoes. The condition may be remedied by excising a section of the lip by a spindle-shaped incision and suturing the skin edges.

In cases in which the nail bed and plate are deformed, the following procedure is advised:

1. Denude the nail from its bed all the way back to the matrix and elevate it.
2. Excise all the subungual hypertrophy.
3. Underscore the skin over the distal end of the distal phalanx.
4. Suture first through the nail at the matrix and out underneath the nail; then pass the needle through the anterior lip, which has been previously freed from the distal phalanx, and then back. Pass the needle through the nail again, from its undersurface to its dorsal surface, where the suture is tied to fold the anterior skin lip under the nail, in which position healing takes place.

REFERENCES

Abramson, D. I.: Diagnosis and treatment of peripheral vascular disorders, New York, 1956, Paul B. Hoeber, Inc.

Aggarwal, N. D., and Singh, H.: Ainhum: Report of an atypical case, J. Bone Joint Surg. **45-B:** 376-378, May 1963.

Aird, I., Johnson, H. D., Lennox, B., and Stansfeld, A. G.: Epithelioma cuniculatum: A variety of squamous carcinoma peculiar to foot, Brit. J. Surg. **42:**245-250, 1954.

Allen, A. C., and Spitz, S.: Malignant melanoma: A clinicopathological analysis of criteria for diagnosis and prognosis, Cancer **6:**1-45, 1953.

Allington, H. V.: Review of the psychotherapy of warts, Arch. Dermatol. Syphilol. **66:**316-326, Sept. 1952.

Allyn, B., and Waldorf, D. S.: Treatment of verruca with vaccinia, J.A.M.A. **203:**807, Feb. 1968.

Anderson, R.: Treatment of intractable plantar warts, Plast. Reconstr. Surg. **19:**384-388, May 1957.

Asboe-Hansen, G., Brodthagen, H., and Zachariae, L.: Treatment of keloids with topical injections of hydrocortisone acetate, Arch. Dermatol. **73:**162-165, Jan.-June 1956.

Ashby, B. S.: Primary carcinoma of the nail-bed, Brit. J. Surg. **44:**216-217, Sept. 1956.

Auckland, G., Ball, J., and Griffiths, D. L.: Ainhum, J. Bone Joint Surg. **39-B:**513-519, Aug. 1957.

Baer, R. L., Rosenthal, S. A., Litt, J. Z., and Rogachefsky, H.: Experimental investigations on mechanism producing acute dermatophytosis of feet, J.A.M.A. **160:**184-190, Jan. 1956.

Bartlett, R. W.: A conservative operation for cure of so-called ingrown toenail, J.A.M.A. **108:**1257-1258, Apr. 1937.

Bean, W. B.: Nail growth: A twenty-year study, Arch. Intern. Med. **111:**476-482, Jan.-June 1963.

Billig, H. E., Jr.: Condylectomy for metatarsalgia: Indications and results, J. Int. Coll. Surg. **25:**220-226, Feb. 1956.

Blair, V. P., Brown, J. B., and Byars, L. T.: Plantar warts, flaps, and grafts, J.A.M.A. **108:**24-27, Jan. 1937.

Blank, H.: Treatment of plantar warts, Arch. Dermatol. Syphilol. **56:**459-461, Oct. 1947.

Bloom, W., and Fawcett, D. W.: A textbook of histology, Philadelphia, 1968, W. B. Saunders Co.

Bonavilla, E. J.: Histopathology of the heloma durum: Some significant features and their implications, J. Amer. Podiatry Assoc. **58:**423-427, Oct. 1968.

Bose, B.: A technique for excision of nail fold for ingrowing toenail, Surg. Gynec. Obstet. **132:** 511-512, Mar. 1971.

Brown, J. B., and Fryer, M. P.: Repair of surface defects of the foot, J.A.M.A. **146:**628-632, June 1951.

Browne, H. J.: Squamous carcinomas of the extremities, Thesis, 1953, University of Minnesota.

Charache, H.: Squamous cell carcinoma of the extremities, Surg. Gynec. Obstet. **68:**1002-1006, June 1939.

Committee on Cutaneous Health and Cosmetics: Treatment of verrucae with small pox vaccine, J.A.M.A. **206:**117, Sept. 1968.

Decker, A. M., and Chamness, J. T.: Melanocarcinoma of the plantar surface of the foot: A review of twenty-five cases, Surgery **29:**731-742, May 1951.

Dickson, J. A.: Surgical treatment of intractable

plantar warts, J. Bone Joint Surg. 30-A:757-760, July 1948.

Dingman, R. O., and Grabb, W. C.: The intractable plantar wart, Mich. State Med. Soc. J. 61:297-299, Jan.-June 1962.

Dolce, F. A.: Shoe dermatitis among soldiers, Mil. Surgeon 95:505-507, Dec. 1944.

Ducourtioux, M.: La verrue plantaire et ses traitements, Presse Med. 58:1116, Oct. 1950.

Dunbar, H. F.: Emotions and bodily changes: A survey of literature on psychosomatic interrelationships, 1910-1953, ed. 4, New York, 1954, Columbia University Press.

Duthie, D. A., and McCallum, D. I.: Treatment of plantar warts with Elastoplast and podophyllin, Brit. Med. J. 2:216-218, July 1951.

DuVries, H. L.: Hypertrophy of ungualabia, Chiropody Rec. 16:11, Nov. 1933.

DuVries, H. L.: Ingrown nail, Chiropody Rec. 27:155-159, 164-166, Oct. 1944.

DuVries, H. L.: New approach to the treatment of intractable verruca plantaris (plantar wart), J.A.M.A. 152:1202-1203, July 1953.

DuVries, H. L.: Verruca plantaris, J.A.M.A. 154:1302, Apr. 1954.

DuVries, H. L.: Treatment of plantar wart, J.A.M.A. 172:642, Feb. 1960.

Dyer, A. M., and Cohen, M. F.: A report on the use of negative galvanic current for the correction of incurvated nails, J. Nat. Assoc. Chiropody 45:21-22, Dec. 1955.

Frost, L.: Root resection for incurvated nail, J. Nat. Assoc. Chiropody 40:19-28, Mar. 1950.

Frost, L.: Atraumatic nail avulsion with a novel ungual elevator, J. Amer. Podiatry Assoc. 48:51-56, Feb. 1958.

Galland, W. I.: An operative treatment for corns, J.A.M.A. 100:880-881, Mar. 1933.

Gathings, J. G.: Treatment of keloids with combination of hyaluronidase and kutapressin, Amer. J. Surg. 88:429-430, 1954.

Gaul, L. E., and Underwood, G. B.: Primary irritants and sensitizers used in fabrication of footwear, Arch. Dermat. Syphilol, 60:649-675, 1949.

Giannestras, N. J.: Shortening of the metatarsal shaft for the correction of plantar keratosis, Clin. Orthop. 4:225-231, 1954.

Gibbs, R. C.: Eccrine poroma, J. Amer. Podiatry Assoc. 58:298-300, July 1968.

Gibson, H. G., Montgomery, H., Woolner, L. B., and Brunsting, L. A.: Melanotic whitlow (subungual melanoma), J. Invest. Dermatol. 29:119-129, 1957.

Graham, H. F.: Ingrown toe nail, Amer. J. Surg. 6:411, 1929.

Haboush, E. J., and Martin, R. V.: Painful interdigital clavus (soft corn): Treatment by skin-plastic operation, J. Bone Joint Surg. 29:756-757, July 1947.

Hauser, E. D. W.: Office management of painful feet, Surg. Clin. N. Amer. 37:75-89, Feb. 1957.

Ignatoff, W. B.: Verruca therapy, J. Nat. Assoc. Chiropody 44:37-47, July 1954.

Jansey, F.: Etiologic therapy of ingrowing toe nail, Northwestern Univ. Med. School Quart. 29:358-362, 1955.

Keyes, E. L.: The surgical treatment of ingrown toenails, J.A.M.A. 102:1458-1460, May 1934.

Kile, R. L.: How communicable are warts? J.A.M.A. 162:1222-1224, Nov. 1956.

King, E. S. J.: Glomus tumor, Aust. N. Z. J. Surg. 23:280-295, May 1954.

Kitlowski, E. A.: The treatment of keloids and keloidal scars, Plast. Reconstr. Surg. 12:383-391, 1953.

Krausz, C. E.: Nail survey: 28th October 1942, to 3rd April 1970, Brit. J. Chiropody 35:117, May 1970.

Lloyd-Davies, R. W., and Brill, G. C.: The aetiology and outpatient management of ingrowing toe-nails, Brit. J. Surg. 50:592-597, May 1963.

Lusskin, R.: Serpentine sinus—a tract leading nowhere, J. Bone Joint Surg. 43-A:118-122, Jan. 1961.

McElvenny, R. T.: Corns: Their etiology and treatment, Amer. J. Surg. 50:761-765, Dec. 1940.

McGee, A. R.: Wart treatment with smallpox vaccine, Appl. Ther., 10:310-311 May 1968.

McKeever, D. C.: Arthrodesis of the first metatarsophalangeal joint for hallux valgus, hallux rigidus and metatarsus primus varus, J. Bone Joint Surg. 34-A:129-134, Jan. 1952.

Montgomery, A. H., and Montgomery, R. M.: Mosaic wart: An unusual type of plantar wart, New York State J. Med. 37:1978-1983, Dec. 1937.

Montgomery, A. H., and Montgomery, R. M.: Mosaic type of plantar wart: Its characteristics and treatment, Arch. Dermatol. Syphilol. 57:397-399, Mar. 1948.

Montgomery, A. H., Montgomery, R. M., and Montgomery, D. C.: The problem of plantar radiodermatitis, New York State J. Med. 49:1664-1667, July 1949.

Montgomery, R. M.: Dermatologic care of the painful foot, J. Bone Joint Surg. 46-A:1129-1136, July 1964.

Montgomery, R. M., and Montgomery, A. H.: Common hyperkeratotic lesions of the foot, J.A.M.A. 124:756-761, Mar. 1944.

Morris, J., Wood, M. G., and Samitz, M. H.: Eccrine poroma, Arch. Dermatol. 98:162-165, Aug. 1968.

Ney, G. C.: An operation for ingrowing toe nails, J.A.M.A. 80:374-375, Feb. 1923.

Niles, H. D.: Dermatitis due to shoe leather, J.A.M.A. 110:363-365, Jan. 1938.

Norton, M. L., Sala, A. M., and Silverstein, M. E.:

Ainhum (dactylosis spontanea), Arch. Surg. **75**:473-478, 1957.

Ottley, C. M.: Glomus tumour, Brit. J. Surg. **29**: 387-391, 1942.

Pack, G. T., and Adair, F. E.: Subungual melanoma: Differential diagnosis of tumors of the nail bed, Surgery **5**:47-72, Jan. 1939.

Pack, G. T., Lenson, N., and Gerber, D. M.: Regional distribution of moles and melanomas, Arch. Surg. **65**:862-870, July-Dec. 1952.

Pardo-Castello, V.: Diseases of the nails, ed. 3, Springfield, Ill., 1960, Charles C Thomas, Publisher.

Pinkus, H., Rogin, J. R., and Goldman, P.: Eccrine poroma: Tumors exhibiting features of the epidermal sweat duct unit, Arch. Dermatol. **74**:511-521, Nov. 1956.

Polokoff, M.: Ingrown toenail and hypertrophied nail lip surgery by electrolysis, J. Amer. Podiatry Assoc. **51**:805-808, Nov. 1961.

Reeves, R. J., and Jackson, M. T.: Roentgen therapy of plantar warts, Amer. J. Roentgenol. Radium Ther. Nucl. Med. **76**:977-978, Nov. 1956.

Rutledge, B. A., and Green, A. L.: Surgical treatment of plantar corns, U. S. Armed Services Med. J. **8**:219-221, Feb. 1957.

Schreiner, B. F., and Wehr, W. H.: Primary malignant tumors of the foot: A report of 37 cases, Radiology **21**:513-521, Dec. 1933.

Smyth, M.: Glomus-cell tumors in the lower extremity: Report of two cases, J. Bone Joint Surg. **53-A**:157-159, Jan. 1971.

Spinzig, E. W.: Ainhum: Its occurrence in the United States, with a report of three cases, Amer. J. Roentgenol. **42**:246-263, Aug. 1939.

Stack, J. K.: Ainhum, J. Bone Joint Surg. **32-A**: 444-445, Apr. 1950.

Steinberg, M. D.: A simplified technique for surgery of ingrowing nails, Surgery **36**:1132-1137, Dec. 1954.

Tauber, E. B., Goldman, L., and Claassen, H.: Pachyonychia congenita, J.A.M.A. **107**:29-30, July 1936.

Treatment of plantar warts (editorial), New Eng. J. Med. **248**:659, 1953.

Tye, M.: Ainhum, New Eng. J. Med. **234**:152-154, Jan. 1946.

Van den Brenk, H. A. S., and Minty, C. C. J.: Radiation in the management of keloids and hypertrophic scars, Brit. J. Surg. **47**:595-605, May 1960.

White, C. J., and Laipply, T. C.: Diseases of the nails: 792 cases, Ind. Med. Surg. **27**:325-327, July 1958.

Whitehill, J. L.: Prophylaxis of surgical keloids, Ariz. Med. **11**:399-402, Nov. 1954.

Winograd, A. M.: A modification in the technic of operation for ingrown toe-nail, J.A.M.A. **92**:229-230, Jan. 1929.

Zadik, F. R.: Obliteration of nail bed of the great toe without shortening terminal phalanx, J. Bone Joint Surg. **32-B**:66-67, Feb. 1950.

Zaias, N.: Onychomycosis, Arch. Dermatol. **105**: 263-274, Feb. 1972.

13

Local affections of the bones and soft tissues of the foot

F. Scott Smyth, Jr.

INFECTIOUS DISORDERS

Osteomyelitis

The term "osteomyelitis" implies infection of bone. Particular subtypes, based on objectively determined variations, are placed within this broad definition. They include acute, subacute, and chronic osteomyelitis, as well as special types of infectious diseases, such as mycotic infections of bone (see Chapter 11).

Acute osteomyelitis. This acute infection of bone may occur at any age by means of either local bacterial invasion or bacteremia with secondary seeding.

An intact bone in a healthy individual is resistant to infection and although bacterial infection of soft tissues will often spare the skeleton, massive tissue injury may lower resistance to bacterial invasion. In some cases this lowered resistance is accompanied by a decreased blood supply to the bones as well. Many systemic illnesses will lower this intrinsic resistance, and subsequent infection of bone, which necessitates radical treatment, may occur.

Acute hematogenous osteomyelitis was encountered more frequently during the preantibiotic era than it is today. Antibiotics have significantly diminished the problems of osteomyelitis. In 1936 Wilson and McKeever reported that they found ten out of ninety foci of infection caused by hematogenous osteomyelitis in the bones of the foot. In the ten cases the infection was distributed in the following sites: the calcaneus, five; the metatarsals, three; and the phalanges, two. The use of antibiotics may alter an acute osteomyelitis. For example, when they are administered in a random manner, a chronic smoldering infection may result and bypass the acute stage of the condition. The most common source of blood-borne bacterial seeding is *Staphylococcus aureus* (Clawson and Dunn, 1967).

The clinical picture of acute osteomyelitis varies according to the causative factors involved. Local bacterial invasion by hematogenous seeding produces a regional tissue response, with adjacent thrombosis, leukocytosis, and an attempted walling of the inoculum. The peculiarity of bone and its resistance to physical deformation render spontaneous drainage and tissue contractability impossible; consequently, the infectious process will develop rapidly by means of intramedullary extension until the entire bone may become involved. Acute hematogenous spread is associated with localized pain, erythema, edema, fever, and systemic signs of toxicity. A positive blood culture will confirm the diagnosis.

Infection caused by local inoculation, or contamination caused by the loss of bony integrity due to a compound fracture, may

371

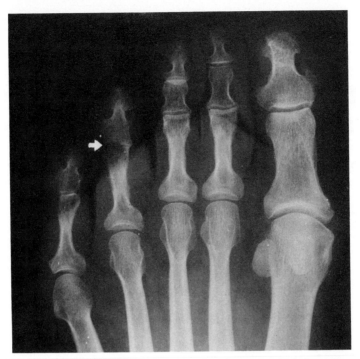

Fig. 13-1. Acute osteomyelitis of head of fourth proximal phalanx (arrow).

not produce the extreme picture of acute hematogenous osteomyelitis because an immediate drainage pathway is available in these instances. However, the attendant tissue destruction and decreased vascularity do provide a medium that perpetuates the acute infection.

The roentgenographic picture of acute osteomyelitis may change. At the time of onset, no positive findings may appear; later, rarefaction caused by hyperemia and disuse, as well as soft-tissue swelling, periosteal thickening, medullary cloudiness, and loss of trabeculation may be evident. Roentgenographic findings may be suggestive of greater bone destruction than actually exists (Fig. 13-1).

If left untreated, acute osteomyelitis will ultimately lead to chronic osteomyelitis or, in some instances, to one of the variant forms of osteomyelitis. The complementary relationship of the resistance of the host and the virulence of the invading agent bear a direct relationship to the ultimate resolution of the condition.

Treatment. The principles of treatment for acute bacterial osteomyelitis are basically the same as those for pyogenic infection in other tissues of the body. Prompt identification of the infecting agent and antibiotic treatment, with correctly timed surgical drainage, are paramount. Needle aspiration through aseptically prepared skin into the suspected area, with immediate culture implantation, has proved to be the most successful technique for identifying the agent of infection. Selection of the antibiotic is best determined by the use of in vitro sensitivity studies and is confirmed by checking bactericidal serum levels with subcultures in the laboratory (Jawetz, 1962). It should be mentioned that in many instances an effective concentration of the antibiotic of choice may be hazardous to other organ systems of the body. Care must be taken to anticipate this danger and to detect such damage promptly (Benner, 1967). Studies of renal function, as well as electrolytic and audiometric studies, may be indicated for debilitated patients be-

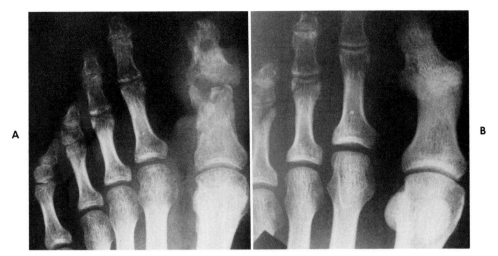

Fig. 13-2. A, Osteomyelitis of entire hallux. B, After healing.

fore antibiotic treatment is initiated. Surgical drainage may be accomplished by direct incision of the abscess, with open packing and delayed closure, or by the insertion of a tube for aspiration. In most areas of infection, tubal aspiration may be performed alternately with topical instillation of the antibiotic (Jergesen and Jawetz, 1963). The primary goals of drainage are to relieve the pressure of the pus and to curtail the spread of the infectious process. Once adequate drainage is established, the systemic findings will regress (Fig. 13-2).

Chronic osteomyelitis. Inadequately treated or untreated acute osteomyelitis, in most cases, will develop into chronic osteomyelitis. At this later stage of bacterial invasion, soft-tissue change, bone destruction, vascular insufficiency, and new bone formation (with or without chronic drainage) characterize the clinical picture. Pain is present, but it is not as severe and incapacitating as it is in the acute form. In the blood smear, leukocytosis may be a finding, but the smear will show relative lymphocytosis or monocytosis, with a normal number of polymorphonuclear leukocytes. Clinically, sites of drainage will appear and a brawny edema will be present. A roentgenogram may show areas of dense sclerotic dead bone, as well as areas of reactive new bone at the periphery.

If chronic osteomyelitis is left untreated, drainage through one or more sinus tracts will eventually occur. Often small bits of dead bone (sequestra) may be seen in the drainage or may be picked out of the sinus tract. In response to the death of bone, the host creates peripheral new bone (involucrum) in order to maintain skeletal integrity. In rare instances the epithelium of the chronic sinus tract undergoes malignant transformation.

Treatment. The treatment of chronic osteomyelitis is inevitably surgical. Bacterial identification, repeated cultures, and prolonged antibiotic therapy, combined with various forms of surgical debridement, may provide arrest of the condition and expedite the return of normal function. Excision of the dead sequestrations as well as the local devitalized soft tissues should be carried out. Local irrigation and suction after debridement may provide good results; muscle pedicle grafts with saucerization may enhance healing (Rowling, 1959). Amputation remains the treatment of choice in some cases involving debility, continued progression of the disease, or both.

Before surgical procedures are performed, contrast studies of the sinus tract (sinograms) should be done in order to expose areas of necrotic tissue not evident

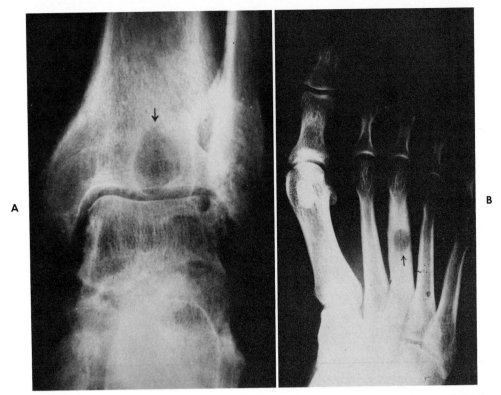

Fig. 13-3. A, Brodie's abscess in lower end of tibia (arrow). **B,** Brodie's abscess of third metatarsal. Note increased density and periosteal thickening of the entire metatarsal shaft.

on the roentgenogram. After surgical procedures have been carried out, the foot should be immobilized until the involucrum is able to withstand strain.

The regenerative power of bone in children is extraordinary; a bone that is nearly destroyed often will become completely regenerated and remodeled, but damage to the growth plate will result in shortening (Trueta, 1959).

Special types of osteomyelitis. Special types of osteomyelitis include Brodie's abscess and Garré's osteomyelitis.

Brodie's abscess. Under particular conditions of host resistance and altered bacterial virulence, the patient with hematogenous osteomyelitis may develop a localized intramedullary abscess that is walled off by reactive bone. Pain is associated with this developing abscess, but little systemic involvement exists. This condition, named

Brodie's abscess, is encountered five times as frequently in adolescent males as it is in the general population. In most of the reported cases, this abscess shows a predilection for the distal tibia. Roentgenograms will demonstrate a well-demarcated, punched-out lesion of the involved bone, with increased cortical density and periosteal thickening (Greenfield, 1969). Roentgenographic findings may not differentiate Brodie's abscess from enchondroma, osteoid osteoma, and bone cyst (Fig. 13-3).

The patient may have acute symptoms, or he may complain of having had mild discomfort for months. In long-standing cases a fusiform swelling may develop adjacent to the bone; the abscess may be sterile at the time of culture. Symptoms may persist for years and then gradually subside with the death of the invading bacteria. No statistics are available on untreated

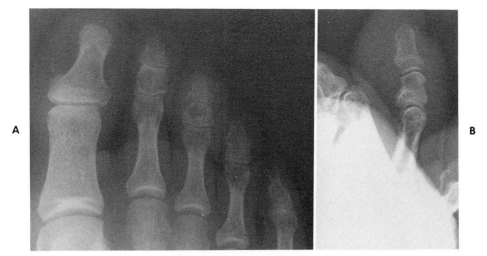

Fig. 13-4. Brodie's abscess invloving middle phalanx in foot of 17-year-old male. **A,** Anteroposterior view. **B,** Lateral view.

cases inasmuch as the diagnosis is only confirmed by treatment.

TREATMENT. Treatment of Brodie's abscess should include culture studies, excision of all necrotic material, and curettage of the bone. In cases in which no abscess is present, primary closure may be considered, but more often excision biopsy, with delayed secondary closure, is most effective. If a minor phalanx is involved, total phalangectomy may be advisable (Fig. 13-4).

Garrés osteomyelitis. In this form of subliminal osteomyelitis, a dense bone reaction occurs without abscess formation or suppuration. The exact reason for this occurrence is unknown. Some authors deny its existence in the antibiotic era (Aegerter and Kirkpatrick, 1968). It is thought to be caused by a low-grade embolic seeding that is transmitted by means of the blood or the lymphatic vessels. More often the tibia is involved, but the tubular bones of the foot may be affected (Fig. 13-5).

The onset of this form of osteomyelitis is either insidious, with pain and edema over the involved bone, or acute, with severe pain and systemic signs of toxicity. If only small bones are involved, the findings may be minimal.

Roentgenographic examination shows an increase in the density of bone trabeculation, as well as cortical thickening caused by periosteal new bone (Greenfield, 1969). A small tubular bone of the foot may become entirely involved in the process. This disease must be differentiated from osteoid osteoma and Paget's disease if the infectious process is localized to an area of a long tubular bone.

TREATMENT. The treatment of Garré's osteomyelitis consists of surgical excision of the dense cortical bone (to allow for medullary exposure), with curettement of any devitalized areas. In order to avoid exacerbation or the spread of infection, cultures should be obtained and antibiotic therapy should be initiated at the time surgical procedures are performed. Initial closure of the wound has been advised by some surgeons who have reported success with this method.

VASCULAR DISORDERS

Before describing particular vascular affections or dysfunctions, it is necessary to clarify the terms as they are presented here. *Aseptic necrosis* signifies bone death in the absence of infection. An *infarct* is an area of necrosis caused by local anemia from an obstruction of circulation (of any origin) to that particular region. *Epiphysitis* is an

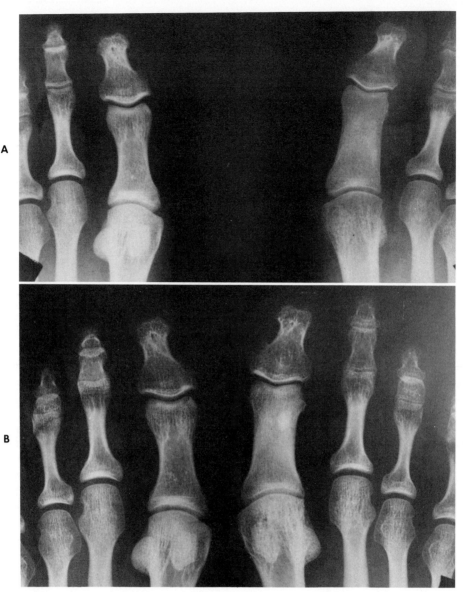

Fig. 13-5. A, Garré's osteomyelitis. *Left,* Normal foot for comparison. *Right,* Sclerosing and periosteal thickening of first proximal phalanx. **B,** One year later. Note the decrease in bone density and the disappearance of periosteal thickening.

inflammatory response of the epiphyseal bone. *Apophysitis* is an inflammatory response of a bony process related to and attached to a bone. *Osteochondrosis* signifies a disease (degeneration, necrosis) of the growth ossification centers, after which regeneration or recalcification occurs. *Osteochondritis* is simply an inflammatory response of bone and cartilage which occurs at any age. *Osteochondritis deformans juvenilis* implies a growth center and is an osteochondrosis; *juvenile deforming tarsal osteochondritis* is an osteochondrosis of the developing tarsal navicular. The above terms are often interchangeable. For example, osteochondritis deformans juvenilis (an

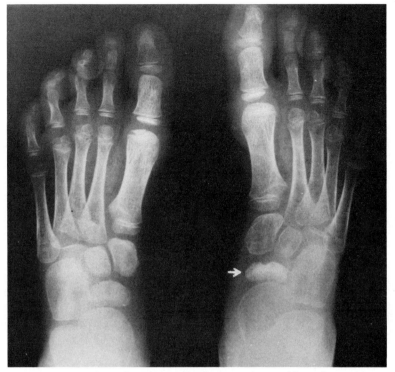

Fig. 13-6. Osteochondrosis of right navicular (Köhler's disease).

osteochondrosis), depending upon the particular ossification center involved, may also be termed an epiphysitis or apophysitis.

Present thinking implies a vascular etiology of these disorders; aseptic necrosis of the tarsal navicular may be the same entity as osteochondrosis or osteochondritis deformans juvenilis.

The osteochondroses

Because of the locomotor and weight-bearing functions of the foot, forces acting upon the growing bones will often play a part in the disruption of the blood supply to the various primary and secondary growth centers. These particular changes and their effect upon function, though often transient, have been given eponyms after those men who first observed and reported them.

Osteochondrosis of the tarsal navicular (Köhler's disease). The average age of onset of this affection of the developing navicular is 5 years. It is an avascular necrosis that is related to the peculiar circinate blood supply of the growing navicular (Waugh, 1958). It is currently thought that compression induces abnormal ossification at a critical stage in development (Fig. 13-6). Further compression from the formation of this additional bone results in the development of ischemia. Roentgenograms will demonstrate sclerotic bone, which resembles a coin or pancake. Reactive hyperemia follows sequentially, along with the development of pain, tenderness, and swelling. Because of the abundant blood supply, the regeneration of bone produces a normal adult tarsal navicular. Reports of the persistence of deformity are rare.

The treatment of osteochondrosis of the tarsal navicular is supportive. Some children experience intense pain, while others may have only vague discomfort. Pain may be reduced by means of plaster immobili-

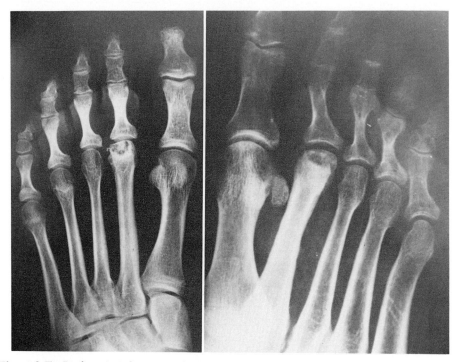

Fig. 13-7. Freiberg's infraction of second metatarsal head in active state, showing sequestration.

zation or a regimen of decreased weight bearing. As has been indicated, the disease is self-limited.

Osteochondrosis of the metatarsal head (Freiberg's infraction). Infraction, meaning incomplete fracture, is not truly an applicable term for this disorder, which is also called Köhler's second disease and, in Europe, Panner's disease. It usually occurs in the head of the second metatarsal and is also an avascular necrosis. Freiberg's infraction most often appears in the second decade of life and is characterized by local tenderness and pain in the area adjacent to the affected bone.

As with other osteochondroses, incidental trauma to the primary growth center at a significant stage of development is thought to cause vascular deprivation and secondary changes. Because the second toe is usually the longest one, it is subject to pressure on its long axis from the wearing of shoes. If this pressure occurs during a critical phase of epiphyseal matura-

tion, an osteochondrosis of this epiphysis may result (Braddock, 1959).

The diagnosis of this disorder, which must be differentiated from a stress fracture, is made roentgenographically (Figs. 13-7 and 13-8). The roentgenogram will show osteosclerosis in the early stages and osteolysis in later stages. Symptoms may vary widely.

The treatment of this disease is directed toward protection and the alleviation of discomfort by various means, including the limitation of activity and the use of a plaster walking cast. In response to healing, excessive bone may develop on the plantar surface of the involved metatarsal head. Instances of surgical intervention to alleviate secondary bone overgrowth have been reported.

Osteochondrosis of the calcaneal apophysis (Sever's disease). This disease is an apophysitis or avascular necrosis of the traction apophysis of the heel (Fig. 13-9). Again, direct trauma from weight bearing

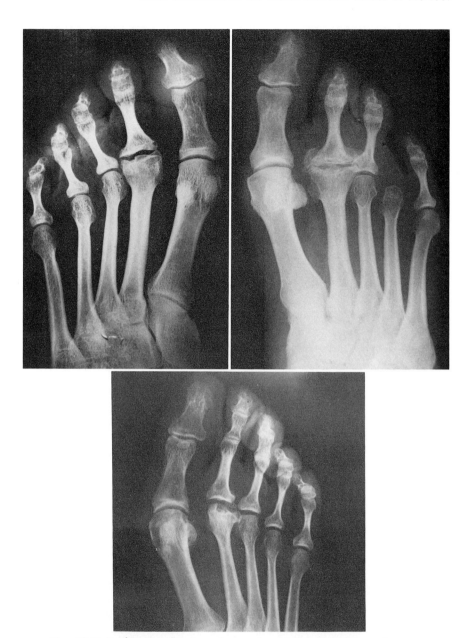

Fig. 13-8. Freiberg's infraction of second metatarsal head in static state.

and the pull of the tendo achillis insertion are thought to be causative factors. It occurs in school-age children bilaterally at times. Its clinical manifestations are progressive heel pain, local tenderness, and antalgic gait.

An initial roentgenogram of the involved apophysis will demonstrate sclerosis and fragmentation. An x-ray taken after res-

olution of the condition will show decreased bone density and atrophy. The epiphyseal line will be irregular. Some patients without this disorder show similar roentgenographic changes but have no symptoms.

Treatment is directed toward protection and the relief of pain and may include decreased physical activity, the wearing of

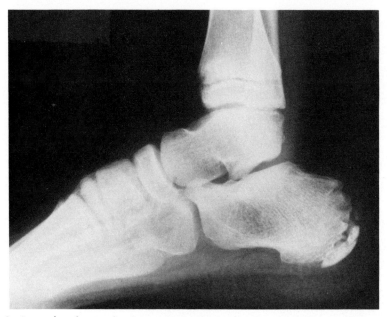

Fig. 13-9. Osteochondrosis of calcaneal apophysis in a 14-year-old boy. Note increased density of the apophysis as well as fragmentation.

sandals, or rigid immobilization. Often a heel pad to hold the foot in equinus is used.

Osteochondrosis of the fifth metatarsal head, the tibial sesamoid of the first metatarsal, the cuboid, the cuneiform, and the talus occur less commonly (Fig. 13-10). In these sites the clinical findings and the aims of treatment are similar.

Aseptic and avascular necrosis; bone infarct

As has been stated, aseptic necrosis refers to the process of bone death in the absence of infection. Aseptic necrosis is an end result; avascular necrosis implies a more distinct cause. If avascular necrosis occurs in a solitary primary growth center, it is classified as an osteochondrosis. At the time of onset, the involved bone exhibits decreased vascularity, marrow necrosis, and at times, calcific deposit on the medullary interstices. The bone becomes roentgenographically dense (with or without fragmentation) in contrast to the remaining bones, which may show signs of osteoporosis of disuse (Aegerter and Kirk-

patrick, 1968). New bone, with a return of reparative vascular invasion and new bone apposition, later causes the roentgenographic picture to change. The bone has a moth-eaten appearance and becomes atrophic with the invasion of granulation tissue, while the new bone apposition causes greater density (Bobechko and Harris, 1960). In the event that many bones are affected with aseptic necrosis, a complete metabolic investigation must be carried out in order to rule out the presence of systemic disease. Care must be taken not to mistake aseptic necrosis for a tumor.

Avascular necrosis of the bones of the foot may occur secondary to trauma, particularly if fracture or dislocation has occurred and the blood supply has been interrupted (Fig. 13-11). The fractured talus is especially vulnerable to aseptic necrosis (see Chapter 6).

In cases of avascular necrosis that cannot be ascribed to metabolic, infectious, or traumatic causes, congenital factors have been cited as etiologic agents. Shaw (1954) reported a particular case of avascular necrosis in which progressive destruction

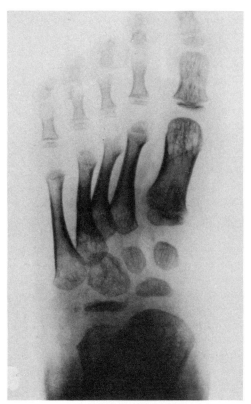

Fig. 13-10. Osteochondrosis of cuboid. (From Khoo, F. Y.: J. Bone Joint Surg. **32-B:**230, 1950.)

of one or more phalanges occurred in six generations of one family. "Idiopathic" avascular necrosis of the metatarsal heads and tarsal bones has been encountered, but reports of such cases are rare (Fig. 13-12).

No rationale exists to explain the arrest of this condition. Except for rare cases in which destruction is permanent, treatment by supportive measures is indicated.

The term "bone infarct" designates a region of circulatory deprivation of bone. It may occur in the metaphyseal or diaphyseal region of a tubular bone and may be asymptomatic. Both bone infarct and aseptic necrosis may describe the same condition.

Osteochondritis

Osteochondritis indicates disruption of the blood supply to mature bone adjacent to cartilage. Trauma, caisson disease, embolism, arteritis obliterans, and heritable predisposing factors may be implicated as causes of osteochondritis (Figs. 13-13 and 13-14). In the event that conditions of osteochondritis cause disruption of the nor-

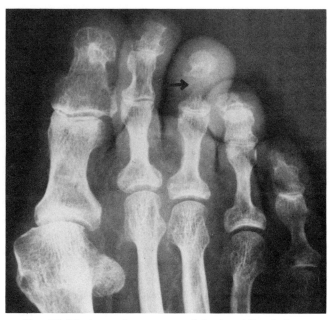

Fig. 13-11. Avascular necrosis of third middle phalanx.

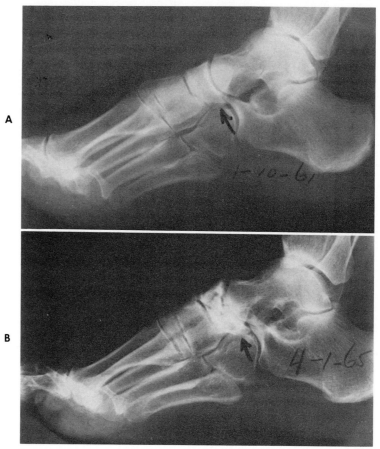

Fig. 13-12. Avascular necrosis of navicular in 42-year-old woman. In 1961, she complained of pain in the talonavicular joint. **A,** Roentgenogram taken at that time. No osseous changes. **B,** Roentgenogram taken 4 years later. Extensive dissolution of this bone had occurred. No underlying cause could be found.

mal continuity of the adjacent convex articular surface of subchondral bone, an osteochondritis dissecans develops (Stillman, 1966).

The talus is the bone of the foot that is most vulnerable to osteochondritis (Figs. 13-15 and 13-16). Berndt and Harty (1959), in a summary of 183 cases, concluded that osteochondritis dissecans of the talus (Fig. 13-15, *B*) most often occurred after transchondral fracture that was initially misdiagnosed or unrecognized or did not immediately appear roentgenographically. Vascular impairment was believed to be perpetuated by the constant shearing of joint action. The ensuing capillary frac-

ture, with failure to revascularize, impeded the normal process of healing. The ultimate result of an unhealed transchondral fractured fragment of the talus is chronic synovitis, which, combined with laxity of the ligaments, will result in ankle-joint degeneration.

Roentgenographic examination, along with the patient's history of recurrent ankle sprain and previous symptoms, confirms the diagnosis. In view of the poor results obtained from conservative measures, treatment of this disorder should be surgical. Even for children surgical extirpation or replacement and fixation of the fragment is advised.

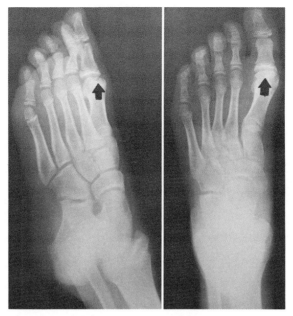

Fig. 13-13. Osteochondritis of left first metatarsal head in foot of 13-year-old female. Her parents had forced her to toe-dance for the 3 previous years.

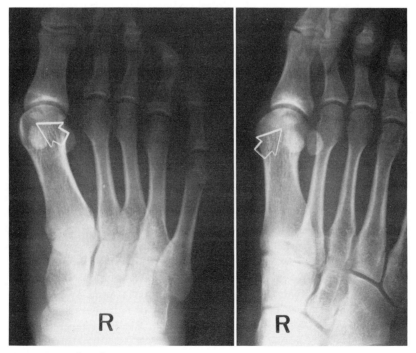

Fig. 13-14. Osteochondritis of first metatarsal head in foot of 15-year-old female. Note threatening sequestration.

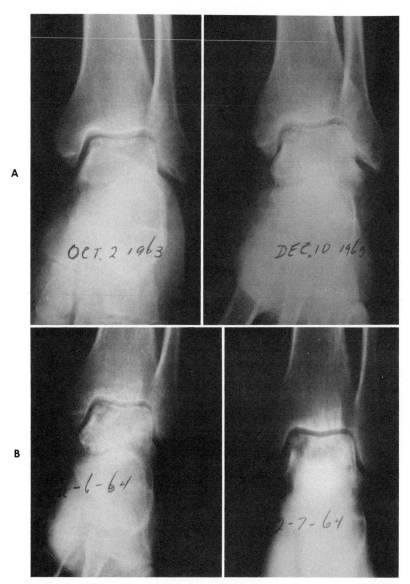

Fig. 13-15. Roentgenograms of ankle of 44-year-old man. In an accident the right foot
was caught, and there was complete inversion ("The bottom of my foot was parallel to
my inner ankle, and I twisted it back in place"). This implies avulsion of the talus and
tearing of the collateral malleolar ligaments. **A,** Roentgenogram taken October 2, 1963.
Left, Negative findings. *Right,* December 10, 1963. Definite evidence of a crushing injury to the trochlear surface of the talus at the medial malleolus. **B,** Roentgenogram
taken February 6, 1964. *Left,* Full-blown osteochondritis dissecans. *Right,* A tomogram of
the same area taken February 7, 1964.

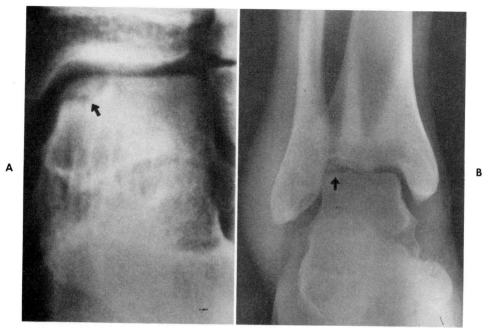

Fig. 13-16. A, Osteochondritis of trochlear surface of talus on tibial side in 13-year-old girl. Note complete separation of bone fragment. **B,** Osteochondritis of trochlear surface of talus on fibular side. Note the edema resulting from it.

TUMOROUS CONDITIONS OF THE SOFT TISSUES AND BONES OF THE FOOT

In this section abnormalities of the cellular derivatives of mesodermal tissue will be stressed. Primary bone tumors are tumors, or neoplasms, comprised of mesodermal tissue elements, which potentially may form any of the component parts of mature bone, with or without further aberrations.

Here again, in classifying tumors, one encounters a problem with nomenclature, for in the past each pathologist created his own particular scheme of classification. Now, under the aegis of F. Schajowicz and the World Health Organization, an effort is being made to institute a common nomenclature. When such world-wide standardization is established, a given name will designate one distinct and specific entity to all pathologists. It is hoped that this effort will soon be completed. Because of the very low incidence of bone tumors (as compared with other neoplasms), the ne-

cessity for the study of bone tumors that relates to a world population is obvious.

Benign tumors of the soft tissues

Fibroma. A fibroma is a tumor of organized, mature, fibrous tissue. It is characterized by mature spindle-shaped cells in whorls, sheets, and bands, which may not be well encapsulated. It is important to differentiate a fibroma from a fibrous reaction to a foreign body. A simple fibroma may occur in any mesenchymal tissue. Variations of fibromas are encountered in the foot, which include keloids, plantar fibromatosis, and neurofibromas.

Keloid. Keloid is the name ascribed to a hypertrophic cutaneous scar in which the normal glandular cutaneous elements are replaced by thin collagen bundles and larger fibroblasts (see also Chapter 12). Some keloids that are associated with skin ulceration and osteomyelitic sinus tracts may undergo carcinomatous degeneration, but most dermal keloids are benign.

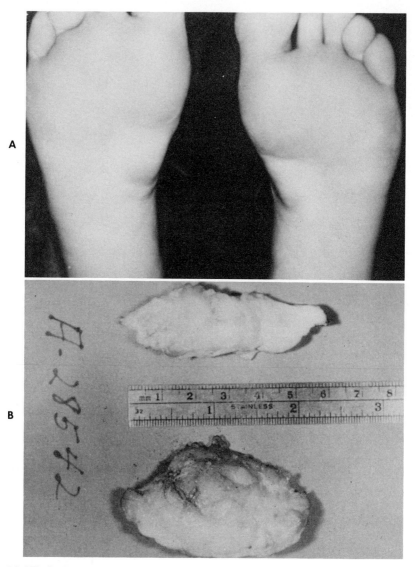

Fig. 13-17. A, Recurrent massive fibromatosis (Dupuytren's contracture) on both feet. **B,** Gross specimen excised. **C,** Postoperative appearance.

Preventive gamma radiation is used in the treatment of keloids. In patients who are known to form keloids, intralesional steroid injection should be used after surgical procedures are performed. Complete excision of the keloid scar will be succeeded by the formation of another keloid and is not advised. A large mature keloid may be removed if the excision is limited to the margin of the fibrous area without encroachment on the normal skin.

Plantar fibromatosis. Plantar fibromatosis, the analogue of proliferative fasciitis of Dupuytren in the hand, is often present but unrecognized in the foot. Fibroblastic collagen proliferation may lead to cutaneous dimpling and progressive encroachment around the tendon sheaths, with secondary flexion contracture and deformity (Figs. 13-17 and 13-18). Fig. 13-19 shows an unusual fibromatosis of the tendo achillis.

C

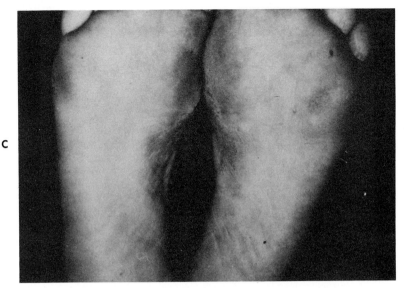

Fig. 13-17, cont'd. For legend see opposite page.

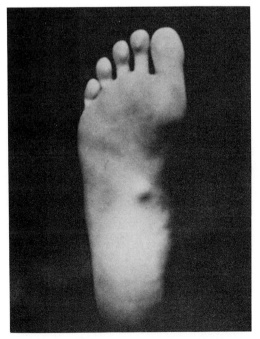

Fig. 13-18. Fibromatosis of plantar fascia in adolescent.

TREATMENT. Local anti-inflammatory steroid injections have proved beneficial in the treatment of nodular lesions in the early stages. Treatment consists of division or excision of the fibroma, depending upon the extent of the involvement (Stoyle, 1964).

TECHNIQUE FOR EXCISION. Pedersen and Day (1954) admonished that unless the entire mass is completely excised, the disease tends to recur.

1. Make an incision along the medioplantar border of the first metatarsal shaft extending to the navicular.
2. Retract the skin, exposing the plantar fascia.
3. Completely excise the mass, which incorporates the fascia in most instances.
4. If a large area of the plantar skin has to be freed, suture it with subdermal catgut to the remaining tissue to avoid hematoma formation.
5. A compression bandage restricts subdermal bleeding. Release the compression in 24 hours and permit the patient to begin mild weight bearing

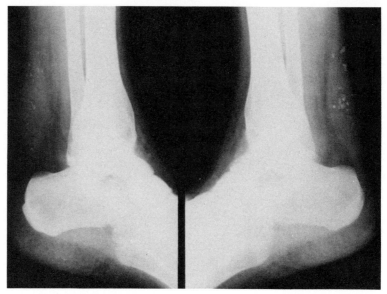

Fig. 13-19. Fibromatosis of tendo achillis with calcification.

on the seventh to the twenty-first post-operative day.

Neurofibroma. Neurofibroma is a proliferation of the fibrous supportive elements of a peripheral nerve. Although they are more often associated with systemic neurofibromatosis, isolated neurofibromas do occur (see Chapter 14, p. 413). The patient will complain of a nodular growth, superficial or deep, that is painful because of its proximity to the nerve.

Excision biopsy will demonstrate nerve fasciculi and increased fibroblastic proliferation of mature perineural supportive fibrous tissue.

Lipoma. Among benign tumors of soft tissue lipomas occur with the greatest frequency and are painless unless secondary pressure is exerted on the adjacent structures. Clinically, a superficial lipoma appears as a soft mass with a characteristic firm, rubber-like consistency. Intramuscular lipomas occur less frequently. Roentgenograms may demonstrate radiolucency, and central calcification has been reported (Greenfield, 1969).

Histologically, a lipoma is an encapsulated mass of mature fat cells with its own vascular stalk. Under conditions of starvation and glyconeogenesis, a loss of body fat will ensue but a lipoma will not decrease in size.

Variations of lipoma include hibernoma, a rare tumor of special fat cells, and lipomatosis associated with Maffucci's syndrome. The treatment of a symptomatic lipoma is excision. Histologic sections will show organized mature fat cells in a well-defined capsule.

"Giant cell" tumors of the tendon sheath. These tumors are xanthomas, which are frequently encountered in tendon sheaths about the fingers, but also occur in the ankles and feet (Jones et al., 1969). These benign tumors are thought to originate from the synovial lining of the sheath (Eisenstein, 1968). The tumors grow slowly; symptoms appear because of the size of the tumors and the pressure they exert on adjacent structures. Recent investigations have produced reports of erosion and invasion of bone in some cases; malignant degeneration does not characteristically occur (Ackerman and Spjut, 1962). Microscopic sections of these well-encapsulated tumors will demonstrate the presence of numerous giant cells in pleomorphic fibrous connective tissue and areas of histiocytes that are richly laden with varying amounts of lipid. The treatment of this tumor is excision.

Pigmented villinodular synovitis. Pigmented villinodular synovitis is another tumor of the mesenchymal-synovial lining of joints. Because of decreased pressure, the tumor tissue may expand into a joint cavity with finger-like projections. In addition to synovial hypertrophy with fibroplasia, lipoid histiocytosis, giant cells, and extracellular and intracellular hemosiderin deposits are prominent features. Pigmented villinodular synovitis occurs mainly in the knee, although some instances of the tumor in the ankle and calcaneocuboid joints have been reported (Ackerman and Spjut, 1962).

Symptoms of pigmented villinodular synovitis are loss of joint function, instability, and enlargement of the joint. Roentgenographic examination may show destruction of bone. The treatment of this tumor is total synovectomy.

Ganglion. A ganglion is an enlarging mucoid fibrous cyst originating in the degenerative vacuoles of the connective tissue adjacent to the lining of a joint or to a tendon sheath. It has been thought to be an extension of the joint itself, probably erroneously, since no communication could be demonstrated to exist (King, 1932; Soren, 1966).

Recently, however, Andrén and Eiken (1971), by arthrographic techniques, were able to demonstrate a tract or duct communicating between the ganglion and joint in over half of the wrist joints studied. It was postulated that a valve mechanism acts to "pump up" the ganglion, causing progressive enlargement, which may explain the necessity for adequate treatment at the time of excision.

Ganglia are most often encountered at the wrist and on the dorsum of the hand; the dorsum of the foot is the next most frequent site. Ganglion cysts of the tendon sheaths about the ankle are common, and they may appear as painless swellings that interfere with shoe comfort. The cyst is soft and can be deformed; it may spontaneously rupture and later recur. Trauma to a ganglion may cause hemorrhage into the cyst, with sudden increase of pain. In these cases diagnosis may be difficult.

To treat ganglion cysts effectively, one must understand their composition. Microscopic examination of the originating basal fibrous tissue adjacent to the cyst will demonstrate numerous small vacuoles and clefts. The cyst accumulates mucinoid material. It enlarges both by direct growth and by the aggregation of other small cystic areas, and it will extend around and deform nerves, arteries, and veins. Needle aspiration may be used for diagnostic purposes. If the aspirate is honey-like, multiple punctures and tearing of the cyst wall may evoke healing by ingrowth of granulation tissue, but recurrence in 70 percent of cases is to be anticipated.

Treatment by excision. All areas of cystic degeneration must be removed, including the fibrous tissue of origin at the base of the cyst. The recommended technique is as follows: An incision is made immediately over the mass. If the ganglion is under a weight-bearing surface, the incision is made on the side of the foot closest to the growth and the ganglion is gently freed from the surrounding tissue. During dissection the sac may rupture, expelling its contents into the wound. In such cases the sac should be grasped, its course followed to its origin, and the sac excised. It may be difficult to follow the course of a ganglion that occurs in a metatarsal interspace. This may necessitate an extended incision or a second incision to extirpate the entire ganglion, as well as a large portion of the base and capsule as necessary. If a small lobe or its source is allowed to remain, usually the condition will recur. All dead spaces left by removal of the ganglion must be obliterated by subdermal suturing. A compression bandage is then applied.

Angioma. Angiomas of the feet are rare. They are tumors of the supportive elements of blood vessels, which may be hamartomatous or neoplastic in origin. Hemangiomas may occur in any tissue. They grow in proportion to the growth of the tissue in which they originate. Hemangiomas more frequently involve muscle or skin; in the latter, the classic port wine stain results. Roentgenograms of larger angiomas may show calcified phleboliths.

Variations of tumors of the supportive tissue of blood vessels are hemangioendothelioma and hemangiopericytoma; which of these tumors will form depends upon the particular element that is undergoing neoplasia. The treatment of angioma is local excision.

Glomus tumor is a variation of vascular supportive element neoplasia, which involves pericytic regulation of the blood flow in normal arteriovenous anastomosis (see also Chapter 12). These tumors are very painful, are often found in the skin of the extremities, and may cause reflex sympathetic dystrophy. Frequently the digits of the hands and feet, particularly the nail beds, are sites of involvement (Smyth, 1971). Erosion of the distal phalanx may occur from pressure. Excision biopsy provides dramatic relief.

Malignant tumors of the soft tissues

Fibrosarcoma. This malignant tumor is of fibrous tissue origin. It may occur at any age, but does so more frequently after the third decade of life. The incidence of fibrosarcoma is 2 percent. It appears as a firm, usually painless mass; its degree of malignancy varies. Histologically, some of these tumors may show plump primitive cell nuclei that bear little similarity to the cells of mature fibrous tissue; others may show spindle cells, with minimal variation from the normal cell. The appearance of multiple mitotic figures, along with minimal collagen organization and poor differentiation, are unfavorable histologic findings. Cystic degeneration and hemorrhage may be characteristic, as well as necrosis and myxomatous change.

Because of the frequency of its local recurrence and later metastasis, this tumor, after biopsy, should be treated by en bloc resection or ablation (Jaffe, 1958). Compared with some mesenchymal sarcomas, fibrosarcoma grows slowly.

Synovioma (synovial sarcoma). The term "synovioma" implies sarcoma of the mesenchymal cells of joints, bursae, and tendon sheaths. It may occur at any age, but the majority of reported cases are in young adults. The knee joint is the joint that is affected predominantly, but involvement of the ankle and the tarsal bones occurs with significant frequency (Stening, 1968). The initial complaint may be an uncomfortable lump that increases in size. These tumors are often mistaken for ganglia; thus, a roentgenographic study is advised before surgical extirpation of any lesion adjacent to a joint is carried out. In the differential diagnosis, spotty calcification may indicate chondroma or hemangioma, as well as synovioma.

Histologic examination will demonstrate malignant fibrous tissue (fibrosarcoma) and anaplastic, plump, synovial tissue cells, which at times appear glandular but are without a true basement membrane. This characteristic differentiates synovioma from pigmented villinodular synovitis. Moreover, only rarely are synoviomas found to occur within the joint space.

The treatment of this tumor must be wide ablation. The mortality rate for persons with this lesion is high, perhaps because of prolonged delay in diagnosis and inadequate initial treatment (Fig. 13-20).

Kaposi's sarcoma (angiosarcoma). The angiosarcoma of Kaposi deserves attention because of its predilection for the skin of the feet and hands, particularly the great toe (Lewis, 1967). This angiosarcoma begins with the appearance of multiple painful red-purple subcutaneous nodules that measure up to 1 cm. in diameter (Fig. 13-21). The lesions may be telangiectatic or verrucose. The tumor enlarges slowly and may cause lymphatic obstruction and edema. Because of the slow growth of this tumor, wide resection with grafting and roentgen treatment provide successful arrest.

Benign tumors and cysts of bone

Because of its weight-bearing function, the foot is subjected to irritation, pressure,

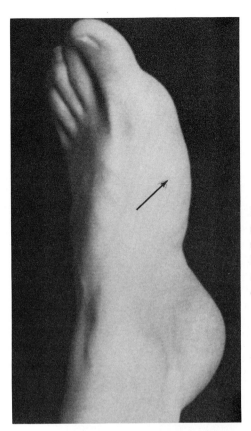

Fig. 13-20. Photograph of foot of 51-year-old man. He noted painless swelling under first metatarsal, increasing gradually for 6 months. It proved to be a synovioma. Four months after above-knee amputation, metastasis to the lungs occurred.

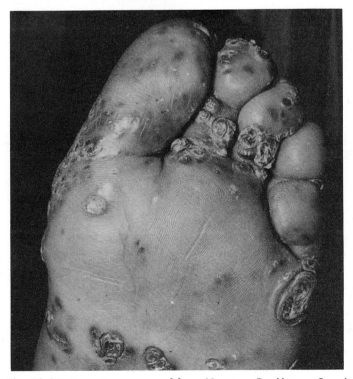

Fig. 13-21. Kaposi's sarcoma of foot. (Courtesy Dr. Marcus Caro.)

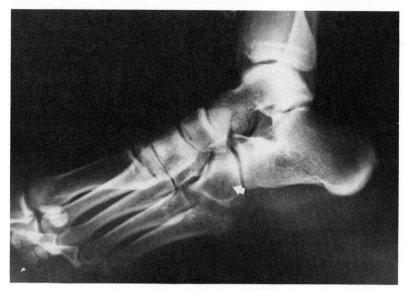

Fig. 13-22. Solitary cyst of cuboid.

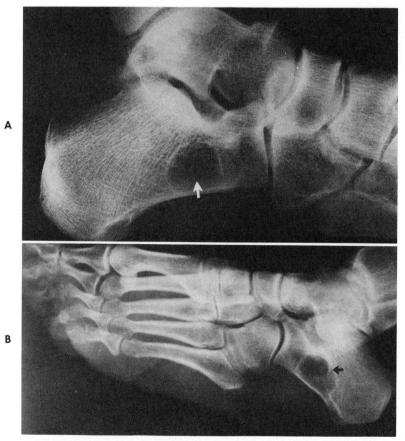

A

B

Fig. 13-23. A, Solitary cyst of calcaneus. **B,** Solitary cyst of calcaneus. Symptomatic.

and repeated strain, and it is often the site of abnormal reactive bone formation. Every abnormal bone mass that appears on the foot should be evaluated.

A cyst of bone is defined as an area that does not contain metaplastic cellular elements; its trabeculation and medullary composition are abnormal. If it is large enough, the cyst may cause cortical thinning and expansion. Fluid may or may not be present. What appears to be a cystic neoplasm on a roentgenogram may in reality be a myxoid fibroma, enchondroma, or other solid tumor. It is well to keep in mind that the diagnosis of bone lesions can be established only by biopsy. Statistics of probability are of academic interest, but they are of little value in the diagnosis of a solitary bone lesion.

Simple bone cyst. Simple bone cysts (unicameral cysts) may occur in all of the bones of the foot (Figs. 13-22 and 13-23). The more typical cyst appears in tubular bone of the metaphysis adjacent to the epiphyseal line. With growth, the cyst will move away from the growth plate and become latent (Jaffe, 1958).

The simple cyst is thought to originate from either a developmental failure of central enchondral ossification or an imperfect vascular function with secondary hemorrhage; or it may occur from both these abnormalities. Cysts of the tarsal bones in the mature foot may also be related to developmental failure.

A simple bone cyst may be asymptomatic. Microfracture and pain may occur if the cyst is present in an area of bone that is subject to repeated strain. Roentgenograms demonstrate sharp demarcation, with or without reactive sclerosis. The microscopic findings of a cellular tumor, with giant cells lining the thin cyst wall, should not cause confusion with giant cell tumor. The giant cell tumor consists of more tumor tissue, and unlike the simple bone cyst, does not contain a large cavity. It is important to differentiate between the simple bone cyst and local rarefaction caused by infection and nonosteogenic metaplasia.

Treatment of the simple bone cyst consists of curettement of the lining and the establishment of medullary continuity, with bone grafting if necessary during the inactive phase.

Aneurysmal bone cyst. This neoplasm, actually a tumor and not a cyst, is an eccentric expansile neoplasm of bone that is named for its characteristic bubble-like roentgenographic appearance (Fig. 13-24). The majority of these tumors occur in the first, second, and third decades of life. They are usually encountered in the metaphyseal area of tubular bones and in the vertebral column, but they may appear in any bone. The symptoms vary in severity from local discomfort to severe pain and abnormal gait, depending upon the area involved; secondary atrophy may occur.

In the years before 1950, much confusion existed between giant cell tumor and vascular cystic giant cell tumor. Many reports of parostealcystic giant cell tumors that appeared in the literature from 1940 to 1950 were actually reports about aneurysmal bone cyst (Lichtenstein, 1950). The microscopic picture of an aneurysmal bone cyst, with its fibrous tissue and multiple vascular clefts or channels into which giant cells seem to protrude and break off, would tend to promote the idea that this lesion is malignant, but it is actually benign. Unlike giant cell tumor, the aneurysmal bone cyst rarely recurs.

The treatment of aneurysmal bone cyst is local excision and bone grafting, if needed. A characteristic of this tumor is marked venous bleeding from the tumor at the time of biopsy.

Osteochondroma and exostosis. These terms are not synonymous. An exostosis is any outcropping or protrusion of bone, while an osteochondroma appears only in bones preformed in cartilage; it is localized to the juxtaepiphyseal region.

Osteochondroma. Osteochondroma is a protrusion of bone covered by a cartilage cap, which continues to grow until epiphyseal enchondral growth is complete (Figs. 13-25 and 13-26). Osteochondroma is

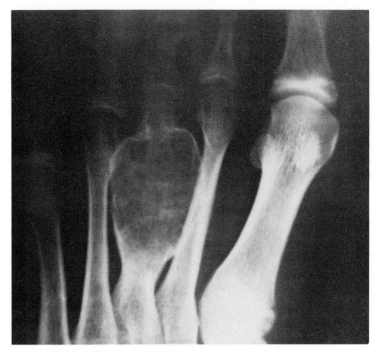

Fig. 13-24. Aneurysmal bone cyst of third metatarsal.

caused by local failure of remodeling, periosteal malfunction, or both; it is the most common benign tumor of bone (Ackerman and Spjut, 1962).

Not all osteochondromas need to be excised, but excision is advisable for those that occur in areas of the foot that are vulnerable to local pressure from the shoe or for those that demonstrate sudden growth. To avoid recurrence, the part excised should include a broad portion of the base. Of all osteochondromas, only 1 percent undergo malignant transformation.

Subungual exostosis of the great toe. Subungual exostosis of the great toe may be classified somewhere between an osteochondroma and a simple exostosis. A cartilaginous cap is present, which gives the subungual tumor an irregular mushroom shape. In spite of its cartilage cap, the subungual exostosis is not related to the epiphyseal line that appears in the proximal portion of the distal phalanx. Another type of exostosis without a cartilaginous cap may be found in the distal phalanges. This exos-

tosis is smoother in appearance. Both forms may cause chronic irritation and pain, which may lead to secondary hypertrophy and nail changes.

Exostoses occur at any age, while osteochondromas develop in children and young adults. The lesser toes may be affected by subungual exostosis, but incidence in these sites is minimal. Roentgenograms will confirm the clincal suspicion of this disorder (Fig. 13-27 and 13-28). The treatment of subungual exostosis is excision.

Exostosis. Exostosis is a bone outcropping that occurs in mature bone and is engendered by mechanical factors, irritation, or trauma. Congenital nonenchondral exostoses have been reported. Exostoses of the talus, heel spurs (see Chapter 8), and pump bumps (see Chapter 7) are types of true exostosis. Exostosis may occur in any of the tarsal bones as well as in the metatarsals and phalanges. It may develop in relation to trauma, or it may be secondary to continual irritation. Exostoses of diseased joints are often found on the dorsal

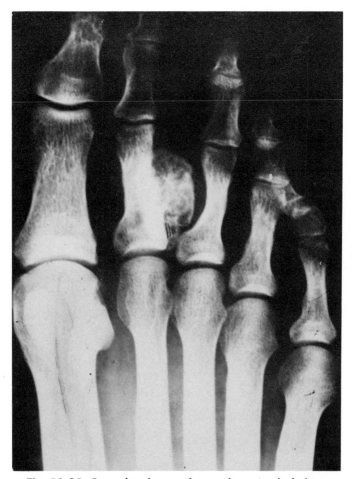

Fig. 13-25. Osteochondroma of second proximal phalanx.

surface of the foot; they may be symptomatic and require excision. Roentgenograms will readily confirm their presence (Figs. 13-29 through 13-34).

The phalangeal metaphyseal area adjacent to the articular surface may enlarge and reactive skin change may occur, producing a soft corn (heloma molle). I have found treatment by "cutaneous syndactylism" (the Kelikian procedure) to be successful.

Osteoid osteoma. This tumor, first described in 1935 by Jaffe, is benign. It is most often cortical or subcortical and is considered to be caused by vascular aberration. It may occur in any region of any bone but occurs with greatest frequency in long tubular bones, particularly in the tibia. The symptoms include mild pain, antalgic gait, and muscular atrophy. The pain is difficult to localize and is often deep, although local tenderness of the bone over the lesion may be present. Night pain relieved by salicylates is considered by some practitioners to be an important diagnostic feature of this tumor, but in my experience this characteristic is not a constant one.

Roentgenographic examination will confirm the presence of this tumor. It appears as a dense area of sclerotic bone with cortical thickening if it is cortical, or as a sclerotic bone island if it is medullary. At the center of this sclerotic bone, a radiolucent nidus may be seen. Tomograms may be used to localize the nidus. Care must be

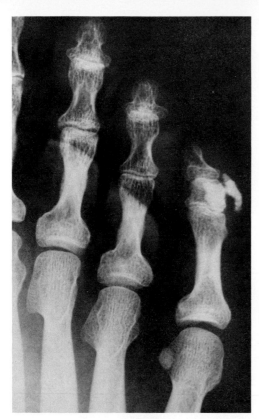

Fig. 13-26. Osteochondroma adjacent to fifth middle phalanx.

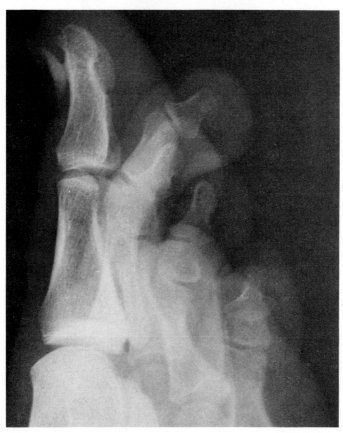

Fig. 13-27. Anvil-shaped subungual exostosis.

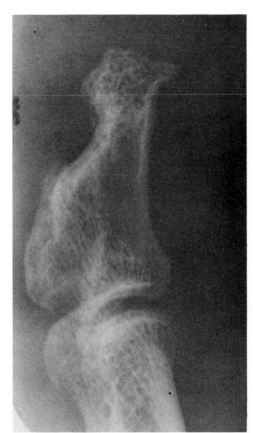

Fig. 13-28. Subungual exostosis at tip of phalanx.

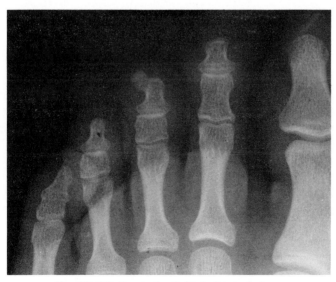

Fig. 13-29. Exostosis of third distal phalanx.

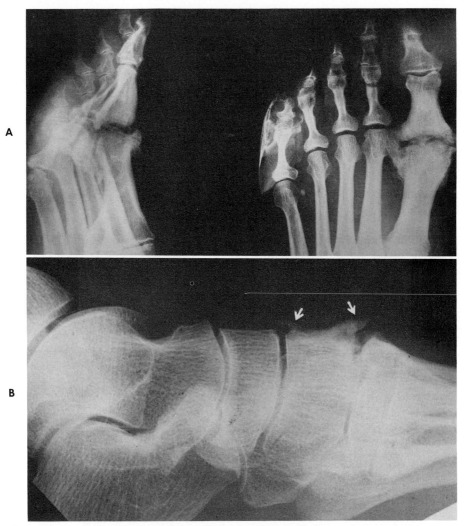

Fig. 13-30. A, Traumatic arthritis of first metatarsophalangeal joint (hallux rigidus), showing extensive reactive bone proliferation. **B,** Traumatic arthritis of first metatarsal–first cuneiform articulation.

taken to differentiate between an osteoid osteoma and a bone island, which has no demonstrable nidus.

The treatment of osteoid osteoma is excision. Rare recurrences have been reported, but these reappearances may be the result of incomplete removal. A roentgenogram of the excised specimen will confirm the adequacy of extirpation. Pathologic examination by microscope will show the central nidus of the osteoid osteoma to consist of vascular, new, woven bone. Here again, the fate of untreated osteoid osteomas is unknown, since the diagnosis is confirmed by treatment. Poulsen (1969) reported successful bloc resection of an osteoid osteoma of the talus.

Osteoblastoma. This tumor, which appears in the first, second, and third decades of life, is described as a giant osteoid osteoma. It occurs most often in the axial skeleton and is less common in the bones of the foot. The talus has been cited as one of the common extra-axial sites (Giannestras and Diamond, 1958; Cowie, 1966).

Roentgenograms show destruction sug-

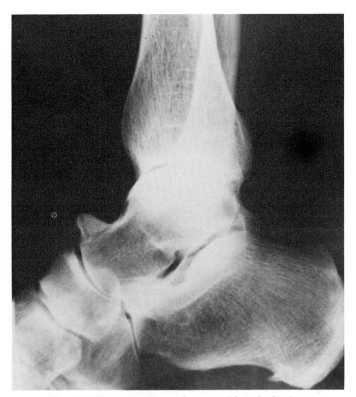

Fig. 13-31. Exostosis on dorsum of head of talus.

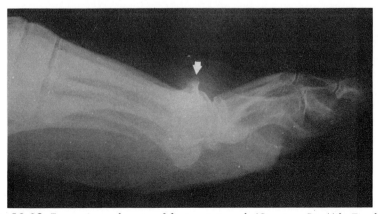

Fig. 13-32. Exostosis on dorsum of first metatarsal. (Courtesy Dr. Milo Turnbo.)

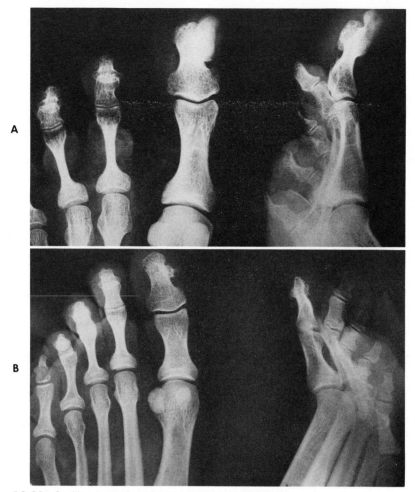

Fig. 13-33. A, Massive subungual exostosis on tibial side of distal phalanx. **B,** Small subungual exostosis on tibial side of distal phalanx.

gestive of malignancy, with new bone formation and extension; thus, it is a tumor that may be mistakenly diagnosed as malignant. The treatment of osteoblastoma is curettement or excision, with bone grafting when it is indicated.

Chondroma. This neoplasm is the most common mesodermal tumor of bone encountered in the foot. More often the chondroma is a type of medullary enchondroma, rather than a parosteal chondroma. Soft-tissue involvement in synovial chondromatosis is rarely encountered.

The solitary enchondroma is seldom painful. It is usually discovered between the second and fifth decades of life, com-

monly in roentgenograms taken after pathologic fracture of the involved bone has occurred. The tarsal bones and the phalanges are the most common sites of this tumor.

The treatment of chondroma is excision, biopsy, and bone grafting. Microscopic tissue examination of a peripheral enchondroma may demonstrate pleomorphism, nests of daughter cells, and other characteristics of a more aggressive tumor. If the site were the ilium, it would be classified as a low-grade sarcoma.

Parosteal chondroma can produce symptoms because its size may impair function. Differential diagnosis between an osteochondroma and a chondroma is shown by

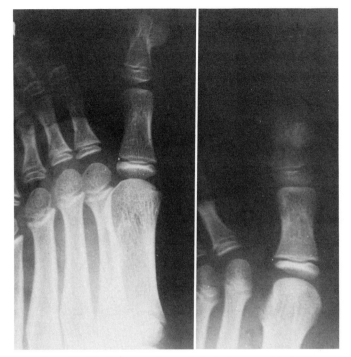

Fig. 13-34. Subungual exostosis in 8-year-old child.

roentgenogram; the former appears as a bone base or stalk, while the latter appears as cartilage with calcification. Chondroma is thought to arise from an aberrant cell rest.

Chondroblastoma. Roentgenograms of this tumor, an affection of growing bones, will show erosion and eccentric destruction. It is important to differentiate between this tumor and giant cell tumor, for the treatment of giant cell tumor must be aggressive, while the treatment of chondroblastoma is simple curettement. A recent large series (Schajowicz and Gallardo, 1971) included reports of several chondroblastomas of the tarsal bones.

Chondromyxoid fibroma. This affection is another cartilage tumor common to the bones of the foot and consists of both cartilage and myxoid cellular elements. It may cause fusiform enlargement of the involved tarsal bone and it may be painful. Roentgenographic findings are an eccentric, well-demarcated, clear area of bone loss, which is circinate and without calcification (Fig.

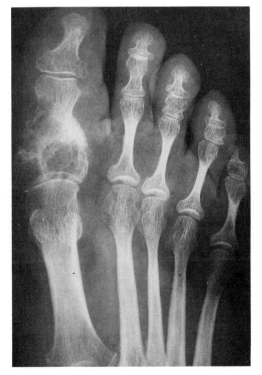

Fig. 13-35. Chondromyxoma of first proximal phalanx. (Courtesy Dr. James Brightwell.)

13-35). Because of its marked cellular variation of cartilage nests and nuclear pleomorphism and its immature mesenchymal tissue in adjacent areas, this tumor has sometimes been misdiagnosed as a sarcoma, with tragic consequences. The possibility of this error must be kept in mind during microscopic examination of this tumor. Successful treatment of the benign chondromyxoid fibroma is curettement.

Benign tumors beneath the nail. The *glomus tumor* (see p. 350 and Chapter 12) is an epithelioid tumor of nerve element. Usually, the glomus body is found in an area adjacent to an arteriovenous anastomosis in the peripheral circulation; it serves to alter the flow of blood. Perhaps after trauma has occurred, glomus bodies enlarge and may encroach upon bone to produce local erosion. The common site is beneath the nail. The pain may be exquisite, with attendant sympathetic radiation. In an altered heat/cold environment, reflex vascular changes may occur. The treatment of glomus tumor is excision biopsy.

The *epidermoid inclusion cyst,* which commonly occurs in the distal phalanges, may be mistaken for an enchondroma (a medullary chondroma). Roentgenograms will disclose erosion of the ungual tuft. Because of pressure on the nail matrix, the nail will be deformed and rippled. The treatment of epidermoid inclusion cyst is excision with curettement and skin grafting.

Malignant tumors of bone

Malignant tumors of bones of the foot, compared with those of other sites, are uncommon; however, the bones of the foot may be affected by the metastatic spread of malignancy that has originated elsewhere.

Osteoclastoma (giant cell tumor). Recently, recorded incidence of osteoclastoma in the foot has increased; it has been reported to occur in the calcaneus, the talus, and the metatarsals (Dahlin, 1967). It is included here as a malignant tumor because without adequate resection, the tumor recurs in more than 30 percent of cases and of these, 10 percent will metastasize (Goldenberg et al., 1970). The presenting symptoms are pain, local tenderness, and swelling. Roentgenograms will show radiolucent bone destruction. The recommended treatment of osteoclastoma is en bloc resection with wide margins. Soft tissue should be included in the excised portion.

Osteosarcoma (osteogenic sarcoma). This neoplasm is a destructive lesion of bone that may occur at any age but most frequently occurs in the second decade of life. Paget's disease may undergo malignant transformation and cause significant secondary incidence of osteosarcoma after the fifth decade of life.

Over 60 percent of osteosarcomas occur in the lower extremities, particularly in the distal femoral and proximal tibial metaphyseal areas. However, enough cases have been reported in the bones of the foot to warrant inclusion of osteosarcoma in the discussion of neoplasms of the foot (Dahlin, 1967).

Symptoms of osteosarcoma include pain, swelling, and local tenderness. A defined mass may or may not be palpable. Roentgenograms will show an area of bone destruction that is without delineation or encapsulation. Expansile new bone formation may produce a sunburst pattern; areas of the tumor may show new bone density. Increased radiodensity of the tumor, with regions of new calcification and tumor bone formation, may be apparent. Microscopic examination may reveal a wide variety of types of cells.

Any anaplastic tumor with osteoid production is classified as an osteosarcoma, even if a predominance of cartilaginous, fibrous, or cystic elements is contained in the primitive mesenchymal tumor tissue (Ackerman and Spiut, 1962).

The treatment of osteosarcoma is prompt ablation. An adequate biopsy is an even more important part of treatment. Before performing an amputation, the clinician should carry out lung scanning; if evi-

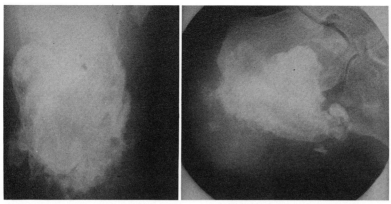

Fig. 13-36. Chondrosarcoma, with malignant degeneration and multiple cartilaginous exostoses.

dence of metastasis is visible, amputation will be hopeless. Doses of radiation, measured to cause necrosis, may be used. This treatment allows time to confirm the presence of metastatic disease, while it arrests local growth of the tumor. Replacement of the foot by a functional prosthetic appliance is likely to be successful.

Chondrosarcoma. This neoplasm is composed of proliferating primitive tissue of cartilaginous origin. Like osteosarcoma, the incidence of this tumor in the bones of the foot is low, but unlike osteosarcoma, chondrosarcoma occurs during the fourth to sixth decades of life and is often slow to metastasize. Moreover, chondrosarcoma differs from osteosarcoma in that its treatment by ablation frequently results in prolonged survival time of the patient. Secondary chondrosarcoma results from malignant metaplasia of a chondroma and occurs in 1 percent of all osteochondromas, including axial enchondromas. Thus the possibility that chondrosarcoma will develop from a solitary osteochondroma or enchondroma, as compared with the possibility of its development from multiple osteochondromas, is remote.

The symptoms of chondrosarcoma are pain and a growing mass. Roentgenograms demonstrate minute calcific stippling of the extraosseous tumor (Fig. 13-36). Osteolysis with cortical expansion will occur. After a histopathologic diagnosis has been made,

which is not an easy task, ablation or wide excision is the treatment of choice (Henderson and Dahlin, 1963).

In other texts, *chondromyxosarcoma,* a variation of chondrosarcoma, is often discussed as a specific entity. I prefer to classify it as a chondrosarcoma in which the metaplastic stroma contains a large amount of mucinoid myxomatous intracellular material. Its behavior is similar to that of chondrosarcoma; a positive mucin reaction is not present. It is important to differentiate this myxomatous chondrosarcoma from chondromyxoid fibroma, which may present a variable histopathologic picture but in reality is benign.

Ewing's sarcoma. Behaviorally, Ewing's sarcoma is the most primitive of mesenchymal tumors. It frequently involves a bone of the lower extremity and appears most often in the first and second decades of life. The patient's initial complaints are pain and swelling. Localized diffuse bone destruction is seen on roentgenogram; the tumor may be mistaken for a local infection. The literature contains reports of Ewing's sarcoma in the phalanges (Fig. 13-37), the calcaneus, the cuneiforms, and the talus (Dahlin, 1967). I have recently seen a case of Ewing's sarcoma in the calcaneus of a 12-year-old boy (Fig. 13-38). Microscopically, the tumor will show packed sheets of small round cells, with areas of necrosis where the rapid growth

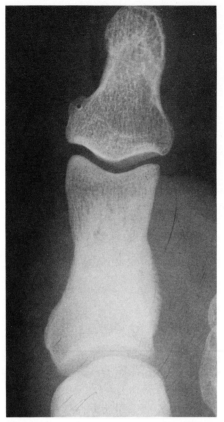

Fig. 13-37. Ewing's sarcoma of toe. (From Andrisek, A. R.: J.A.M.A. **170:**189, 1959.)

of the tumor has exceeded the available blood supply.

The treatment of Ewing's sarcoma, after biopsy, is irradiation. This treatment will result in local resolution of the tumor process, but further widespread metastasis is the rule. The 5-year survival rate is dismally low.

Reticulum cell sarcoma. This neoplasm is another small round-cell tumor that is often confused with Ewing's sarcoma. It differs importantly from Ewing's sarcoma in that the 5-year survival rate of patients with this tumor is a favorable 50 percent. Reticulum cell sarcoma occurs in patients who are usually older than those afflicted with Ewing's sarcoma. The argentaffin quality of the reticulin will provide an aid in the diagnosis of this tumor; the nucleus is indented and is shaped like a catcher's mitt. Reports of its occurrence in the tarsal bones exist in the literature (Dahlin, 1967). After biopsy, the treatment of this tumor is ablation.

LOCALIZED BONE ATROPHY (OSTEOPOROSIS)

Local osteoporosis is commonly seen in patients during routine roentgenographic

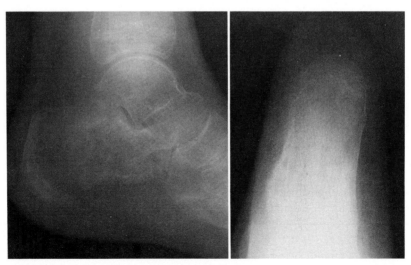

Fig. 13-38. Ewing's sarcoma in calcaneus of 12-year-old child. (Courtesy G. Beattie.)

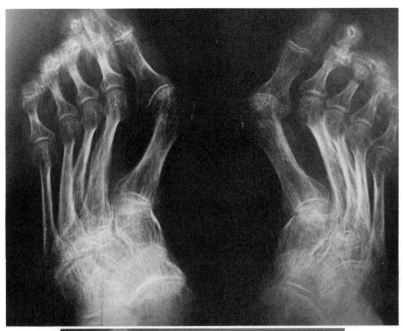

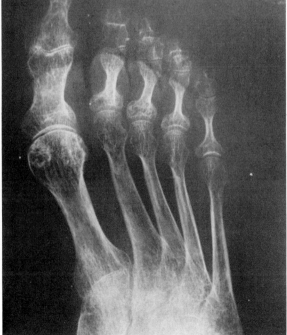

Fig. 13-39. Extensive osteoporosis in two patients. Note the generalized decalcification.

examination of the foot after prolonged immobilization and absence of weight bearing (Fig. 13-39). In such patients the lack of stress and inactivity have resulted in loss of normal osteoblastic activity (Geiser and Trueta, 1958).

It is important to differentiate localized bone atrophy from systemic forms of bone atrophy and to distinguish other generalized metabolic bone disease from osteoporosis. Additional films as well as appropriate laboratory studies are indicated if any question of the etiology of the condition exists or if there is no improvement after the patient resumes normal activities.

The localized osteoporosis, or atrophy of disuse, will slowly reverse its course when the patient resumes his normal activity. The density of the involved bone, as compared with that of the unaffected bone, will return to normal. During this transitional period, edema, discoloration of the skin, and subjective heat or cold sensation may be evident, along with pain. The intensity of this pain may equal the pain experienced at the time of the original injury.

Sudeck's atrophy (reflex dystrophy)

In cases in which pain, edema, and loss of function do not improve within several weeks, it is probable that reflex dystrophy may be present (Trueta, 1963). Characteristically, the onset of reflex dystrophy is slow and insidious; the symptoms progress for a month or two and then climax in severe intractable pain. In some patients this reflex dystrophy is transient; in others, the condition may persist and may be unresponsive to all modes of treament. Sudeck's atrophy has been reported to be present in patients after they have experienced mild trauma without fracture (Arieff et al., 1963).

The etiology of Sudeck's atrophy is thought to be vascular (due to either arteriolar spasm or venous stasis), in combination with muscular disuse. The hysterical origin of this disorder has also been considered. Roentgenograms will show a marked loss of bone substance, particularly

in secondary trabeculations throughout the osseous structures of the foot (Fig. 13-40, *B*). Spontaneous fracture may occur (Fig. 13-41).

Treatment of this disorder varies according to the individual case. It consists of active and assistive physical therapy to promote muscular and joint motion, even though the patient may experience pain. Elastic stockings, progressive weight bearing, and whirlpool and contrast baths have been proved to be effective means of conservative treatment. In prolonged cases in which conservative measures are ineffective, local or paravertebral block and lumbar sympathectomy have produced improvement. The usefulness of hypnosis or acupuncture in the treatment of Sudeck's atrophy has not been confirmed.

DISEASES OF THE SESAMOIDS

The medial and lateral sesamoids of the distal first metatarsal are the most constant sesamoid bones of the foot. They may be congenitally absent; also, additional sesamoid bones may occur in the lesser toes.

Sesamoid bones, named for their similarity in appearance to sesame seeds, do not contain periosteum. They are intimately related to the fibrous tissue of the tendon. The superior (dorsal) surface of the sesamoid is composed of cartilage, which articulates with the cartilaginous projection of the metatarsophalangeal joint surface. The plantar surface of the sesamoid bone is covered by the thick fibrous tissue of the ball of the foot. The medial (tibial) sesamoid is larger than the lateral sesamoid, and it lies more directly under the metatarsal head. The smaller, lateral sesamoid articulates with the outer fibular side of the distal first metatarsal (Colwill, 1969).

Bipartite and multipartite sesamoids (Fig. 13-42) occur in approximately 10 percent of all feet; the tibial sesamoid is more often the divided one. Three-fourths of bipartite sesamoids are unilateral. Most bilateral sesamoids are symmetrical; thus, the differentiation between a fractured ses-

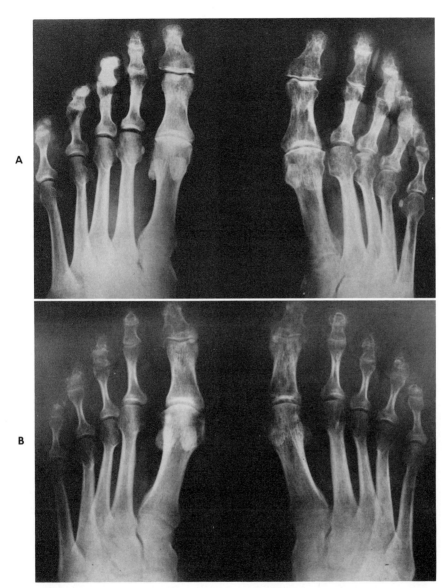

Fig. 13-40. Sudeck's atrophy. **A,** Normal foot for comparison. **B,** Note generalized decalcification and mottling of bones.

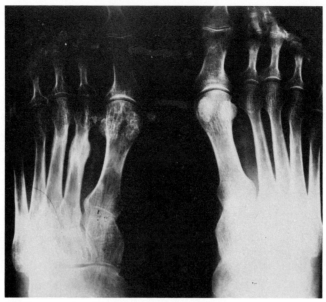

Fig. 13-41. Sudeck's atrophy of left foot with fatigue fracture of second metatarsal, resulting from softening of bone.

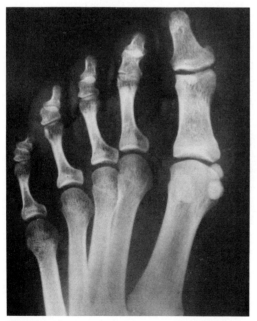

Fig. 13-42. Dorsoplantar view of dislocation of distal half of bipartite sesamoid into first metatarsophalangeal joint.

amoid and a multipartite sesamoid may not be confirmed by comparison with the sesamoid of the opposite member (Colwill, 1969). Fractures are confirmed by healing and decreased pain (Devas, 1963).

Simple sesamoiditis

Anatomic malformation, caused either by an enlarged sesamoid bone impinging upon the joint articulation distally or by excessive displacement from singular or recurrent trauma, may result in simple sesamoiditis. Symptoms include pain both during weight bearing and during passive dorsiflexion of the great toe. The term of onset of simple sesamoiditis may vary from a week to 6 months or longer. Its severity may vary also, depending upon the cause of the condition. Local tenderness is present, and an adventitious bursa may develop (Figs. 13-43 and 13-44).

Treatment should be directed toward elimination of weight bearing by means of rest, padding, and casts. Injections (sterile) of local anesthetic and anti-inflammatory cortisone derivatives may be of help in confirming the diagnosis. The degree of dis-

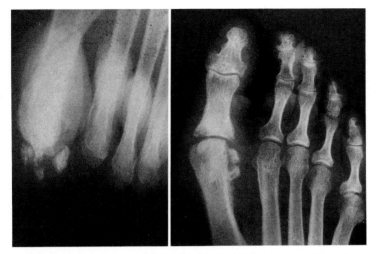

Fig. 13-43. Nonpyogenic osteomyelitis of both sesamoids with complete disorganization. The process was local in origin and of 5 months' duration. Sanguineous material was obtained on drainage.

A

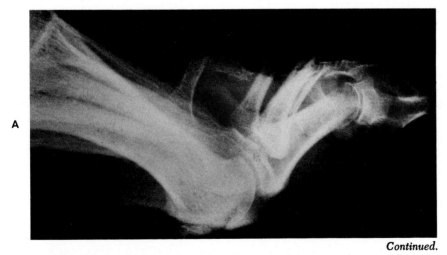

Continued.

Fig. 13-44. A, Medial view. Aseptic necrosis of the tibial sesamoid secondary to diabetes mellitus. **B,** Dorsoplantar view also showing degenerative changes of fibular sesamoid.

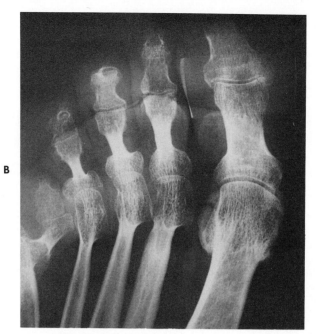

B

Fig. 13-44, cont'd. For legend see p. 409.

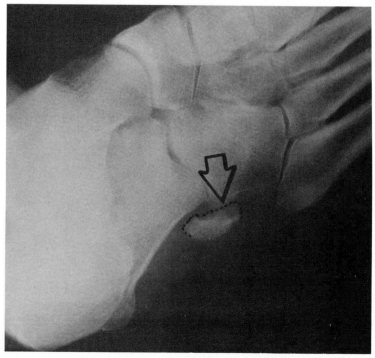

Fig. 13-45. Osteochondritis of os peroneum. It became painful, and excision was necessary.

placement and the amount of excess longitudinal growth of the sesamoid may be determined roentgenographically. Axial views with tomography may be of use. In recalcitrant cases, surgical excision may be indicated.

Chondromalacia, osteochondritis deformans juvenilis, and avascular necrosis of the sesamoids. These disorders are varieties of so-called sesamoiditis. Osteochondritis deformans juvenilis usually affects adolescents and young adults; the pain is chronic and is often relieved by a metatarsal bar. Roentgenographically, fragmentation and changes similar to those that occur in osteochondritis deformans juvenilis of any other bone may be seen. The pain caused by this condition is treated by means of protective padding until it subsides. Repair and secondary bone changes may result in a beaking of the sesamoid or in other deformities. Osteochondritis may also occur in accessory bones (Fig. 13-45).

Chondromalacia is thought to be another cause of simple sesamoiditis. No abnormality or displacement exists in this disorder, but local tenderness persists over the articular surface. Degeneration of the sesamoid may result in hallux rigidus; the metatarsophalangeal joint appears normal but the metatarsal joint, which articulates with the sesamoid, shows the abnormality (Gervis, 1960).

Avascular necrosis of the sesamoids may occur after an acute osteomyelitis or may be a presenting feature of developmental vascular change. If the deformity is severe and the symptoms persist after conservative treatment has been carried out, excision may be necessary (Golding, 1960).

REFERENCES
Infectious disorders—osteomyelitis

Aegerter, E., and Kirkpatrick, J. A., Jr.: Orthopedic diseases, ed. 3, Philadelphia, 1968, W. B. Saunders Co.

Benner, E. J.: Use and abuse of antibiotics, J. Bone Joint Surg. **49-A**:977-988, July 1967.

Clawson, D. K., and Dunn, A. W.: Management of common bacterial infections of bones and joints, J. Bone Joint Surg. **49-A**:164-182, Jan. 1967.

Greenfield, G. B.: Radiology of bone diseases, Philadelphia, 1969, J. B. Lippincott Co.

Jawetz, E.: Assay of antibacterial activity in serum, Amer. J. Dis. Child. **103**:81-84, Jan. 1962.

Jergesen, F., and Jawetz, E.: Pyogenic infections in orthopedic surgery: Combined antibiotic and closed wound treatment, Amer. J. Surg. **106**:152-162, Aug. 1963.

Rowling, D. E.: The positive approach to chronic osteomyelitis, J. Bone Joint Surg. **41-B**:681-688, Nov. 1959.

Trueta, J.: The three types of acute haematogenous osteomyelitis: A clinical and vascular study, J. Bone Joint Surg. **41-B**:671-680, Nov. 1959.

Wilson, J. C., and McKeever, F. M.: Bone growth disturbance following hematogenous osteomyelitis, J.A.M.A. **107**:1188-1192, Oct. 1936.

Vascular disorders

Aegerter, E., and Kirkpatrick, J. A., Jr.: Orthopedic diseases, ed. 3, Philadelphia, 1968, W. B. Saunders Co.

Berndt, A. L., and Harty, M.: Transchondral fractures (osteochondritis dissecans) of the talus, J. Bone Joint Surg. **41-A**:991-1020, Sept. 1959.

Bobechko, W. P., and Harris, W. R.: The radiographic density of avascular bone, J. Bone Joint Surg. **42-B**:626-632, Aug. 1960.

Braddock, G. I. F.: Experimental epiphysial injury and Freiberg's disease, J. Bone Joint Surg. **41-B**:154-159, Feb. 1959.

Shaw, E. W.: Avascular necrosis of the phalanges of the hands (Thiemann's disease), J.A.M.A. **156**:711-713, Oct. 1954.

Stillman, B. C.: Osteochondritis dissecans and coxa plana: Review of the literature, J. Bone Joint Surg. **48-B**:64-81, Feb. 1966.

Waugh, W.: The ossification and vascularisation of the tarsal navicular and their relation to Köhler's disease, J. Bone Joint Surg. **40-B**:765-777, Nov. 1958.

Benign tumors of soft tissues

Ackerman, L. V., and Spjut, H. J.: Tumors of bone and cartilage, Washington, D. C., 1962, Armed Forces Institute of Pathology.

Andrén, L., and Eiken, O.: Arthrographic studies of wrist ganglions, J. Bone Joint Surg. **53-A**:299-302, Mar. 1971.

Eisenstein, R.: Giant-cell tumor of tendon sheath, J. Bone Joint Surg. **50-A**:476-486, Apr. 1968.

Greenfield, G. B.: Radiology of bone diseases, Philadelphia, 1969, J. B. Lippincott Co.

Jones, F. E., Soule, E. H., and Coventry, M. B.: Fibrous xanthoma of synovium (giant-cell tumor of tendon sheath, pigmented nodular synovitis), J. Bone Joint Surg. **51-A**:76-86, Jan. 1969.

King, E. S. J.: The pathology of ganglion, Aust. N. Z. J. Surg. 1:367-381, Mar. 1932.

Pedersen, H. E., and Day, A. J.: Dupuytren's disease of the foot, J.A.M.A. 154:33-35, Jan. 1954.

Smyth, M.: Glomus-cell tumors in the lower extremity: Report of two cases, J. Bone Joint Surg. 53-A:157-159, Jan. 1971.

Soren, A.: Pathogenesis and treatment of ganglion, Clin. Orthop. 48:173-179, Sept.-Oct. 1966.

Stoyle, T. F.: Dupuytren's contracture in the foot, J. Bone Joint Surg. 46-B:218-219, May 1964.

Malignant tumors of soft tissues

Jaffe, H. L.: Tumors and tumorous conditions of the bones and joints, Philadelphia, 1958, Lea & Febiger.

Lewis, G. M.: Practical dermatology, ed. 3, Philadelphia, 1967, W. B. Saunders Co.

Stening, W. S.: Primary malignant tumours of calcaneal tendon, J. Bone Joint Surg. 50-B:676-677, Aug. 1968.

Benign tumors and cysts of bone

Ackerman, L. V., and Spjut, H. J.: Tumors of bone and cartilage, Washington, D. C., 1962, Armed Forces Institute of Pathology.

Cowie, R. S.: Benign osteoblastoma of the talus, J. Bone Joint Surg. 48-B:582-583, Aug. 1966.

Giannestras, N. J., and Diamond, J. R.: Benign osteoblastoma of the talus: A review of the literature and report of a case, J. Bone Joint Surg. 40-A:469-478, Apr. 1958.

Jaffe, H. L.: "Osteoid osteoma": A benign osteoblastic tumor composed of osteoid and atypical bone, Arch. Surg. 31:709-728, 1935.

Jaffe, H. L.: Tumors and tumorous conditions of the bones and joints, Philadelphia, 1958, Lea & Febiger.

Lichtenstein, L.: Aneurysmal bone cyst: A pathological entity commonly mistaken for giant-cell tumor and occasionally for hemangioma and osteogenic sarcoma, Cancer 3:279-289, Mar. 1950.

Poulsen, J. O.: Osteoid osteoma, Acta Orthop. Scand. 40:198-204, 1969.

Schajowicz, F., and Gallardo, H.: Chondromyxoid fibroma (fibromyxoid chondroma) of bone: A clinico-pathological study of 32 cases, J. Bone Joint Surg. 53-B:198-216, May 1971.

Malignant tumors of bone

Ackerman, L. V., and Spjut, H. J.: Tumors of bone and cartilage, Washington, D. C., 1962, Armed Forces Institute of Pathology.

Dahlin, D. C.: Bone tumors, ed. 2, Springfield, Ill., 1967, Charles C Thomas, Publisher.

Goldenberg, R. R., Campbell, C. J., and Bonfiglio, M.: Giant cell tumor of bone, J. Bone Joint Surg. 52-A:619-664, June 1970.

Henderson, E. D., and Dahlin, D. C.: Chondrosarcoma of bone: A study of two hundred eighty-eight cases, J. Bone Joint Surg. 45-A:1450-1458, Oct. 1963.

Localized bone atrophy (osteoporosis)

Geiser, M., and Trueta, J.: Muscle action, bone rarefaction and bone formation, J. Bone Joint Surg. 40-B:282-311, May 1958.

Sudeck's atrophy

Arieff, A. J., Bell, J. L., Tigay, E. L., and Kurtz, J. F.: Reflex physiopathic disturbances, J. Bone Joint Surg. 45-A:1329-1330, Sept. 1963.

Trueta, J.: The role of vessels in osteogenesis, J. Bone Joint Surg. 45-B:402-418, May 1963.

Diseases of the sesamoids

Colwill, M.: Osteomyelitis of the metatarsal sesamoids, J. Bone Joint Surg. 51-B:464-468, Aug. 1969.

Devas, M. B.: Stress fractures in children, J. Bone Joint Surg. 45-B:528-540, Aug. 1963.

Gervis, W. H.: Hallux valgus and hallux rigidus, J. Bone Joint Surg. 42-B:158, Feb. 1960.

Golding, C.: Museum pages: V. Sesamoids of the hallux, J. Bone Joint Surg. 42-B:840-843, Nov. 1960.

14

Diseases of the nerves of the foot

Roger A. Mann

Most neurologic disorders of the foot stem from changes in the cerebrospinal system, with secondary changes in the lower extremity. Except for connective-tissue changes in the digital branches of the plantar nerve, intrinsic diseases of the nerves of the foot are rare. Some discussion of them, however, is pertinent here.

INTERDIGITAL PLANTAR NEUROMA

Histologically, plantar neuroma is a neurofibroma, which is an accumulation of collagenous material in the neurilemma (sheath of Schwann). Neurilemma is present only in peripheral nerves; therefore, such changes occur only in peripheral nerves, as pointed out by both Boyd (1943) and Ewing (1942). Winkler and associates (1948) reviewed microscopic sections of twenty specimens of presumed neurofibroma of the foot but did not find evidence of active proliferation of either nerve or neurilemma. They found instead that the enlargement was caused by a deposition of hyaline and collagenous material.

In 1876 Morton described the entity known as Morton's neuralgia or Morton's metatarsalgia. He suggested that the condition was probably caused by neuritis of the third branch of the medial plantar nerve. Textbooks on anatomy describe the medial plantar nerve as having four digital branches. The most medial branch is the proper digital nerve to the medial aspect of the great toe. The next three branches are

named the first, second, and third common digital nerves. They are distributed to both the medial and lateral aspects of the first, second, and third interspaces respectively. The lateral plantar nerve gives off a superficial branch, which splits into a proper digital nerve to the lateral side of the small toe, and it also gives off a common digital nerve to the fourth interspace. The common digital nerve frequently gives rise to a communicating branch, which passes to the third digital branch of the medial plantar nerve in the third interspace (Fig. 14-1).

Tubby (1912) treated a series of patients who had so-called Morton's neuralgia by excising the head of the fourth metatarsal. He stated: "On occasion when the nerve was seen, it was resected and it often showed small nodular masses." Nissen (1948) remarked that before 1940 several English surgeons who had noticed nodular masses on the plantar digital nerve in the course of surgical procedures involving the plantar surface thought that fibrous changes were taking place. Betts (1940) was the first to demonstrate histologically the extensive connective-tissue enlargement of the third digital branch of the medial plantar nerve. He observed this enlargement in nineteen cases in which he and his colleagues performed resections of the nerve because of so-called Morton's neuralgia. McElvenny (1943) and McKeever (1952) reported independently that they found the presence of a thickened digital

413

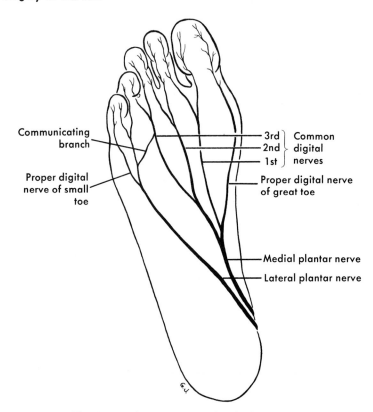

Fig. 14-1. Plantar nerves of right foot.

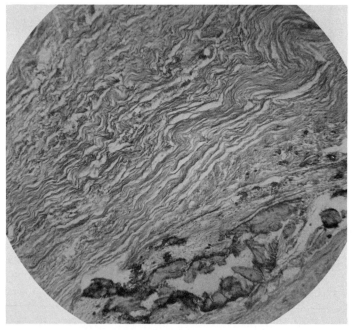

Fig. 14-2. Palisade arrangement of cells typical of neurofibroma, with inert deposits in lower part of field (× 85).

nerve in the third metatarsal interspace about the same time as Betts. Since then, Baker and Kuhn (1944), Bickel and Dockerty (1947), Watson-Jones (1949), and others have substantiated Betts' observations. Pincus (1950) thoroughly reviewed publications concerning neurofibroma of the foot. The reported cases of neurofibroma of the foot refer to the third metatarsal interspace involving the third digital branch of the medial plantar nerve. Apparently the only exception is a case reported by Hauser (1943), who described the excision of a massive neurofibroma of the first digital branch. In 1952 DuVries and Cascino reported a case involving the first digital nerve. The observations in that case were confusing because the growth contained a large amount of radiopaque material (Fig. 14-2).

Neuroma is somewhat more prevalent in women. The ratio reported by investigators varies (Scotti, 1957), but in a series of 200 cases reported by Bovill (1965) the ratio was found to be 4 to 1. The lesion occurs at all ages but more often between 30 and 50 years, especially in a narrow, flaccid-type foot.

Etiology. The cause of neuroma as related to the foot is not entirely clear. Nissen (1948) believed it to be a result of degeneration of the digital vessels in the cleft between the third and fourth toes. Winkler and colleagues (1948) postulated that the predisposition of the third digital nerve to the disease was related to its receiving a filament from the lateral plantar nerve (Fig. 14-1), although the third digital nerve is essentially a branch of the medial plantar nerve. It is possible that neuromas of the digital plantar nerve branches result from chronic irritation. Irritating factors include the wearing of faulty footwear, walking on hard floors, standing for long periods, the proximity or touching of metatarsal heads as a result of metatarsal fractures, and anatomic variations of bones and nerves on the plantar surface.

From the standpoint of the biomechanics of the foot, more motion appears to occur in the third interspace than in the other interspaces—probably because of the joining of the medial and longitudinal arch systems at the third interspace. DuVries feels that of the five metatarsals, the fourth is least securely anchored at its base. This weak attachment permits a floating action of the distal end of the fourth metatarsal when the foot is in motion. The anatomic instability of this metatarsal head may well cause a constant grating against the terminal portion of the third digital nerve. Prolonged irritation of living tissue caused by mechanical friction can induce proliferation of connective tissue or collagenous material in the involved area. Furthermore, the three digital branches of the medial plantar nerve lie between the heads and shafts of the metatarsals and are subject to constant friction. In response to friction, collagenous connective tissue accumulates in the neurilemma. Increased thickness subjects it to greater friction. The overwhelming predilection to thickening of the third digital branch seems to give credence to the fact that the contributing causes of neuroma are increased motion and friction in the area of the third interspace.

The third digital nerve is the one that is by far the most frequently affected. The second is sometimes affected; the first is rarely affected.

Dissection and sectioning of digital plantar nerves taken at random from cadavers and from freshly amputated feet show that microscopically, asymptomatic nerves and neuromas have a similar appearance.

Symptoms. When the second or third digital branch is affected, the early symptoms may be varying degrees of pain about the metatarsophalangeal joint and pain in the third metatarsal interspace, which may become burning in nature. Occasionally the pain may retrogress along the foot upward into the calf, and it is often aggravated by weight bearing. The symptoms gradually worsen and in some cases become intractable.

Diagnosis. Palpation of the plantar as-

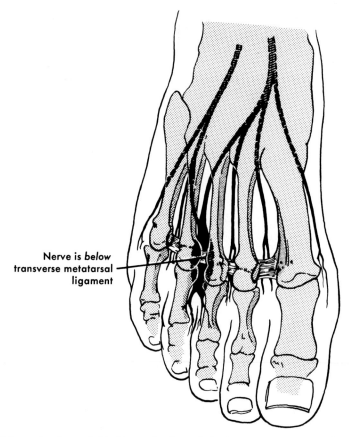

Nerve is *below*
transverse metatarsal
ligament

Fig. 14-3. Schematic view of third branch of medial plantar nerve. Note that it courses plantarward, under the transverse metatarsal ligament.

pect of the involved interspace often causes a sharp stabbing pain similar to that which occurs when the patient bears weight on the foot. The growth is ordinarily too small to be palpated (Fig. 14-3). The diagnosis must be made on the basis of clinical observation, since neither roentgenograms nor laboratory tests offer clues. Occasionally the toes associated with the involved interspace demonstrate hyperesthesia to pinprick.

In the differential diagnosis of plantar neuroma, the possibility of tarsal-tunnel syndrome (p. 419) should always be kept in mind. Sometimes bony abnormalities involving the lesser metatarsophalangeal joints produce similar symptoms (Fig. 14-4).

Neuroma of the first digital nerve, be-

cause it is massive, is readily palpated immediately under the first metatarsal interspace in which it occurs. Pain is at least as severe in this area as it is in the lesser branches.

Treatment. Conservative treatment includes such palliative measures as metatarsal bars and pads, but these appliances usually afford only temporary relief. Intractable pain in the interspace between the third and fourth metatarsal head, which cannot be relieved by mechanical measures, justifies a diagnosis of operable neuroma.

Excision of the entire nerve gives complete relief. European surgeons excise the nerve of the second or third digital branch through a plantar approach, as described by Betts (1940) and by Nissen (1948). In this country the approach generally is

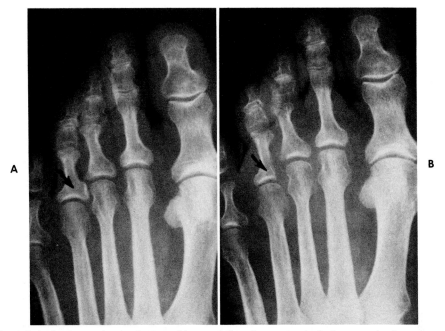

Fig. 14-4. A, Anomalous relation of base of fourth proximal phalanx to third metatarsal head in foot of 54-year-old woman. Twice she had undergone surgical procedures for neuroma, without relief. **B,** Correction of anomaly. Symptoms were alleviated.

through the dorsum, as described by Mc-Elvenny (1943) and by McKeever (1952). The American approach has advantages, the most important being prevention of scar formation on the plantar surface. Furthermore, this approach does not pass through important fascial planes as does the plantar incision. The nerve is easily pressed into the metatarsal interspace and does not present obstacles to grasping and excision.

Operative technique for neuroma commonly involving second or third digital nerve. In twenty-five referred surgical cases of presumed neuroma of the digital branch of the lateroplantar nerve in the fourth metatarsal interspace, the pathologist reported that the characteristic palisade arrangement of neuroma was absent. In two cases the pathologist observed glomus cells, indicating a glomus tumor. Operation did relieve symptoms in most cases.

1. Under hemostasis, make an incision over the dorsum of the metatarsal interspace, extending it from the center point in the web of the toes proximally to about the middle of the metatarsal interspace.
2. Carry the incision down into the lower depth of the interspace.
3. Spread apart the heads of the adjacent metatarsals by means of a Weitlander or mastoid retractor.
4. Apply pressure with a finger on the plantar surface of the toe web; this will bring dorsally an encapsulated lobular mass (Fig. 14-5, *A*). Grasp the mass, which includes the nerve ending. Dissect it proximally and plantarward under the transverse metatarsal ligament. Excise the nerve proximal to the transverse metatarsal ligament (Fig. 14-5, *B*).
5. Instill 5 mg. hydrocortisone in the wound.
6. Suture the skin and fascia in layers.
7. Apply a compression bandage and release it in 24 hours, at which time ambulation may begin.

The procedure is the same when the

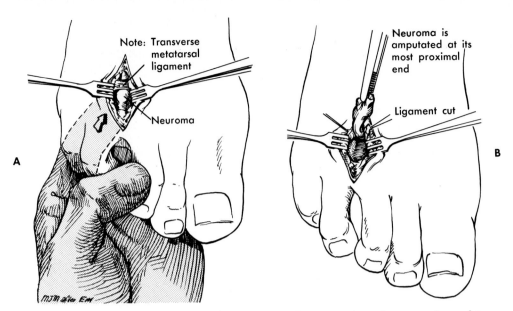

Fig. 14-5. A, Application of pressure, with index finger against plantar surface of toe web space. **B,** Neuroma dissected proximally under transverse metatarsal ligament and amputated proximally to this ligament.

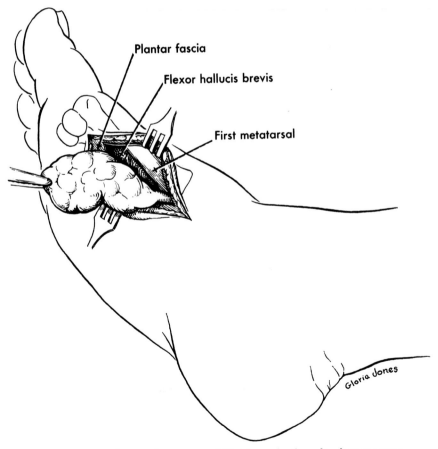

Fig. 14-6. Delivery of neuroma of first branch of medioplantar nerve.

lesion is in the second metatarsal inter-space. In rare instances a neuroma develops at the first digital branch of the medial plantar nerve. When such a neuroma does form it is usually massive and must be excised on the medial border of the forefoot (Fig. 14-6).

CAUSALGIA

Etiology. Causalgia results when a nerve trunk is incorporated in a surgical or fracture scar, or when a sensory nerve receives a direct injury, as by penetrating wounds, or prolonged pressure by casts. The pain is over or distal to the area of the nerve lesion and may correspond to cutaneous distribution of the nerve. Pressure or palpation of the area where the nerve is included in a scar accentuates the pain. The region may show trophic and vasomotor changes. In amputees pain is experienced in the region of the stump or as phantom pain in structures already amputated.

With reference to the foot, causalgia is a postoperative complication in many cases. De Takats (1945) calls attention to other painful conditions in the extremities from injuries to the peripheral nerve. Cullen (1948) reported twenty-four cases of causalgia, five involving the foot. Severe osteoporosis, resembling Sudeck's atrophy, developed in all the bones of the foot in one patient 12 months after injury. Causalgia in all five cases resulted from injuries to the internal popliteal nerve. The distribution of pain in all instances was in the sole of the foot. In cases observed by Bovill (1965) the pain was along the course of the lateral dorsal cutaneous nerve from the lateral malleolus to the fifth toe. The lateral dorsal cutaneous nerve in that area is superficial, so that its inclusion in a scar along its course is understandable. Stroking the area gave rise to an unbearably sharp burning sensation, mainly distal to the nerve lesion.

Symptoms. Causalgia is a neuralgia characterized by constant, intense local pain and burning, which may be accompanied by local skin changes such as rubor, in-

creased perspiration, and coolness. It is a clinical syndrome that can result from accidental or surgical trauma to a peripheral nerve containing sensory fibers.

Treatment. The treatment discussed here relates only to the foot. Injection of procaine hydrochloride or alcohol has been recommended, but satisfactory results are doubtful. Roentgen therapy has also been suggested, but its efficacy has not been proved. In cases of causalgia of the foot as a result of a severe injury to the posterior tibial or common peroneal nerve, sympathetic block is a valuable therapeutic measure as well as a diagnostic and prognostic test, because it foretells whether sympathectomy will give permanent relief.

When causalgia is the result of direct injuries of the foot, neurolysis or neurectomy offers best results. The sensory nerve trunk involved should be freed of all entanglements of scar tissue. If that is not possible, the trunk should be exposed proximally to the area where it is entwined in scar tissue and about 1 cm. of the nerve excised.

Nerve entrapment (tarsal-tunnel) syndrome

The nerve entrapment syndrome in the upper extremity, particularly in the wrist, has been well documented in recent years. The analogous abnormality involving the posterior tibial nerve underneath the flexor retinaculum at the ankle was described in 1962 by Keck and, later in the same year, by Lam as the tarsal-tunnel syndrome (Fig. 14-7). The literature now contains several excellent reviews on this subject.[*]

Etiology. Entrapment of the nerves of the foot occurs more often than is generally realized. The major cutaneous nerve trunks are close to the surface, and any surface trauma (accidental or surgical) may trap such a nerve in its course. Transverse incisions over the foot necessarily involve the

---

[*]See Goodgold et al., 1965; Lam, 1967; Marinacci, 1968; Edwards et al., 1969; Gretter and Wilde, 1970; and Lincheid et al., 1970.

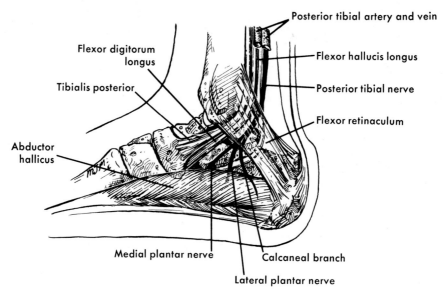

Posterior tibial artery and vein

Flexor digitorum longus

Flexor hallucis longus

Tibialis posterior

Posterior tibial nerve

Flexor retinaculum

Abductor hallicus

Medial plantar nerve

Calcaneal branch

Lateral plantar nerve

Fig. 14-7. Anatomy of tarsal tunnel.

cutaneous nerves that course horizontally and, therefore, often entrap them. Likewise, heavy objects falling on the dorsum of the foot may produce subcutaneous scarring that will envelop the cutaneous nerves. Most commonly affected are the terminal branches of the superficial peroneal nerve, but branches of the sural or medial plantar nerves may be involved.

Commonly encountered are cases of severe disability from intractable pain and paresthesia of the foot caused by nerve entrapment secondary to injury or operative procedures.

Symptoms. As a rule, the symptom complex is a burning sensation in the plantar aspect of the foot, usually in the distribution of the medial plantar nerve. The pain is often constant and may radiate along the inner side of the calf upward to the knee. The symptoms increase during walking or exercising and sometimes diminish when the patient is at rest. Pain frequently occurs during the night.

Diagnosis. The diagnosis is made by eliciting a positive Tinel's sign over the posterior tibial nerve as it passes behind the medial malleolus. Occasionally, Tinel's sign may persist along the course of the medial or lateral plantar nerves. Motor and sensory

deficit may or may not be elicited. Nerve conduction tests that demonstrate an abnormal latency period or delayed conduction time confirm the diagnosis. Electromyographic studies of the abductor hallucis or the abductor digiti quinti may demonstrate fibrillation potentials.

Treatment. The flexor retinaculum, which decompresses the posterior tibial nerve, must be released. The medial and lateral plantar branches should be followed to make certain that a more distal entrapment has not occurred.

Surgical technique. The tarsal tunnel is approached through a curved incision, which begins about 1 cm. posterior to the medial margin of the tibial shaft and is then carried downward parallel to the tibia and behind the medial malleolus. Once the incision passes the plane of the tip of the medial malleolus, it is curved gradually plantarward. The retinaculum is identified and carefully released in its entirety. The posterior tibial nerve is identified in the proximal portion of the dissection and traced distally. Care must be taken to avoid cutting the calcaneal branch, which may be small and surrounded by fatty tissue. The medial and lateral plantar nerves are identified and traced distally. The medial plantar branch should be followed along the superior margin of the abductor hallucis and flexor sheath of the flexor hallucis longus. The lateral plantar nerve is followed into the substance of the abductor hallucis. Any fibrous bands within this muscle that seem to be constricting the nerve should be released. At the conclusion of the dissection, the three terminal branches of the posterior tibial nerve should be lying free. One milliliter of hydrocortisone is instilled into the wound around the nerve. A sterile compression dressing is applied. The patient should not bear weight on the operated foot for a period of 3 weeks.

REFERENCES

Interdigital plantar neuroma

Baker, L. D., and Kuhn, H. H.: Morton's metatarsalgia: Localized degenerative fibrosis with neuromatous proliferation of the fourth plantar nerve, South. Med. J. 37:123-127, Mar. 1944.

Betts, L. O.: Morton's metatarsalgia: Neuritis of the fourth digital nerve, Med. J. Aust. 1:514-515, Apr. 1940.

Bickel, W. H., and Dockerty, M. B.: Plantar neuromas, Morton's toe, Surg. Gynec. Obstet. 84:111-116, Jan.-June 1947.

Bovill, E. G., Jr.: Diseases of nerves. In DuVries, H. L.: Surgery of the foot, ed. 2, St. Louis, 1965, The C. V. Mosby Co.

Boyd, W.: A textbook of pathology, ed. 4, Philadelphia, 1943, Lea & Febiger, p. 906.

DuVries, H. L., and Cascino, J. P.: Massive neurofibroma (neurinoma) of the foot with calcification, J. Int. Coll. Surg. 17:688, 1952.

Ewing, J.: Neoplastic diseases, Philadelphia, 1942, W. B. Saunders Co.

Hauser, E. D. W.: Neurofibroma (neurinoma) of the foot, J.A.M.A. 121:1217-1219, Apr. 1943.

McElvenny, R. T.: The etiology and surgical treatment of intractable pain about the fourth metatarsophalangeal joint (Morton's toe), J. Bone Joint Surg. 25:675-679, July 1943.

McKeever, D. C.: Surgical approach for neuroma of plantar digital nerve (Morton's metasarsalgia), J. Bone Joint Surg. 34-A:490, Apr. 1952.

Morton, T. G.: A peculiar and painful affection of fourth metatarsophalangeal articulation, Amer. J. Med. Sci. 71:37-45, Jan. 1876.

Nissen, K. I.: Plantar digital neuritis: Morton's metatarsalgia, J. Bone Joint Surg. 30-B:84-94, Feb. 1948.

Pincus, A.: Intractable Morton's toe (neuroma), J. Nat. Assoc. Chiropod. 40:19, 1950.

Scotti, T. M.: The lesion of Morton's metatarsalgia (Morton's toe), Arch. Pathol. 63:91-102, Jan.-June 1957.

Tubby, A. H.: Deformities, including diseases of the bones and joints, ed. 2, vol. 1, London, 1912, Macmillan and Co., Ltd., p. 721.

Watson-Jones, R.: Leri's pleonosteosis, carpal tunnel compression of the median nerves and Morton's metatarsalgia, J. Bone Joint Surg. 31-B: 560-571, Nov. 1949.

Winkler, H., Feltner, J. B., and Kimmelstiel, P.: Morton's metatarsalgia, J. Bone Joint Surg. 30-A:496-500, Apr. 1948.

Causalgia

Cullen, C. H.: Causalgia: Diagnosis and treatment, J. Bone Joint Surg. 30-B:466-477, Aug. 1948.

de Takats, G.: Causalgic states in peace and war, J.A.M.A. 128:699-704, July 1945.

Bovill, E. G., Jr.: Diseases of nerves, In DuVries, H. L.: Surgery of the foot, ed. 2, St. Louis, 1965, The C. V. Mosby Co.

Nerve entrapment (tarsal-tunnel) syndrome

Edwards, W. G., Lincoln, C. R., Bassett, F. H., III, and Goldner, J. L.: The tarsal tunnel syndrome: Diagnosis and treatment, J.A.M.A. 207: 716-720, Jan. 1969.

Goodgold, J., Kopell, H. P., and Spielholz, N. I.: The tarsal-tunnel syndrome: Objective diagnostic criteria, New Eng. J. Med. 273:742-745, Sept. 1965.

Gretter, T. E., and Wilde, A. H.: Pathogenesis, diagnosis, and treatment of the tarsal-tunnel syndrome, Cleve. Clin. Quart. 37:23-29, Jan. 1970.

Keck, C.: The tarsal-tunnel syndrome, J. Bone Joint Surg. 44-A:180-182, Jan. 1962.

Lam, S. J. S.: A tarsal-tunnel syndrome, Lancet 2:1354-1355, Dec. 1962.

Lam, S. J. S.: Tarsal tunnel syndrome, J. Bone Joint Surg. 49-B:87-92, Feb. 1967.

Linscheid, R. L., Burton, R. C., and Fredericks, E. J.: Tarsal-tunnel syndrome, South. Med. J. 63:1313-1323, Nov. 1970.

Marinacci, A. A.: Neurological syndromes of the tarsal tunnels. Bull. Los Angeles Neurol. Soc. 33:90-100, 1968.

Part three

15

Conservative treatment and office procedures

Roger A. Mann

Prior to discussing conservative means of treating some disorders of the feet, it is appropriate to say a word or two about footwear and its influence upon the functioning of the feet. As has been emphasized in Chapter 8, shoes, especially women's shoes, have been responsible for a majority of the toe deformities physicians commonly encounter. Although men and women have worn and suffered the consequences of improper footwear since antiquity, contemporary society continues to perpetuate the use of ill-fitting shoes. As we have seen, the deforming effects of improper shoes on a normal foot can readily cause such deformities as hallux valgus, hammertoes, hard corns, and plantar keratoses.

Properly fitted footwear should not crowd the forefoot but should allow the toes to extend fully as the person walks (see Fig. 8-2, *C*). To ensure adequate length and width, shoes should always be fitted to the weight-bearing foot.

MODIFICATIONS OF THE SHOE

Numerous modifications can be made in the heel, shank, or sole areas of the basic shoe (separately or in combination) to correct specific disorders of the foot. Rather than recommend an "orthopaedic shoe" for all symptomatic feet, the clinician should prescribe shoe modifications that suit the individual needs of the patient.

Wedges and pads are used to accomplish shoe modifications. A wedge is usually made of leather and is placed on the exterior walking surface of the shoe or within the construction of the shoe itself. Its purpose is to alter the weight-bearing pattern of the foot. Unlike the wedge, the pad acts on a specific site. It is used for therapeutic purposes and is in direct contact with the foot. It is usually made of felt or leather, but occasionally it is made of rubber.

The heel

Thomas heel. The most common heel modification is the Thomas heel (Fig. 15-1). This heel was originally designed to bring the calcaneus from a valgus position to a more neutral one and to support the medial aspect of the foot. Its use is indicated in cases of symptomatic flatfoot. It provides a varus tilt to the calcaneus and gives mechanical support to the collapsing talonavicular joint as well. In cases of hindfoot valgus it can be used to keep the calcaneus in a varus position. A Thomas heel should not be used if the calcaneus is in a varus position.

Unfortunately, today most Thomas heels are not properly fitted. To be effective, a Thomas heel should extend from the midportion of the navicular bone on the medial side to a line that intersects the longitudinal axis of the fibula on the lateral side. The

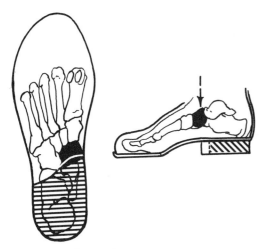

Fig. 15-1. Thomas heel. Note that the Thomas heel extends to the midportion of the navicular in order to provide support.

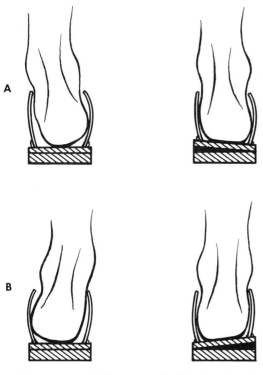

Fig. 15-2. Heel lifts. **A,** Medial heel wedge for correction of valgus heel deformity. **B,** Lateral heel wedge for correction of varus heel deformity.

Thomas heel may be combined with an inner heel lift in order to help accomplish inversion of the calcaneus.

Heel lifts. A medial or lateral lift of 0.3 to 0.6 cm. may be used in order to bring the heel out of a varus or valgus position (Fig. 15-2). Such a lift will transfer weight to the medial or lateral aspect of the foot.

Widened heels. Heels that have been widened are used to stabilize and thereby diminish painful subtalar motion. They are beneficial in the treatment of degenerative changes in the subtalar joint.

The shank

The shank of the shoe can be either flexible or rigid. In attempting to correct a postural abnormality of the foot by means of an external modification of the heel or sole, one usually recommends that the shank be flexible so that the foot will respond to the areas that have been corrected. Conversely, if an appliance is to be placed within the shoe, the shank should be more rigid.

The sole

The sole of the shoe can be modified through the use of lifts to affect the regions of the great toe, the metatarsals, and the medial and lateral aspects of the foot.

Lifts in the region of the great toe. Lifts in this area make the great toe less flexible and restrict the motion of the joint. This modification in the sole of the shoe is useful in the treatment of hallux rigidus (Fig. 15-3). A rocker-bottom shoe will also diminish the motion in the metatarsophalangeal joint of the great toe.

Lifts in the region of the metatarsals. This area of the sole is often modified by a metatarsal bar. It is used to transfer the weight usually borne by the metatarsal heads to a more proximal plantar area. The bar should be placed proximal to the metatarsal heads and may be either straight or curved (Fig. 15-4). Improper placement of the bar in relation to the metatarsal heads is the most common error made in using this type of appliance. If the bar is placed too far forward, the painful metatarsal con-

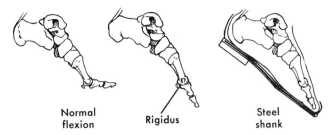

Normal flexion   Rigidus   Steel shank

Fig. 15-3. Sole modification for treatment of hallux rigidus. A steel shank is incorporated in order to diminish motion at the metatarsophalangeal joint.

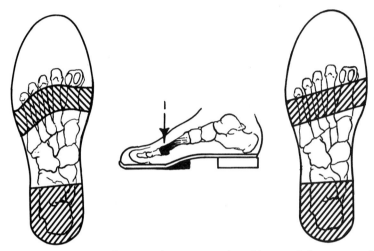

Fig. 15-4. Metatarsal bars. These appliances may be either straight or curved but must be placed proximal to the metatarsal heads.

dition will be aggravated. The sole of the patient's shoe should be examined to determine the weight-bearing area; marks should then be made on the sides of the sole just proximal to the metatarsal heads. In this way proper placement of the bar by the shoemaker is assured. The bar can be from 0.3 to 1 cm. thick, depending upon the clinical picture.

The anterior heel is also effective in relieving pressure on the metatarsal region and is preferred by some clinicians to the metatarsal bar. Both of these appliances are used to relieve metatarsalgia caused by atrophy of the plantar fat pad, intractable plantar keratosis, Morton's neuroma, trauma to the metatarsal heads, and other conditions that affect the metatarsal heads.

Lifts in the medial and lateral regions of the foot. Medial and lateral sole lifts (0.3 to 0.6 cm. thick) may be used either alone or combined with a heel modification to help correct imbalances of the foot. A medial lift will transfer the weight to the outer border and can be used to accommodate forefoot varus or to help realign the foot after trauma. A lateral lift will transfer weight to the inner border of the foot, may be used to treat forefoot valgus, and will also help to realign the foot after trauma (Fig. 15-5). In the treatment of flatfoot it is used to help correct the forefoot varus that often accompanies the hindfoot valgus. A lateral lift is often combined with a Thomas heel in order to help correct a flatfoot deformity (Fig. 15-6).

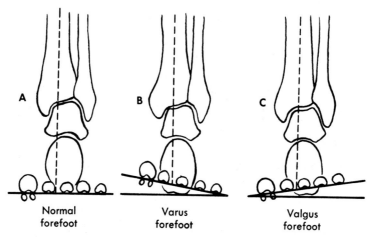

Normal forefoot

Varus forefoot

Valgus forefoot

Fig. 15-5. Forefoot alignment. **A,** Normal forefoot. **B,** Fixed varus forefoot. The condition may be treated with a medial sole lift. **C,** Fixed valgus forefoot. The condition may be treated with a lateral sole lift. (From Sgarlato, T. E.: A compendium of podiatric biomechanics, San Francisco, 1971, California College of Podiatric Medicine.)

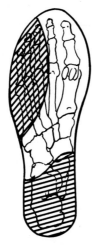

Fig. 15-6. Combination of Thomas heel, which corrects heel valgus and supports navicular, and lateral sole lift, which corrects forefoot varus. This combination is used in the treatment of flatfoot deformity.

Appliances

Felt pads. Felt pads are used primarily to relieve areas of abnormal pressure, usually upon the plantar aspect of the foot. They may also be used to support the longitudinal arch during the period when the clinician is attempting to determine which configuration of supports is best suited to his patient. The pads may be cut by the physician (Fig. 15-7) or ready-made adhesive-backed pads may be purchased in various sizes. In treating an area of abnormal wear or in attempting to ascertain exactly where to place permanent pads, we have found placing pads in the shoe or taping them to the patient's foot useful.

The main disadvantage of felt pads for permanent use is their tendency to pack down; to be most effective, they should be used in a shoe that has a fairly rigid sole. Correct placement and the indications for the most commonly used shoe pads are illustrated in Fig. 15-8.

Once felt pads have provided relief to the patient, a more permanent type of insert can be substituted. Leather appliances, metal arch supports (e.g., the Whitman support), a UC-BL type of insert, or a functional orthotic appliance to correct imbalance of the foot may be prescribed.

Leather appliances. The leather appliance is well adapted simply to elevate a metatarsal in order to redistribute the weight upon the plantar aspect of the foot. This type of modification will allow the affected area to carry less weight and will

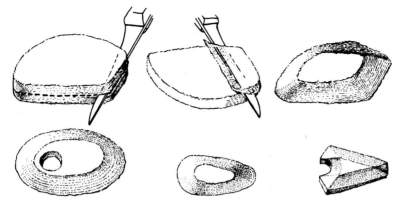

Fig. 15-7. Felt pads. Such pads may be shaped by the physician in order to relieve abnormal pressure on the plantar aspect of the foot.

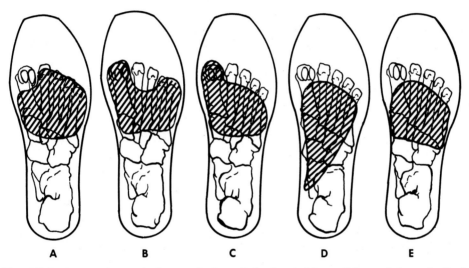

A   B   C   D   E

Fig. 15-8. Commonly used shoe pads for relief of painful conditions of foot. **A,** Pad designed to relieve pressure on sesamoids. **B,** Pad to support various metatarsal heads (in this case, for treatment of Morton's neuroma). **C,** Pad to support short first metatarsal and relieve pressure on lesser metatarsal heads. **D,** Pad to support longitudinal arch and relieve pressure on metatarsal heads. **E,** Pad to relieve pressure on metatarsal heads.

thus relieve the symptoms. Examples of commonly used leather appliances are shown in Fig. 15-9. The use of these appliances is indicated in the treatment of plantar callosities, metatarsalgia, Morton's neuroma, and for treating various afflictions of the metatarsal heads.

Metal appliances. Appliances made of metal are useful to support a symptomatic foot in which there is a structural weakness (as in flatfoot) or a distortion such as is caused by fracture-dislocation. The adult foot with a residual structural abnormality (such as partially corrected clubfoot) or with advanced arthritis may be helped by a metal appliance. All such feet require well-molded metal supports to achieve the mechanical stability that the ligamentous and

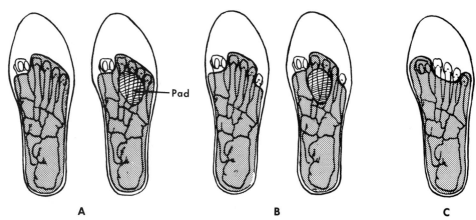

Fig. 15-9. Commonly used leather appliances for relief of painful conditions of foot. A pad (striped area) may be incorporated into the appliance for greater support. **A,** For relief of painful sesamoids. **B,** For relief of painful callosities under first and fifth metatarsal heads. **C,** For relief of metatarsalgia in second, third, and fourth metatarsals.

bony structures cannot provide. This type of appliance must be fabricated over an accurate mold of the foot.

The UC-BL type of insert. The UC-BL type of insert helps to correct structural abnormalities of the foot through control of the hindfoot and is based upon the premise that the hindfoot controls the forefoot. The heel is placed in a corrected position; the correction is maintained with a laminated fiber glass heel cup (Fig. 15-10). Although the applications of the UC-BL type of insert are still being explored, it has been proved to be useful in the treatment of symptomatic flatfoot, hallux valgus aggravated by an associated flatfoot deformity, calcaneal spurs with associated fasciitis of the plantar aponeurosis, and various other postural problems of the foot (Henderson and Campbell, 1967).

Orthotic appliances. Functional orthotic appliances are used in an attempt to balance a foot in which an anatomic disorder is present (e.g., forefoot varus or valgus as illustrated in Fig. 15-5, hindfoot varus or valgus, or a combination of these disorders). These appliances are fitted to a plaster mold of the foot held in a corrected position and are generally fabricated from a rigid plastic material (Fig. 15-11). Heel

and forefoot posts are added to the appliance to give the needed correction.

FOOT STRAPPING

Foot strapping is advantageous for the treatment of specific disorders. Only those strappings used most commonly are discussed.

Acute injuries. Acute injuries that result in foot strain, sprain, or undisplaced fracture may be treated with foot strapping and a wooden shoe. The strapping consists of circular rings of tape that are wrapped around the forefoot and basically support it. When treating the fresh injury, care must be taken to allow for edema to occur.

Symptomatic calcaneal spurs and plantar fasciitis. In these disorders, bow strapping (Fig. 15-12, *A*) relieves pressure, thereby reducing discomfort. A felt pad relieves pressure on the plantar tubercle of the calcaneus (Fig. 15-12, *B*).

Acute sesamoiditis. In the treatment of this disorder the hallux should be taped in a plantar-flexed position in order to relax the tendons containing the sesamoids.

Symptomatic hammertoe. A hammered toe can often be treated by passing tape around the normal toe on each side of the hammered toe, thus making a sling of the

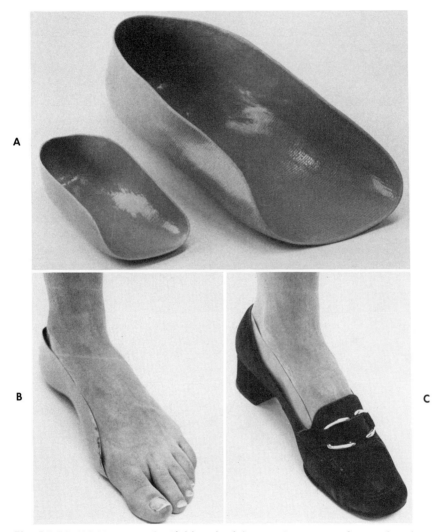

Fig. 15-10. UC-BL inserts. **A,** Child and adult sizes. **B,** Insert on foot and in shoe.

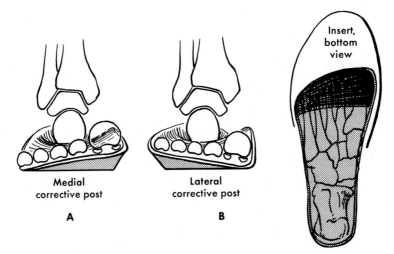

Fig. 15-11. Orthotic appliances. **A,** Fixed varus forefoot treated by supporting medial side of foot. **B,** Fixed valgus forefoot treated by supporting lateral side of foot.

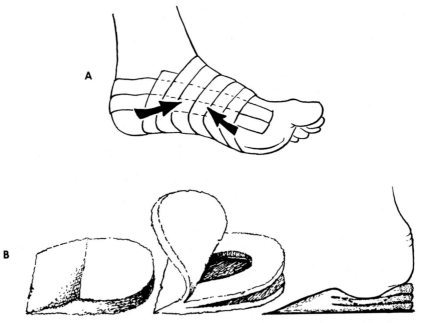

Fig. 15-12. A, Bow strapping. This strapping relieves pressure on the plantar fascia by shortening the medial side of the foot. **B,** Cut-out felt pad to relieve pressure on plantar tubercle of calcaneus.

tape (Fig. 15-13). In addition, pads placed underneath the toe are helpful (Fig. 15-14).

PHYSICAL THERAPY

Physical therapy of the foot and ankle is directed toward the reestablishment of full range of motion in the foot and the strengthening of its muscles. Its use is indicated after the foot has been injured or after a surgical procedure has been performed on the foot.

Sprains and fractures of the ankle. Extension and flexion exercises for the ankle and inversion and eversion ones for the subtalar joint may be prescribed for the treatment of healed ankle sprains or fractures. The patient should begin these exercises without bearing weight and then progress to bearing weight when functional motion has been reestablished.

Toes. Toe-gripping exercises using marbles and jacks help increase the range of motion of the toes.

Tendo achillis. Stretching exercises for the tendo achillis are best performed as follows: The patient stands erect, approximately 60 to 90 cm. away from the wall. He extends his arms to the wall and gently leans forward until his hands touch it, keeping his body erect and his heels firmly on the floor. When the patient first begins this exercise, his feet should be parallel; as progress is made, he should internally ro-

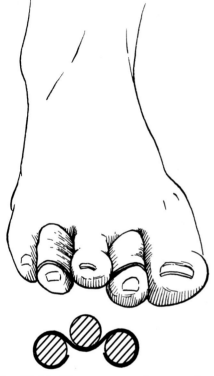

Fig. 15-13. Sling to support hammered toe.

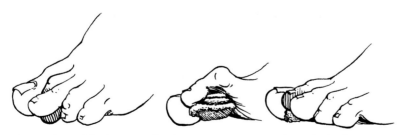

Fig. 15-14. Felt pad built up under hammertoe. It provides relief of pressure on the tip of the toe.

tate his foot 15 to 30 degrees in order to produce increased stretching of the tendon.

REFERENCES

Brachman, P. R.: Mechanical foot therapy, Danville, Ill., 1966, Interstate Printers and Publishers.

Cailliet, R.: Foot and ankle pain, Philadelphia, 1968, F. A. Davis Co.

Henderson, W. H., and Campbell, J. W.: UC-BL shoe insert: Casting and fabrication. The Biomechanics Laboratory, University of California, San Francisco and Berkeley. Technical Report 53, Aug. 1967.

Lewin, P.: The foot and ankle: Their injuries, diseases, deformities and disabilities, ed. 4, Philadelphia, 1959, Lea & Febiger.

Swanson, M. J. M.: Textbook of chiropody, ed. 2, Baltimore, 1954, The Williams & Wilkins Co.

16

Operative principles and requirements

Michael W. Chapman

PREOPERATIVE CONSIDERATIONS

Surgeons acknowledge that to obtain the best results from surgical procedures performed upon the hand, wise preoperative judgment, proper surgical instruments, skilled atraumatic surgical technique, and intensive, conscientious postoperative care are required. That these requisites are also mandatory for surgical operations upon the foot may not be as well recognized. Moreover, training in procedures especially for the foot is also necessary to ensure successful surgical treatment.

Pick (1949) described the surgical operation as a "premeditated, measured and ingenious form of trauma, with the respectable purpose of ablating certain diseases and bodily defects in man or animal."[*] All surgical intervention is in some degree traumatic, and one must strive to keep this trauma and its resultant morbidity minimal. More importantly, one must always keep the risks of surgical operations in mind and balance against them the expected gain from surgical intervention, particularly when operating for cosmetic reasons. When considering surgical correction of a mildly symptomatic bunion, for example, one should be aware that fitting the foot to the shoe may not be as successful as fitting the shoe to the foot.

---

[*]Pick, J. F.: Surgery of repair, vol. 1, Philadelphia, 1949, J. B. Lippincott Co., p. 109.

Suitable office procedures

Surgical procedures performed on the foot may be divided into those of the forefoot (metatarsals and phalanges), which comprise 90 percent of cases, and those of the hindfoot (tarsals), which comprise the remainder. Some minor disorders, such as warts, small benign growths, and minor nail diseases, may be treated in the office, provided the office is equipped with an autoclave, appropriate instruments, dressing materials, linens, and all other armamentaria essential for procedures of a minor nature. Proper preparation and asepsis must be as rigidly controlled in the office as in the hospital. If local anesthetics are employed, resuscitation equipment should be available in the event that the patient suffers an adverse reaction.

Instructions to the patient

The following specific instructions to the patient who is to undergo a surgical operation as an outpatient will prevent misunderstandings and are helpful to the surgeon:

1. Shave all hair from the foot and leg, taking care to avoid nicks.
2. Clip toenails.
3. Scrub the foot, especially around the nails, with soap and brush for 10 minutes shortly before leaving for the office or hospital outpatient department.

4. Bring along white socks and laced oxfords that may be cut if necessary to allow for swelling and dressings.

The diabetic patient needs special attention but is not denied necessary operation because of his disease. It is generally conceded that a controlled diabetic patient, properly prepared, is not a greater surgical risk than is a nondiabetic patient; however, it is safer to consider all diabetic patients as poor surgical risks. As illustrated by disorders associated with diabetes mellitus, foot problems often reflect systemic disease. Surgeons should therefore not undertake surgical operations on the foot unless they are capable of caring for the whole patient. Even for minor operations, the diabetic patient should be hospitalized where adequate laboratory facilities are available. He should be observed carefully by a physician experienced in the treatment of diabetes.

INSTRUMENTS

Surgical procedures done on the foot require instruments that are small, sharp, capable of being used in restricted space, and yet sufficiently tough to handle heavy fibrous tissues. Rhinologic, otolaryngologic, and hand surgery instruments are well

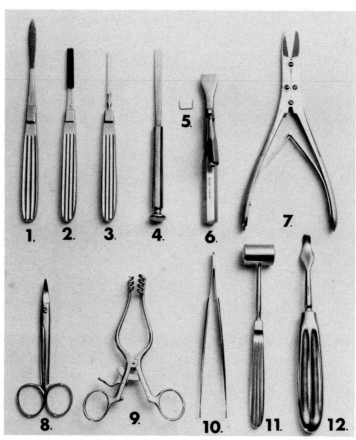

Fig. 16-1. *1,* Joseph nasal rasp; *2,* Maltz rasp; *3,* nasal saw with short neck; *4,* 8 mm. and 10 mm. osteotome, Stille pattern; *5,* 1 cm. staple; *6,* stapler; *7,* 19 cm. double-action bone forceps, DuVries modification; *8,* Sistrunk scissors, DuVries modification; *9,* Weitlander self-retaining retractor; *10,* Brown grasping forceps; *11,* mastoid mallet; and *12,* small Chandler elevator.

suited for foot surgery. The surgeon who specializes in procedures of the foot must see that suitable armamentaria are provided by the hospital, or he must supply his own.

Essential instruments and materials. The instruments shown in Fig. 16-1, in addition to the routine instrument tray, are sufficient for most surgical procedures on the forefoot. The number of each instrument available will vary with the operation. Of particular value in forefoot operative procedures are the modified Sistrunk scissors shown in Fig. 16-1.

Suturing needles. Needles, like other instruments, should be small but tough. Technical difficulties in foot surgery are very often caused by needles that are too large or too flimsy or both. Tendon repairs are best carried out with 4-0 synthetic suture swedged on double-ended Bunnell needles. Nerve repairs in the foot should be made with 7-0 to 8-0 black silk or synthetic suture swedged onto appropriately sized needles. The following needles fulfill most of the needs in foot surgery: No. 1848 Anchor brand surgical needles, sizes 1 and 2; 5 cm. Bunnell needles; and No. 1834 Anchor brand surgical needles, sizes 8 and 9.

Sutures. Suture materials are selected according to the preference of the surgeon, but they should be nonreactive and of the most minimal size acceptable.

Dressing materials. The following dressing materials should be at hand in an office or hospital surgical dressing room:

1. A 2.5 cm. gauze roller for bandaging the toes
2. A 4 cm. gauze roller for bandaging the forefoot
3. Sterile gauze sponges
4. Telfa squares, to be applied over incisions or raw surfaces to prevent the dressing from adhering to the wound
5. Sponge-rubber sheets, 1 cm. and 1.3 cm. for padding
6. 1 cm. piano felt for padding.
7. Paraffined lace mesh for draining ulcers
8. Lamb's wool for protection between the toes
9. Fine-mesh gauze
10. Materials for plaster casting

Tourniquets. When the surgeon performs procedures on the digits while the patient is under digital block anesthetic, the use of a tourniquet at the base of the toe is acceptable. The pressure should be broadly distributed, however; a medium or small Penrose drain held with a hemostat works well (Fig. 16-2). Rubber bands or similar

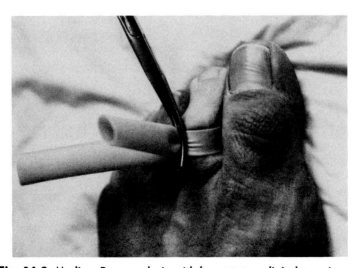

Fig. 16-2. Medium Penrose drain with hemostat as digital tourniquet.

small-caliber devices should not be used since they may generate high localized pressures which could cause irreversible damage to the digital neurovascular bundle. Digital tourniquets are contraindicated in persons with diabetes or peripheral vascular disease.

Unless its use is contraindicated because of peripheral vascular disease, a limb tourniquet is indispensable. Sterling Bunnell's aphorism, "Could a jeweler repair a watch immersed in ink?"* is as applicable to surgical operations on the foot as it is to those on the hand. The pneumatic tourniquet is the safest and most effective type of tourniquet and should always be applied to the proximal third of the thigh. Application to the distal thigh or to the leg may result in neurovascular injury.

It is usually practical to exsanguinate the extremity before inflating the tourniquet; however, elevation of the extremity during surgical preparation will allow some blood to remain in the veins and is often adequate to obtain good hemostasis, particularly if a bipolar electrode forceps is employed.

The amount of tourniquet pressure required is proportional to the circumference of the limb. For adults from 400 to 500 mm. of mercury is usually adequate. Less pressure is used for children; usually from 150 to 300 mm. of mercury is sufficient. When it is applied to normal limbs, the tourniquet can usually remain inflated for 1 hour. After 1½ hours of inflation, posttourniquet paresthesia will occasionally occur, but permanent residua are rarely if ever encountered. If 2 hours of tourniquet time is required, it is best to deflate the tourniquet after 1 hour for a 20-minute period and then reinflate it. When prolonged procedures are performed, it is often convenient to employ a tourniquet for the first 90 minutes and then proceed without an inflated tourniquet.

---

*Bunnell's surgery of the hand, ed. 4 (revised by J. H. Boyes), Philadelphia, 1964, J. B. Lippincott Co., p. 132.

OPERATIVE CONSIDERATIONS
Anesthesia

Most major operations on the foot need to be done under general or spinal anesthesia, but most minor procedures of the foot can be done under local anesthesia administered by the surgeon. Local infiltration and peripheral nerve blocks at the ankle work well. However, a thigh tourniquet cannot be used, since there is no anesthetic in the area of the tourniquet and most patients experience severe tourniquet pain. Blocks of the common digital nerve in the metatarsal area are useful when not contraindicated and when no more than three toes are to be operated upon.

Anesthetic agents containing epinephrine should not be used in digital blocks. Digital nerves are most effectively blocked as follows: With a small-gauge needle, enter the dorsum of the web space and place from 2 to 5 ml. of a 1 percent solution of a local anesthetic around the common digital nerve between the metatarsal heads. The use of digital nerve blocks in the toes should be avoided.

Technique for ankle block anesthesia. To block the deep peroneal nerve, introduce the needle lateral to the tendon of the tibialis anterior and advance it until contact is made with bone. Inject 10 ml. of a 1 percent procaine hydrochloride solution. The posterior tibial nerve may be reached just medial to the tendo achillis. Insert the needle through the deep fascia until it impinges on bone behind the medial malleolus. Withdraw the needle slightly and inject 5 to 10 ml. of 1 percent procaine hydrochloride. Block the sural nerve by injecting 5 to 10 ml. of 1 percent procaine hydrochloride on the lateral side of the tendo achillis. Insert the needle horizontally until it strikes the bone and then withdraw it slightly. Adjacent to each of the nerves is a large vessel that must be avoided in order not to introduce the drug directly into the bloodstream.

General and special precautions. Question the patient regarding known sensitivity to the drug or class of drugs to be administered. For the vast majority of cases, however, it is unnecessary to use more than 20 ml. of a 1 percent solution (200 mg.), a dose well within the usual limits of toxicity. Authenticate labels of all solutions before administering the drug.

Skin incisions of the foot

The anatomic structures and skin cleavages of the foot run longitudinally. If the incision must be made at a distance from the field of operation, it is usually better to make a longitudinal incision to follow those structures. It is true, however, that the scar of a longitudinal incision, if it is located over a moving joint, may restrict motion or produce contracture of the part (see Chapter 18).

Suturing. The importance of dexterity and atraumatic handling of tissue cannot be overemphasized (Tauber, 1955; Partipilo, 1957; Bunnell, 1964). In general, the technique to be used for operations on the foot should simulate that for operations on the hand. Particular attention should be paid to the preservation of viable skin cover.

POSTOPERATIVE CARE

To prevent postoperative edema and bleeding during the early postoperative period, the patient should be placed at bed rest, and his limb should be elevated. The patient's peripheral and neurovascular status should be carefully observed. Severe postoperative pain may occur because of an excessively tight circumferential dressing; circumferential plaster casts are sometimes slit in order to allow for swelling.

Weight bearing. As a rule, operations on the forefoot primarily involve soft tissue. It requires from 6 to 10 weeks for this tissue to gain sufficient strength to withstand stress. The part must be protected by adequate dressings during this period. Premature excessive weight bearing or wearing a shoe that has not been cut away from the operative site may produce a worse postoperative deformity than was present originally.

A moderate amount of weight bearing may be permitted between 24 and 72 hours, depending upon the procedure. In 3 or 4 days the complete original dressing should be changed. At that time the sutures should be examined carefully. Should there be signs of strangulation, the offending sutures should be removed; under normal conditions sutures are removed at 14 days postoperatively. After the third or fourth day a cutout oxford may be worn over a heavy white sock. This supports the foot without restricting the area of operation. An uncut shoe should not be worn until the edema and inflammatory process have subsided. This requires from 3 to 8 weeks.

Operations involving bony fusion must be followed by plaster immobilization for such time as is required for bony union to take place.

COMPLICATIONS OF SURGICAL PROCEDURES ON THE FOOT

Possible complications of surgical procedures on the foot are:
1. Unequal weight distribution
2. Delayed healing and infection
3. Recurrence of the deformity or production of a new deformity
4. Reaction to suture material
5. Wound dehiscence
6. Osteoporosis
7. Traumatic aneurysm
8. Postoperative anesthesia and paresthesia
9. Bone nonunion

Weight distribution. Extensive surgery of the foot may permanently alter weight distribution. When healing has been completed, weight distribution should be studied. Weight bearing should be balanced as required with the use of proper support, such as inlays, wedging of shoes, or the application of bars on the soles of the shoes.

Delayed healing and infection. Delayed healing and infection are ordinarily caused by any one or a combination of the following factors: vascular deficiency; abuse of tissue during surgical procedures; excessive subdermal postoperative bleeding producing diffused thrombotic blood (this type of bleeding can be prevented by always applying a compression dressing for the first 12 to 24 hours postoperatively); secondary infection, either fungal or bacterial; debilitating general disease; and premature use or movement of the affected part.

Spores of *tinea pedis* (dermatophytosis, also variously called trichophytosis, Hong Kong foot, athlete's foot, epidermophytosis) may invade the surgical incision and produce delayed healing. This type of infection differs from a pyogenic infection in that the symptoms of a pyogenic infection are violent and the entire wound may be disrupted and exude pus. Trichophytic infection affects only the surface, disrupts only the skin margins, and produces only mild symptoms. It is well to apply a dye type of fungicide when trichophytic infection is anticipated (see Chapter 12).

The symptoms of bacterial infection often appear within 72 hours but may also appear at a later time. Extraordinary systemic symptoms, signs of infection, or unusual wound pain should prompt the surgeon to inspect the operative site early. Rest, with elevation of the foot; establishment of wound drainage and culture and sensitivity studies; and the use of specific antibiotic therapy as indicated are employed to treat infections if they occur.

Although problems of bacterial carriers among hospital personnel, maintenance of sanitary operating room conditions, and development of antibiotic resistance have justifiably received much attention, it is our feeling that improper surgical technique is the single factor most responsible for postoperative infection.

Recurrence of deformity or appearance of new deformity. An improperly applied dressing may allow recurrence of the original deformity or produce a new deformity. If correction is accomplished before the tenth postoperative day, the correction can be maintained. If the deformity persists after that time, it may continue to do so.

Reaction to suture material. Occasionally a reaction to suture material used subder-

mally produces a sterile suture abscess. Symptoms may not appear for weeks or months postoperatively. When they do appear, the surface over the suture becomes soft and fluctuant and has a bluish discoloration. When the area is punctured, a sanguineous material is discharged, often containing the offending suture, or the suture is readily removed. Healing occurs after removal of the suture or sutures.

Wound dehiscence. Dehiscence may take place immediately after removal of skin sutures or may occur a few days later. This complication is more common in the foot than in other parts of the body. It may be caused in part by hematomas in or under the incision or by excessive handling of tissue during the operation. If dehiscence occurs, cleanse the wound with a mild antiseptic. Coaptation of the skin margins with butterfly adhesive tapes will approximate the skin margins until union occurs.

Postoperative osteoporosis. An infrequent complication of surgical operations on the foot is a generalized osteoporosis in the area of operation. Usually the entire foot becomes involved, although in some cases only one bone may be affected. The condition is a form of Sudeck's atrophy. The symptoms appear about 6 to 8 weeks after an apparently uneventful postoperative course. The disease manifests itself by pain, swelling, rubor, and often by cool, damp, and blotchy skin of the foot. Roentgenograms of both feet disclose loss of bone substance in one or more bones of the operated foot (Fig. 16-3). Although its cause is unknown, this disorder is probably best thought of as a sympathetic dystrophy caused by disuse. No uniformly effective treatment is known, but as the patient resumes normal activity, most of the symptoms eventually disappear.

Traumatic aneurysm. Aneurysm as a complication of surgery of the foot is uncommon. When it happens, it is caused by injury to a vessel during surgical procedures, especially when a tourniquet has been applied. If an artery has been completely divided, it will retract in its sheath and close

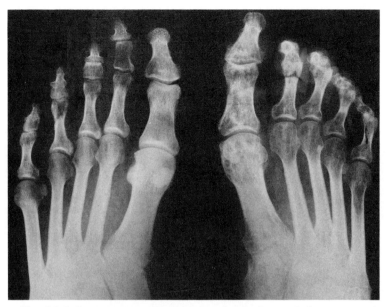

Fig. 16-3. Postoperative osteoporosis of right foot. Left foot is normal.

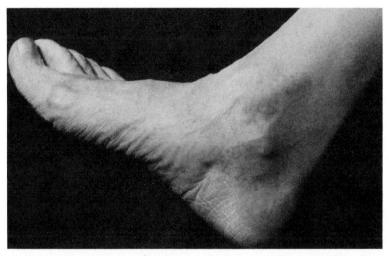

Fig. 16-4. Traumatic aneurysm of posterior tibial artery after operation along medial malleolus. (Courtesy Dr. Ronald Tanner.)

with little ill effect; however, if it has been only nicked and not divided, a hematoma forms and eventually becomes a false aneurysm (Fig. 16-4). If an adjacent vein is also nicked, development of an arteriovenous aneurysm may be anticipated. Scott (1955), Webb-Jones (1955), and Coughlin (1951) have reported such cases. In most cases of aneurysm a second surgical procedure is necessary to extirpate the aneurysm and ligate the vessels.

Postoperative anesthesia and paresthesia. Anesthesia or paresthesia caused by injury to a sensory nerve is a complication sometimes encountered after a surgical procedure performed on the foot. It may be unrecognized for some time postoperatively. In most instances sensation returns in 3 or 4 months. In a few instances patients become accustomed to the loss of sensation and are not disturbed by it. In those cases in which postoperative paresthesia is disabling, it may be necessary to resect a sensitive neuroma. The avoidance of surgical intrusion upon the major sensory nerves will usually prevent the occurrence of this complication.

Bone nonunion. Osteotomies occasionally are followed by delayed union or nonunion of bone. These difficulties can be avoided by restricting osteotomies to areas of cancellous bone if possible, by avoiding the distraction of the bone ends, and by providing adequate internal or external fixation or both until roentgenographic examination shows evidence of healing.

If nonunion does occur, a clinical trial should be undertaken before bone grafting is performed. Some fibrous unions are stable and free of pain and thus require no treatment.

REFERENCES

Bunnell's surgery of the hand, ed. 4 (revised by J. H. Boyes), Philadelphia, 1964, J. B. Lippincott Co., p. 5.

Coughlin, J. J.: Arterio-venous aneurysm of the foot following plantar fasciotomy, Northwest Med. **50:**772-773, Oct. 1951.

Howe, C. W.: Prevention and control of postoperative wound infections owing to Staphylococcus aureus, New Eng. J. Med. **255:**787-794, Oct. 1956.

Partipilo, A. V.: Surgical technique and principles of operative surgery, ed. 6, Philadelphia, 1957, Lea & Febiger, pp. 125-142.

Scott, J. H. S.: Traumatic aneurysm of the peroneal artery, J. Bone Joint Surg. **37-B:**438-439, Aug. 1955.

Tauber, R.: Basic surgical skills, Philadelphia, 1955, W. B. Saunders Co.

Webb-Jones, A.: Aneurysm after foot stabilization, J. Bone Joint Surg. **37-B:**440-442, Aug. 1955.

17

Amputations

Michael W. Chapman

Amputation is the (usually surgical) removal of a limb, portion of a limb, or other part. Disarticulation is amputation at a joint. For accuracy of description, these terms will both be employed in this chapter, along with a designation of the anatomic level of severance. Amputation as a collective term will be used as such.

Beyond the immediate consideration of treating the primary disease that has led to an amputation of all or part of the foot, the secondary consideration in performing an amputation should be to provide a successful weight-bearing stump. During weight bearing, the stump is subject to considerable pressure and to multiple minor episodes of trauma. For the amputation of a foot to be successful, the remaining stump should be pain free, stable, mobile, and neither vulnerable to skin infirmities and ulceration caused by pressure nor subject to the development of static deformities. If possible, it should be adaptable to the fitting of a prosthesis, standard shoes, or both.

Anatomic prerequisites for successful weight-bearing stumps are: (1) trabeculated bone, (2) skin and soft tissue that can be adapted to weight bearing, (3) good muscular control, and (4) mechanical leverage (Tooms, 1971).

INDICATIONS FOR AMPUTATION

Because modern medical advances have led to the extended survival of aged persons, geriatric disorders such as peripheral vascular disease are becoming more prevalent. Thus, today the leading indication for amputations of the foot is peripheral vascular disease. It should be noted that ischemia caused by major vessel occlusion due to arteriosclerosis differs from that caused by vasculitis or diabetes mellitus; in the latter the small-vessel disease present may make healing much more difficult. In fact, gangrene in diabetes mellitus often occurs in the absence of major vessel disease. A useful fact to keep in mind is that a wound is healed only by the patient's own blood supply.

Vascular disorders and diabetes mellitus are systemic disorders that require meticulous preoperative evaluation and preparation of the whole patient. Postoperative management should likewise be holistic. Practitioners who are not prepared to care for the whole patient should not undertake the performance of amputation procedures.

Selection of the level of amputation and the timing of such procedures require careful judgment and are beyond the scope of this discussion.

Chronic pyogenic infection, particularly osteomyelitis, is a frequent precursor of amputation, especially in the diabetic, the atherosclerotic, and the neurotrophic foot. Unusual chronic infections such as Madura foot, tuberculosis (particularly of the hindfoot), and coccidioidomycosis, if unresponsive to medical treatment, may be best treated by an amputation or a ray resection.

Acute infections are usually responsive to customary medical and surgical measures. Severe, acute, life-threatening infections such as gas gangrene may demand immediate amputation through normal tissue. However, the introduction of hyperbaric oxygen therapy may lead to a reevaluation of the role of amputation in this disease.

Our mechanized civilization has made trauma the second most frequent cause for amputations in the foot, and most amputations performed because of trauma are actually revisions of traumatic amputations. Until recently, the only absolute indication for amputation has been deprivation of the blood supply. Present and future developments in microvascular surgery will require reevaluation of this principle. Crush or mutilating injuries of such severity as to make the preservation of a satisfactory functional part impossible may lead to amputation. In cases in which open injuries lead to amputation, the surgeon's first responsibility is to prevent infection by carrying out adequate debridement and copious irrigation. Open amputation provides the most effective and safe way to prevent infection and to manage tissue of marginal viability.

In cases of partial traumatic amputation or severe crush or mutilating injury in which the viability of the distal segment is questionable, it is best to employ conservative measures initially. Similarly, if viability of the distal segment is questionable in patients with burns and frostbite, conservative treatment should be pursued until demarcation occurs. If infection is avoided, with time the nonviable portions will become apparent and elective amputation can then be carried out, often at a more distal level than one would have anticipated initially.

Congenital deformities such as supernumerary digits are corrected by amputation in infancy for cosmetic reasons. At a later age, pain and limitation of physical performance constitute the principal indications for amputation of such digits.

Tumors of the foot, both benign and malignant, may make amputation necessary for adequate control.

GENERAL OPERATIVE PRINCIPLES

No special procedures other than those outlined in Chapter 17 are usually required for the preoperative preparation of a patient who is to undergo an elective amputation of the foot. Amputations on the ischemic and neurotrophic limb, especially in the presence of infection, warrant special consideration and necessitate variations of technique.

To ensure surgical success, adequate preoperative preparation is important. Infection should be controlled by confining the patient to bed for a period that may last several weeks. During this time, antibiotics, surgical drainage, debridement, and dressing changes are employed. In diabetic patients with gangrene amputation can be contemplated after gangrene is localized and infection is controlled. However, rest pain, edema, and rubor proximal to the line of incision must be absent before amputation can be successfully accomplished.*

The key to uncomplicated healing of an amputation stump, beyond assuring that an adequate blood supply is present at the level of amputation, is gentle, atraumatic operative technique. The blood supply to the skin of the foot is usually damaged by rough handling and by closure under tension. Primary wound healing, so important in facilitating immediate prosthetic fitting and early ambulation, can be obtained by observing the following principles:

1. Elective incisions should be designed to preserve the plantar surface of the toe or foot, since the skin in this area is especially adapted for weight bearing.

2. In the foot, good coverage with skin capable of withstanding weight-bearing trauma is generally more important than the preservation of stump length.

3. Except under special circumstances,

*See Collens and Wilensky, 1953; Pedersen and Day, 1954; Wheelock et al., 1957; and Wheelock, 1961.

skin grafts should not be used in weight-bearing areas.

4. Scars should not be placed on the ends of stumps or on weight-bearing portions of stumps. (Traumatic amputations, however, usually require some ingenuity and must often be carried out with less orthodox placement of the skin flaps.)

If possible, the thin subcutaneous tissue in the forefoot should be preserved, as well as the vertical septae between the skin and the underlying deep fascia, particularly in the heel pad. Nerves are pulled distally without excessive traction. They are cut sharply with a fresh blade so that they will retract proximal to the line of bone division. This technique will prevent the formation of a neuroma under a weight-bearing bone. Particular attention should be paid to the subcutaneous sensory nerves, which are often ignored by less meticulous surgeons. It is unnecessary and inadvisable to ligate or coagulate nerves in the foot. Tendons are pulled down and divided, thus permitting them to retract. Vessels are ligated and hemostasis is accomplished prior to closure. If a tourniquet is employed for hemostasis during amputation, it should be released before closure to assure that hemostasis has again been secured. Tourniquets should not be used in the presence of vascular disease. If bones are transected, their distal ends should be smoothed and shaped so as to provide the best weight-bearing surface. This practice is particularly important in transmetatarsal amputations.

The sine qua non for surgery of ischemic tissue is aseptic, atraumatic, meticulous technique. Sharp dissection, effective hemostasis, obliteration of dead space at the time of closure, and skillful approximation of skin edges without tension are mandatory. Skin margins should not be squeezed by forceps.

Open amputations should have skin flaps formed in such a manner as to facilitate secondary closure. Because some skin retraction almost always occurs, these flaps are usually fashioned somewhat longer than they would be if primary closure were to be undertaken. Some means of dressing the wound postoperatively to prevent skin retraction should be employed. A useful dressing may be made by placing the usual bulky dressing material about the stump and then adhering tubular stockinette to the foot and skin flaps by means of either tincture of benzoin or ace adherent.

Forefoot amputations are almost never drained. Hindfoot amputations, particularly the Syme's amputation, often require drainage, which is usually best managed with suction through plastic tubing (Hemovac). Care should be taken not to apply excessive suction to stumps that have open bone ends. Drains are generally removed when bleeding has ceased (at 48 to 72 hours).

Skin sutures should be of small caliber (4-0 to 5-0), nonreactive suture material (e.g, steel or the synthetic materials such as nylon). In amputations in which secondary closure of a stump is anticipated or complete closure without tension is initially impossible, wire sutures are often useful. They can be tightened at a later time, thus eliminating the need for the placement of additional suture material. Mattress sutures should not be employed because of their deleterious effect upon the blood supply to the skin. If accurate approximation of skin edges presents a problem, it is well to use one row of widely placed, interrupted sutures and then a second row of small-caliber sutures in the skin edge. Some surgeons believe that the use of small sutures placed in an interrupted fashion permits better adjustment of skin tension.

The postoperative dressings function primarily to prevent edema and to provide tissue rest. Hence, it is advisable to use bulky compression dressings that incorporate some form of splintage to immobilize the ankle. Postoperatively the patient should be kept at bed rest, with the extremity moderately elevated.

PROSTHESES

Those prostheses that are employed following amputations distal to the ankle are relatively simple. Amputations of toes may require only sponge rubber or lamb's wool

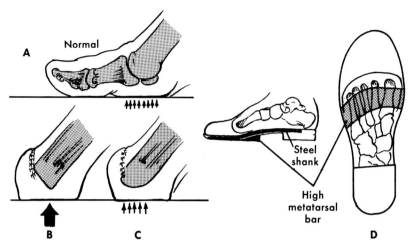

Fig. 17-1. Weight bearing in forefoot amputation. **A,** Normal foot. There is a wide area of weight-bearing surface in stance and in gait. **B,** Transmetatarsal amputation. After sharp transection of the metatarsal shaft (cortical bone), the sharp lower edge becomes a pivot point in gait, resulting in exaggerated local pressure. **C,** Transmetatarsal amputation. Contouring the cancellous metatarsal head provides a broad weight-bearing surface parallel to the ground. **D,** Forefoot amputation. Shoeing the foot with a rigid sole and a high metatarsal bar prevents pivoting on the forefoot, thus reducing the high pressures under the ends of the metatarsals. This technique is especially valuable in the neurotrophic foot.

inserted into the tip of the shoe. A spring steel shank in the sole will prevent deformity of the shoe and will provide assistance with push-off. If a sole shank is deemed necessary, it should be carried out at least to the metatarsal heads. In amputations of the second toe, a spacer composed of any firm but pliable material may be inserted into the space between the first and third toes in order to prevent hallux valgus. Transmetatarsal amputations should be fitted with a filler for the toe of the shoe, and a steel sole shank should always be fitted to protect the end of the stump. A metatarsal bar that employs the principle illustrated in Fig. 17-1, *D* is often necessary. For the Syme's amputation, the Canadian prosthesis with the SACH (solid ankle cushion heel) foot is employed (Wilson, 1961).

AMPUTATION LEVELS

Forefoot amputations, through the metatarsals or distal to the metatarsals, are classified as minor procedures and usually satisfy the aforementioned anatomic prerequisites for providing successful weight-bearing stumps. Generally, the length of the toes and the metatarsal bones should be preserved as far as possible. While disarticulation through the interphalangeal joints or amputation of any of the toes distal to the metatarsophalangeal joint have only a minimal effect on function, amputation of the great toe creates functional difficulties. Loss of this toe has only a moderate effect on stance or slow gait; however, loss of length impairs push-off and causes limping during rapid gait or running. Moreover, some diminution of the weight-bearing function of the metatarsophalangeal joint of the great toe can create excessive pressures on the lateral metatarsal heads, and as a result plantar calluses may form.

Complete amputation of the second toe may result in migration of the great toe into the space previously occupied by the second toe, causing a hallux valgus deformity.

Amputation of the lesser toes, although producing little disability in most individuals, can be disabling to athletes. Impairment in athletic maneuvers in which spring and resilience of the foot are required can present a problem (Flint and Sweetnam, 1960; Slocum, 1949).

The metatarsal area is the next proximal level at which satisfactory function may be obtained after amputation. Again, as much length of the metatarsal as possible should be preserved. The usual and most acceptable amputation level is just proximal to the metatarsal heads. Transmetatarsal amputation proximal to this level may produce mechanical difficulties in the stump and cause complications from pressure.

The disability resulting from transmetatarsal amputations increases as the level of amputation moves proximally. Loss of toe push-off and the absence of an effective fulcrum at the ball of the foot are chiefly responsible for the impairment of gait.

The tarsometatarsal joint is the highest level at which adequate function of the foot may be retained after amputation, but the awkwardness in walking occasioned by the loss of support in push-off is frequently disabling. Amputation at this level is in disrepute because the patient often develops severe equinovalgus deformity (Slocum, 1949; Stack, 1958; Thompson, 1963; Tooms, 1971). This deformity is caused by muscle imbalance, with the gastrocnemius and the soleus muscles pulling the foot down into equinus because of the absence of the foot and toe dorsiflexors.

The next most proximal amputation frequently employed is the Syme's amputation, which is essentially an amputation slightly proximal to the articulating surface of the tibia at the ankle joint. Amputations between this level and the transmetatarsal level are mentioned mainly for historical reasons.

Tarsometatarsal disarticulation is known as Lisfranc's (1790-1847) amputation. Chopart (1743-1795) described a midtarsal disarticulation in which a long plantar flap was used. Neither of these amputations is currently employed because of the disadvantages of midfoot amputations previously described.

The amputations of Pirogoff, Boyd, and Vasconcelos involve the hindfoot. They incorporate partial resection of portions of the talus and calcaneus and fusion of the remaining segments. Pirogoff (1810-1881) disarticulated the ankle with a talectomy and a resection of the anterior two-thirds of the calcaneus. The remaining calcaneus was then fused to the distal tibia. Weight bearing occurred on the normal heel. This amputation is not recommended, as it offers little advantage over the Syme's amputation, and one is faced with the possibility of failure of fusion.

Boyd (1939) described talectomy with calcaneotibial arthrodesis. In this amputation a larger segment of the calcaneus is preserved than in the Pirogoff procedure, and it has the advantage of providing a serviceable weight-bearing stump with minimal shortening. The calcaneus is used for direct weight bearing and a prosthesis is not required. This procedure is rarely used, however, as it offers minimal advantage over the Syme's amputation, and again one is faced with the problem of obtaining bony fusion.

The Vasconcelos amputation (midtarsal disarticulation; tibiotalar and subtalar arthrodesis and section of the inferior surfaces of the calcaneus) produces a similar end result to that of the Boyd amputation and is technically more difficult.

OPERATIVE TECHNIQUE
Partial amputation of the distal phalanx of the hallux (subtotal phalangectomy)

Subtotal phalangectomy is indicated for extreme deformity of the nail and distal phalanx of the hallux (Fig. 17-2). The procedure is as follows:

1. Make a semilunar incision starting on either side, about 0.5 cm. proximal to the eponychium, over the dorsum of the toe. Carry the incision down to the bone and extend it on both sides to about one-third of the way to the plantar surface.
2. Begin a second semilunar incision at either end of the initial incision and continue it completely around the

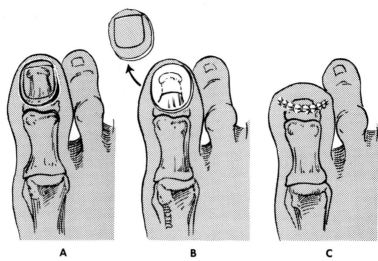

Fig. 17-2. Partial amputation of distal phalanx of great toe. **A,** Incision to remove skin, nail, and matrix. **B,** Excision of skin, fat, and shaded bone. **C,** Approximation of distal skin flap to proximal skin edge with multiple fine sutures.

distal end of the toe until it meets both ends of the first incision.

3. Free and remove the entire dorsal flap, including the nail and the nail bed, from the dorsum of the distal phalanx.
4. Undermine the remaining intact tissue around the distal phalanx.
5. Amputate the distal half of the distal phalanx.
6. Round and smooth the stump with a Joseph nasal rasp.
7. At this point the distal flap approximates the initial semilunar incision. Enough bone should be removed so that the flap can be sutured without tension. If the distal skin flap is sutured under tension, the suture line may slough.

Amputation of the distal phalanx (total phalangectomy)

Total phalangectomy is required primarily for the first and second toes and occasionally for the three lesser toes. When amputation of the distal phalanx of one of the three lesser toes is indicated, it is often more practical to amputate the entire toe. The second toe, however, should not be ampu-

tated unless it is absolutely necessary. Once the second toe has been removed, hallux valgus is almost certain to ensue, even in a previously normal foot. Toe amputation for ischemic gangrene is often unsuccessful and transmetatarsal amputation becomes necessary. However, amputation for chronic ulceration, often associated with osteomyelitis of the phalanx, may be undertaken with an excellent prospect of success.

The procedure for amputation of the distal phalanx of the lesser toes is the same as that described for partial amputation of the distal phalanx of the great toe.

Disarticulation of the phalangeal joint of the great toe

The principal indications for disarticulation of the phalangeal joint of the great toe are the presence of osteomyelitis, neoplasm, or a severe crush injury of the distal phalanx.

1. Make a semielliptical incision over the dorsum of the hallux, beginning on the side of the head of the proximal phalanx and ending at the same point on the opposite side of the phalanx. The uppermost curve of the el-

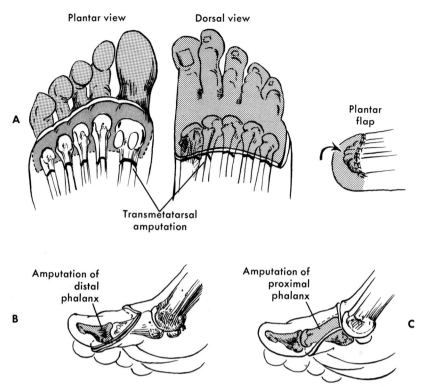

Fig. 17-3. Amputations using long plantar flap. **A,** Transmetatarsal amputation. **B,** Amputation of distal phalanx of great toe. **C,** Amputation of proximal phalanx of great toe.

lipse should course just proximally to the head of the proximal phalanx.

2. Begin a second semielliptical incision at the starting point of the first incision and continue the incision plantarward and distally to meet at the end of the first incision (Fig. 17-3, *B*). Note that the plantar flap is the longest.

3. Disarticulate the distal phalanx and bring the plantar flap forward to cover the head of the proximal phalanx, suturing the flap to the dorsal margin. The plantar flap always must be of sufficient length to permit suturing without tension; otherwise the suture line will slough and a wide scar will result.

4. The long flexor and extensor tendons may or may not be sutured to each other; the choice is that of the surgeon. The sheaths of the tendons ad-

here to the shaft of the proximal phalanx by circular fibers and retain their function after healing, even though not sutured.

Disarticulation at the metatarsophalangeal joint of the lesser toes

When a lesser toe must be amputated, it is best to remove it at the metatarsophalangeal joint. Amputation through the proximal phalanx leaves a small, useless stump, which is subject to friction and pressure. The stump is so close to the web that it looks no better than a metatarsophalangeal disarticulation. (Fig. 17-4.)

1. Make a teardrop (racket) incision completely around the base of the toe to be amputated, with the apex of the incision pointing proximally on the dorsum.

2. Plantar flex the toe, opening the dor-

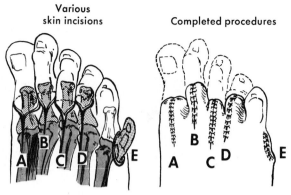

Various
skin incisions   Completed procedures

Fig. 17-4. Incisions for amputations of single toes and metatarsals. **A,** Closed amputation of great toe (disarticulation at metatarsophalangeal joint or amputation through proximal phalanx). **B,** Closed amputation through proximal phalanx. **C,** Closed metatarsophalangeal disarticulation. **D,** Open amputation with longer medial-lateral flaps to facilitate drainage and later closure. Incisions are designed to leave loosely gaping wounds without sutures. **E,** Supernumerary digit. Elliptical incision and excision of a convexity of tissue permits closure of the skin and soft tissue.

sal incision and permitting the metatarsophalangeal joint to be incised on the dorsum and carried around both sides of the joint. The extensor tendon will also be transected with this cut.

3. On dorsiflexion of the toe, section the plantar capsule to permit complete removal of the toe. Identify the neurovascular bundles. Isolate and transect the nerve; ligate the vessels. It is not an advantage to suture the flexor and extensor tendons to each other; their removal does not impair the function of the foot.

4. Suture the skin margins from side to side and apply a compression bandage. Ambulation may begin the next day. Healing is usually uneventful.

Disarticulation at the metatarsophalangeal joint of the great toe

Contrary to the advice regarding the lesser toes, the base of the proximal phalanx of the hallux should be saved whenever possible because of the important intrinsic muscles that insert into it. This is especially true of the flexor hallucis brevis, which, when deprived of its insertion, retracts the

sesamoids proximal to the middle of the shaft of the first metatarsal.

1. Make a dorsal semilunar incision, starting just behind the head of the first metatarsal (Fig. 17-4, A).

2. Make a second plantar horseshoe incision with its uppermost crest distally, beginning in the first toe web and ending on the medial side of the base of the proximal phalanx. This forms a plantar flap that should be made as wide and as long as possible to permit covering the stump without tension.

3. If the base of the proximal phalanx can be saved, saw the bone at its proximal epiphyseal line and smooth and round it with a rasp. Cover the stump with the plantar flap and suture it into place. In the event that the entire proximal phalanx must be removed, after the horseshoe incision has been made, sever the extensor and flexor hallucis longus tendons just proximal to their insertion into the distal phalanx and hold them aside. Section the dorsal metatarsophalangeal capsule transversely. Plantar flex the toe. Separate the tendons of the

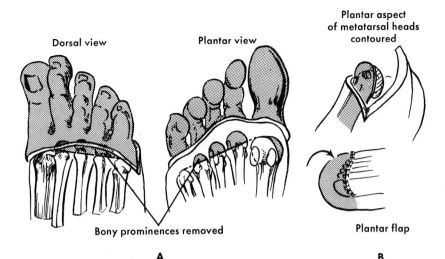

Dorsal view Plantar view Plantar aspect of metatarsal heads contoured

Bony prominences removed Plantar flap

A **B**

Fig. 17-5. Amputation of all toes. **A,** Disarticulation of all toes permitted by skin incision. **B,** Division of soft tissue and contouring of plantar aspect of metatarsal heads. **C,** Distal ends of metatarsals freed of bony prominences. (After Flint, M., and Sweetnam, R.: J. Bone Joint Surg. **42-B:**90-96, Feb. 1960; Fowler, A. W.: J. Bone Joint Surg. **41-B:** 507-513, Aug. 1959.)

adductor, abductor, and flexor hallucis brevis from the base of the proximal phalanx. Remove the entire toe.
4. Suture the flexor hallucis brevis tendon to the long flexor tendon; suture the long flexor tendon to the long extensor tendon. This forms a cover on the articular surface of the first metatarsal head. The abductor and adductor hallucis tendons usually can be sutured to each other or to the long tendons.
5. Bring up the plantar skin flap to cover the stump and suture it into place.

Weight bearing should not be permitted for about 3 weeks. Because the great toe has an important balancing function in walking or running and its loss can affect weight bearing seriously, a shoe with a rigid sole or a rigid inlay, extending the full length of the shoe, should be prescribed.

Amputation of all toes

Amputation of all toes may be indicated in severe deformities, congenital anomalies,

gangrene of the tips of the toes as a result of frostbite, and cases of previous amputation of all but one or two toes, rendering these especially subject to trauma (Fig. 17-5). Healing and resultant function are usually good in such cases (Fowler, 1959; Flint and Sweetnam, 1960; London, 1969).

Amputation of a metatarsal (ray resection)

Ray resection is most commonly performed on the fifth ray. It is most frequently employed in cases of congenital deformity involving supernumerary rays and for neoplasms or severe chronic infections involving a single metatarsal. In the event that ray resection is elected for removal of a supernumerary ray and if six completely normal rays are present, one usually elects to resect the fifth ray, leaving the sixth ray on the lateral border of the foot intact. In so doing, a surgical scar on the lateral aspect of the foot is avoided.

Except for the resection of a supernumerary ray, a single metatarsal rarely needs to be amputated. Gangrene or extensive traumatic mutilation usually involves all or multiple metatarsals. It is possible, however, for a single metatarsal to be diseased or to be destroyed by injury. Removal is then indicated.

1. Begin an incision on the dorsum of the foot at the base of the metatarsal to be removed and carry the incision distally to the web space, thence through the web, and loop it around the flexor crease of the toe to be removed.
2. Continue the course of the incision, through the alternate web, and extend the incision proximally to the starting point of the incision.
3. Retract the skin margins and carry the incision down into the intermetatarsal space on both sides of the metatarsal. Next, identify the neurovascular bundles and handle in the usual fashion. Take care to avoid injury to the neurovascular bundles of the adjacent toes.
4. Divide the tendons and allow them to retract.
5. Using extraperiosteal dissection, work distally to proximally and disarticulate the metatarsal.
6. Close the resulting dead space as much as possible.
7. Approximate the skin margins.

The most difficult problem encountered in ray resection in the foot is closure of the dead space at the proximal portion of the wound where the base of the metatarsal was present. This area should be closed as much as possible. A drain is not customarily employed, but the wound should be watched carefully for proper healing.

Transmetatarsal amputation

Transmetatarsal amputation is indicated occasionally for severe crush injuries of the toes and metatarsal heads, for tumors, and for infection and gangrene. Transmetatarsal amputation in diabetic peripheral vascular disease may be indicated in preference to below-knee amputations for ulceration and gangrene, providing that extension of gangrene to the dorsal or plantar skin is not present proximal to the line of incision. The most reliable signs of viability of the proximal portion of the foot are the presence of warmth to palpation and a line of demarcation. Transmetatarsal amputation is the procedure of choice when amputation of the second toe is required, when one or more toes are gangrenous, and even when extension involves the first or fifth metatarsal head.

Before World War II and the widespread use of antibiotics, blood transfusions, and vascular surgery, high amputation was often done for gangrenous toes in the diabetic limb. Since that time, more conservative amputations have been successful without increased morbidity and mortality. Pedersen and Day (1954) reported only two gross failures in a group of twenty-three transmetatarsal amputations for gangrene as a result of peripheral vascular disease. Wheelock et al. (1957) reported 69 percent of their transmetatarsal amputation cases as functional 1 year after surgery. In 1961, Wheelock reported that 63 percent were functional 2 years after surgery. Of 428 amputations in diabetics, 162 had angiography and 49 were subjected to arterial surgery for localized obstruction. Adequate collateral circulation was frequently evident without pulsation. Indeed, with no pulsation distal to the aorta, 44 percent of the amputations needed no further surgical treatment for 2 years. However, delayed venous filling was associated with a high rate of failure. The importance of preoperative preparation and meticulous technique cannot be overemphasized.

The amputation level is just proximal to the metatarsal heads at the level of the dorsal skin incision (Fig. 17-3, A). When the amputation has been completed, only bone remains between the dorsal and plantar skin flaps. If the saw level is more proximal, it will pass through the deep structures of the foot, including relatively ischemic muscle that increases the risk of infection and necrosis.

1. Begin the dorsal incision midway between the dorsal and plantar surfaces

on the side of the hallux. Continue the incision at the level of the amputation, in a straight line across the dorsum, cutting sharply down to the bone to the midpoint on the side of the fifth toe.

2. Begin the plantar incision at either end of the dorsal incision, incising sharply down to the bone; parallel the flexion crease of the toes 1 cm. proximally and carry the incision to the opposite side.

3. Dissect the plantar flap to the level of the bone amputation.

4. With a saw remove the metatarsal heads singly, beginning with the first, and form an even stump. The metatarsals should be rongeured smooth; the first or fifth may require resectioning or beveling. Especially in ischemic feet, the metatarsals should be divided at the level of the dorsal skin incision, care being taken to avoid dissection of the dorsal flap.

5. Divide the plantar tendons at the bone level and remove the sesamoids. Identify the neurovascular structures and treat in the usual fashion.

6. Close in one layer, using fine steel wire. The dog ears are not removed, since they provide vital blood supply to the plantar flap.

7. Apply a bulky dressing. Immobilize the foot and ankle with a padded splint. Especially in those cases of borderline viability, bed rest should be continued until the sutures are removed in 2 or 3 weeks. If an occasional suture appears tight, it may be removed earlier. Buerger's exercises should be begun in 10 to 14 days after surgery. Full weight bearing is allowed only after complete healing has occurred; this may require 4 to 6 weeks.

Syme's amputation

The distinguishing features of the operation described by Syme (1799-1870) are disarticulation at the ankle joint, re-

section of the malleoli, and coverage with plantar skin alone. This amputation provides a satisfactory weight-bearing stump that can be used without a prosthesis even though approximately 5 to 8 cm. of shortening may be present. Following this procedure, a prosthesis is customarily employed that provides superior full end–weight-bearing function, superb control, and excellent proprioception. If cosmesis is of great concern, this amputation is generally not recommended. The bulbous nature of the stump necessitates a thick-ankled prosthesis which cannot be matched to the normal side and which may be unattractive in women who wear skirts.

In peripheral vascular disease, the Syme's amputation occasionally is successful even after the failure of a transmetatarsal amputation.

If sufficient distal infection is present at the operative site to cause considerable risk, one of two alternatives can be chosen: A two-stage Syme's amputation can be performed in which the ankle is disarticulated but the malleoli are not resected. By using this type of procedure, one limits possible postoperative infection to the soft tissues and will probably avoid involvement of the tibia, the fibula, or both. The stump may be left open or may be closed over two plastic tubes, which function to decompress the dead space in the heel flap and are also used as routes for local antibiotic irrigation. When the wound is well healed and no evidence of infection has been present for a number of weeks, a second procedure to resect the malleoli and to shape the stump properly can then be carried out.

Some surgeons will undertake an alternative method even in the presence of gross infection in the foot: The classic Syme's amputation is performed and the stump is closed over two plastic tubes. Wound suction and irrigation with local antibiotics may then be instituted and systemic antibiotics of the appropriate type may also be employed.

A modified version of the classic Syme's technique is as follows:

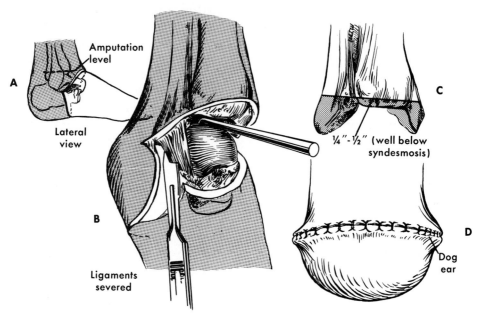

Fig. 17-6. Syme's amputation. **A,** Incisions and bone level. **B,** Exposure of ankle joint and severance of ligaments. **C,** Saw line 0.6 to 1 cm. above ankle joint and parallel to ground. **D,** Completed amputation. (Modified from Crenshaw, A. H., editor: Campbell's operative orthopaedics, ed. 5, vol. 1, St. Louis, 1971, The C. V. Mosby Co.)

1. Position the foot at a right angle and make two incisions (Fig. 17-6, *A*). The plantar incision extends from the tip of the lateral malleolus across the sole of the foot and curves slightly forward to a point one finger's width below the medial malleolus. Carry the incision to the bone. The dorsal incision joins the ends of the previous incision, running upward and forward. Care should be taken not to carry the apex of these two incisions posterior to the malleoli. Deepen the dorsal incision and enter the ankle joint. Cut the tendons sharply and allow them to retract. Handle the neurovascular structures in the usual manner.

2. Divide the tibial and fibular collateral ligaments by placing a knife in the joint and drawing it inferiorly.

3. Dislocate the talus forward by placing a bone hook in its posterior aspect; proceed with excision of the talus and calcaneus.

4. With sharp dissection, enter the sub-periosteal plane on either side of the calcaneus and extend this dissection inferiorly. Continue the dissection until the entire calcaneus is free posteriorly and the tendo achillis has been divided (Fig. 17-6, *B*).

5. Place the bone hook into the tuberosity and deliver the calcaneus forward into the wound. Apply careful, sharp dissection close to the calcaneus and remove the foot, leaving the heel flap.

6. Turn the heel flap proximally in a gentle fashion and free the malleoli and the distal 0.6 cm. of the tibia. Then transect the malleoli and a portion of the tibia with a single saw cut so that the plane of section will parallel the ground when the patient is standing (Fig. 17-6, *C*). Strive to achieve the greatest cross-sectional area possible. Round and smooth all sharp corners with a rasp.

7. If a tourniquet has been employed, release it and obtain hemostasis. Care should be taken at this point

to assure that all nerves have been transected so as to lie proximal to the distal tibial surface. Ligate the blood vessels at the level of the skin flaps, taking particular care to preserve the posterior tibial blood supply to the heel flap.

8. Obliterate the dead space with a Penrose or Hemovac suction drain, which exits at either corner of the wound.
9. To close the wound, center the heel pad and begin to suture anteriorly midway between incision ends, using fine catgut for the subcutaneous tissue and nonreactive synthetic or wire suture for the skin. Approximate the margin of the heel pad to the margin of the dorsal incision. Use interrupted everting skin sutures and *never* trim the dog ears, since doing so may compromise the circulation (Fig. 17-6, *D*).
10. Secure the position of the heel flap, which is freely movable, with two strips of adhesive tape wide enough to hold it securely without overlapping or creating excess pressure. Center one strip on the heel pad and then apply the ends to the lateral and medial aspects of the leg. Apply the second strip in the same manner but at right angles, securing the ends on the anterior and posterior aspects of the leg. (Some surgeons prefer to stabilize the flap by inserting a Steinmann pin into the distal tibia.)
11. Apply a bulky compression dressing. (We prefer a hard dressing and apply a well-molded, well-padded short leg cast. This type of dressing usually assures maintenance of the proper position of the heel pad and minimizes edema.)

Postoperative care. Remove the drains when drainage has ceased for 24 hours (or from 48 to 72 hours.) Keep the limb elevated.

The cast and dressing are changed at weekly intervals. At approximately 3 weeks, when the sutures are out and healing is adequate, a walking heel may be added to the cast and weight bearing can be started. The cast at this point should be well molded according to the patellar-tendon–bearing principle. Prosthetic fitting is carried out when stump shrinkage has stabilized.

Complications. Slough of the heel flap may result from injury to the posterior tibial artery. A distorted heel pad may result from disruption of the fibroadipose septa of the heel pad or from misplacement of the plantar flap. Shifting of the heel pad on weight bearing can occur if the cut surface on the tibia is not parallel to the ground during weight bearing.

A painful stump may be caused by neuroma formation on the posterior tibial nerve. Defective skin coverage in atypical flaps and bony spurs and callous formation in defective heel pads also produce pain (Harris, 1956, 1961; Slocum, 1949; Wilson, 1927; Wilson, 1961; Tooms, 1971).

REFERENCES

Boyd, H. B.: Amputation of the foot with calcaneotibial arthrodesis, J. Bone Joint Surg. **21:** 997-1000, Oct. 1939.

Collens, W. S., and Wilensky, N. D.: Peripheral vascular diseases, ed. 2, Springfield, Ill., 1953, Charles C Thomas, Publisher.

Flint, M., and Sweetnam, R.: Amputation of all toes: A review of forty-seven amputations, J. Bone Joint Surg. **42-B:**90-96, Feb. 1960.

Fowler, A. W.: A method of forefoot reconstruction, J. Bone Joint Surg. **41-B:**507-513, Aug. 1959.

Harris, R. I.: Syme's amputation: The technical details essential for success, J. Bone Joint Surg. **38-B:**614-632, Aug. 1956.

Harris, R. I.: The history and development of Syme's amputation, Artif. Limbs **6:**4-43, Apr. 1961.

London, P. S.: Amputations of the fingers and toes. In Rob, C., and Smith, R., editors: Operative surgery, ed. 2, London, 1969, Butterworth & Co.

Pedersen, H. E., and Day, A. J.: The transmetatarsal amputation in peripheral vascular disease, J. Bone Joint Surg. **36-A:**1190-1199, Dec. 1954.

Slocum, D. B.: An atlas of amputations, St. Louis, 1949, The C. V. Mosby Co.

Stack, J. K.: Technical essentials in amputation, Surg. Clin. N. Amer. **38:**301-305, Feb. 1958.

Thompson, R. G.: Amputation in the lower extremity, J. Bone Joint Surg. **45-A**:1723-1734, Dec. 1963.

Tooms, R. E.: Amputations. In Crenshaw, A. H., editor: Campbell's operative orthopaedics, ed. 5, vol. 1, St. Louis, 1971, The C. V. Mosby Co., pp. 838-900.

Wheelock, F. C., Jr.: Transmetatarsal amputations and arterial surgery in diabetic patients, New Eng. J. Med. **264**:316-320, Feb. 1961.

Wheelock, F. C., Jr., McKittrick, J. B., and Root, H. F.: Evaluation of the transmetatarsal amputation in patients with diabetes mellitus, Surgery **41**:184-189, Feb. 1957.

Wilson, A. B., Jr.: Prostheses for Syme's amputation. Artif. Limbs, **6**:52-101, Apr. 1961.

Wilson, P. D.: Amputations. In Whipple, A. O., editor: Nelson loose-leaf living surgery, New York, 1927, T. Nelson & Sons.

18

Surgical approaches to the deep structures of the foot and ankle

Verne T. Inman

Identical skin incisions may be employed for a variety of surgical procedures on the deep structures of the foot and ankle. The selection of a particular incision should have two objectives. The first and most important is to provide an adequate exposure of the anatomic parts so that the surgeon can accomplish his task with dispatch and facility. The second objective is to select an incision that will minimize functional losses. To achieve this objective, the surgeon should keep in mind the following principles:

1. Deprivation of the blood supply may cause a delay in healing and increase the probability of infection.

2. Contractures of surgical scars may limit motion if they are present across normal skin creases.

3. The presence of scars over bony prominences or weight-bearing surfaces where they are subjected to pressures may prove distressing to the patient.

4. The sectioning of small cutaneous nerves often results in areas of anesthesia. These may be in themselves of little significance but when a painful neuroma develops in the proximal end of the nerve, annoying and often incapacitating symptoms result. This is particularly true when the nerve is caught within the incision and the scar is subjected to the external pres-

sure of a shoe or to distortion during the normal movements of walking.

5. Incisions on the weight-bearing surfaces of the foot should be avoided.

It appears proper at this time to enunciate several anatomic and physiologic principles:

1. Peripheral nerves and blood vessels generally are found to be contiguous; the larger nerves accompany arteries and their venae comites, and the smaller nerves accompany veins. When clamping these vessels, the surgeon should be aware that there may be small nerves adjacent to them. If a nerve is included in the tie, the patient later may have complaints that will prove annoying to him and embarrassing to the surgeon.

2. Undermining the skin must be avoided. If flaps are to be extended, the superficial and, if possible, the deep fascia should be included so as to preserve the blood supply.

3. It is preferable to make a longer incision than to employ forceful retraction on the skin. One should remember that incisions heal from side to side and not from end to end.

4. Within a physiologic range, the metabolism of cells changes with temperature. When operating without a tourniquet, the surgeon may employ warm wet sponges,

but hot sponges with temperatures above 60° C. (140° F.) will kill cells. When operating under a tourniquet, the surgeon should use cold sponges exclusively. It is harmful to warm the tissues; to do so increases their metabolic requirements and simultaneously deprives them of circulation.

5. It may be redundant to emphasize that tissues should be handled atraumatically. However, it does no harm to emphasize that tissues should not be crushed, stretched, or permitted to dry or be burned with hot sponges.

6. Removal of the tourniquet and control of bleeding is advisable before closure. A "dry" operative wound will heal better than a "soupy" one.

In the following pages, various surgical approaches to the structures of the foot and ankle are briefly described. Some are classic approaches that have been employed routinely over many years; others are special incisions described by individual surgeons for specific purposes. An attempt will be made in the descriptions to present the advantages and disadvantages of each approach. In addition, the various reconstructive or surgical procedures that may be performed through a particular incision will be enumerated. For a more detailed description of each approach, the reader will find at the end of the chapter a list of references that includes material of the originating surgeons.

EXPOSURE OF THE ANKLE JOINT
Medial approaches

Simple medial approach. This approach may be employed for reduction and internal fixation of fractures of the medial malleolus. It provides only an exposure of the fracture. It is inadequate to permit exploration of the ankle joint or repair of the deltoid ligament, and it places the scar over a bony prominence. The tendon of the

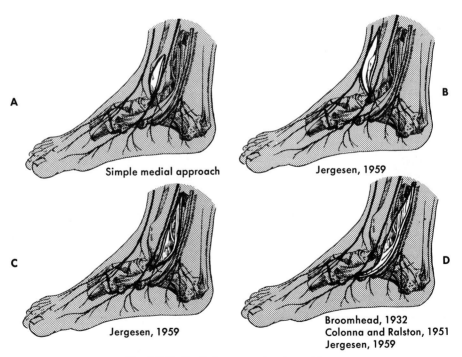

A   Simple medial approach

B   Jergesen, 1959

C   Jergesen, 1959

D   Broomhead, 1932
Colonna and Ralston, 1951
Jergesen, 1959

Fig. 18-1. Medial approaches to ankle.

tibialis posterior grooves the malleolus, and if the incision is made carelessly the sheath of the tendon may be opened or the tendon may be cut. If care is not exercised, the incision may divide the saphenous vein and nerve, which cross superficial to the malleolus. Care should be exercised to preserve the saphenous nerve.

A straight longitudinal incision is made that extends from a point 5 cm. above the tip of the malleolus and is carried distally to the tip of the malleolus. The skin is retracted slightly to expose the malleolus extraperiosteally (Fig. 18-1, A).

Medial anterior approach (Jergesen, 1959). This incision not only permits exposure of the medial malleolus but also has the added advantage of permitting inspection of the medial side of the ankle joint. Such exposure is important in internal fixation of fractures of the medial malleolus. Using this approach, one can determine the adequacy of the reconstitution of the articular surfaces as well as detect the presence of small bone fragments or the interposition of soft tissue. Furthermore, the surgeon can check whether the fixation devices (screws or pins) have traversed the joint cavity. The deltoid ligament can be readily exposed for inspection or repair through this incision.

The incision begins anterior to the medial malleolus (approximately 5 to 6 cm. above its tip), proceeds distally to the joint level, and then curves backward, passing 1 to 2 cm. below the tip of the malleolus, and stopping directly below the posterior margin of the malleolus. The saphenous vein and the saphenous nerve are exposed and retracted posteriorly. The superficial fascia is divided in the direction of the skin incision. The fascia is undermined to expose the malleolus and the superficial fibers of the deltoid ligament. The sheath of the posterior tibial tendon, covered by the flexor retinaculum, is found deep in the distal extremity of the incision. A longitudinal incision of the anterior joint capsule along the anterior margin of the del-

toid ligament generally permits adequate exposure of the anteromedial compartment of the ankle joint (Fig. 18-1, B).

Posteromedial approach (Jergesen, 1959). This is an excellent approach for the open reduction and internal fixation of fractures that involve both the medial malleolus and the posterior lip of the tibia, with or without posterior displacement of the talus in the mortise.

The patient is placed in prone lateral decubitus. The longitudinal extent of the incision is determined by the location of the fracture. The incision parallels the posterior aspect of the tibia, curves forward gently to pass 2 cm. below the tip of the malleolus, and ends at the level of its anterior margin. The tibial periosteum may be incised directly beneath the longitudinal component of the skin incision. In this way the posteromedial aspect of the distal extremity of the tibia is exposed subperiosteally without entering the deep portion of the muscle compartment. To preserve the periosteal attachment of the fracture fragments, one may accomplish extraperiosteal exposure by entering the deep posterior muscle compartment. Proximally the intermuscular septum is divided close to its attachment to the tibia. Distally the flexor retinaculum ligament and the sheath of the posterior tibial tendon are incised. The dissection should be developed close to the periosteum. The foot is plantar flexed to facilitate retraction of the posterior tibial tendon and to expose the posterior talotibial ligament as well as the adjacent joint capsule (Fig. 18-1, C).

Posteromedial approach (Colonna and Ralston, 1951). The incision begins 6 cm. proximal and 2 cm. posterior to the medial malleolus. It curves anteriorly and inferiorly across the center of the medial malleolus. The medial malleolus is then exposed by reflecting the periosteum, with care being taken to preserve the deltoid ligament. The flexor retinaculum is then divided, and the flexor hallucis longus tendon and the neurovascular bundle are retracted laterally. The posterior tibial and

flexor digitorum longus tendons are retracted medially and anteriorly to expose
the posterior tibial fracture (Fig. 18-1, *D*).

**Medial approach to the posterior mal-
leolus (Broomhead, 1932).** This approach
is of particular value in fractures of the
medial tip of the posterior tibia. The incision begins midway between the posterior border of the tibia and the medial border of the tendo achillis. It then curves inferior to the medial malleolus, continuing
to the medial margin of the foot; thus, exposure of both the medial and posterior lip
of the tibia is accomplished. The distal
tibia is exposed by reflecting the capsule
and periosteum and then retracting posteriorly the tendons of the tibialis posterior,
flexor digitorum longus, and flexor hallucis longus muscles, along with the neurovascular bundle (Fig. 18-1, *D*).

**Exposure of the medial aspect of the
ankle by osteotomy of the medial malleolus (Banks and Laufman, 1953).** Once the
medial malleolus has been exposed through
either an anterior or posterior medial approach, it may be osteotomized at the level
of its junction with the shaft of the tibia.
By abducting the foot, the entire superior
surface of the talus and the articular surface of the tibia may be exposed.

In closure, the medial malleolus is accurately replaced and maintained by a
screw or pin.

This addition to the medial or posteromedial approaches permits treatment of
osteochondritis dissecans or other benign
lesions within the ankle joint.

Lateral approaches

**Simple lateral approach (McLaughlin and
Ryder, 1949).** The incision begins over the
distal third of the fibula and curves gently
forward to run just in front of the anterior
end of the bone and to end just below the
tip of the malleolus. The peroneal tendons
are retracted posteriorly and the extensor
digitorum longus tendon is retracted anteriorly to expose the tibiofibular syndesmosis and the lateral fibular lip. The distal
end of the malleolus is exposed by longi-

tudinally splitting the fibers of the fibular
collateral ligament. The lateral malleolar
fracture can be readily visualized and reduced with this approach; however, access
to the joint itself is limited (Fig. 18-2, *B*).

Anterolateral approach (Jergesen, 1959).
This approach gains access to the tibiofibular joint and the anterolateral aspect
of the ankle joint. The proximal origin of
the incision depends on the site and extent
of the fracture.

The incision begins along the anterolateral margin of the distal fibular shaft, proceeds distally to the level of the ankle
joint, curves back to pass a scant finger-
breadth below the malleolar tip, and ends
at a point directly below the posterior margin of the malleolus. The lateral branch of
the superficial peroneal nerve lies in the
subcutaneous fat in the anterior portion of
the incision. A smaller, inconstant branch
separates from the main trunk distal to the
point at which it perforates the fascia in
the middle third of the ligament. This small
branch lies in fat and courses distally, parallel to the lower shaft of the fibula, to ram-
ify in the area of the malleolus. Injury to
this branch, after a longitudinal incision
over the center of the lower fibula has been
made, may lead to a sensitive scar.

Dissection of the skin posteriorly exposes
the lateral malleolus. The fibular attachment of the transverse crural ligament and
the crural fascia are divided to free the
tendons of the peroneus tertius and the extensor digitorum longus. The sural nerve
and the lesser saphenous vein are located
in the lower part of the incision. To gain
access to the calcaneal attachment of the
calcaneofibular ligament, the inferior retinaculum is incised and the peroneal tendons are retracted (Fig. 18-2, *C*).

**Posterolateral approach (Gatellier and
Chastang, 1924).** This approach makes use
of the fact that the fibula in many cases
is fractured. The incision begins at a point
10 to 12 cm. proximal to the tip of the lateral malleolus and proceeds distally along
the posterior margin of the fibula to the
malleolar tip. Then it curves anteriorly for

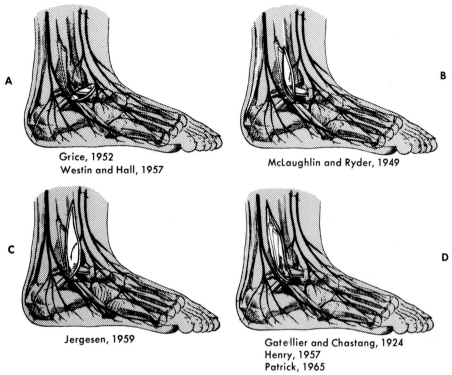

Grice, 1952
Westin and Hall, 1957

McLaughlin and Ryder, 1949

Jergesen, 1959

Gatellier and Chastang, 1924
Henry, 1957
Patrick, 1965

Fig. 18-2. Lateral approaches to ankle.

2 to 5 cm., in line with the peroneal tendons. The fibula and the lateral malleolus are exposed subperiosteally; the sheaths of the peroneal retinacula and tendons are incised, and the tendons are displaced anteriorly. If no fibular fracture is present, the malleolus is osteotomized from 8 to 10 cm. proximal to the malleolar tip. The interosseous membrane as well as the anterior and posterior malleolar ligaments are divided; the calcaneofibular and talofibular ligaments are preserved as a hinge. The distal fibula is turned laterally on the hinge to expose the lateral and posterior distal tibia and the lateral ankle joint. Unsuspected fragments can be removed from the joint and anatomic reduction of the posterior fragment can be accomplished. This approach also permits access to the entire lateral surface of the talus.

To close, the fibula is replaced and fixed with a long screw into the tibia. The tendons are replaced and the tendon sheaths and retinacula are repaired. The cross screw is removed when the patient is ambulatory (Fig. 18-2, D). This approach has been reemphasized by Patrick (1965).

Posterolateral approach (Henry, 1957). This approach is similar to that described by Gatellier and Chastang (1924). The patient is prone with a sandbag beneath the instep, the knee is bent, and the foot is plantar flexed. The incision begins approximately 2 cm. below the lateral malleolus and extends from 10 to 12 cm. proximally and 1 cm. anterior to the lateral border of the tendo achillis. The fascia is incised in line with the incision. Approximately 2 to 3 cm. above the calcaneus, a branch of the peroneal artery is encountered and the underlying fat is opened. The interval is then sought between the flexor hallucis longus and the peroneus brevis. By blunt dissection the interval is enlarged as far proximally as possible. The flexor hallucis longus is retracted medially to expose the posterolateral aspect of the tibia (Fig. 18-2, D).

Posterior approach

The posterior approach, originally described by Picot (1923), has now become a standard one. A 12 cm. incision begins along the posterolateral border of the tendo achillis to the level of its insertion. The superficial and deep fascia are divided. A Z-plastic division and reflection of the tendo achillis is carried out. The fat and areolar tissue in the space between the flexor hallucis longus and the peroneus brevis tendon are retracted medially to expose the distal tibia, the posterior ankle joint, and the posterior surface of the talus (Fig. 18-3, *D*).

Anterior approach

In the approach described by Colonna and Ralston (1951), the incision begins along the anterior aspect of the ankle approximately 8 to 10 cm. proximal to the joint line; it continues distally to a point approximately 5 cm. below the joint. The deep fascia is divided in line with the skin incision. The approach is usually developed in the interval between the extensor hallucis longus and extensor digitorum longus tendons; however, Scaglietti (1940) and Nicola (1945) advised using the interval between the tendons of the tibialis anterior and the extensor hallucis longus. The anterolateral, malleolar, and lateral tarsal arteries must be identified, isolated, and ligated. The dorsalis pedis artery and the deep peroneal nerve are carefully exposed and retracted. The periosteum, capsule, and synovium are incised in line with the skin incision, and the full anterior width of the ankle joint is exposed by subcapsular and subperiosteal dissection (Fig. 18-4, *A*).

EXPOSURE OF THE ANKLE JOINT INCLUDING THE SUBTALAR AND TRANSVERSE TARSAL ARTICULATIONS
Anterolateral approach

Exposure of the ankle, the talocalcaneal, the talonavicular, and the calcaneocuboid articulations is best accomplished through an anterolateral approach. Boyd (1971), who has described this approach, has sug-

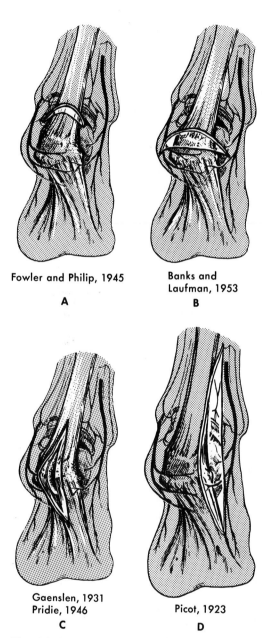

Fowler and Philip, 1945

A

Banks and Laufman, 1953

B

Gaenslen, 1931
Pridie, 1946

C

Picot, 1923

D

Fig. 18-3. Posterior approaches to calcaneus and its adjacent structures.

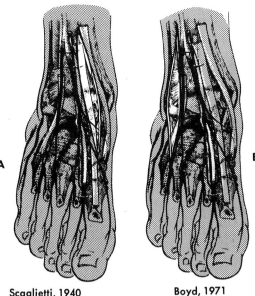

Scaglietti, 1940
Nicola, 1945
Colonna and Ralston, 1951

Boyd, 1971

Fig. 18-4. Anterior approaches to ankle and its adjacent structures.

gested that it may well be called a "universal incision" for many surgical procedures on the foot and ankle. It avoids major vessels and nerves, and it can be extended proximally to reveal the distal tibia or distally to expose the articulations between the cuboid and the fourth and fifth metatarsals. Through such an incision arthrodesis of the tarsal joints may be carried out. Excision of the talus as well as various talar coalitions may be performed.

The skin incision extends from a point 5 cm. above the ankle joint and 1 cm. in front of the anterior edge of the fibula and proceeds distally toward the base of the fourth metatarsal.

The skin in this area is an overlap area supplied by twigs from the intermediate dorsal cutaneous peroneal branch and the superficial branches of the sural nerve. If the intermediate dorsal cutaneous branch is exposed, it should be carefully preserved and retracted medially. The anterolateral malleolar artery will be encountered proximally and the lateral tarsal artery distally in the incision. Both may be sacrificed.

The fascia and crural ligaments are incised, exposing the capsule of the ankle. The extensor digitorum brevis muscle may be detached from its origin and reflected to uncover the talonavicular and calcaneocuboid regions and the region of the sinus tarsi (Fig. 18-4, *B*).

Lateral approaches to the subtalar joint and adjacent structures

Approach to the subtalar and talonavicular joints (Kocher, 1911). This is a classic approach to the subtalar and talonavicular joints for subtalar or triple arthrodesis. It was, at one time, widely used.

The incision begins about 2 cm. proximal to the tip of the lateral malleolus, proceeds in a gentle curve around and below the malleolus, and terminates at the level of the talonavicular joint. The small saphenous vein and nerve should lie posteriorly, and the intermediate dorsal cutaneous nerve crosses the anterior portion of the incision. Both should be protected. The deep fascia is incised to expose the peroneal tendons. They may be retracted posteriorly; if it is necessary to gain a wider field, they may be divided by a Z-plasty and later resutured. The calcaneofibular ligament must be cut in order to gain access to the posterior facet of the subtalar articulation. If the lateral side of the ankle is to be explored, the anterior talofibular ligament must also be cut to permit dislocation of the talus medially (Fig. 18-5, *C*).

The disadvantage of this incision is that it necessitates the cutting of tendons and ligaments. Also, it is notorious for its poor healing. An anterolateral incision is preferable.

Lateral approach to the sinus tarsi (Grice, 1952; Westin and Hall, 1957). Exposure of the sinus tarsi is readily performed through a short, lateral, curvilinear incision. This is the approach typically used in extra-articular arthrodesis of the subtalar joint in children.

The incision is approximately 3 to 4 cm. in length. It follows the skin creases from the tip of the lateral malleolus upward and

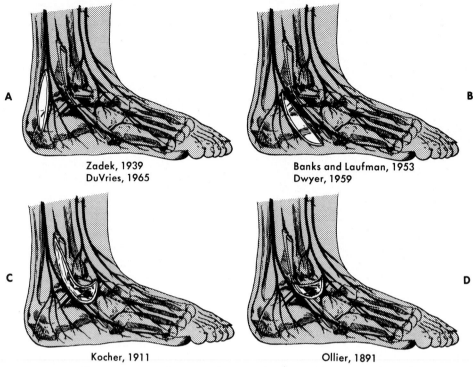

A

Zadek, 1939
DuVries, 1965

B

Banks and Laufman, 1953
Dwyer, 1959

C

Kocher, 1911

D

Ollier, 1891

Fig. 18-5. Lateral approaches to calcaneus and subtalar joint.

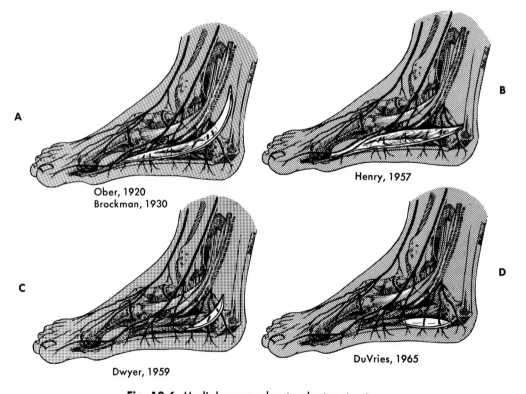

A

Ober, 1920
Brockman, 1930

B

Henry, 1957

C

Dwyer, 1959

D

DuVries, 1965

Fig. 18-6. Medial approaches to plantar structures.

forward and lies directly over the sinus tarsi. The peroneal tendons are located in the posterior extremity of the incision. Care should be taken to avoid cutting the intermediate dorsal cutaneous branch of the superficial peroneal nerve, which lies just at the anterior end of the incision. The cruciate ligament is incised and preserved to facilitate closure. The fat and the loose connective tissue are removed to expose the upper bony borders of the sinus tarsi. The origin of the extensor digitorum brevis and the attachments of the interosseous talocalcaneal ligament appear at the floor of the sinus (Fig. 18-2, A).

Approach to the subtalar joint (Ollier, 1891). This is an approach that essentially uses only the anterior portion of the Kocher incision. It is slightly longer than the limited approach employed by Grice (1952) and Westin and Hall (1957) for extra-articular arthrodesis (Fig. 18-2, A). The approach is adequate for a subtalar or triple arthrodesis.

The incision commences 1 cm. below the tip of the lateral malleolus and curves gently upward to terminate over the talonavicular joint. The intermediate dorsal cutaneous nerve crosses the anterior extremity of the incision and should be preserved. The peroneus tertius and long extensor tendons are exposed and must be retracted medially. The peroneal tendons lie distal and posterior to the lateral malleolus. They may be retracted inferiorly. The origin of the extensor digitorum brevis must be detached from its calcaneal attachment and is reflected distally (Fig. 18-5, D).

EXPOSURE OF THE CALCANEUS AND ADJACENT STRUCTURES
Medial approach to the calcaneus (Dwyer, 1959)

This approach can be used to expose the medial side of the calcaneus for osteotomy. It is also available for exposure of the soft-tissue structures posterior to the medial malleolus. This incision is applicable for decompression of the posterior tibial nerve in patients with tarsal tunnel syndrome or rupture of the posterior tibial tendon.

The incision begins at the superior aspect of the calcaneus and 1 cm. posterior to the medial malleolus. It curves around and slightly distal to the malleolus and terminates at the tuberosity of the navicular. If the incision has been made properly, the saphenous vein and nerve will lie anterior to the incision. The posterior artery and its venae comites and the posterior tibial nerve are located beneath the retinaculum; they lie between the tendons of the tibialis posterior and flexor digitorum muscles anteriorly and the flexor hallucis posteriorly. In exposing the medial side of the calcaneus, the dissection may be carried down superficial to the retinaculum. The retinaculum must be incised in order to expose the tendons or neurovascular structures for exploration (Fig. 18-6, C).

Lateral approach to the calcaneus (Banks and Laufman, 1953)

The lateral surface of the calcaneus is readily exposed through a curvilinear incision. This approach may be used for wedge osteotomies of the calcaneus (Dwyer, 1959), for osteomyelitis, or for excision of benign tumors.

The skin incision is approximately 8 to 10 cm. in length and parallels the underlying peroneal tendons. It begins at a point approximately 1 cm. behind the lateral malleolus, curves with an upward concavity (just distal to the tip of the lateral malleolus), and terminates proximal to the base of the fifth metatarsal. Since the incision follows the course of the sural nerve, which lies in the subcutaneus tissue, the nerve should be sought, exposed, and protected. The thick subcutaneous tissue may be undercut and reflected to expose the underlying bone (Fig. 18-5, B).

Posterior approaches to the calcaneus

Circumferential heel incision (Banks and Laufman, 1953). This approach exposes the entire posterior aspect of the calcaneus. It may be employed in open reduction of avulsion fractures, for osteotomies, or for partial excision of the calcaneus.

With the patient prone, a transverse incision approximately 15 cm. long is made along one of the skin creases, extending equally on either side of the midpoint of the heel. Skin flaps are undercut to permit wide separation of the wound. The entire posterior and inferior aspects of the calcaneus may be exposed (Fig. 18-3, B).

Split heel approach (Gaenslen, 1931; Pridie, 1946). This approach has been employed for the complete or partial extirpation of the calcaneus in cases of osteomyclitis (Gaenslen, 1931) or in markedly comminuted fractures (Pridie, 1946).

The incision is made in the midline of the heel and begins 2 to 3 cm. above the attachment of the tendo achillis to the calcaneus. It extends to the plantar surface of the heel and ends at the level of the calcaneocuboid articulation. The tendo achillis is split in line with the skin incision for a distance of 2 to 3 cm. as is the plantar aponeurosis. With an osteotome or saw, the calcaneus is cut longitudinally and the two halves are separated. Curettement of abscesses can be carried out, or excision of the calcaneus may be accomplished by shelling out the fragments of bone. The superficial fibers of the tendo achillis and periosteum, which pass over the bone to become continuous with the plantar fascia, should be preserved (Fig. 18-3, C).

Exposure of the tendo achillis

Exposure of the tendo achillis can be readily accomplished by a straight linear incision placed medially, laterally, or directly posteriorly. However, a medial approach is generally recommended, since cosmetically a scar on the medial side is less apparent.

Exposure of the Achilles bursae

Normally a bursa is present at the attachment of the tendo achillis to the calcaneus, which lies between the tendon and the posterosuperior edge of the calcaneus. An adventitious bursa may be present between the skin and the tendon. The superficial bursa is readily approached through a transverse or longitudinal incision. A curved transverse incision located above the edge of the counter of the shoe is perhaps the preferable approach.

Resection of the deep bursa, without an osteotomy of the calcaneus, may be carried out through a mediolateral or a posterior approach.

Posterior approach (Fowler and Philip, 1945). A curved transverse incision is made with an upward convexity that is sufficiently high to prevent pressure from the counter of the shoe. The flap is reflected downward. A superficial bursa is readily exposed; if a deeper bursa is to be resected, the upward skin flap may be undermined and retracted upward to expose the tendo achillis. The tendon is split for a distance of 4 cm. and is separated to expose the bursa. A sharp posterior edge of the calcaneus can be rounded, but a transverse osteotomy cannot be performed with ease through this incision (Fig. 18-3, A).

Posterolateral approach (Zadek, 1939). A longitudinal incision from 5 to 6 cm. in length is made lateral and parallel to the tendo achillis. The bursa is readily isolated and removed. In addition, any sharp edge of the calcaneus can be smoothed off. If an excisional wedge is to be removed from the calcaneus, the wedge can be taken by extending this incision distally (Fig. 18-5, A).

EXPOSURE OF THE PLANTAR STRUCTURES
Medial approaches to the plantar structures

Henry (1957). Since the foot is essentially a half-hemisphere that is open medially, structures in the plantar surface are most conveniently approached from the medial side. The skin incision should be located in the overlap area between the medial dorsal cutaneous and the saphenous nerves. The incision begins at the first metatarsophalangeal articulation, proceeds in a smooth curve, passes just below the tuberosity of the navicular, and terminates anterior to the attachment of the tendo achillis to the calcaneus. The key to the exposure of all the deep structures is the abductor hallucis. By isolating its tendon distally and following it proximally, the surgeon carefully detaches the muscle from its attachments extending from the navicular tuberosity to the inner tuberosity of the calcaneus. The nerve supply to the abductor enters the muscle on its deep side and should be exposed and preserved. The muscle is hinged downward with the plantar flap, thus exposing most of the deep structures in the foot (Fig. 18-6, *B*).

DuVries (1965). This is a simple and direct approach to expose the tuber portion of the calcaneus and the attachment of the plantar aponeurosis. It may be employed for a fasciotomy of the aponeurosis, the removal of a calcaneal spur, or the resection of benign tumors.

An incision approximately 5 cm. long begins at a point just short of the heel and is carried forward along the line of the junction of the thick plantar skin and the side of the heel. The skin with its fascia is slightly undermined to permit retraction, and the deep fascia is exposed. The deep fascia is incised, and the abductor hallucis, the plantar fascia, and the anterior inferior aspect of the calcaneus are exposed (Fig. 18-6, *D*).

Combined posteromedial and plantar exposure (Ober, 1920; Brockman, 1930). It is sometimes necessary to expose the posterior aspect of the ankle and subtalar articulation together with structures on the medial and plantar surfaces of the midfoot. An approach with such exposure is appropriate for a posterior and medial release in resistant clubfoot. The incision is a combination of the posteromedial and the medial exposures of the plantar structures.

The incision begins approximately 5 to 6 cm. proximal to the medial malleolus and midway between the border of the tibia and the tendo achillis. It is carried distally, curves around the medial malleolus and along the medial side of the foot, and terminates in the region of the medial cuneiform. The saphenous vein and the saphenous nerve lie anteriorly. The posterior flap is reflected to expose the tendo achillis; the anterior flap is reflected to expose the posterior tibial tendon beneath the deep fascia. From this stage on, the extent of the deep dissection depends upon the surgical procedure to be performed. In any case, the posterior tibial nerves and vessels must be carefully exposed and retracted if the surgeon wishes to expose the posteromedial aspect of the ankle and subtalar joints. To expose the deep plantar structures, the abductor hallucis must be dissected free from its attachments to the fascia, the navicular, and the calcaneus (Fig. 18-6, *A*).

EXPOSURE OF THE STRUCTURES OF THE FOREFOOT

Many incisions are available for the exposure of specific structures on the dorsum of the foot. Since most of these are essentially subcutaneous, only cutaneous nerves, tendons, and certain vessels need to be considered. Surgeons generally agree that surgical exposure of the extensor tendons and the metatarsals can be adequately obtained through longitudinal incisions overlying and roughly paralleling the appropriate structures (Fig. 18-7, *B*).

The choice of a surgical approach when dealing with abnormalities in the area of the metatarsophalangeal articulations is not unanimously agreed upon among surgeons. Some express grave misgivings concerning the placement of a skin incision on the weight-bearing surface of the foot; others recommend such approaches with impunity, stating that surgical exposure is the important criterion. Neither group has presented unequivocal evidence to cause the widespread adoption of a standard approach. Therefore, the individual surgeon must base his choice upon his own experience and upon reports in the literature.

The most common indications for the use of surgical procedures in this area of the foot are such disorders of the forefoot as dislocation of the metatarsophalangeal ar-

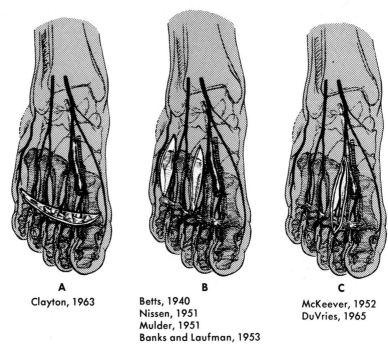

A	B	C
Clayton, 1963	Betts, 1940 Nissen, 1951 Mulder, 1951 Banks and Laufman, 1953	McKeever, 1952 DuVries, 1965

Fig. 18-7. Dorsal approaches to structures of forefoot.

ticulations (hammertoes), metatarsalgias, and perineural fibromas.

Approaches to the metatarsal heads for resection

Resection of the metatarsal heads is a procedure that has proved of value in cases of marked deformities of the forefoot caused by the ravages of rheumatoid arthritis. These deformities consist of depression of the metatarsal heads, dorsal luxations at the metatarsophalangeal articulations, and hammertoes. The indication for surgical correction is incapacitating pain on weight bearing. Originally, most surgeons approached the metatarsal heads through multiple dorsal incisions, but at present most surgeons prefer a single transverse incision, which may be located on either the plantar or dorsal surface of the foot.

Transverse plantar approach (Hoffmann, 1911). Hoffmann was one of the first surgeons to perform resections of the metatarsal heads. After experimenting with dorsal approaches, he proposed a plantar incision. A single transverse curved plantar incision

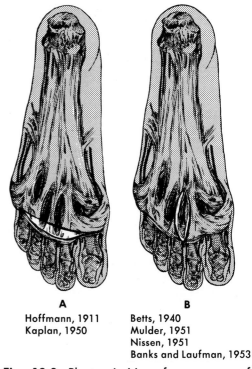

A	B
Hoffmann, 1911 Kaplan, 1950	Betts, 1940 Mulder, 1951 Nissen, 1951 Banks and Laufman, 1953

Fig. 18-8. Plantar incisions for exposure of structures in area of metatarsophalangeal articulations.

is made just proximal to the web of the toes. A plantar flap of fascia and skin is reflected proximally, immediately exposing the metatarsal heads.

The same approach has been recommended by Kaplan (1950) for exposure of the plantar digital nerves as they lie between the metatarsal heads. The advantage of this incision is its exposure of digital nerves in several interspaces through a single incision (Fig. 18-8, *A*).

Transverse dorsal approach (Clayton, 1963). Clayton, after trying many dorsal incisions, proposed a single tranverse dorsal approach to the metatarsal heads. The skin incision is made over the metatarsal heads and curves slightly proximally on the medial side to overlie the first metatarsophalangeal joint. The extensor tendons are exposed. They may be retracted or, if markedly contracted, they may be cut in the line of the incision. The incision is opened by depressing the toes and the bases of the proximal phalanges; the metatarsal heads are thereby delivered into the wound. The metatarsals are osteotomized at the junction of the shaft to the head, and the metatarsal heads are dissected free. Only subcutaneous tissue and skin are sutured. If the tendon of the extensor hallucis has been cut, it is resutured (Fig. 18-7, *A*).

Approaches to the digital nerves for removal of perineural fibromas

Longitudinal plantar approach (Betts, 1940). This incision was originally proposed as a direct approach to the digital nerves for the removal of perineural fibromas. It offers an excellent view of the digital nerve and preserves the transverse metatarsal ligament. The disadvantages of the incision are (1) that it places the scar on the weight-bearing surface and (2) that it provides an exposure that is limited to a single metatarsal interspace. This incision is recommended by Nissen (1951), Mulder (1951), and Banks and Laufman (1953).

A straight longitudinal incision is made on the plantar surface of the foot that extends from the web between the toes proximally for 3 cm. The incision is placed midway between the metatarsal heads (Fig. 18-8, *B*).

Transverse plantar approach (Kaplan, 1950). To avoid placing the scar over the metatarsal pads and to permit exposure of more than a single digital nerve without section of the transverse metatarsal ligament, a transverse incision was proposed for the removal of perineural fibromas. This approach is similar to the one suggested by Hoffmann (1911) for excision of the metatarsal heads.

The incision is placed transversely, slightly distal to the interdigital folds, and may extend from the medial side of the first toe to the lateral side of the fifth toe. The subcutaneous plantar fat is cut in the line of the skin incision to expose the digital extensions of the plantar fascia. The skin with superficial fascia is retracted, exposing the flexor tendon sheaths that lie superficial to the tendons of the lumbricales muscles and transverse metatarsal ligament (Fig. 18-8, *A*).

Longitudinal dorsal approach (McKeever, 1952; DuVries, 1965). Because of antipathy for plantar incisions, many surgeons employ a dorsal approach. While this approach avoids placing a scar on the weight-bearing surface, the exposure of the nerve requires deeper dissection and the cutting of the transverse metatarsal ligament.

A skin incision is made between the proper metatarsals, extending from the web proximally for 3 cm. With a hemostat, blunt dissection is carried out between the metatarsal heads. To separate the metatarsal heads adequately in order to expose the digital nerve, the transverse metatarsal ligament must be incised. Firm pressure under the metatarsals will present the nerve. To permit sufficient proximal sectioning of the nerve, it may be necessary to grasp the nerve with a hemostat to deliver it into the wound (Fig. 18-7, *C*).

REFERENCES

Banks, S. W., and Laufman, H.: An atlas of surgical exposures of the extremities, Philadelphia, 1953, W. B. Saunders Co.

Betts, L. O.: Morton's metatarsalgia: Neuritis of the fourth digital nerve, Med. J. Aust. 1:514-515, Apr. 1940.

Boyd, H. B.: Surgical approaches. In Crenshaw, A. H., editor: Campbell's operative orthopaedics, ed 5, vol. 1, St. Louis, 1971, The C. V. Mosby Co., p. 60.

Brockman, E. P.: Congenital club-foot (talipes equinovarus), Bristol, 1930, J. Wright and Sons, Ltd.

Broomhead, R.: Discussion on fractures in the region of the ankle-joint, Proc. Roy. Soc. Med. 25:1082-1087, May 1932.

Clayton, M. L.: Surgery of the lower extremity in rheumatoid arthritis, J. Bone Joint Surg. 45-A:1517-1536, Oct. 1963.

Colonna, P. C., and Ralston, E. L.: Operative approaches to the ankle joint, Amer. J. Surg. 82:44-54, July 1951.

DuVries, H. L.: Surgery of the foot, ed. 2, St. Louis, 1965, The C. V. Mosby Co., p. 226.

Dwyer, F. C.: Osteotomy of the calcaneum for pes cavus, J. Bone Joint Surg. 41-B:80-86, Feb. 1959.

Fowler, A., and Philip, J. F.: Abnormality of the calcaneus as a cause of painful heel: Its diagnosis and operative treatment, Brit. J. Surg. 32:494-498, 1945.

Gaenslen, F. J.: Split-heel approach in osteomyelitis of os calcis, J. Bone Joint Surg. 13:759-772, Oct. 1931.

Gatellier, J., and Chastang: La voie d'accès juxta-rétro-péronière dans le traitement sanglant des fractures malléolaires avec fragment marginal postérieur, J. Chir. (Paris) 24:513-521, Nov. 1924.

Grice, D. S.: An extra-articular arthrodesis of the subastragalar joint for correction of paralytic flatfeet in children, J. Bone Joint Surg. 34-A:927-940, Oct. 1952.

Henry, A. K.: Extensile exposure, ed. 2, Baltimore, 1957, The Williams & Wilkins Co.

Hoffmann, P.: An operation for severe grades of contracted or clawed toes, Amer. J. Orthop. Surg. 9:441-448, 1911.

Jergesen, F.: Open reduction of fractures and dislocations of the ankle, Amer. J. Surg. 98:136-150, Aug. 1959.

Kaplan, E. B.: Surgical approach to the plantar digital nerves, Bull. Hosp. Joint Dis. 11:96-97, Apr. 1950.

Kocher, T.: Textbook of operative surgery, ed. 3, (translated by H. J. Stiles and C. B. Paul), London, 1911, A. and C. Black.

McKeever, D. C.: Surgical approach for neuroma of plantar digital nerve (Morton's metatarsalgia), J. Bone Joint Surg. 34-A:490, Apr. 1952.

McLaughlin, H. L., and Ryder, C. T.: Open reduction and internal fixation for fractures of the tibia and ankle, Surg. Clin. N. Amer. 29:1523-1534, 1949.

Mulder, J. D.: The causative mechanism in Morton's metatarsalgia, J. Bone Joint Surg. 33-B:94-95, Feb. 1951.

Nicola, T.: Atlas of surgical approaches to bones and joints, New York, 1945, The Macmillan Co.

Nissen, K. I.: The etiology of Morton's metatarsalgia, J. Bone Joint Surg. 33-B:293, May 1951.

Ober, F. R.: An operation for the relief of congenital equino-varus deformity, J. Orthop. Surg. 2:558-565, Oct. 1920.

Ollier, L.: Traité des résections et des opérations conservatrices qu'on peut praticquer sur le système osseux, vol. 3, Paris, 1891, G. Masson.

Patrick, J.: A direct approach to trimalleolar fractures, J. Bone Joint Surg. 47-B:236-239, May 1965.

Picot, G.: L'intervention sanglante dans les fractures malléolaires, J. Chir. (Paris) 21:529-542, 1923.

Pridie, K. H.: A new method of treatment for severe fractures of the os calcis: A preliminary report, Surg. Gynec. Obstet. 82:671-675, June 1946.

Scaglietti, O.: Tecnica e risultati dell'artrodesi della tibio-tarsica, Chir. Organi Mov. 26:244-254, Nov. 1940.

Westin, G. W., and Hall, C. B.: Subtalar extra-articular arthrodesis: A preliminary report of a method of stabilizing feet in children, J. Bone Joint Surg. 39-A:501-511, June 1957.

Zadek, I.: An operation for the cure of achillobursitis, Amer. J. Surg. 43:542-546, Feb. 1939.

19

Major surgical procedures for disorders of the ankle, tarsus, and midtarsus

Verne T. Inman

THE ANKLE

Open reduction of fractures about the ankle

If closed reduction fails to reposition all the articular surfaces of the mortise of the ankle joint accurately, open reduction and internal fixation are indicated.

Fractures of the internal malleolus. The saphenous nerve crosses the medial malleolus midway between its anterior and posterior borders. The nerve can be palpated by passing one's fingernail across the skin. The nerve is felt as a taut cord that passes between the fingernail and the underlying bone. The nerve should be avoided, since its injury or section may produce annoying symptoms. To avoid the nerve, either a posteromedial or an anteromedial approach can be used (see Chapter 18). In the posterior approach care should be taken not to open the sheath of the posterior tibial tendon or to lacerate the tendon. The posterior approach will avoid the saphenous nerve, but it affords a less satisfactory view of the interior of the ankle joint. The anteromedial approach, if extended distally, is more likely to interrupt the saphenous nerve, but this approach provides a better view of the interior of the ankle joint and enables the surgeon to check the accuracy of the reduction.

The distal fragment of the medial malleolus is usually slightly displaced anteri-orly. After the fracture site is exposed, soft-tissue imposition should be looked for and the tissue should be removed. The malleolar fracture can be reduced and fixed with a towel clip while a screw or pin is placed through the distal tip of the malleolus into the shaft of the tibia.

Fractures of the lateral malleolus. The sural nerve passes along the posterior border of the lateral malleolus and can be palpated beneath the skin between the examiner's fingernail and the underlying bone. Preliminary palpation will help avoid interruption of this nerve. The lateral malleolus can be exposed through a direct longitudinal incision placed over the malleolus. Fractures of the lateral malleolus are usually spiral in nature and occur at the level of the joint or above the joint in the distal shaft. In the latter case, one should be suspicious of a possible tibiofibular diastasis. The fracture can usually be reduced with ease and fixed with an intermedullary pin or screw.

Fractures of the posterior lip of the tibia (trimalleolar fracture or Cotton's fracture). An isolated fracture of the posterior lip of the tibia occurs infrequently; however, it is a common fracture in conjunction with fractures of the malleoli with a posterior dislocation of the ankle joint. More than any other type of fracture, it is one that requires open reduction and an accurate realignment of the fragments. Usually the fracture occurs on the lateral side of the plafond; the talus is rotated and is displaced backward and laterally.

The posterior aspect of the ankle joint can be approached through a posterolateral or posteromedial incision. A 10 cm. linear incision is made just medial or lateral to the tendo achillis. The tendon is retracted either laterally or medially. The dissection is carried down through the loose fatty areolar tissue until the posterior aspect of the joint is encountered. The flexor hallucis longus tendon is located as it crosses the posterior capsule from the lateral side toward the medial side. The tendon is retracted medially and the posterior aspect of the ankle joint is exposed. By keeping lateral to the tendon of the flexor hallucis longus, the posterior tibial vessels and the nerve are avoided. The fracture can be readily located, and the upwardly displaced posterior lip of the tibia is corrected with a towel clip. After visual confirmation of the reduction, the surgeon may fix the reduction by the insertion of a stainless steel nail or a screw. Since accurate alignment is mandatory, roentgenograms should be taken after reduction and before closure.

Fractures of the anterior lip of the tibia. These fractures require accurate reduction. The anterior aspect of the tibia is best exposed through an anteromedial approach. The incision is made in the space between the anterior tibial tendon and the extensor tendons; the tendons are displaced medially to expose the anterior aspect of the joint.

After reduction is carried out, the fragments may be fixed with stainless steel pins or screws.

Arthrodesis of the talocrural (ankle) joint

Many methods to arthrodese the ankle have been reported in the literature. The selection of one particular procedure over others has been influenced by such factors as the type of pathologic process present, the preconceived ideas of individual surgeons, and the kind of fusion that is indicated. Extra-articular fusions have been done for septic arthritis, particularly for tuberculous destruction of the joint. They have also been used for cases in which the surgeon has felt that simultaneous fusion of the ankle and subtalar joints was necessary because of the presence of lesions involving both articulations. Such cases fall into a special category and are discussed separately.

In arthrodeses of the ankle joint alone, the objective of all reported procedures is to accomplish a snug fit between the body of the talus and the mortise, which, after removal of the articular cartilage from the surfaces of the joint, is loose and sloppy. To ensure firm contact between the bony surfaces and to stabilize the joint during the period of time required for union, various procedures have been employed. These include the packing of bone chips into the space between the bones, the use of bone grafts to span the joint, and the performance of osteotomies of one or both of the malleoli in order to narrow the mortise. Any combination of these methods has been used, with or without additional internal fixation with metal pins, rods, and screws.

Most of the basic operations were introduced by the pioneers in orthopaedic surgery at the beginning of this century. An excellent historical review with an extensive bibliography of earlier operative procedures has been published by Schwartz (1946). Only minor modifications have been introduced by individual surgeons who felt that their contributions either improved the chances of fusion or decreased the time that was required to achieve a firm union.

The methods used to arthrodese the ankle joint may be divided into the four categories listed below. Figs. 19-1 through 19-4 offer a pictorial summary of the various procedures.

1. Intra-articular bone grafts. The ankle joint has been exposed through various incisions, which include a lateral J-shaped incision (Schwartz, 1946), the anterolateral

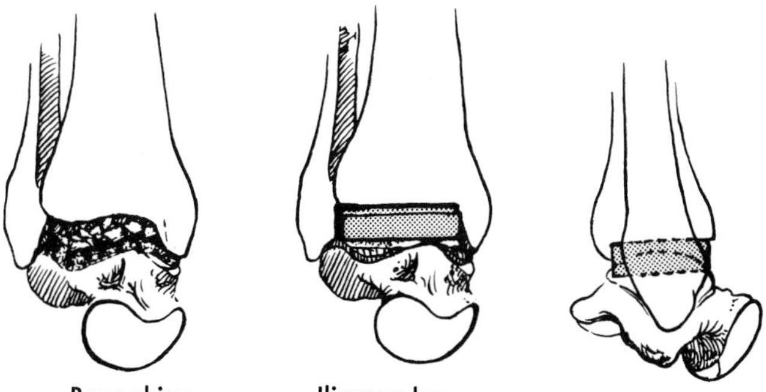

Internal bone graft

Bone chips

Cramer, 1910
Lasker, 1923
Hallock, 1945
Anderson, 1945
Schwartz, 1946
Barr and Record, 1953
Vahvanen, 1969

Iliac wedge
Chuinard and Peterson, 1963

Fig. 19-1. Arthrodeses of talocrural joint using intra-articular bone grafts. **A,** Denuding articular surfaces of cartilage and packing interval with bone chips. **B,** Insertion of single bone graft between plafond and talus.

approach (Cramer, 1910; Lasker, 1923; Hallock, 1945; Anderson, 1945; Vahvanen, 1969), and the approach that employs two linear incisions, one along the anterior border of the lateral malleolus and a second along the anterior margin of the medial malleolus (Barr and Record, 1953). After denuding all cartilage from the articular surfaces to expose bleeding bone, the joint space is filled with bone chips either "fish-scaled" from the tibial and talar surfaces (Hallock, 1945) or secured from the iliac crest or the anterior surface of the tibia (Fig. 19-1, A). Chuinard and Peterson (1963) inserted a wedge graft taken from the iliac crest between the plafond of the tibia and the talus (Fig. 19-1, B). This method of arthrodesis is particularly applicable to young individuals whose epiphyses are still open.

2. Malleolar osteotomies. The need to achieve a snug fit between the trochlea of the talus and the mortise after removal of the articular cartilage was recognized early. Goldthwait (1908) proposed narrowing the mortise by performing an osteotomy of the fibula and displacing the fibula medially.

Several modifications of this procedure have appeared (Horwitz, 1942; Adams, 1948). Glissan (1949) and Cordebar (1956) osteotomized the medial malleolus. Mead (1951) osteotomized both malleoli. Wilson (1969) osteotomized only the anterior halves of both malleoli in order to avoid possible injury to or malfunction of the tendons of the peroneal and tibialis posterior muscles (Fig. 19-2).

Various incisions were employed by the several surgeons, depending upon the required exposure.

3. Anterior tibial graft. This procedure has been an old and popular method of arthrodesis (Fig. 19-3). It appears to have been first employed by Cramer (1910), Lasker (1923), and Campbell (1929). The ankle joint is exposed through an anterior approach. After denuding the articular cartilage from the joint surfaces and correcting the deformity, the surgeon cuts a bone graft from the anterior aspect of the tibia, places it across the joint, and affixes it to the talus and the tibia with screws (Fig. 19-3, A). A modification of this procedure proposed by Hatt (1940) was popularized

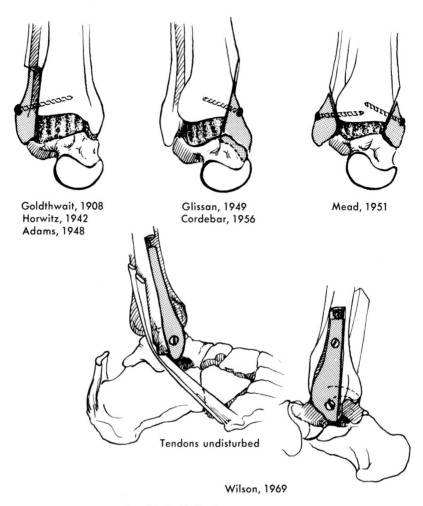

Goldthwait, 1908
Horwitz, 1942
Adams, 1948

Glissan, 1949
Cordebar, 1956

Mead, 1951

Tendons undisturbed

Wilson, 1969

Fig. 19-2. Malleolar osteotomies.

by Brittain (1942), in which the tibial graft is embedded into the body of the talus through a hole in the plafond (Fig. 19-3, *B*).

4. Compression arthrodesis. While Anderson (1945) used an external metal appliance to retain the bones in position and White, in discussing Hallock's paper (1945), stated that he had been placing pins through the tibia and the calcaneus which were connected by rubber bands to maintain compression, it was Charnley (1959) who popularized compression arthrodesis (Fig. 19-4). He employed a transverse incision across the anterior aspect of the ankle joint which extended 1 cm. above the tip of each malleolus. The

extensor tendons were divided, the vessels were ligated and cut, and the nerves were severed. The extensor tendons were resutured during closure. Ratliff (1959), in a review of fifty-five ankles repaired by Charnley's technique, reported a high percentage of fusion. However, minor complications and disabilities also occurred. These residual conditions included extensor tendons adherent to the scar, persistent mild edema of the foot distal to the incision, persistent numbness over the dorsum of the foot, and a decrease in the power of dorsiflexion of the toes.

Jansen (1962) approved the concept of compression arthrodesis but felt that the transverse incision was unnecessary. He

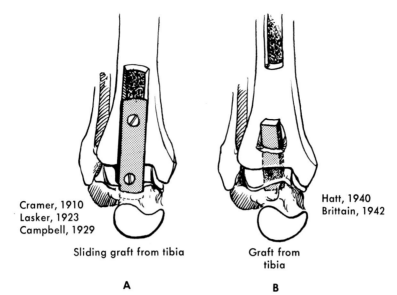

Cramer, 1910
Lasker, 1923
Campbell, 1929

Sliding graft from tibia

Hatt, 1940
Brittain, 1942

Graft from
tibia

A   B

Fig. 19-3. Anterior tibial bone grafts. An anterior bone graft supplements the intra-articular fusion.

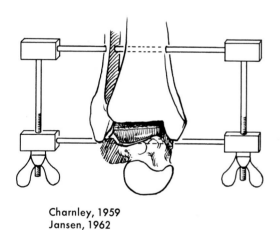

Charnley, 1959
Jansen, 1962

Fig. 19-4. Compression arthrodesis. After removal of articular cartilage from joint surfaces, joints are continuously compressed by means of pins, threaded rods, and wing nuts.

combined compression with the medial and lateral approach of Anderson (1945) and reported twenty-four out of twenty-five solid fusions. Dahmen and Meyer (1965) published an extensive and critical review of their experience with the various methods of fusion of the talocrural joint.

Posterior bone blocks

Posterior bone blocks have been employed as supplementary techniques for the stabilization of the foot. The procedures of Campbell (1923, 1925) and Gill (1933) are illustrated in Fig. 19-5. A case of paralytic dropfoot treated by means of the Gill procedure is illustrated in Fig. 19-6. Indications for these procedures as well as the Inclan (1949) procedure have been recorded in detail by Wheeldon and Clark (1936), Branch (1939), Inclan (1949), and Ingram and Hundley (1951). When used in conjunction with triple arthrodesis and a laterally stable talotibial joint, the posterior bone block limits plantar flexion by contact with the inferior and posterior articular surfaces of the tibia.

Soft-tissue procedures

Surgical repair of the ligaments of the ankle. Severe ligamentous injuries of the ankle often masquerade as sprains. For adequate evaluation, roentgenograms of the ankle in stressed position must be taken; occasionally, arthrograms are necessary as well.

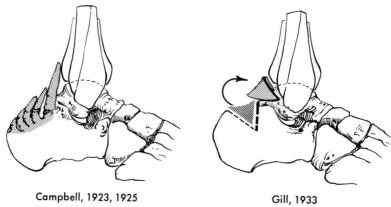

Campbell, 1923, 1925   Gill, 1933

Fig. 19-5. Posterior bone blocks of ankle joint for stabilization of foot.

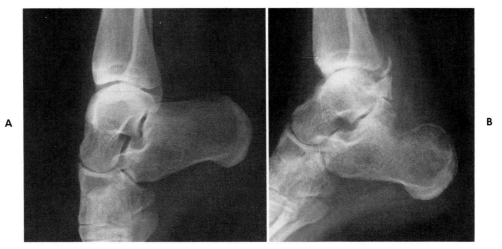

Fig. 19-6. Treatment of paralytic dropfoot. **A,** Preoperative roentgenogram of right foot of 25-year-old female. She had poliomyelitis in childhood. **B,** Postoperative roentgenogram of same foot. A Gill procedure was performed.

The collateral ligaments. Complete tears of the collateral ligaments necessitate surgical exploration and repair. In acute cases direct surgical repair of the torn ligaments is possible (Ruth, 1961) (Fig. 19-7). In old cases with instability of the ankle, however, reconstruction of the collateral ligaments is necessary.

RECONSTRUCTION OF THE LATERAL COLLATERAL LIGAMENT. The lateral collateral ligament of the ankle is composed of three separate structures. With forceful inversion of the ankle the susceptibility to rupture of each component appears to be as follows (Francillon, 1962): The anterior talofibular ligament is most likely to be torn. With further inversion, disruption of the fibulocalcaneal ligament occurs in addition to the tear of the anterior talofibular ligament (Ruth, 1961). Isolated tears of the fibulocalcaneal ligament are infrequent and occur only if the foot is inverted while it is in a position of full dorsiflexion. Tears of the posterior talofibular ligament seem to occur rarely if at all (Ashhurst and Bromer, 1922; Anderson and LeCocq, 1954).

Various procedures for the reconstruction of the lateral collateral ligament have been employed. Elmslie (1934) attempted to replace the injured ligaments anatomically with a strip of fascia lata (Fig. 19-8). His procedure demonstrated an appreciation of the mechanical relationships that obtain between the arrangement of the ligaments and the axes of motion of the ankle and subtalar joints. Some surgeons have questioned the durability of fascia for the repair and have preferred to use tendon. The obvious availability of the peroneal tendons led to their use in these procedures, which differed only according to the personal ingenuity of the surgeon who employed the handy structures. Unfortunately, the anatomic arrangements that resulted from these procedures placed the newly formed collateral ligaments in such a position that subtalar motion was always compromised.

Other procedures that have been used for reconstruction of the lateral collateral ligaments in unstable ankle joints are depicted in Fig. 19-9. The surgeons advocating each procedure are referred to, and these references are to be found in a list at the end of the chapter.

RECONSTRUCTION OF THE MEDIAL COLLATERAL (DELTOID) LIGAMENT. Isolated tears of this ligament are rare. In cases in which the foot has been forcibly everted, the medial malleolus is more likely to be fractured or the ligament is more apt to be avulsed from the tibia. Small fragments of bone are seen on roentgenograms.

Watson-Jones (1955) has warned that in suspected injuries to the medial collateral ligament, one should be alert to the possibility of a diastasis of the distal tibiofibular syndesmosis. Because of the nature

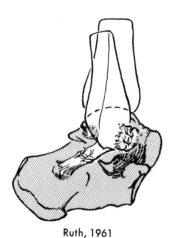

Ruth, 1961

Fig. 19-7. Procedure for reconstruction of lateral collateral ligament. Resuturing of the ligament is readily accomplished if performed immediately after the injury has occurred.

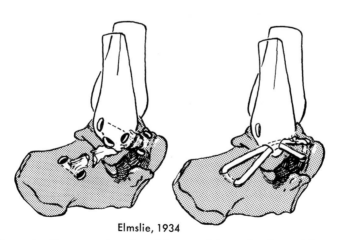

Elmslie, 1934

Fig. 19-8. Reconstructive procedure for old tears of lateral collateral ligament of ankle using fascia lata.

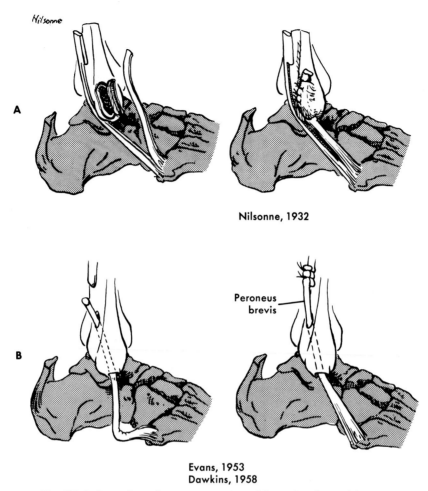

Nilsonne, 1932

Peroneus
brevis

Evans, 1953
Dawkins, 1958

Fig. 19-9. Procedures for reconstruction of lateral collateral ligament.

of the pathologic findings, direct repair of the ligament in acute cases is indicated, and tightening of the structure for chronic instability of the ankle has been reported.

The technique of Schoolfield (1952) has been adapted to repair recurrent sprains of the deltoid ligament. The anterior skin flap is deflected to expose the deltoid ligament, which is detached from the medial malleolus and freed to its insertions. The foot is inverted at this point to permit suturing the deltoid ligament to the periosteal and ligamentous tissues over the medial malleolus just above the natural origin of the deltoid ligament (Fig. 19-10).

For recurrent sprains of the deltoid ligament, DuVries (1965) found that crucial incision and cross-shaped scar formations gave preferable results. A vertical incision is bisected by a horizontal incision, forming a cross of equal arms. The margins are sutured together to leave a cross-shaped scar that is strong enough to act successfully as a stabilizer of the ankle (Fig. 19-11).

Tendon transfers about the hindfoot. Since the talus has no muscular attachments, the stability of this bone within its skeletal compartment is in constant jeopardy. During weight bearing and locomotion, all the muscles that act between the leg and the remaining skeletal structures in the foot play varying roles in keeping the talus properly aligned within the ankle

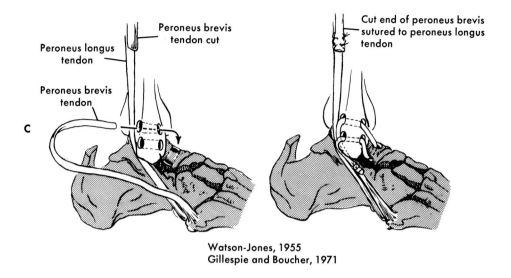

Peroneus longus
tendon

Peroneus brevis
tendon

Peroneus brevis
tendon cut

Cut end of peroneus brevis
sutured to peroneus longus
tendon

C

Watson-Jones, 1955
Gillespie and Boucher, 1971

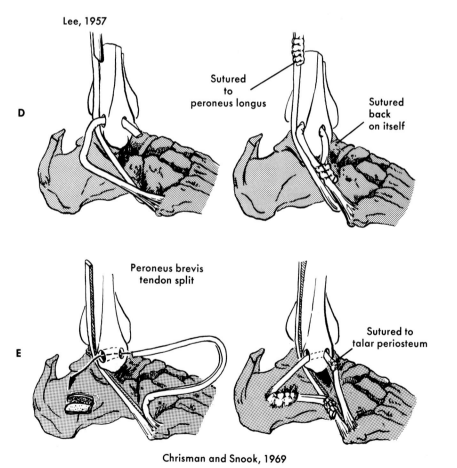

Lee, 1957

D

Sutured
to
peroneus longus

Sutured
back
on itself

Peroneus brevis
tendon split

E

Sutured to
talar periosteum

Chrisman and Snook, 1969

Fig. 19-9, cont'd. Procedures for reconstruction of lateral collateral ligament.

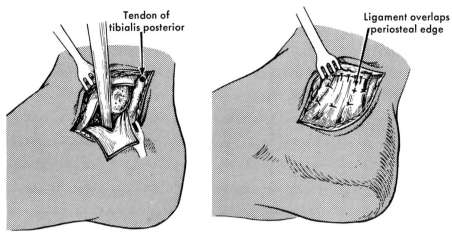

Schoolfield, 1952

Fig. 19-10. Schoolfield's technique. **A,** Deltoid ligament stripped from above, downward over medial malleolus. **B,** Foot held in inversion. The upper margin of the deltoid ligament is sutured to the periosteal edge, which it overlaps.

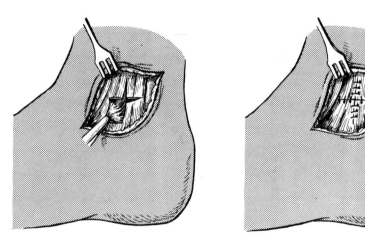

DuVries, 1965

Fig. 19-11. DuVries' technique. **A,** Vertical incision into deltoid ligament bisected at center by transverse incision. The resulting four right-angular flaps of the ligament are denuded and freed from the bone. **B,** Four flaps sutured to form cross-shaped scar which stabilizes ankle.

mortise above, in maintaining the alignment of the articular surfaces of the calcaneus below, and in preserving functional contact with the navicular in front. Synovitis of tendon sheaths, dislocations and ruptures of tendons, and paralysis or spasticity of muscles may alter the forces so that stability is impaired and deformity

results. In attempts to rebalance these forces, many tendon transfers have been carried out. It is impossible to enumerate them all; however, when considering the performance of a tendon transference, the surgeon should consider the following questions:

1. What is the etiology of the functional

loss? Is the condition static or progressive? In the child, what effect will growth have upon the function of the transfer?

2. Is the muscle of the tendon to be transferred sufficiently strong, and is its fiber length such that adequate excursion is assured? Will the tendon be long enough to reach the area into which it is to be implanted?

3. Is the phasic action of the donor muscle the same as that of the diseased one which it will replace? Close and Todd (1959) have indicated that a complete change in phasic action of muscles in the lower extremity is not likely to occur.

4. What will be the consequences of the loss of the normal function of the donor tendon?

5. Should arthrodesing procedures be performed along with the tendon transfer?

Certain principles should be followed in tendon transfers. As has been indicated above, a muscle having approximately the same phasic action should be selected for transfer. The line of pull of the muscle and its tendon should be as straight as possible from its origin to the new insertion. If at all possible, the tendon should be firmly fixed to bone through a drill hole or an osteoperiosteal tunnel.

The length-tension relationship in striated muscle is such that maximal tension can only be developed if the muscle is at its rest length. If the muscle is activated when it is shorter or longer than its rest length, it will generate less force. Rest length can be determined by gently pulling the tendon and estimating the increase in passive resistance to further stretching. The rest length is that point at which passive resistance can first be determined by the surgeon. Thus, the tendon should be implanted in bone with only minimal tension, with the skeletal part in the position of maximal function.

Because of the multiplicity of factors that must be considered, each case presents a unique problem that the surgeon must consider carefully before he attempts a solution by means of a tendon transfer.

Synovectomies. Synovectomies have had a long and variegated history. Those interested in an excellent historical review are referred to the article by Geens (1969). London (1955) rekindled enthusiasm for synovectomy of the knee in rheumatoid arthritis, and the literature since that time has become copious. With the increasing popularity of synovectomy of the knee, the procedure has been applied to almost every joint. This operation is useful for relieving pain in the active stages of the disease before joint destruction has occurred. Whitefield (1967), Heywood (1967), Vahvanen (1968), Jakubowski (1970), and Murray (1972) have reported on the use of this procedure on the ankle joint.

The most satisfactory approach is the anterolateral incision, which permits excision of most of the synovial membrane lining at the front and sides of the joint. As much of the synovial membrane in the posterior part of the joint as possible is removed with a pituitary rongeur.

Tendon dislocations and subluxations in the region of the ankle. There are several tendons in the region of the ankle that are often subject to partial or complete dislocation. These dislocations usually result from twisting injuries to the ankle, but they have been reported to occur spontaneously. The peroneals are by far the most frequently injured tendons; reports of single cases as well as relatively large series of cases are contained in the literature. Mounier-Kuhn and Marsan (1968) published a careful review of forty-four cases, dividing them into five groups according to etiology, pathology, and treatment. In readily reducible acute dislocations that are stable after reduction, conservative treatment consisting of reduction and immobilization of the foot in a cast for 6 to 8 weeks may be used. If the reduction is unstable, as is the case in osteoperiosteal avulsions (Murr, 1961; Murr, comments on Folschveiller's article, 1967) and in complete tears of the tendon sheath, surgical repair is indicated.

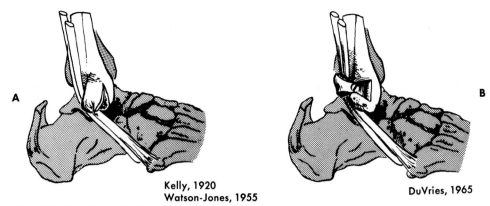

A

B

Kelly, 1920
Watson-Jones, 1955

DuVries, 1965

Fig. 19-12. Method of deepening sulcus for prevention of recurrent dislocations of peroneal tendons.

Several surgical procedures have been employed. Plication and resuturing of the tendon sheath has been used (Mounier-Kuhn and Marsan, 1968; Diamant-Berger, 1971). Weigert (1969) tightened the sheath by suturing its border to the fibula through drill holes in the malleolus. Folschveiller (1967) and Bogutskaia (1970) reinforced the sheath with a flap of periosteum, which was reflected from the fibula and sutured over the repaired tendon sheath. In chronic dislocations and habitually dislocating tendons, osteotomies of the malleolus are required. Kelly (1920) and Watson-Jones (1955) displaced an osteoperiosteal graft from the malleolus posteriorly (Fig. 19-12, *A*). DuVries (1965) cut a wedge-shaped bone graft from the malleolus, displaced it posteriorly, and fixed it with a screw (Fig. 19-12, *B*). These procedures deepened the sulcus and prevented recurrences of the dislocation.

The posterior tibial tendon may be dislocated from its sulcus behind the medial malleolus, although such occurrences appear to be very rare. Muralt (1956) was the first to describe such a case. Scheuba (1969), in reporting two cases, felt that a habitually dislocating posterior tibial tendon may be more common than is indicated from the literature. He pointed out that when individuals complain of instability and pain in the area of the medial malleolus, it is well to keep in mind the possibility of this condition, for it is easily overlooked.

Because of the lack of reported cases, no standard operative procedure has emerged. Based upon the experience gained from peroneal dislocations, an osteoperiosteal flap from the medial malleolus, similar to that in the procedure used by Kelly and Watson-Jones on the lateral malleolus, seems indicated.

THE TARSUS
The posterior tarsus

Subtalar and triple arthrodeses. During the first two decades of this century the problem of treatment of the deformed or flail foot, which occurred as a sequela to poliomyelitis, occupied the attention of the orthopaedist. The necessity of stabilizing the articulations of the posterior tarsus was apparent. The surgical solution to this problem was attempted with two ideas in mind: One was to achieve greater stability by obliterating or limiting ankle and subtalar motion; the other was to displace the foot posteriorly so that the body weight passed more nearly through the midfoot. A variety of surgical procedures were proposed and carried out by different surgeons, ranging from talectomy to pantalar arthrodesis. The majority of the operations were intended to correct pes cavus and to stabil-

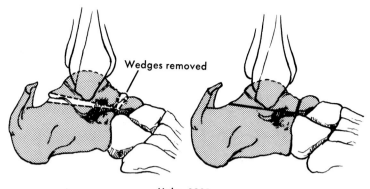

Hoke, 1921

Fig. 19-13. Classic Hoke arthrodesis.

ize the subtalar and the transverse tarsal articulations.* Numerous modifications, with adjuvant procedures such as tendon transfers, have been used. Some of these procedures have withstood the test of time, while many have been abandoned.

Subtalar and triple arthrodeses are now carried out less frequently, since the deformities resulting from poliomyelitis no longer constitute a major part of the practice of orthopaedics. Excellent reviews and discussions concerning surgical arthrodeses, particularly in poliomyelitis, have been presented.†

While the need for a variety of procedures to deal with the multiplicity of disabilities resulting from poliomyelitis is presently not so great, indications for subtalar and triple arthrodeses in specific cases still remain. From the numerous methods employed in the past, two have proved useful and have become accepted as standard procedures. The first is the Hoke arthrodesis, with numerous modifications (Fig. 19-13). It is an intra-articular arthrodesis and is useful for painful arthritic processes involving the subtalar and transverse tarsal articulations.

The second is the extra-articular arthrodesis of Grice (Fig. 19-14), which is use-

ful in blocking subtalar motion in those patients who have no gross skeletal deformities but have instability of the hindfoot. The Grice arthrodesis is particularly applicable in children, since there is little interference with future growth of the foot.

In the Grice extra-articular arthrodesis, the operative technique is relatively simple. The region of the sinus tarsi is exposed through a short, curvilinear incision that extends from the peroneal tendons to the extensor tendons. The ligamentous structures and adipose tissue are removed from the sinus tarsi. The origin of the extensor digiti brevis is dissected from the calcaneus and is reflected distally, allowing complete visualization of the interval between the talus and calcaneus. With an osteotome slots are cut in the inferior surface of the talus and in the superior surface of the calcaneus. The surgeon should recall the direction of the axis of the subtalar joint; the graft, to provide adequate stabilization, must lie in a plane that is perpendicular to this axis (Fig. 19-14.) Thus, the graft should run distally and anteriorly; otherwise, it will not block motion of the subtalar joint and may become displaced. The graft may be taken from the anterior superior surface of the tibia or from the iliac crest.

There are several other surgical methods of arthrodesing the articulations of the hindfoot. These procedures were formerly

---

*See Jones, 1908; Davis, 1913; Hoke, 1921; Ryerson, 1923; Dunn, 1928.
†See Hart, 1937; Hallgrímsson, 1943; Schwartz, 1946; and Crego and McCarroll, 1938.

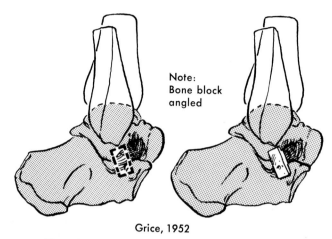

Note:
Bone block
angled

Grice, 1952

Fig. 19-14. Grice extra-articular arthrodesis.

employed for paralytic deformities and are depicted in Fig. 19-15. The surgeons advocating each procedure are indicated, and their works are to be found in the list of references at the end of the chapter.

Combined talonavicular, talocrural, and pantalar arthrodesis. Orthopaedic surgeons disagree as to the indications for an arthrodesis of the joints of the posterior tarsus. Furthermore, once the decision has been made to carry out such an extensive fusion, there is further disagreement as to which is the best procedure to follow. Lorthioir (1911), who originally reported the results of such an operation, extirpated the entire talus and replaced it as a free graft in order to achieve a pantalar arthrodesis. The same procedure (Fig. 19-16) has been reported by Crainz (1924), and Hunt and Thompson (1954); however, most orthopaedic surgeons appear to be fearful of the possibility of necrosis of the talus when it is employed as a free graft and have used other methods (Marek and Schein, 1945). While Lorthioir (1911), Steindler (1923), Crainz (1924), Hamsa (1936), Hunt and Thompson (1954) and Waugh et al. (1965) carried out their fusions in a single stage, Liebolt (1939) and Patterson et al. (1950) felt that fewer complications resulted when the fusion was performed in two stages, with either the subtalar or the talocrural joint being fused first.

Various approaches have been recommended, depending upon the surgical procedure to be used. If a single stage arthrodesis is to be performed, the most popular surgical incisions appear to be the anterolateral or the Kocher incisions. In cases in which an anterior bone graft, a posterior bone graft, or both are being considered, the preferred combination seems to be the anterolateral and posterolateral incisions.

The methods employed to achieve bony stabilization of both the talocrural and subtalar articulations may be divided into two general categories: (1) those that are essentially intra-articular, in which the cartilage is denuded from all articular surfaces of the respective joints, and (2) those that are extra-articular, which depend upon various types of bone grafts that span the joints. The procedures employed by various surgeons are summarized in Fig. 19-17. Names of the surgeons are indicated under each drawing, and the specific references may be found at the end of the chapter.

Talectomy (astragalectomy). Talectomy is a surgical procedure that has been performed for many years. The first talectomy was done in 1608, probably by Fabricus of Hilden, for a compound fracture. After that time the procedure was mainly used for fracture or disease. In 1901 Whitman published a report of thirteen cases

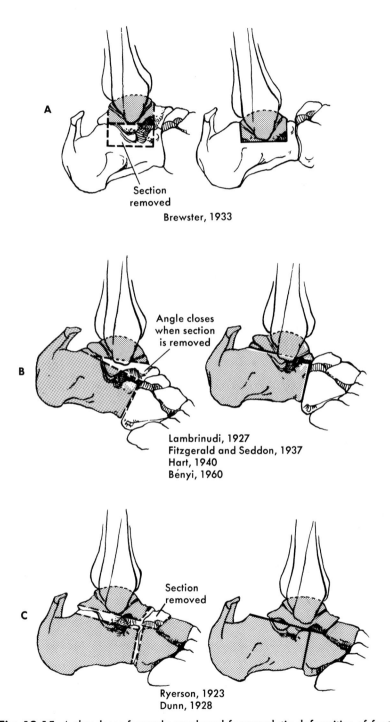

A

Section removed

Brewster, 1933

B

Angle closes when section is removed

Lambrinudi, 1927
Fitzgerald and Seddon, 1937
Hart, 1940
Bényi, 1960

C

Section removed

Ryerson, 1923
Dunn, 1928

Fig. 19-15. Arthrodeses formerly employed for paralytic deformities of foot.

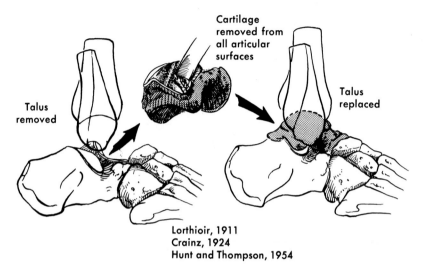

Cartilage
removed from
all articular
surfaces

Talus
removed

Talus
replaced

Lorthioir, 1911
Crainz, 1924
Hunt and Thompson, 1954

Fig. 19-16. Pantalar arthrodesis accomplished by removal of entire talus, denuding it of all its articular catilage, and reinserting it as graft.

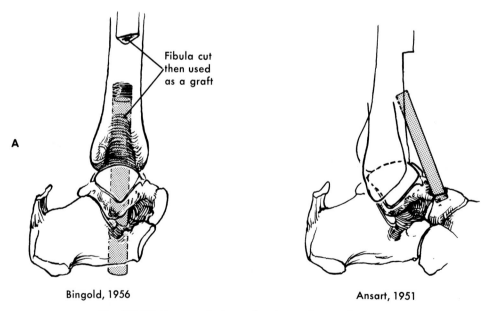

A

Fibula cut
then used
as a graft

Bingold, 1956

Ansart, 1951

Fig. 19-17. Extra-articular arthrodeses of posterior tarsus.

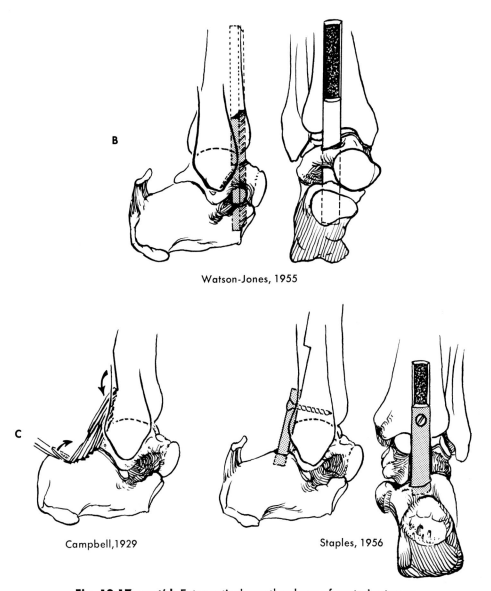

B

Watson-Jones, 1955

C

Campbell, 1929

Staples, 1956

Fig. 19-17, cont'd. Extra-articular arthrodeses of posterior tarsus.

of paralytic talipes of the calcaneus type that he had treated by talectomy. For 20 years the procedure gained popularity in the treatment of calcaneus and calcaneovalgus feet. It was also found useful in flail feet, especially those secondary to poliomyelitis and not associated with varus or equinus deformities. The reason for the apparent success of talectomy was that it provided enough laxity of the tissues in both the equinus and varus deformities to permit correction without tension. Furthermore, the false joint between the mortise and the calcaneus was sufficiently stable when the foot was plantigrade to permit weight bearing.

Following a peak of popularity during the late 1920s, the enthusiasm for this procedure began to wane. Dunn (1930) stated that "the operation of astragalectomy should not now be taught or practised for the treatment of any type of paralytic deformity of the foot."* However, commendatory reports continued to appear in the orthopaedic literature. Thompson (1939), in an excellent review, surveyed 2,066 records and reported on a sample of 100 patients who had undergone talectomies. His conclusions were that the foot can be corrected and stabilized by removal of the talus, that in children the deformity is apt to recur with growth, and that disabling pain is likely to occur in patients over 15 years of age. Tompkins et al. (1956) stated that "astragalectomy does not deserve either wholesale condemnation or unqualified praise."†

With proper application and indications, talectomy remains an excellent procedure. Besides having been used for the correction of paralytic deformity, it has also been employed for diverse pathologic conditions such as osteoblastoma or osteoid osteoma, osteogenic sarcoma, giant-cell tumor, Ewing's sarcoma, tuberculosis, fracture and posttraumatic arthritis, and occasionally for osteomyelitis. Excision of the talus for traumatic fracture or fracture-dislocation is a procedure that has been used for many years. It has also been used in spina bifida and arthrogryposis multiplex congenita (Menelaus, 1971), for the correction of untreated clubfoot in the adult, and in rheumatoid arthritis (Murray, 1972).

With the increasing interest in prosthetic replacement of skeletal parts, talectomy for aseptic necrosis following fractures of the talus has been carried out. Sohier (1952, 1953), Boron and Viarnaud (1958), and Queinnec and Queinnec (1971) have replaced the excised talus with a plastic replica and have reported favorable results.

The criteria for a good result with talectomy are: (1) even weight distribution on the plantar surface in both stance and gait; (2) good lateral stability; (3) an ankle axis that is forward and at a right angle to the long axis of the foot; (4) limited ankle motion, especially in dorsiflexion; (5) no pain; (6) no necessity for external support; and (7) a good appearance of the foot.

A talectomy may be performed by one of several methods. Whitman (1901) approached the talus through a curved posterolateral incision, which extended from the attachment of the tendo achillis, passed below the lateral malleolus, and terminated over the head of the talus. The two peroneal tendons were freed and were either retracted distally or divided. The lateral collateral ligaments of the ankle were cut and the foot was inverted, exposing the talus, which was extracted with comparative ease after the inferior talocalcaneal (interosseous) ligament was severed.

More recently, as talectomy has been employed in avascular necrosis and rheumatoid arthritis, the anterolateral approach has been widely used. In such an approach the talus is readily extirpated with minimal disruption of the supporting soft-tissue structures. After detaching the dorsal capsule and cutting the inferior talocalcaneal ligament in the sinus tarsi, the talus is scooped out totally with a curved gouge. To achieve a better fit between the mortise and the superior surface of the calcaneus in cases in which no prosthetic replacement is being considered, it may be necessary to remove a portion of the malleoli and to reshape the posterior facet of the calcaneus so that the tibial plafond contacts the calcaneus below and the navicular in front.

Although many surgeons prefer arthrodeses, tendon transfers or both for stabilization of a paralytic foot, these procedures are not universally accepted because they often give unpredictable results. The method of talectomy as described by Whitman was once judged the best procedure for the stabilization of a paralytic foot by the American Orthopaedic Surgery Committee.

---

*Dunn, N.: Reconstructive surgery in paralytic deformities of the leg, J. Bone Joint Surg. **12**:299-308, 1930.

†Tompkins, S. F., Miller, R. J., and O'Donoghue, D. H.: An evaluation of astragalectomy, South. Med. J. **49**:1128, Oct. 1956.

External rotation of the foot not compensated for by internal rotation of the leg in gait can be corrected by osteotomy of the tibia as a secondary procedure, but it is rarely necessary. An important point in the surgical technique is to avoid aligning the foot with the patella, as doing so may lead to an unstable foot with a varus deformity.

The calcaneus

Open reduction and bone grafting for fractures of the calcaneus. It is well known that the prognosis for fractures involving the articular surfaces of the calcaneus is unfavorable. Accurate realignment of the displaced fragments is mandatory and often can only be achieved under direct vision by an open reduction. Palmer (1948) stated that in approximately 50 percent of cases a major longitudinal fracture line through the calcaneus occurs. It extends from the medial side upward and laterally, splitting the calcaneus into two major fragments. The fracture passes through the posterior facet of the calcaneus. The lateral fragment is usually found displaced, and a "ledge" or "step" is produced in the articular surface of the posterior facet. Such fractures are amenable to open reduction and bone grafting. To select the proper cases for such a procedure requires the closest cooperation between the surgeon and radiologist.

Widén (1954), Vestad (1968), and Hazlette (1969) have reported favorable results with open reduction and bone grafting for suitable cases.

The surgical procedure is relatively simple. The calcaneus is approached through a curvilinear incision approximately 15 cm. long, which extends from the back of the calcaneus, passes just below the lateral malleolus, and terminates at the calcaneocuboid articulation. The sheath of the peroneal tendons is incised and the tendons are displaced forward. The talocalcaneal ligament is divided, and the posterior facet of the talocalcaneal (subtalar) joint is exposed. The heel is carefully inverted to reveal the articular surface of the calcaneus; this allows inspection and assessment of the extent of the injury. With a traction pin through the tuber of the calcaneus and with judicious use of an elevator, the joint surfaces may be realigned. However, the reduction is usually very unstable and a large defect, formed by compression of the cancellous bone, is present. A bone graft from the iliac crest is shaped and driven into the defect, and this graft acts as a key to hold the reduction. Hazlette (1969) found it necessary in some cases to use screws to supplement the graft and to secure the reduction of major fragments. The degree of stability of the reduction should indicate to the surgeon whether or not the transfixing pin should be incorporated into the cast in order to ensure that the reduction is maintained during the early stages of healing.

Osteotomies of the calcaneus. In the so-called normal or average foot, the superincumbent body weight is transmitted through a vertical plane to the talus and thence to the tuberosity of the calcaneus. The axes of the subtalar and ankle joints, when projected onto a transverse plane, intersect in the center of the trochlea (Isman and Inman, 1969). The body of the calcaneus has a medial curve, which brings the tuberosity under the weight-bearing line of the leg. With such an arrangement a metastable state is created that requires minimal muscular effort to maintain. The variations in the position of the axis of the subtalar joint and the variability of the anatomic structure of the calcaneus may cause the weight-bearing line of the leg to fall outside the reaction point on the heel. A moment is thus created that, if not resisted by muscular effort, will cause the foot either to pronate or to supinate. This situation has been recognized for many years and has led to the development and use of shoe modifications and different types of appliances. Surgical procedures designed to bring the weight-bearing line of the leg within the reaction point on the heel and thus improve alignment were also

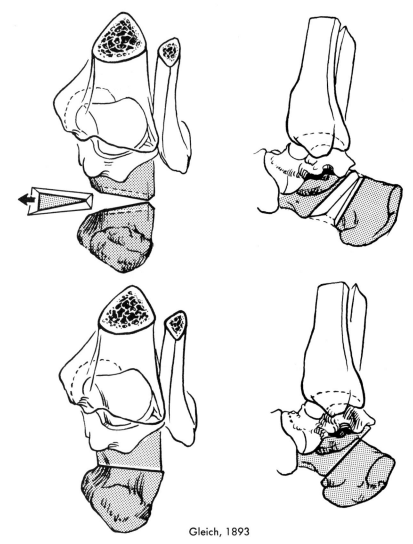

Gleich, 1893

Fig. 19-18. Original osteotomy of calcaneus for correction of flatfoot.

devised and are of interest historically. Trendelenburg (1889), in cases of flatfoot, moved the weight-bearing line of the leg laterally by carrying out a supramalleolar varus osteotomy of the tibia and fibula. Gleich (1893) osteotomized the calcaneus, moving its posterior segment downward and medialward so as to retain the motions of joints and preserve the elasticity of the foot (Fig. 19-18). Operations that fused the midtarsal region of the foot, popular at that time, sacrificed these elements.

Since the pioneering efforts of these surgeons, osteotomy of the calcaneus has been used for a variety of deformities of the foot, including cosmetic improvement in cases of flatfoot, treatment of congenital flaccid flatfoot, and correction of deformities resulting from spastic or paralytic states. Osteotomy has been employed in both pes cavus and pes planus and has consisted of both closing and opening wedges, with and without lateral or medial displacement of the posterior portion of the calcaneus. While the purpose of all the osteotomies is to improve the alignment of the weight-bearing structures of the hindfoot, one should be aware that

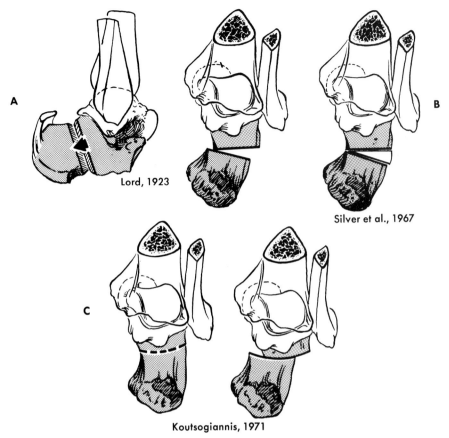

Fig. 19-19. Displacement osteotomies for treatment of flatfoot.

these procedures may also alter the function of the effective lever arms of the muscles that act upon the calcaneus. Unfortunately, these effects have not been adequately studied, but in the reported cases supplementary tendon lengthening and transplants have often been necessary.

The calcaneus may be easily approached from either the medial or the lateral side. Gleich (1893) used a "stirrup" incision, which passed under the heel to expose the inferior aspect of the calcaneus. Few surgeons have employed it, however, since it places a scar on the weight-bearing surface. An opening wedge tends to increase the normal posterior projection of the heel slightly and may make skin closure more difficult. In employing an opening wedge, many surgeons felt it necessary to fill the defect with some type of bone graft. Clos-

ing wedges that retain a precise contact of the surfaces are technically a little more difficult to achieve. Furthermore, a closing wedge tends to shorten the heel slightly.

The various types of osteotomies of the calcaneus may be roughly divided into three categories: (1) those that are used to treat valgus deformities (Figs. 19-18 through 19-20), (2) those that are employed to improve cavus feet (Fig. 19-21), and (3) those that are used for specific pathologic conditions.

Surgical treatment of Haglund's disease. Undue prominence of the posterior superior portion of the calcaneus may lead to painful symptoms in the area of the attachment of the tendo achillis. The majority of these painful heels are seen in adolescent patients, and the condition may be bilateral. To relieve the symptoms, re-

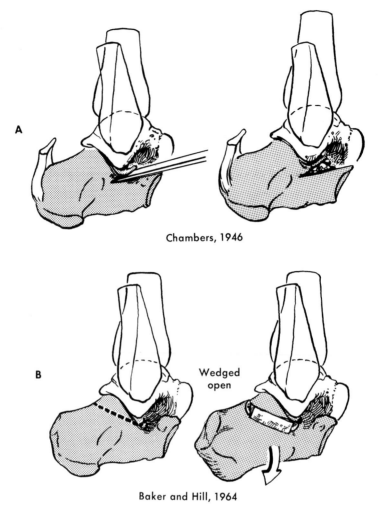

A

Chambers, 1946

B   Wedged
     open

Baker and Hill, 1964

Fig. 19-20. Procedures to restrict pronatory motion, without resorting to arthrodesis.

duction of the prominent posterior projection of the calcaneus is indicated. This has been accomplished by direct extirpation of the offending bony projection or by the performance of a rotational osteotomy of the calcaneus. The former procedure must be done with considerable care. Nissen (1957) has warned that removal of too small a piece of bone may not cure the condition and the removal of too large a piece may weaken the attachment of the tendo achillis and lead to subsequent rupture. Heller (1971) has reported such a case.

To remove the posterior superior projec-

tion of the calcaneus surgically, Fowler and Philip (1945) employed a transverse curvilinear skin incision and split the tendo achillis; however, most surgeons prefer a para–tendo achillis approach. DuVries has successfully employed this method in many cases. He utilizes a lateral approach and removes a wedge of bone, being careful to avoid any injury to the attachment of the tendo achillis (Fig. 19-22). Preoperative and postoperative roentgenograms of a correctly performed osteotomy are shown in Fig. 19-23.

Keck and Kelly (1965) preferred a cuneiform osteotomy of the calcaneus. In this

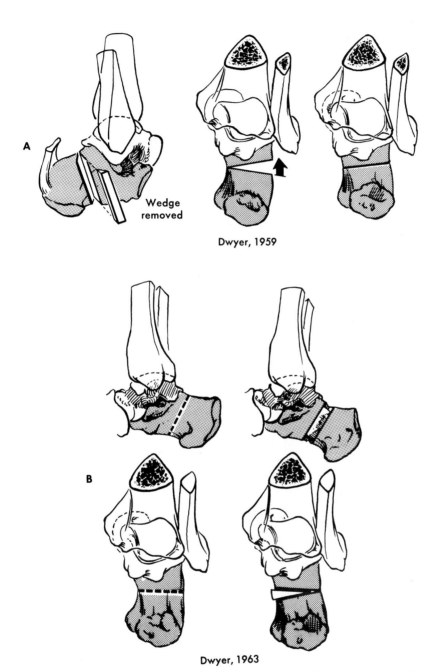

Dwyer, 1959

Dwyer, 1963

Fig. 19-21. Osteotomies for inverted heel and pes cavus. **A,** Original procedure: closing osteotomy on lateral side. **B,** Opening wedge with graft on medial side. The procedure was proposed by Dwyer to replace a closing osteotomy, which shortened the heel.

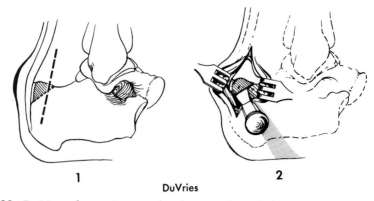

DuVries

Fig. 19-22. Excision of prominence of calcaneus through lateral incision. *1,* Skin incision. *2,* Osteotomizing superior prominence.

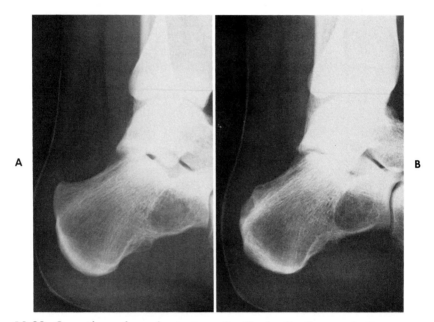

Fig. 19-23. Correctly performed osteotomy for Haglund's disease. **A,** Roentgenogram of prominent superior tuberosity of calcaneus of 16-year-old female. **B,** Roentgenogram 1 year after excision of prominence.

procedure the posterior portion of the calcaneus is rotated, and the prominence of its posterior superior margin impinging on the tendo achillis is reduced (Fig. 19-24).

Surgical treatment of calcaneal spurs. Several operative procedures have been devised for this condition. All of them consist of osteotomies of parts of the calcaneus. Griffith (1910) and Chang and Miltner

(1934) exposed the plantar surface of the calcaneus through a circular flap. A U-shaped incision was made completely around the heel, and the skin flap was reflected to expose the plantar surface of the heel at the origin of the plantar fascia (Fig. 19-25). The fascia was severed at its origin, and amputation of the spur was carried out. Blokhin and Vinogradova (1937)

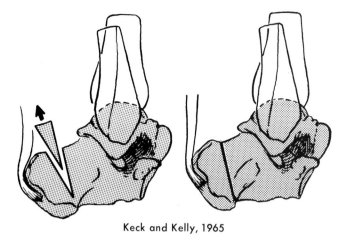

Keck and Kelly, 1965

Fig. 19-24. Osteotomy to decrease prominence of calcaneus.

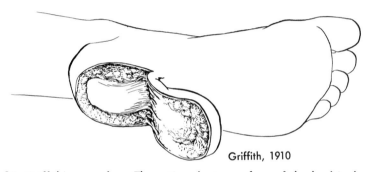

Griffith, 1910

Fig. 19-25. Griffith's procedure. The entire plantar surface of the heel is denuded as a flap, the spur is removed, and the flap is sutured into place. (From DuVries, H. L.: Arch. Surg. **74:**536, 1957.)

reported thirty-three cases in which they used a modified Chang and Miltner technique successfully in the seventeen patients whom they followed for 1 to 4 years postoperatively.

Steindler and Smith (1938) reported the use of a rotational osteotomy of the entire tuberosity of the calcaneus which required lengthening of the tendo achillis. Such an extensive surgical procedure, in most cases, seems unwarranted (Fig. 19-26).

DuVries (1957) recommended a simple medial approach to the plantar surface of the calcaneus, with sectioning of the plantar aponeurosis at its calcaneal attachment and excision of the spur with a small osteotome (Fig. 19-27). A roentgenogram of a painful spur (Fig. 19-28, A) that was successfully treated in this manner is shown in Fig. 19-28, B.

THE MIDTARSUS

The surgical correction of some deformities of the foot has been achieved by means of wedge osteotomies or fusions in the area of the midtarsus. Such procedures have been employed in cases of marked pes cavus or pes planus, with or without accompanying adduction or abduction of the forefoot, as well as in cases in which operative procedures on the hindfoot are not indicated because of the absence of any appreciable varus or valgus of the heel.

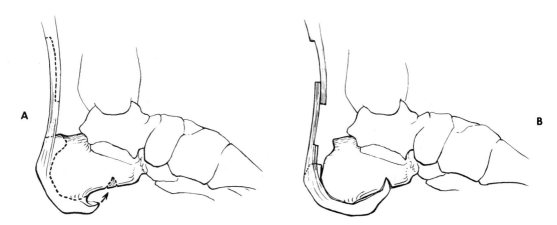

Fig. 19-26. Steindler's rotation osteotomy for heel spur. **A,** Tendo achillis lengthened and osteotomy performed in posterior portion of calcaneus. **B,** Posterior portion rotated. The spur fits into a previously prepared notch in the plantar surface of the body of the calcaneus. (From DuVries, H. L.: Arch. Surg. **74:**536, 1957.)

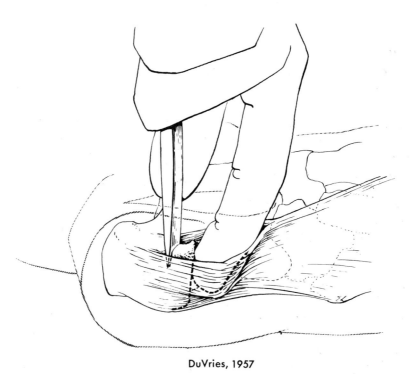

DuVries, 1957

Fig. 19-27. Removal of spur with osteotome through short medial incision.

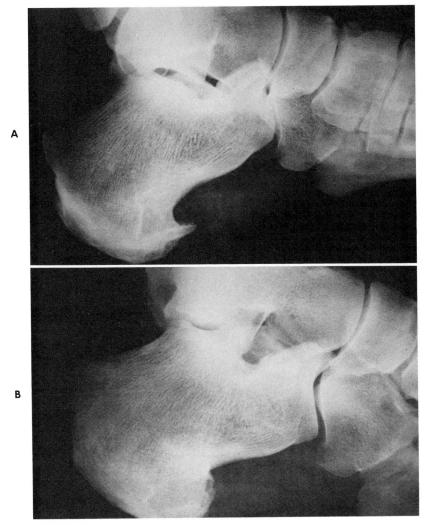

Fig. 19-28. Painful calcaneal spur. **A.** Roentgenogram taken preoperatively. **B,** Same foot 3 years postoperatively. Symptom free.

Pes cavus

Cole (1940) employed a transverse midtarsal osteotomy to treat pes cavus in those patients for whom all types of conservative treatment (e.g., soft-tissue releases, manipulations, tendon transfers, casts, and external appliances) had failed. This procedure consisted of the removal of a wedge of bone from the navicular, the cuneiforms, and the cuboid (Fig. 19-29, A); closing of the wedge led to the correction of the deformity. In those cases in which adduction of the forefoot accompanied the cavus deformity, as in persistent or untreated clubfoot, the direction of the wedge of bone could be changed to correct this added deformity (Fig. 19-29, B).

Pes planus

One should recall that there are two types of flatfoot—rigid and flexible. The term peroneal spastic flatfoot has been loosely applied to the type of flatfoot in which passive correction of the deformity is resisted by contracture and reflex spasm of the peroneal muscles. Such resistance is

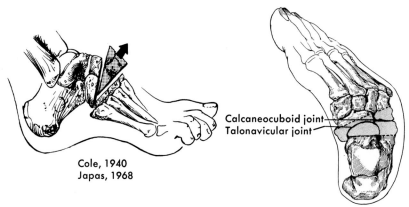

Calcaneocuboid joint
Talonavicular joint

Cole, 1940
Japas, 1968

Fig. 19-29. Midtarsal osteotomies. **A,** Midtarsal osteotomy for correction of pes cavus. **B,** Midtarsal osteotomy for correction of pes cavus with adduction of forefoot. (From Crenshaw, A, H., editor: Campbell's operative orthopaedics, ed. 5, vol. 2, St. Louis, 1971, The C. V. Mosby Co.)

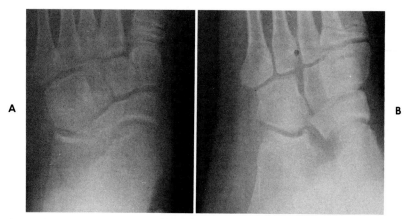

Fig. 19-30. Excision of calcaneonavicular bar. **A,** Preoperative roentgenogram. **B,** Postoperative roentgenogram.

indicative of an irritative lesion in the hindfoot or midfoot. These lesions are frequently found in arthritic processes involving the subtalar and transverse articulations and in various types of tarsal coalitions. Since the proper remedial procedure must be based upon the precise pathologic condition, a careful physical and roentgenographic examination of the foot is mandatory.

If the condition is caused by the presence of a calcaneonavicular bar, DuVries has found that excision of the bar through a lateral approach to the sinus tarsi will often relieve the disorder, especially in adolescents (Fig. 19-30). Should arthritic changes in the subtalar or transverse tarsal articulations be the etiologic factor, subtalar or triple arthrodesis may be the indicated treatment.

The only kind of flexible flatfoot that requires treatment is symptomatic flatfoot. The cosmetic appearance of the foot is not an indication for surgical procedures. Conservative measures (appliances such as heel wedges, higher heels, and shoe inserts)

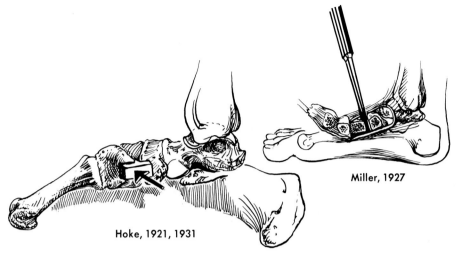

Miller, 1927

Hoke, 1921, 1931

Fig. 19-31. Stabilization procedures. **A,** Stabilization of naviculocuneiform joint by means of bone graft. **B,** Arthrodesis of talonavicular joint and of cuneiform and first metatarsal without graft.

may be employed to improve the appearance of the foot and to reduce the concommitant deformation of the shoe.

In most cases of flexible flatfoot, an accompanying valgus position of the hindfoot is usually present. Since inversion of the heel by various means both improves the appearance of the foot and relieves symptoms, most surgical procedures have been carried out on the hindfoot (e.g., osteotomies of the calcaneus and subtalar fusions). However, in some individuals pes planus appears to manifest itself as a vertical collapse of the longitudinal arch without a valgus heel, and in these individuals stabilization procedures of the midfoot are indicated.

Hoke (1921, 1931) and Miller (1927) found that the instability of the medial side of the longitudinal arch appeared to be caused by the malfunctioning of a series of individual articulations between the first metatarsal, the first cuneiform, the navicular, and the head of the talus. They believed that stability of the longitudinal arch could be restored without undue loss of mobility by arthrodesing some of these articulations. Hoke arthrodesed the naviculocuneiform articulation, using an inlay tibial

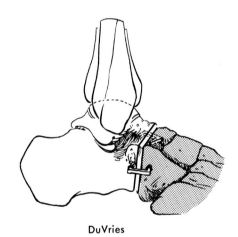

DuVries

Fig. 19-32. Arthrodesis of talonavicular and calcaneocuboid articulations for treatment of flatfoot with no osseous anomalies.

graft after removing the articular cartilage (Fig. 19-31, *A*). Miller resected the articular cartilage between the navicular and the first cuneiform and, in more severe cases, also between the first cuneiform and the base of the first metatarsal. In such a procedure any abduction of the forefoot could be corrected by removing various sizes of wedges of bone (Fig. 19-31, *B*).

L'Episcopo and Sabatelle (1939) re-

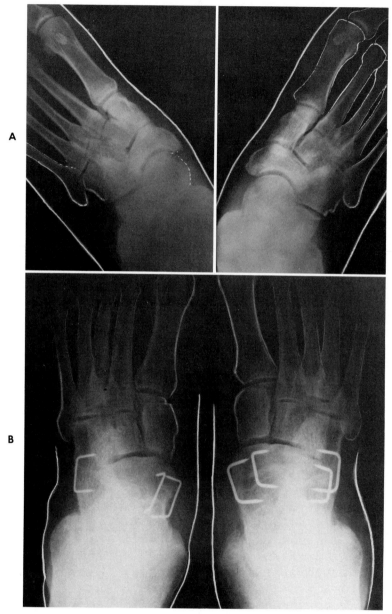

Fig. 19-33. Treatment of bilateral flatfoot by double arthrodesis. **A,** Roentgenogram of feet of 41-year-old male with bilateral painful flatfoot. Note extreme pronation of both feet. A double arthrodesis was performed November 1963. **B,** Anteroposterior view of both feet taken February 1972. **C,** Lateral view taken at same time. Patient's feet were completely asymptomatic.

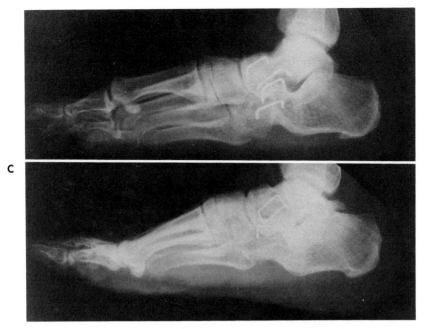

Fig. 19-33, cont'd. For legend see opposite page.

ported their observations of sixteen patients with flatfoot after operation by Hoke's procedure; 68 percent had obtained good results and 32 percent fair results. Butte (1937) reported on seventy-six feet operated on by Hoke's procedure; results were satisfactory in about 50 percent. Jack (1953) performed Hoke's operation for flatfoot in forty-six cases and obtained satisfactory results in 82 percent.

For the treatment of symptomatic flexible flatfoot with no osseous anomalies, DuVries has used an arthrodesis of the talonavicular and calcaneocuboid articulations (Fig. 19-32). He reports good results in more than forty cases (Fig. 19-33). His technique consists of two curvilinear incisions, one to expose the talonavicular joint and the other the calcaneocuboid joint. Cartilage is removed from all articular surfaces and the bones are trimmed so that they may be closely coapted. They are fixed with small staples.

Special mention should be made concerning the possible role played by an accessory navicular in painful flatfoot. Kidner (1929, 1933) presented evidence that the presence of an accessory navicular or an abnormal prolongation of the tuberosity of the navicular resulted in a medial displacement of the attachment of the tendon of the tibialis posterior muscle. Such an anatomic arrangement caused the tibialis posterior muscle to act more as an adductor of the forefoot than a supinator and elevator of the longitudinal arch. The so-called Kidner procedure consists of careful excision of the accessory navicular and transposition of the tendon so that it lies more laterally and beneath the navicular. Unfortunately, no large series or long-term follow-up of individuals who have undergone the Kidner procedure has been found in the literature; thus no evaluation of its efficacy can be given.

REFERENCES

Adams, J. C.: Arthrodesis of the ankle joint: Experiences with the transfibular approach, J. Bone Joint Surg. 30-B:506-511, Aug. 1948.

Anderson, K. J., and LeCocq, J. F.: Operative treatment of injury to the fibular collateral ligament of the ankle, J. Bone Joint Surg. 36-A:825-832, July 1954.

Anderson, R.: Concentric arthrodesis of the ankle joint: A transmalleolar approach, J. Bone Joint Surg. 27:37-48, Jan. 1945.

Ansart, M. B.: Pan-arthrodesis for paralytic flail foot, J. Bone Joint Surg. 33-B:503-507, Nov. 1951.

Ashhurst, A. P. C., and Bromer, R. S.: Classification and mechanism of fractures of the leg bones involving the ankle: Based on a study of three hundred cases from the Episcopal Hospital, Arch. Surg. 4:51-129, Jan. 1922.

Baker, L. D., and Hill, L. M.: Foot alignment in the cerebral palsy patient, J. Bone Joint Surg. 46-A:1-15, Jan. 1964.

Barr, J. S., and Record, E. E.: Arthrodesis of the ankle joint, New Eng. J. Med. 248:53-56, Jan. 1953.

Bényi, P.: A modified Lambrinudi operation for drop foot, J. Bone Joint Surg. 42-B:333-335, May 1960.

Bingold, A. C.: Ankle and subtalar fusion by a transarticular graft, J. Bone Joint Surg. 38-B:862-870, Nov. 1956.

Blokhin, V. N., and Vinogradova, T. P.: Shpory pyatochnykh kostey [Calcaneal spurs], Ortop. Travmatol. Protez. 11:96-113, 1937.

Bogutskaia, E. V.: Privychnyy vyvikh sukhzuliy malobyertsovykh myshts u sporsmyenov [Habitual dislocation of fibular muscles of athletes], Khirurgiia (Mosk) 46:83-85, Sept. 1970.

Boron, R., and Viarnaud. E.: Une observation de prothèse astragalienne en acrylique, Mem. Acad. Chir. 84:549-550, June 1958.

Branch, H. E.: Drop-foot: End results of a series of bone-block operations, J. Bone Joint Surg. 21:141-147, Jan. 1939.

Brewster, A. H.: Countersinking the astragalus in paralytic feet, New Eng. J. Med. 209:71-73, July 1933.

Brittain, H. A.: Architectural principles in arthrodesis, Baltimore, 1942, The Williams & Wilkins Co.

Butte, F. L.: Navicular-cuneiform arthrodesis for flat-foot: An end-result study, J. Bone Joint Surg. 19:496-502, Apr. 1937.

Campbell, W. C.: An operation for the correction of "drop-foot," J. Bone Joint Surg. 5:815-824, Oct. 1923.

Campbell, W. C.: End-results of operation for correction of drop-foot, J.A.M.A. 85:1927-1929, Dec. 1925.

Campbell, W. C.: An operation for the induction of osseous fusion in the ankle joint, Amer. J. Surg. 6:588-592, May 1929.

Chambers, E. F. S.: An operation for the correction of flexible flat feet of adolescents, West. J. Surg. Obstet. Gynec. 54:77-86, Mar. 1946.

Chang, C. C., and Miltner, L. J.: Periostitis of the os calcis, J. Bone Joint Surg. 16:355-364, Apr. 1934.

Charnley, J.: Compression arthrodesis of the ankle and the shoulder, J. Bone Joint Surg. 33-B:180-191, May 1959.

Chrisman, O. D., and Snook, G. A.: Reconstruction of lateral ligament tears of the ankle: An experimental study and clinical evaluation of seven patients treated by a new modification of the Elmslie procedure, J. Bone Joint Surg. 51-A:904-912, July 1969.

Chuinard, E. G., and Peterson, R. E.: Distraction-compression bone-graft arthrodesis of the ankle: A method especially applicable in children, J. Bone Joint Surg. 45-A:481-490, Apr. 1963.

Close, J. R., and Todd, F. N.: The phasic activity of the muscles of the lower extremity and the effect of tendon transfer, J. Bone Joint Surg. 41-A:189-208, Mar. 1959.

Cole, W. H.: The treatment of claw-foot, J. Bone Joint Surg. 22:895-908, Oct. 1940.

Cordebar, J.: Reconstitution de la mortaise tibio-tarsienne, Presse Méd. 64:774, Oct. 1956.

Crainz, S.: L'artrodesi del piede per mezzo dell' astragalectomia seguita de reimpianto parziale o totale dell'astragalo, Policlinico (Chir.) 31:1-7, 1924.

Cramer, K.: Beitrag zur Arthrodese des Talo-cruralgelenkes, Zentralbl. Chir. mechan. Orthop. 4:113-116, 1910.

Crego, C. H., Jr., and McCarroll, H. R.: Recurrent deformities in stabilized paralytic feet: A report of 1100 consecutive stabilizations in poliomyelitis, J. Bone Joint Surg. 20:609-620, July 1938.

Dahmen, G., and Meyer, H.: Über die verschiedenen Methoden zur Arthrodese des oberen Sprunggelenkes, Arch. Orthop. Unfallchir. 58:265-281, 1965.

Davis, G. G.: The treatment of hollow foot (pes cavus), Amer. J. Orthop. Surg. 11:231-242, Oct. 1913.

Dawkins, A.: The unstable subtalar joint. Proceedings and reports of councils and associations, J. Bone Joint Surg. 40-B:357, May 1958.

Diamant-Berger, L.: La luxation des tendons péroniers latéraux, Presse Méd. 79:17, Jan. 1971.

Dunn, N.: Suggestions based on ten years' experience of arthrodesis of the tarsus in the treatment of deformities of the foot. In The Robert Jones birthday volume: A collection of surgical essays, London, 1928, Oxford University Press.

DuVries, H. L.: Heel spur (calcaneal spur), Arch. Surg. 74:536-542, 1957.

DuVries, H. L.: Surgery of the foot, ed. 2, St. Louis, 1965, The C. V. Mosby Co.

Dwyer, F. C.: Osteotomy of the calcaneum for pes cavus, J. Bone Joint Surg. 41-B:80-86, Feb. 1959.

Dwyer, F. C.: The treatment of relapsed club foot by the insertion of a wedge into the calcaneum, J. Bone Joint Surg. 45-B:67-75, Feb. 1963.

Elmslie, R. C.: Recurrent subluxation of the ankle-joint, Ann. Surg. 100:364-367, Aug. 1934.

Evans, D. L.: Recurrent instability of the ankle: A method of surgical treatment, Proc. Roy. Soc. Med. 46:343-344, May 1953.

Fitzgerald, F. P., and Seddon, H. J.: Lambrinudi's operation for drop-foot, Brit. J. Surg. 25:283-292 ,1937.

Folschveiller, J.: Abriss des Retinaculum Musculi fibularium proximale und seine Folgen, Hefte Unfallheilkd. 92:98-100, Oct. 1967.

Fowler, A., and Philip, J. F.: Abnormality of the calcaneus as a cause of painful heel: Its diagnosis and operative treatment, Brit. J. Surg. 32:494-498, 1945.

Francillon, M. R.: Distorsio pedis with an isolated lesion of the ligamentum calcaneo-fibulare, Acta Orthop. Scand. 32:469-475, 1962.

Geens, S.: Synovectomy and débridement of the knee in rheumatoid arthritis. Part I. Historical review, J. Bone Joint Surg. 51-A:617-625, June 1969.

Gill, A. B.: An operation to make a posterior bone block at the ankle to limit foot-drop, J. Bone Joint Surg. 15:166-170, Jan. 1933.

Gillespie, H. S., and Boucher, P.: Watson-Jones repair of lateral instability of the ankle, J. Bone Joint Surg. 53-A:920-924, July 1971.

Gleich, A.: Beitrag zur operativen Plattfussbehandlung, Arch. klin. Chir. 46:358-362, 1893.

Glissan, D. J.: The indications for inducing fusion at the ankle joint by operation, with description of two successful techniques, Aust. N. Z. J. Surg. 19:64-71, Aug. 1949.

Goldthwait, J. E.: An operation for the stiffening of the ankle joint in infantile paralysis, Amer. J. Orthop. Surg. 5:271-275, Jan. 1908.

Grice, D. S.: An extra-articular arthrodesis of the subastragalar joint for correction of paralytic flat feet in children, J. Bone Joint Surg. 34-A:927-940, Oct. 1952.

Griffith, J. D.: Osteophytes of the os calcis, Amer. J. Orthop. Surg. 8:501-506, Feb. 1910.

Hallgrímsson, S.: Studies on reconstructive and stabilizing operations on the skeleton of the foot. With special reference to subastragalar arthrodesis in the treatment of foot deformities following infantile paralysis, Acta Chir. Scand. (Suppl. 78) 88:1-215, 1943.

Hallock, H.: Arthrodesis of the ankle joint for old painful fractures, J. Bone Joint Surg. 27:49-58, Jan. 1945.

Hamsa, W. R.: Panastragaloid arthrodesis: A study of end results in eighty-five cases, J. Bone Joint Surg. 28:732-736, July 1936.

Hart, V. L.: Arthrodesis of the foot in infantile paralysis, Surg. Gynec. Obstet. 64:794-805, Apr. 1937.

Hart, V. L.: Lambrinudi operation for drop-foot, J. Bone Joint Surg. 22:937-941, Oct. 1940.

Hatt, R. N.: The central bone graft in joint arthrodesis, J. Bone Joint Surg. 22:393-402, Apr. 1940.

Hazlette, J. W.: Open reduction of fractures of the calcaneum, Canad. J. Surg. 12:310-317, July 1969.

Heller, W.: Achillessehnenausriss nach Operation einer Haglund-Ferse, Z. Orthop. 109:534-537, Mar.-Nov. 1971.

Heywood, A. W. B.: Rheumatoid arthritis—the orthopaedic contribution. III. The trunk and lower limb, S. Afr. Med. J. 41:267-271, Mar. 1967.

Hoke, M.: An operation for stabilizing paralytic feet, Amer. J. Orthop. Surg. 3:494-505, 1921.

Hoke, M.: An operation for the correction of extremely relaxed flat feet, J. Bone Joint Surg. 13:773-783, Oct. 1931.

Horwitz, T.: The use of the transfibular approach in arthrodesis of the ankle, Amer. J. Surg. 55:550-552, Mar. 1942.

Hunt, W. S., Jr., and Thompson, H. A.: Pantalar arthrodesis: A one-stage operation, J. Bone Joint Surg. 36-A:349-362, Apr. 1954.

Inclan, A.: End results in physiological blocking of flail joints, J. Bone Joint Surg. 31-A:748-754, Oct. 1949.

Ingram, A. J., and Hundley, J. M.: Posterior bone block of the ankle for paralytic equinus: An end-result study, J. Bone Joint Surg. 33-A:679-690, July 1951.

Isman, R. E., and Inman, V. T.: Anthropometric studies of the human foot and ankle, Bull. Prosthetics Res. BPR 10-11:97-129, Spring 1969.

Jack, E. A.: Naviculo-cuneiform fusion in the treatment of flat foot, J. Bone Joint Surg. 35-B:75-82, Feb. 1953.

Jakubowski, S.: Synowektomia stawv skokowo-goleniowego goś ćcu przewleklym postepujacym (Ankle joint synovectomy in rheumatoid arthritis), Chir. Narzadow Ruchu Ortop. Pol. 35:683-689, 1970.

Jansen, K.: Arthrodesis of the ankle joint, Acta Orthop. Scand. 32:476-484, 1962.

Japas, L. M.: Surgical treatment of pes cavus by tarsal V-osteotomy: Preliminary report, J. Bone Joint Surg. 50-A:927-944, July 1968.

Jones, R.: An operation for paralytic calcaneo-cavus, Amer. J. Orthop. Surg. 5:371-376, Apr. 1908.

Keck, S. W., and Kelly, P. J.: Bursitis of the posterior part of the heel: Evaluation of surgical treatment of eighteen patients, J. Bone Joint Surg. 47-A:267-273, Mar. 1965.

Kelly, R. E.: An operation for the chronic dislocation of the peroneal tendons, Brit. J. Surg. 7:502-504, 1920.

Kidner, F. C.: The prehallux (accessory scaphoid) in its relation to flat-foot, J. Bone Joint Surg. 11:831-837, Oct. 1929.

Kidner, F. C.: The prehallux in relation to flat-foot, J.A.M.A. **101**:1539-1542, Nov. 1933.

Koutsogiannis, E.: Treatment of mobile flat foot by displacement osteotomy of the calcaneus, J. Bone Joint Surg. **53-B**:96-100, Feb. 1971.

Lambrinudi, C.: New operation on drop-foot, Brit. J. Surg. **15**:193-200, 1927.

Lasker, W.: Spätresultate der Arthrodesenopera-tion nach Cramer, zugleich ein Beitrag zur Frage der Knochentransplantation, Bruns Beitr. klin. Chir. **128**:499-514, 1923.

Lee, H. G.: Surgical repair in recurrent dislo-cation of the ankle joint, J. Bone Joint Surg. **39-A**:828-834, July 1957.

L'Episcopo, J. B., and Sabatelle, P. E.: The Hoke operation for flat feet, J. Bone Joint Surg. **21**: 92-97, Jan. 1939.

Liebolt, F. L.: Pantalar arthrodesis in poliomye-litis, Surgery **6**:31-34, July 1939.

London, P. S.: Synovectomy of the knee in rheu-matoid arthritis: An essay in surgical salvage, J. Bone Joint Surg. **37-B**:392-399, Aug. 1955.

Lord, J. P.: Correction of extreme flatfoot: Value of osteotomy of os calcis and inward displace-ment of posterior fragment (Gleich operation), J.A.M.A. **81**:1502-1506, Nov. 1923.

Lorthioir, J.: Huit cas d'arthrodèse du pied avec extirpation temporaire de l'astragale, J. Chir. Ann. Soc. Belge Chir. **11**:184-187, 1911.

Marek, F. M., and Schein, A. J.: Aseptic necro-sis of the astragalus following arthrodesing pro-cedures of the tarsus, J. Bone Joint Surg. **27**: 587-594, Oct. 1945.

Mead, N. C.: Arthrodesis of the ankle joint: A simple efficient method, Northwestern Univ. Med. School Quart. Bull. **25**:248-250, 1951.

Menelaus, M. B.: Talectomy for equinovarus de-formity in arthrogryposis and spina bifida, J. Bone Joint Surg. **53-B**:468-473, Aug. 1971.

Miller, O. L.: A plastic flat foot operation, J. Bone Joint Surg. **9**:84-91, Jan. 1927.

Mounier-Kuhn, A., and Marsan, C.: Le syndrome des tendons péroniers, Ann. Chir. **22**:641-649, 1968.

Muralt, R. H.: Luxation der Peronäalsehnen, Z. Orthop. **87**:263-274, 1956.

Murr, S.: Dislocation of the peroneal tendons with marginal fracture of the lateral malleolus, J. Bone Joint Surg. **43-B**:563-565, Aug. 1961.

Murray, W. R.: Personal communication, 1972.

Nilsonne, H.: Making a new ligament in ankle sprain, J. Bone Joint Surg. **14**:380-381, Apr. 1932.

Nissen, K. I.: Remodelling of the posterior tuber-osity of the calcaneum. In Rob, C., and Smith, R., editors: Operative surgery, vol. 5, London, 1957, Butterworth & Co., pp. 315-317.

Palmer, I.: The mechanism and treatment of frac-tures of the calcaneus, J. Bone Joint Surg. **30-A**: 2-8, Jan. 1948.

Patterson, R. L., Jr., Parrish, F. F., and Hathaway, E. N.: Stabilizing operations on the foot: A study of the indications, techniques used, and end results, J. Bone Joint Surg. **32-A**:1-26, Jan. 1950.

Queinnec, A., and Queinnec, J.: Résultats éloi-gnés de deux cas de prothèse de l'astragale par des pièces en "plastique," Chirurgie **97**:193-196, 1971.

Ratliff, A. H. C.: Compression arthrodesis of the ankle, J. Bone Joint Surg. **41-B**:524-534, Aug. 1959.

Ruth, C. J.: The surgical treatment of injuries of the fibular collateral ligaments of the ankle, J. Bone Joint Surg. **43-A**:229-239, Mar. 1961.

Ryerson, E. W.: Arthrodesing operations on the feet, J. Bone Joint Surg. **5**:453-471, July 1923.

Scheuba, G.: Die Luxation der Tibialis posterior-Sehne, Monatsschr. Unfallheilkd. **72**:540-543, 1969.

Schoolfield, B. L.: Operative treatment of flatfoot, Surg. Gynec. Obstet. **94**:136-140, Jan. 1952.

Schwartz, R. P.: Arthrodesis of subtalus and mid-tarsal joints of the foot: Historical review, pre-operative determinations and operative proce-dure, Surgery **20**:619-635, July-Dec. 1946.

Silver, C. M., Simon, S. D., Spindell, E., Litchman, H. M., and Scala, M.: Calcaneal osteotomy for valgus and varus deformities of the foot in cere-bral palsy: A preliminary report on twenty-seven operations, J. Bone Joint Surg. **49-A**:232-246, Mar. 1967.

Sohier, H. M. L.: Astragale en acrylic employée comme prothèse après astragalectomie pour frac-ture, Mém. Acad. Chir. **78**:666-667, June-July 1952.

Sohier, H. M. L.: Astragales en matière plastique, Bull. Méd. Ec. prepar. Med. Pharm. Dakar **1**: 132-144, 1952-1953.

Staples, S.: Posterior arthrodesis of the ankle and subtalar joints, J. Bone Joint Surg. **38-A**:50-58, Jan. 1956.

Steindler, A.: The treatment of flail ankle: Panas-tragaloid arthrodesis, J. Bone Joint Surg. **5**:284-293, Apr. 1923.

Steindler, A., and Smith, A. R: Spurs of the os cal-cis, Surg. Gynec. Obstet. **66**:663-665, Jan.-June 1938.

Thompson, T. C.: Astragalectomy and the treat-ment of calcaneovalgus, J. Bone Joint Surg. **21**: 627-647, July 1939.

Trendelenburg, F.: Ueber Plattfussoperationen, Arch. klin. Chir. **39**:751-755, 1889.

Vahvanen, V.: Synovectomy of the talocrural joint in rheumatoid arthritis, Ann. Chir. Gynaecol. Fenn. **57**:576-582, 1968.

Vahvanen, V.: Arthrodesis of the TC or pantalar joints in rheumatoid arthritis, Acta Orthop. Scand. **40**:642-652, 1969.

Vestad, E.: Fractures of the calcaneum: Open reduction and bone grafting, Acta Chir. Scand. **34:**617-625, 1968.

Watson-Jones, R.: Fractures and joint injuries, ed. 4, Baltimore, 1955, The William & Wilkins Co.

Waugh, T. R., Wagner, J., and Stinchfield, F. E.: An evaluation of pantalar arthrodesis: A follow-up study of one hundred and sixteen operations, J. Bone Joint Surg. **47-A:**1315-1321, Oct. 1965.

Weigert, M.: Ein einfaches Verfahren zur operativen Behandlung der habituellen Peronaeal-sehnenluxation, Z. Orthop. **105:**273-274, July 1968–Jan. 1969.

Wheeldon, T. F., and Clark, M. M.: The Gill bone block operation for foot drop, J.A.M.A. **106:**447-449, Feb. 1936.

Whitefield, G. A.: Surgical management of rheumatoid arthritis, Scott. Med. J. **12:**107-113, Mar. 1967.

Whitman, R.: The operative treatment of paralytic talipes of the calcaneus type, Amer. J. Med. Sci. **122:**593-601, 1901.

Widén, A.: Fractures of the calcaneus: A clinical study with special reference to the technique and results of open-reduction, Acta Chir. Scand. (Suppl. 188) **108:**78-79, 1954.

Wilson, H. J.: Arthrodesis of the ankle: A technique using bilateral hemimalleolar onlay grafts with screw fixation, J. Bone Joint Surg. **51-A:** 775-777, June 1969.

20

Major surgical procedures for disorders of the forefoot

Henri L. DuVries

THE FIRST METATARSOPHALANGEAL JOINT

Surgical procedures for hallux valgus

It has become apparent that since the causative factors and the pathologic changes in hallux valgus vary from case to case, no single procedure can be successful in all cases. Reports of operative procedures for its correction (Fig. 20-1) are numerous (Galland and Jordan, 1938). The surgeon must study each individual case of hallux valgus and apply a procedure or combination of procedures that suits that particular case.

Simple and modified condylectomies. Simple condylectomy, or exostosectomy, of the tibial side of the first metatarsal head is one of the most common procedures advocated for hallux valgus because it is simple and seldom disabling. It produces disability only when performed in cases of severe dislocation of the great toe joint or when too much of the tibial side of the head of the first metatarsal has been removed. McElvenny and Thompson (1940) and Levine (1938) also removed the tibial condylar lip of the base of the first proximal phalanx; however, that is of value only when the protuberance is caused entirely by an unusually wide first metatarsal head. It is of little or no value when there is ex-

treme hallux valgus and it may even worsen the deformity.

Stanley and Breck (1935) reported the results in 211 cases in which they removed the tibial condylar side of the head of the first metatarsal exostosis through a unique web incision (Fig. 20-2).

Arthrodesis. Girdlestone and Spooner (1937) and Joplin (1950) considered splayfoot a forerunner of hallux valgus. Girdlestone and Spooner aimed to correct the condition by arthrodesis of the base of the proximal phalanx to the head of the first metatarsal (Fig. 20-3), thereby making use of the adductor hallucis to pull the metatarsal heads together. Wilson (1967) reported his use of a cone arthrodesis of the first metatarsophalangeal joint. His procedure consisted of making a cone fit between the metatarsal head and the base of the proximal phalanx of the great toe. He stated that by careful positioning of the reamers, it was possible to fuse the joint in as much as 10 to 15 degrees of dorsiflexion or valgus.

Moynihan (1967) recommended arthrodesing the first metatarsophalangeal joint of the great toe by two similar procedures: a peg and socket arthrodesis, and a procedure in which the cartilage, subchondral bone, and exostosis were excised. In both

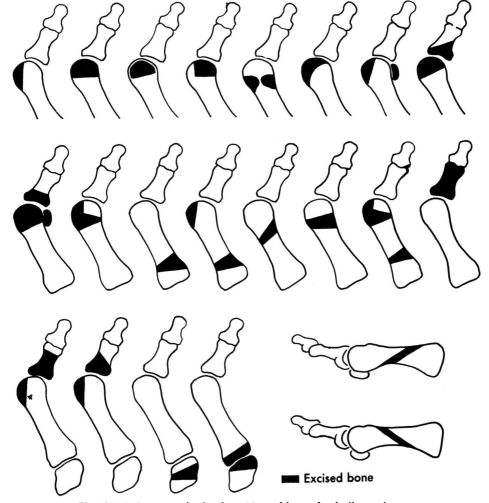

Fig. 20-1. Some methods of excision of bone for hallux valgus.

procedures the arthrodesed joint was fixed with a screw. He performed these operations on 108 patients, with good results in 86 percent of cases.

Plantar sling. Joplin (1950) fashioned a transverse plantar sling of the extensor digitorum longus tendon from the fifth toe (Fig. 20-4), which he brought under the metatarsal arch and passed through a drill hole in the first metatarsal head with the freed adductor hallucis tendon. He then sutured it to the capsule on the tibial side of the first metatarsophalangeal joint. The procedure combines some of the features of an operation that laces a strip of fascia lata around the metatarsal heads to bind them for splayfoot, as reported by Krida (1939). McBride (1928) also employs fascia lata lacing as part of his procedure.

These procedures have value in severe splayfoot. Blosser (1964) performed a modified Krida procedure on forty cases of hallux valgus with good results. It would appear that a strip of fascia lata would bind and hold the distal part of the metatarsals together more securely than would the long extensor, which is a very thin tendon.

Condylectomy combined with step-down osteotomy. Hawkins and associates (1945) and Mitchell and co-workers (1958), in ad-

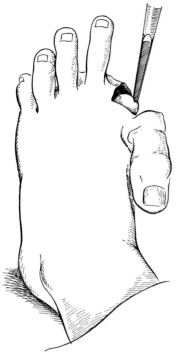

Fig. 20-2. Stanley and Breck's technique for correction of hallux valgus.

dition to removing the tibial condylar side of the first metatarsal head, performed a step-down osteotomy on the first metatarsal shaft (Fig. 20-5). They reported excellent results in a large series of cases.

This procedure has much to recommend it in the uncommon cases of hallux valgus accompanied by a first metatarsal that is longer than the lesser metatarsals (Fig. 20-6, *A*). However, when the first metatarsal is shorter than the second, the resultant additional shortening places an excessive amount of weight bearing on the head of the second metatarsal, and often a new problem is produced (Fig. 20-6, *B*).

Subcapital amputation. Hueter (1870) was one of the first to advise subcapital amputation of the first metatarsal head. The procedure was later modified by Mayo (1908) and Soresi (1931), among others. It is a commonly practiced procedure (Fig. 20-7). Rix (1968) reported good results with his modification of the Mayo proce-

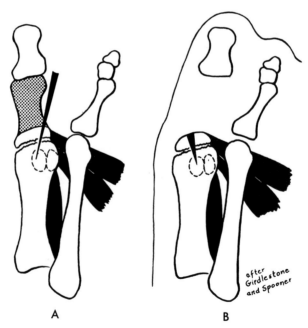

A   B

Fig. 20-3. Girdlestone and Spooner's technique for correction of hallux valgus. **A,** Excision of distal seven-eighths of the proximal phalanx. **B,** Anchoring of base of the proximal phalanx to head of first metatarsal.

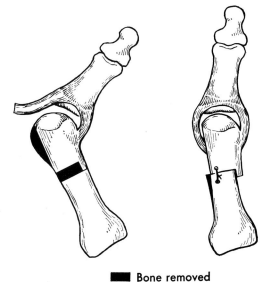

■ Bone removed

Fig. 20-5. Hawkins' step-cut osteotomy of first metatarsal shaft for hallux valgus.

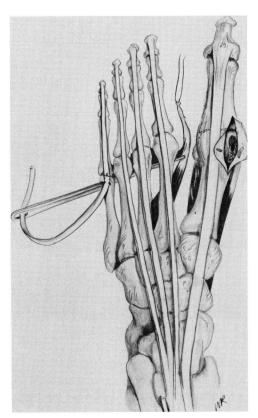

Fig. 20-4. Joplin's plantar sling technique for hallux valgus. Extensor tendon of the fifth digit is threaded under the metatarsal heads and, together with the tendon of the adductor hallucis, is threaded through a drill hole in the first metatarsal head and sutured to capsule on the tibial side. (Courtesy American Academy of Orthopaedic Surgeons, Inc.)

dure. The modification consisted of altering the skin incision, reversing the base of the soft-tissue flap, and in some cases transplanting the abductor hallucis tendon.

In all first metatarsal subcapital amputations, the base of the proximal phalanx moves by the pull of the flexor hallucis brevis and abductor hallucis into the space formerly occupied by the head, thereby straightening the toe and producing excellent cosmetic results. However, the functional results are limited, because the weight-bearing surface of the first metatarsal head has been destroyed. A review of

100 cases of severe disability resulting from subcapital amputation emphasizes that function of the first metatarsal is as important as the weight bearing of all the other four metatarsals; thus, subcapital amputation is deplored.

The distal half of the shaft of the first metatarsal receives its blood supply from the epiphyseal head. Therefore, the ever-present danger of destroying the blood supply by subcapital amputation, which will lead to atrophy of the distal half of the shaft (Figs. 20-8 and 20-9), must always be kept in mind. False ankylosis of the first metatarsophalangeal joint may ensue if the head is not rounded during subcapital amputation. When the head is angulated by amputation, the articular surface of the head is left pinpointed and a gouging action into the base of the proximal phalanx is produced (Fig. 20-10).

I have seen no static deformity of the first metatarsophalangeal joint in which this procedure is indicated. Such a procedure destroys the most important weight-bearing surface of the forefoot, and it is gratifying that the operation has generally been abandoned, although it is still practiced. It re-

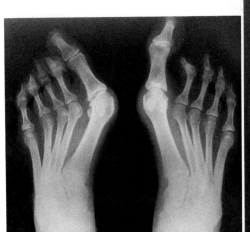

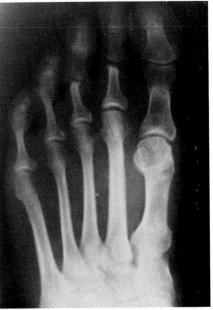

Fig. 20-6. **A,** Hallux valgus with abnormally long first metatarsal. Hawkins-Mitchell step-down osteotomy is the procedure of choice in this case. **B,** Result of step-down osteotomy for hallux valgus. The first metatarsal of this 24-year-old woman was shorter than the second before the operation. A painful plantar keratosis ensued caused by excessive weight bearing on the second metatarsal, requiring a Giannestras step-down osteotomy on the second metatarsal.

quires heroic measures to treat those who have become severely disabled as a result of this procedure (Fig. 20-11).

Seeburger (1964) reported ninety-five cases of metallic implants into the metatarsal heads, some for postsurgical subcapital amputations (Fig. 20-12), and he states that results were from good to excellent.

Amputation of the base of the proximal phalanx. Keller described his operation for amputating the proximal half of the first proximal phalanx for hallux valgus correction in 1904; later (1912) he reported refinements. His procedure has acquired support, notably by Brandes (1929), Galland and Jordan (1938), Schein (1940), and Cleveland and Winant (1950). It is probably the most widely used procedure in the United States.

Keller's technique. An elliptical incision, having its base dorsally, is made over the great toe joint. A U-shaped incision with its base about 1 cm. distal to the base of the proximal phalanx is made in the tibial capsule of the great toe joint. The flap is dissected distally to expose the medial surface of the head of the first metatarsal and the base of the proximal phalanx. The tibial condyle of the first metatarsal is amputated. The attachments to the base of the proximal phalanx are freed. Approximately 1 to 1.5 cm. or the proximal third of the base of the proximal phalanx is amputated and smoothed with a rasp. The toe is brought into alignment, and the U-shaped flap is sutured to the periosteum just behind the tibial side of the head of the first metatarsal. This is done under mild tension, with the toe in a slightly overcorrected position. The skin is then sutured (Fig. 20-13).

The Keller method is perhaps the most common procedure practiced for the surgi-

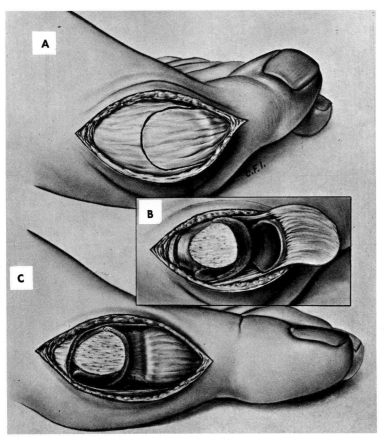

Fig. 20-7. Mayo operation. **A,** Incisions through skin, fascia, and bursa. **B,** Flap of bursa reflected distally, exostosis resected from metatarsal head, and head remodeled. **C,** Flap turned into joint space and sutured to lateral part of capsule. (From Crenshaw, A. H., editor: Campbell's operative orthopaedics, ed. 5, vol. 2, St. Louis, 1971, The C. V. Mosby Co.)

cal treatment of hallux valgus, probably because of its simplicity and the fact that it usually gives excellent cosmetic results. However, the great toe is always shortened, its function in walking is diminished, and in some cases the toe becomes a useless appendage. That happens because the important action of the great toe is controlled by the intrinsic muscles that are inserted into the base of the proximal phalanx, and in this procedure that part of the bone is amputated, thereby destroying the function of these muscles.

The sesamoids usually recede proximally (Figs. 20-14 and 20-15), because the flexor hallucis brevis insertion has been destroyed and the weight-bearing function of the sesamoids has been lost. Hallux extensus may also follow this procedure as a result of the severance of the flexor hallucis brevis, which reduces the counteraction against the extensor hallucis longus and brevis and produces the disabling deformity.

Pain in the first metatarsocuneiform joint occurs occasionally after the Keller procedure, because the removal of the base of the proximal phalanx reduces the stability

Text continued on p. 517.

A

B

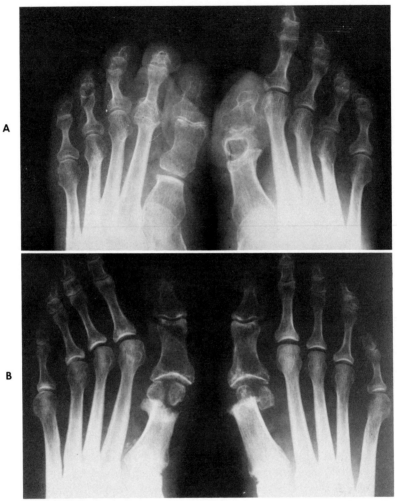

Fig. 20-8. End results of subcapital amputation of first metatarsal head for hallux valgus.

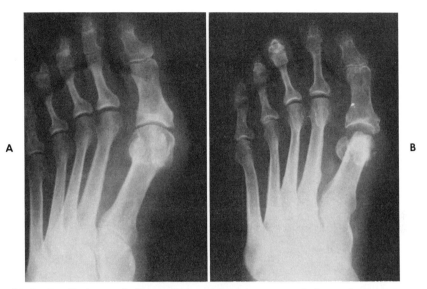

Fig. 20-9. A, Moderate hallux valgus. Roentgenogram of foot of this 55-year-old woman shows the subcapital amputation that was performed in 1961. **B,** Roentgenogram taken 2 years after operation. Severe disability ensued after subcapital amputation. This disability was bilateral because both feet had been operated upon.

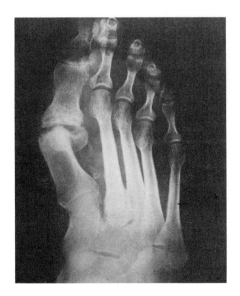

Fig. 20-10. Pointed articulation of head of first metatarsal with base of proximal phalanx after subcapital amputation. Patient was in constant pain during walking.

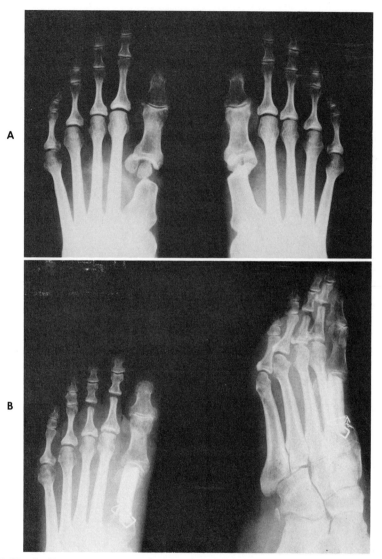

Fig. 20-11. A, Roentgenograms taken in 1954 showing subcapital amputation of first metatarsal heads for hallux valgus. The operation was performed elsewhere. In 1960 this 38-year-old woman sought relief for disability caused by sesamoids wedged between the base of the proximal phalanx and the remains of the first metatarsal of the left foot. A fibular bone graft was performed. **B,** Roentgenograms taken 1 year postoperatively. **C,** Roentgenograms taken 4 years (1964) postoperatively. The foot has remained asymptomatic.

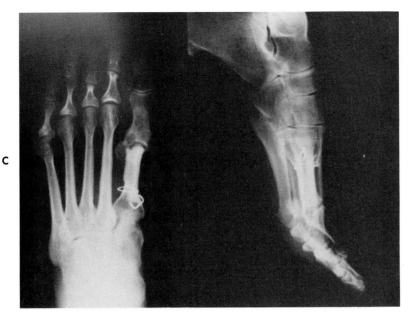

Fig. 20-11, cont'd. For legend see opposite page.

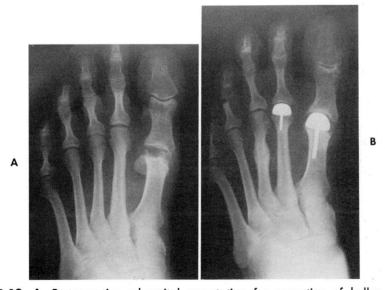

Fig. 20-12. A, Postoperative subcapital amputation for correction of hallux valgus. The foot was symptomatic. **B,** Metallic prosthesis inserted for better articular surface of metatarsal head. Note fatigue fracture of the third metatarsal. (Courtesy Dr. R. H. Seeburger.)

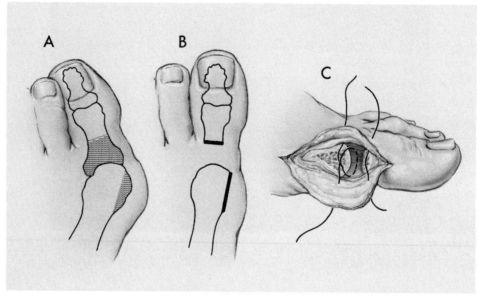

Fig. 20-13. Keller's operation for correction of hallux valgus.

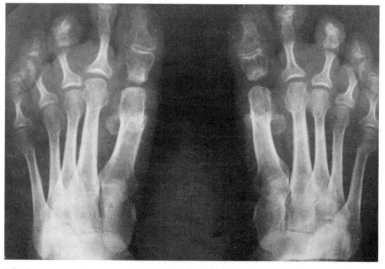

Fig. 20-14. Recession of sesamoids to middle of first metatarsal shaft. The flexor hallucis brevis insertion had been destroyed during the Keller procedure.

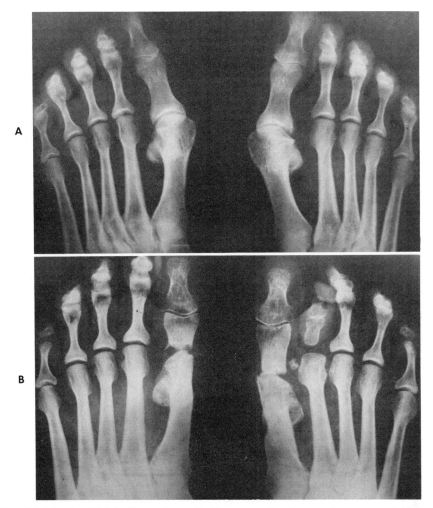

Fig. 20-15. A, Mild hallux valgus. **B,** Same as **A** after performance of Keller procedure. The patient was in constant pain because of the roughening of the proximal surface of what remained of the proximal phalanx. Amputation of the base of the right second proximal phalanx made that digit frail and unstable.

of the first metatarsal head, thereby putting extra stress at the base of this ray (Fig. 20-16).

Over 150 cases have come into my hands because of disability after Keller's procedure. In my experience, a larger group seeks help for postoperative disability resulting from this procedure than from any other operation employed in the alleviation of this deformity. Unfortunately, once the base of the proximal phalanx has been destroyed, little can be done to restore normal function. It is difficult to visualize a static

deformity of the first metatarsophalangeal joint in which this procedure is indicated.

Silver (1923) was one of the first to call attention to muscle imbalance, especially imbalance of the intrinsic muscles, in the etiology of hallux valgus. He considered those muscles basic in producing the deformity.

Silver's technique for reduction of hallux valgus. A semilunar incision is made over the medial surface of the great toe joint, with its vertex placed dorsally. A **Y**-shaped incision is made in the capsule to form

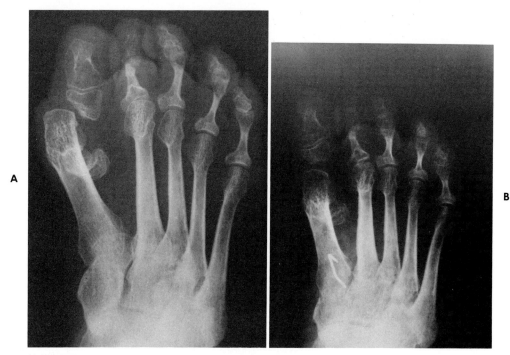

Fig. 20-16. A, Roentgenogram taken after postoperative Keller procedure for pain in first metatarsocuneiform joint. **B,** Roentgenogram taken 18 months after stabilization of first metatarsocuneiform joint. Symptoms have disappeared.

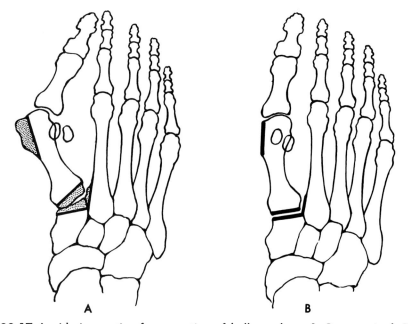

Fig. 20-17. Lapidus' operation for correction of hallux valgus. **A,** Bone excised. **B,** Deformity corrected.

three flaps: one distal, one dorsal, and one plantar. The flaps are dissected so that the head of the metatarsal is exposed. While the great toe is plantar flexed, a tenotome is inserted just above the plantar capsule of the joint and a longitudinal incision is made on the fibular side of the capsule. With the toe dorsiflexed, a longitudinal incision is made in the dorsal margin of the capsule on the fibular side. The toe is strongly adducted. A vertical incision is made on the fibular capsule between the two longitudinal incisions. This capsulotomy releases the tension on the fibular side of the joint. The toe is overcorrected and the distal flap on the medial side is sutured to the periosteum just behind the head of the first metatarsal. The dorsal and plantar flaps are sutured over the distal flap.

Lapidus (1934) believed that the varus of the first metatarsal shaft was an extremely important factor in hallux valgus deformity. He advised arthrodesis of the first metatarsocuneiform joint and the tibial side of the base of the second metatarsal. He also excised the tibial condyle of the first metatarsal head (Fig. 20-17).

The procedure is of definite value in cases of juvenile hallux valgus and also in adult patients in whom the first metatarsal is in extreme varus.

McBride (1928, 1935, 1954) supported Silver regarding the influence of the intrinsic muscles on the deformity, particularly the adductor hallucis, whose conjoined tendon inserts into the base of the proximal phalanx of the great toe (see Fig. 8-12, A). He further called attention to the usual displacement of the fibular sesamoid into the space between the first and second metatarsal heads.

McBride's technique. Through an incision over the first metatarsal interspace the conjoined tendon of the adductor hallucis is detached from its insertion and the fibular sesamoid is excised. The medial margin of the incision is retracted over the tibial side of the great toe joint, and the tibial side of the head of the first metatarsal is amputated. The conjoined tendon of the

adductor hallucis is transferred onto the dorsum of the head of the first metatarsal bone.

McBride was the first to suggest a procedure for the correction of hallux valgus that aimed at the correction of the underlying pathologic-anatomic disorder. His procedure, although scientific and rewarding when properly performed, has not been favored. It is too difficult to accomplish without training and practice.

Recommended procedures for reduction of hallux valgus. For the purpose of surgical correction, hallux valgus is classified by type as follows:

1. The common adult type, without congenital or hereditary abnormalities or abnormalities from disease, comprises about 80 percent of the cases.
2. The juvenile type, seen occasionally, has congenital predisposing factors that are present to a severe degree and cause the patient to develop deformity in childhood (Fig. 20-18).
3. There is an infrequently seen type in which the first metatarsal is markedly longer than the second metatarsal (Figs. 8-11 and 20-6, A).
4. Hallux valgus is sometimes accompanied by severe splayfoot.
5. Hallux valgus occurs in the rheumatoid foot.

The following procedures have proved effective for those types listed.

TYPE 1. DuVries' modified McBride technique is indicated for the common adult type of hallux valgus. In a series of 2,400 cases of hallux valgus over a 37-year span, reduction by means of a modified McBride procedure proved excellent in 90 percent of the cases; fair in 8 percent, and poor in 2 percent, with postoperative deformities (see p. 528).

1. Under hemostasis (by means of a rubber tourniquet or pneumatic cuff) make an incision over the first metatarsal interspace, extending from the web proximally and medialward, crossing the tendon of the extensor hallucis longus, and terminating at a

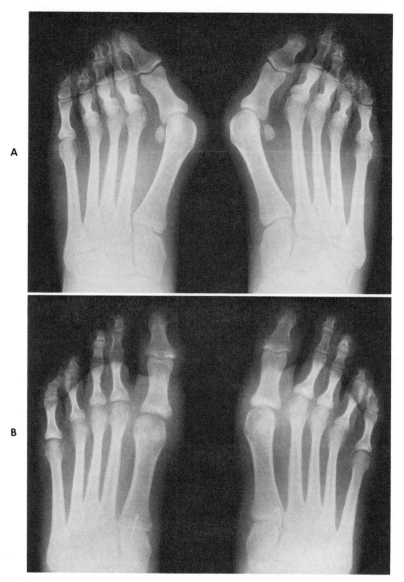

Fig. 20-18. A, Roentgenogram showing hallux valgus in 16-year-old girl. **B,** Roentgenogram 1 year postoperatively after modified McBride procedure with stabilization of the base of the first metatarsocuneiform joints. Note staple, which aids in arthrodesis.

point near the mediodorsal aspect of the base of the first metatarsal (Fig. 20-19, *1*).

2. Retract the skin; spread the first and second metatarsal heads by means of a Weitlander or mastoid retractor (Fig. 20-19, *2*).

3. Carry the distal end of the incision downward in the interspace until the tendon of the adductor hallucis comes plainly into view. The dorsal cutaneous branch of the deep peroneal nerve lies in the center of the incision. Free it and retract it with the fibular margin of the incision. If this nerve is severed, the patient will experience numbness of the great toe, in which case sensation either

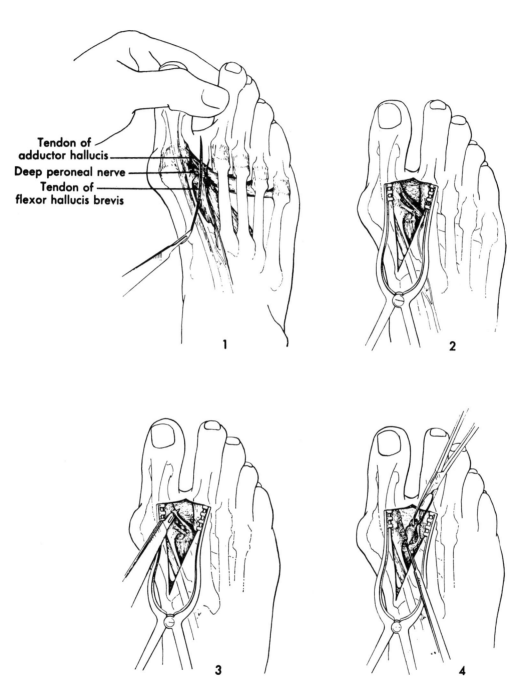

Tendon of
adductor hallucis
Deep peroneal nerve
Tendon of
flexor hallucis brevis

1

2

3

4

Fig. 20-19. DuVries' technique for hallux valgus reduction.

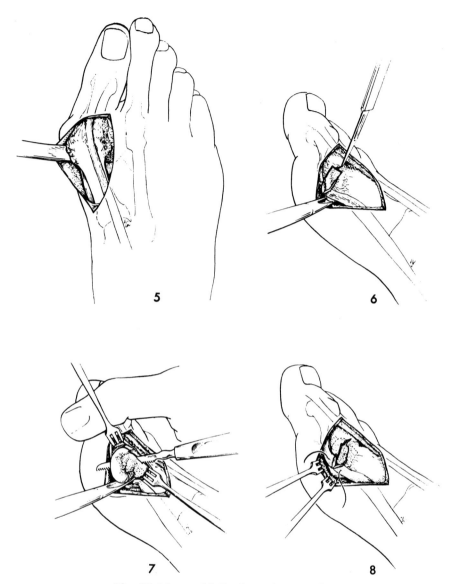

5   6

7   8

Fig. 20-19, cont'd. For legend see p. 521.

returns in 3 or 4 months or the patient ceases to be aware of anesthesia.

4. Detach the adductor hallucis tendon from its insertion into the base of the proximal phalanx (Fig. 20-19, 3).

5. Grasp the freed tendon by means of Allis forceps, and with a slight pull on the tendon, bring the fibular sesamoid a little farther into the metatarsal interspace. The stub of this tendon, which is conjoined with the tendon of the flexor hallucis brevis, can be used as a guide in excising the sesamoid (Fig. 20-19, 4).

6. Completely denude and remove the sesamoid by means of sharp dissection against the body of the sesamoid.

7. At this point the great toe joint can usually be aligned in a straight position. In a few cases some capsular fi-

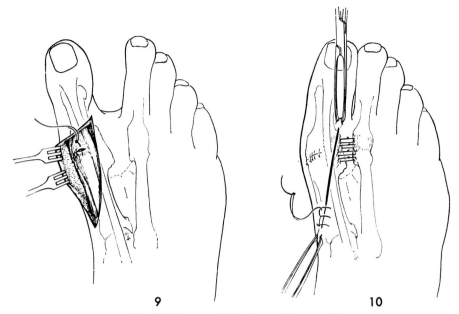

9   10

Fig. 20-19, cont'd. For legend see p. 521.

bers on the fibular side of the great toe joint may still hold the joint in deformity; if so, section them.

8. As soon as the great toe joint has been aligned, dissect and free the tibial margin of the incision and retract over the tibial side of the great toe joint by means of a periosteal or Chandler elevator placed between the skin and the plantar surface of the first metatarsophalangeal joint. The capsule of the tibial side of the first metatarsophalangeal joint and the tendon of the abductor hallucis thus will have been completely exposed (Fig. 20-19, 5).

9. Excise a vertical section about 0.5 cm. wide from the tibial capsule of the first metatarsophalangeal joint; include the tendon of the abductor hallucis.

10. After removal of this section, carry the vertical incision dorsally to about the medial margin of the extensor hallucis longus tendon (Fig. 20-19, 6).

11. Dissect and denude from the bone

the distal and proximal margins of the capsule, which will expose the tibial condylar process of the first metatarsal head.

12. By means of a nasal saw or osteotome amputate the tibial condylar process of the first metatarsal head, beginning with the condylar groove on the articular surface of the head (see Fig. 20-19, 7).

13. Round the head with a Joseph nasal rasp.

14. Suture the capsule and tendon of the abductor hallucis in their shortened position (Fig. 20-19, 8 and 9). Suture the capsule on the fibular side of the first metatarsophalangeal joint to the capsule of the second metatarsophalangeal joint, incorporating the freed adductor hallucis tendon in the sutures (Fig. 20-19, 10). This brings the two heads together.

15. Instill 10 mg. hydrocortisone acetate into the first metatarsophalangeal joint.

16. If the taut tendon of the extensor

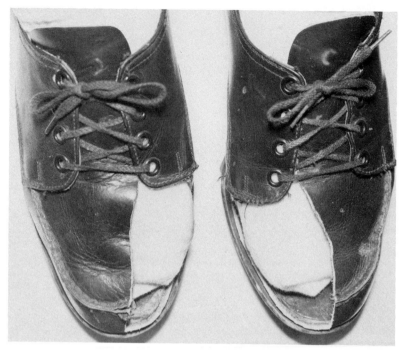

Fig. 20-20. Cutout shoes worn postoperatively after hallux valgus operation.

hallucis longus holds the great toe dorsiflexed, lengthen the tendon by means of a Z-plasty. The tourniquet placed over the calf instead of the thigh may cause a reflex spasm that may be mistaken for a contracted tendon.

17. Suture the skin margins.

18. While the great toe joint is immobilized in a normal position, apply a snug compression bandage by binding it with the second and third toes.

19. Remove the tourniquet. Examine the foot for bleeding through the dressing. If bleeding is present, apply an additional snug compression bandage.

20. After 12 to 24 hours, release but do not remove the compression bandage. Apply additional gauze to keep the foot snugly bandaged. After 3 or 4 days change the dressing completely. The patient may be ambulatory at this stage but must wear cutout shoes (Fig. 20-20) or postoperative wooden-soled shoes.

21. Remove the sutures between the seventh and tenth day. Apply a new snug bandage, with the great toe joint partly immobilized by a snug bandage and adhesive tape (Fig. 20-21).

22. Redress the foot every 7 to 10 days. Be sure that the great toe joint is maintained in a straight position for about 2 months, because until that time the tibial capsular structures that have been sutured are still fragile; any deviation of the toe or any pressure against the toe forces this capsule to give and elongate again. Wedges of gauze or sponge rubber may be needed between the first and second toes to maintain the straight position (Fig. 20-22). The patient wears the postoperative shoe during the 2 months, after which he is fitted with a new shoe, appropriately designed with a well-rounded toe. The patient wears the new shoe for an additional 3 months or until other types of shoes can be worn comfort-

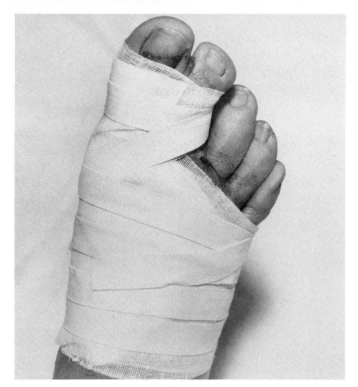

Fig. 20-21. Postoperative dressings for hallux valgus. The second toe serves as a splint. Sometimes the third digit is also included as a splint.

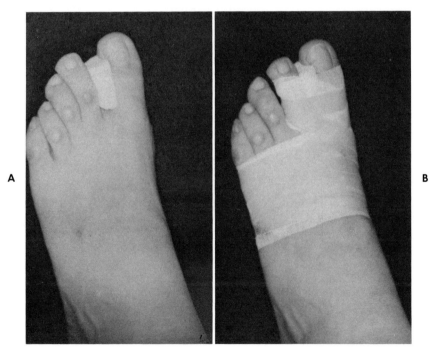

Fig. 20-22. A, Sponge rubber inserted between first and second toes. **B,** Bandaging of foot with sponge rubber between first and second toes. Dressing fits snugly over the metatarsals but is neutral over the digit. This is important so that when the patient bears weight the sutures between the first and second metatarsal heads will not spread apart.

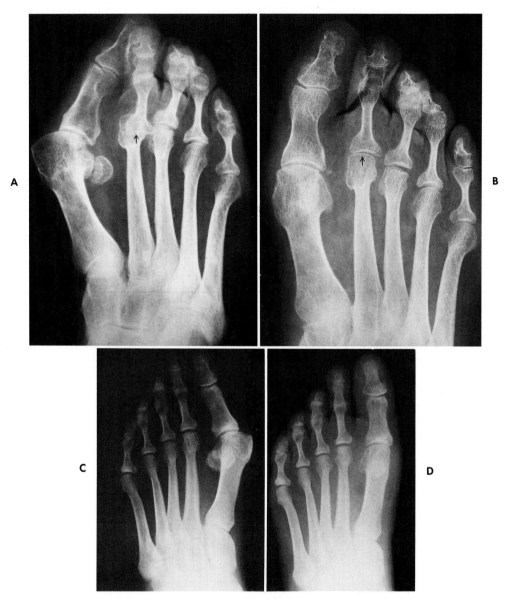

Fig. 20-23. A, Hallux valgus and second metatarsophalangeal dislocation. **B,** Three years postoperatively. Note second metatarsophalangeal dislocation reduced without bone excision. (See static second metatarsophalangeal dislocation in Fig. 8-43.) **C,** Roentgenogram taken preoperatively of another hallux valgus. **D,** Roentgenogram of same foot 2 years postoperatively.

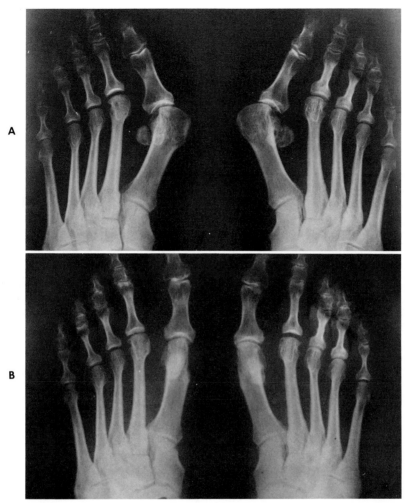

Fig. 20-24. A, Severe hallux valgus. **B,** Roentgenogram 12 years postoperatively.

ably. Results are illustrated in Figs. 20-23 and 20-24.

The postoperative care of hallux valgus is about as important as the surgical procedure itself. The soft tissues that have been repaired around the reduced deformity remain fragile for about 2 months, during which time they will not resist new deforming forces. Therefore, unless it is maintained in a neutral position throughout that time, the great toe can go back into valgus or move into a varus position.

In most cases these secondary deformities can be avoided if the surgeon watches carefully to see that the hallux remains in a neutral position for the 2-month postoperative period. If the great toe tends to go back into valgus, a sponge rubber plug should be placed between it and the second toe, and the deformity should be overcorrected slightly into varus by means of adhesive strips applied around the plug and anchored on the tibial side of the first metatarsal shaft. If the great toe tends to go into a varus position and the tibial side of the joint capsule seems tight when the hallux is passively pushed into valgus, the foot should be dressed without a plug between the toes. The hallux should be slightly overcorrected into valgus, incorporated with the second, third, or even fourth toe, and taped with additional adhesive.

Complications are uncommon. When pyogenic infection is present, both local and general symptoms arise within 72 hours. A broad-spectrum antibiotic is indicated at the least suggestion of infection. It is administered under extreme vigilance until control is assured.

The spores of tinea infection are common invaders of the skin of the foot. Tinea infection is characterized by low-grade inflammation of the wound. It may be mistaken for part of the normal healing process until it produces an avulsion of the incision when the sutures are removed. The surgical area should be painted with a fungicide and the margins maintained with adhesive butterfly dressings. Healing is ordinarily uneventful.

The common postoperative deformities of this procedure which I have seen are (1) recurrent hallux valgus; (2) postoperative hallux varus; and (3) dorsal contracture of the hallux, often accompanied by a hammered interphalangeal joint of the great toe. I believe that most of these deformities are caused by inefficient surgical technique, poor postoperative care, or both. Dorsal contracture of the hallux with a hammered interphalangeal joint of the great toe probably occurs in many cases as a result of excessive injury of the flexor hallucis brevis at its insertion.

To correct recurrent hallux valgus, a repetition of the original procedure will usually suffice. For correction of postoperative hallux varus, see p. 224, and for treatment of dorsal contracture of the hallux, see Jones' tendon transfer, p. 535.

Occasionally a reaction to subdermal sutures (stitch abscess) may not appear until 4 to 8 weeks postoperatively. A small bluish fluctuating area appears over the subdermal suture. Usually the tissues expel the fluid spontaneously, leaving an aperture through which the suture can be extracted; but occasionally the suture must be removed surgically.

TYPE 2. The adolescent type of hallux valgus is seen in patients between the ages of 10 and 20 years, and the deformity is caused, to a marked degree, by the presence of congenital and hereditary predisposing factors. The procedure described for the common adult type alone will result in a large percentage of recurrence. However, if in addition to that procedure the base of the first metatarsocuneiform joint is arthrodesed, results will prove more satisfactory. Results in over 150 cases have been uniformly satisfactory (Figs. 20-18 and 20-25, A and B). Stabilization is accomplished by extending the incision proximally to a point over the first cuneiform–navicular joint. The capsule of the first metatarsocuneiform joint is opened transversely over the dorsum, and the integuments on the tibial side of this joint are freed. The articular surface of the joint is then excised with an osteotome. The denuded bone surfaces are readily coapted; a small staple will maintain this coaptation. The capsular and tendinous structures in the operated area near the first metatarsophalangeal joint are sutured in the same manner as they are in the adult type of procedure. The staple is inserted in the metatarsocuneiform joint, the fascia is sutured, and the skin is closed in the usual manner.

A non–weight-bearing cast is applied and maintained for about 2 weeks and is then changed to a walking cast which is worn for about 6 weeks.

Wilson (1963) reported the use of an oblique osteotomy of the distal third of the first metatarsal, combined with trimming of the exostosis. The distal fragment was displaced laterally, the metatarsal shortened, and the position stabilized by placing the great toe into a position of overcorrection. He believed that this operation was particularly useful for active adolescents, since it did not interfere with the efficiency of the foot.

TYPE 3. For the abnormally long first metatarsal with hallux valgus, the Hawkins-Mitchell step-cut osteotomy (Fig. 20-5) offers the most rational approach.

TYPE 4. Hallux valgus with marked splayfoot should be treated as is the adolescent type (Fig. 20-25, C and D).

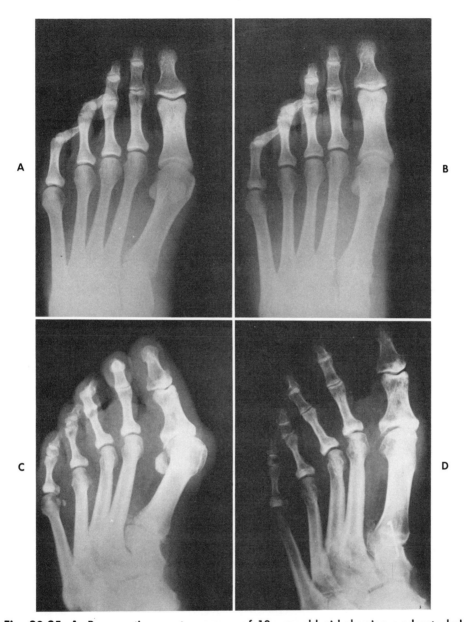

Fig. 20-25. A, Preoperative roentgenogram of 18-year-old girl showing moderate hallux valgus and metatarsus primus varus of left foot. **B,** Roentgenogram taken 2 years postoperatively. It was not necessary to excise the fibular sesamoid; the three middle metatarsals have assumed normal alignment. **C,** Roentgenogram of 58-year-old woman with marked left hallux valgus and splayfoot. **D,** Roentgenogram taken 2 years postoperatively.

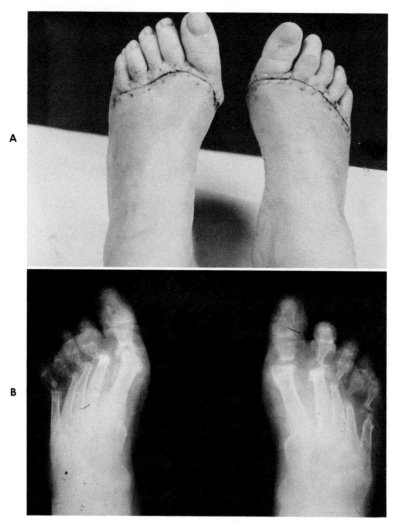

Fig. 20-26. Rheumatoid arthritis. **A,** Clayton's incision for correction of rheumatoid forefoot. **B,** Postoperative films of rheumatoid feet. (Courtesy Dr. M. L. Clayton.)

TYPE 5. The treatment of hallux valgus in the rheumatoid foot is discussed in the next paragraphs.

CLAYTON PROCEDURE (FIG. 20-26). One of the most thorough investigations of the rheumatoid foot and the techniques of its care was reported by Clayton (1960), who outlined an operative procedure which he has used with success. Marmor (1964) has used the Clayton procedure with slight modification and found it to be efficacious.

Clayton's basic procedure is metatarso-phalangeal joint resection as outlined by

Hoffmann (1912). The degree of deformity determines the extent of excision: In severe cases all the metatarsal heads and bases of the proximal phalanges are excised, whereas in lesser deformities modification of bone excision is practiced. Kates and associates (1967) used a modification of an operation described by Hoffmann (1912) and Fowler (1957, 1959) for fixed clawing of the toes in rheumatoid arthritis. Through a plantar incision curved convex proximally from the neck of the first to that of the fifth metatarsal, the five metatarsal heads were removed and a Kirschner wire was inserted to hold the great toe in line. They reported satisfactory results.

In the last 18 years we have reduced 100 rheumatoid feet with very satisfactory results by arthrodesing the first metatarsophalangeal joint and excising the bases of the proximal phalanges of the lesser toes, which are deformed at the metatarsophalangeal joint. One advantage of this approach is that the first ray is lengthened and can more nearly assume its normal weight-bearing responsibility. The first ray retains its flexibility and motion after the arthrodesis from the movement of the interphalangeal and the first metatarsal–medial cuneiform joints. The lesser metatarsal heads are released from their fixed, ankylosed plantarward position by excision of the bases of the lesser proximal phalanges, thus eliminating the fixed severe plantar depressions of the metatarsal heads which are characteristic of this disease. These heads, freed by the operation, now can bear weight without gouging into the soft tissues under their plantar surface.

An equally important advantage is that less bone is excised, and in rheumatoid foot operations, as in many other operations to correct forefoot deformities, the less excision of the osseous components of the articular surfaces of the metatarsophalangeal joints, the greater the opportunity the surgeon has to correct cases that may require additional procedures.

Since the operation requires that the first metatarsophalangeal joint be arthrodesed and the foot be immobilized in a plaster boot for 8 weeks, many patients elect to have correction made in two stages, one foot at a time. To date 90 percent of our patients have returned within 1 year to have correction on the unoperated foot.

DUVRIES-DICKSON PROCEDURE. The DuVries-Dickson procedure is as follows:

1. Make an incision over the first metatarsal interspace (Fig. 20-27) from the first web, proximally and tibialward, to a point over the base of the first metatarsal.

2. Carry the distal end of the incision downward to the insertion of the adductor hallucis.

3. Detach the tendon from its insertion. If the fibular sesamoid maintains the usually present hallux valgus deformity, excision of the fibular sesamoid will release the deformity.

4. Dissect and retract the tibial skin margin to expose the first metatarsophalangeal joint.

5. Incise the capsule of this joint longitudinally along the extensor hallucis longus tendon; dissect and retract its margins to expose the entire joint.

6. Remove any hypertrophic bone that may be present around the head of the first metatarsal (Fig. 20-28, A).

7. Remove the articular surface of the head of the first metatarsal and the base of the proximal phalanx. Coapt and maintain the two remaining flat surfaces with a small staple.

8. Close the capsule over this joint with a few fine gut sutures.

9. Retract the fibular skin margin of the incision to expose the second metatarsophalangeal joint. Through an incision in the capsule of this joint excise the base of the proximal phalanx.

10. Through a second linear incision over the third metatarsal interspace excise the bases of the third and fourth proximal phalanges. If the base of the fifth proximal phalanx requires it, excise through the last incision. (This can usually be done.)

11. Suture the capsular structures between the first and second metatarsal heads to each other with fine chromic gut. When healed, the sutured heads will aid in the stabilization of this part of the forefoot. The capsular structures in the third metatarsal interspace may also be sutured to each other.

12. Close the skin as usual and apply a cast. The cast may or may not need

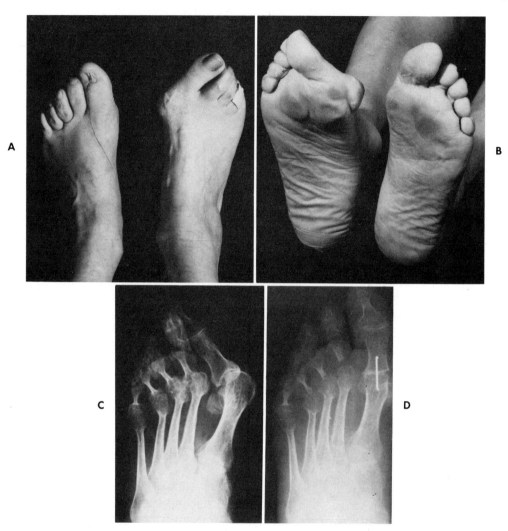

Fig. 20-27. A, Dorsal view of left rheumatoid foot taken 1 year postoperatively, showing lines of incisions. The right foot has since also been corrected. **B,** Same patient, plantar view. **C,** Preoperative and postoperative roentgenograms of same patient's left foot.

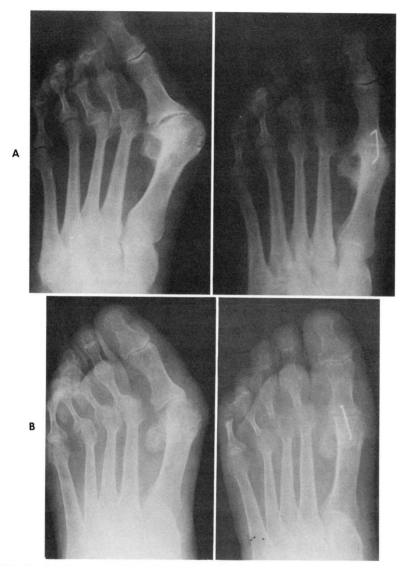

Fig. 20-28. A, Rheumatoid left foot of 52-year-old woman preoperatively and post-operatively. Note hypertrophic changes around the first metatarsal head, which has been remodeled. **B,** Preoperative and postoperative films of left foot. This 56-year-old woman had severe rheumatoid arthritis of the feet. The staple was removed 1 year post-operatively when she returned for correction of the right foot.

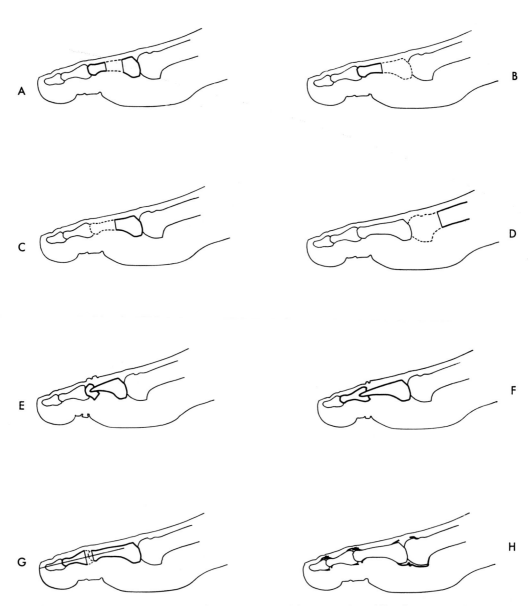

Fig. 20-29. Various operations for correction of hammered middle three toes. **A,** Excision of middle third of proximal phalanx. **B,** Excision of proximal half of proximal phalanx. **C,** Excision of distal half of proximal phalanx. **D,** Excision of head of metatarsal. **E,** Shaft of proximal phalanx sharply pointed and fixed into its own head. **F,** Distal end of proximal phalanx cupped into base of middle phalanx. **G,** Proximal phalangeal joint denuded of cartilage. A Kirschner wire is passed through three phalanges. **H,** All contracted capsules sectioned and elongated capsules shortened.

to be changed before a walking heel is applied (10 days later—to be removed about 2 months later).

13. Should the staple become loose and irritating after fusion of the joint has taken place, it can easily be removed under local anesthesia.

DEFORMED TOES
Surgical procedures for the correction of hammertoes

Many complex procedures have been offered for the correction of hammertoes, especially of the middle three toes (Fig. 20-29). Taylor (1940) and Selig (1941) suggested drawing a Kirschner wire through all the phalanges. Tierney (1937) and Young (1938) advised forming a cup and ball of the distal end of the proximal joint. Borg (1950), Michele and Krueger (1948), Lapidus (1939), and Lorenz (1929) excised different parts of the phalanges. Wagner (1934) and Forrester-Brown (1938) advocated tendon transplantation to correct the hammered great toe. Sgarlato (1970) discussed two methods of transferring the flexor digitorum longus tendon to a primary attachment at the base of the proximal phalanx.

Recommended procedures for reduction of hammered great toe. The procedure outlined here is intended for mild cases in which the deformity is not fixed and can be reduced passively, although it cannot be held in reduction.

1. From the dorsal aspect of the interphalangeal joint, remove a transverse spindle-shaped section, about 0.5 cm. in width, of skin, capsule, and tendon of the extensor hallucis longus.
2. Remove 2 or 3 mm. of the head of the proximal phalanx and round it with a nasal rasp.
3. Suture the dorsal capsule and the tendon of the extensor hallucis longus in the shortened position and suture the skin.
4. Partly immobilize the toe by adhesive splinting for 2 to 3 weeks. The splinting may be achieved by bandaging the great toe to the three adjacent

toes and carrying the bandage over all the metatarsophalangeal joints.

Jones' tendon transfer. In congenital hammered great toe (see Fig. 4-23, *B*) the articular surface of the interphalangeal joint is abnormal and soft-tissue repair alone will not permanently reduce the deformity. Arthrodesis of the joint as described in Jones' technique without transference of the extensor hallucis longus will usually best correct this condition. (Fig. 20-30, *B*).

For fixed, rigid cases, especially when there is marked dorsal contracture at the metatarsophalangeal joint, Jones' technique for transference of the tendon of the extensor hallucis longus and arthrodesis of the interphalangeal joint still offers the best results.

1. Make a transverse incision over the hallux phalangeal joint (Fig. 20-31, *A* and *B*).
2. Detach the extensor hallucis longus tendon from its insertion.
3. Make a second longitudinal incision along the border of the extensor hallucis longus tendon, beginning over the base of the proximal phalanx, extending proximally to the middle of the first metatarsal shaft (Fig. 20-31, *A*).
4. Pull out the extensor hallucis longus tendon at the proximal end of this incision.
5. Drill a transverse hole through the first metatarsal just behind and at the upper part of the neck.
6. Thread a 1-0 silk suture through the end of the previously freed tendon with a small, fine, curved needle; then thread both ends of the suture through the eye of a 2.5-cm. curved needle. Pass the eye of the needle through the drill hole and guide the tendon through it (Fig. 20-31, *B*).
7. Suture the end of the tendon to the body of the tendon on the dorsum of the first metatarsal shaft.
8. Denude the interphalangeal joint of cartilage and flatten the articular surface so that they fit perfectly.

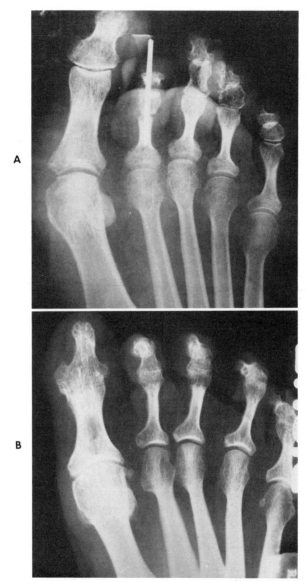

Fig. 20-30. A, Hammered second toe. Arthrodesis of both interphalangeal joints was performed and the pin was inserted elsewhere by another surgeon. One year postoperatively the digit was entirely rigid and in a dorsiflexed position, requiring further surgical intervention. **B,** Arthrodesed interphalangeal joint for hammered great toe. (Not the same patient as in **A.**)

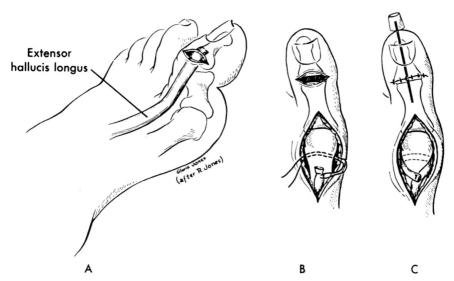

Extensor
hallucis longus

A   B   C

Fig. 20-31. Jones' reduction for static clawed great toe. **A,** Incision for cut and release of tendon. **B,** Phalangeal joint denuded of cartilage and tendon threaded through drill hole. **C,** Tendon sutured to itself and pin inserted into arthrodesed phalangeal joint. The exposed pin is covered with cork.

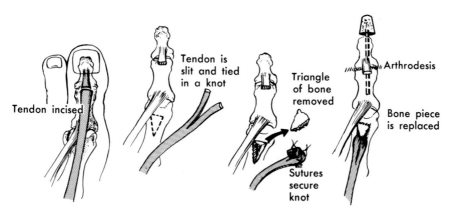

Tendon incised

Tendon is
slit and tied
in a knot

Triangle
of bone
removed

Arthrodesis

Bone piece
is replaced

Sutures
secure
knot

Fig. 20-32. DuVries' modification of Jones' tendon transfer. The extensor hallucis longus is severed at the interphalangeal joint and spliced longitudinally about 3 cm. The extensor hallucis brevis is left inserted (unless severely contracted). A triangular section of cortical bone is removed from just behind the neck of the first metatarsal with an osteotome. The spliced extensor hallucis longus is tied in a knot. Nonabsorbable knot sutures are employed to prevent untying. The knot is forced into the medullary canal of the metatarsal. The triangular portion of bone is replaced. The interphalangeal joint is arthrodesed as in Jones' procedure.

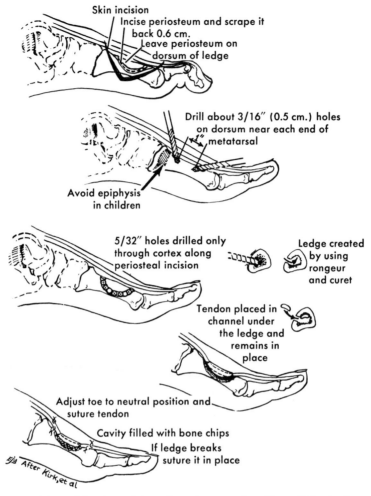

Skin incision
Incise periosteum and scrape it
back 0.6 cm.
Leave periosteum on
dorsum of ledge

Drill about 3/16" (0.5 cm.) holes
on dorsum near each end of
metatarsal

Avoid epiphysis
in children

5/32" holes drilled only
through cortex along
periosteal incision

Ledge created
by using
rongeur
and curet

Tendon placed in
channel under
the ledge and
remains in
place

Adjust toe to neutral position and
suture tendon

Cavity filled with bone chips
If ledge breaks
suture it in place

After Kirk, et al

Fig. 20-33. Kirk's modification of Jones' tendon transfer. (From Kirk, A. A., and others: J. Bone Joint Surg. **53-A**:774, June 1971.)

9. Pass a threaded Kirschner wire through the distal phalanx and halfway through the shaft of the proximal phalanx. Then fit a cork over the exposed part of the Kirschner wire to protect it (Fig. 20-31, *C*).

10. Close the skin as usual and apply a plaster splint.

11. In 10 days remove the splint and sutures. Apply a boot cast with a walking heel, which the patient wears for 6 weeks.

The DuVries modification (Fig. 20-32) of Jones' tendon transfer is as follows:

1. Remove a triangular section of cortical bone the sides of which are about 1 cm. from the dorsum of the first metatarsal, just behind the head.

2. Divide the distal end of the freed extensor hallucis longus longitudinally, for about 2.5 cm.

3. Tie the divided ends into a knot and pass a few 3-0 silk sutures through this knot to keep it permanently.

4. Excise the distal remnant of the tendon at the knot.

5. Force the knot into the triangular aperture and probe it into the prox-

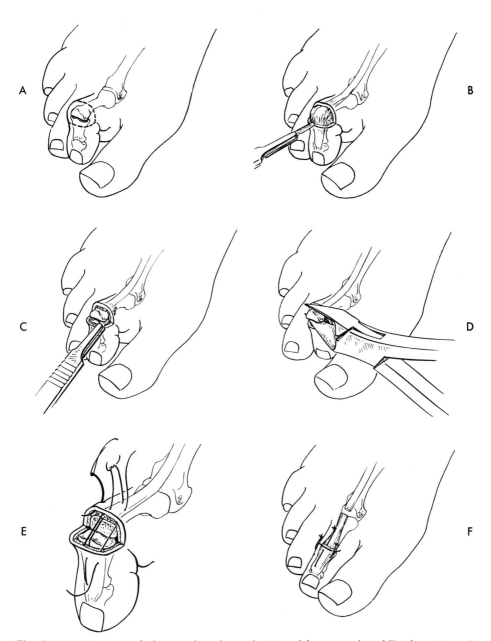

Fig. 20-34. Recommended procedure for reduction of hammered middle three toes. **A,** Elliptical incision made over dorsum of head of proximal phalanx. **B,** Like sections of tendon and capsule removed. **C,** Capsule incised on both sides of head of proximal phalanx. **D,** Head of proximal phalanx amputated. **E** and **F,** Skin, tendon, and capsule sutured.

imal portion of the medullary canal.

6. Replace the previously excised triangular section of cortical bone.
7. Suture the fascia over the tendon transference.
8. Arthrodese the phalangeal joint as in Jones' procedure.

Kirk and associates (1971) devised a method they called ledge tenodesis for transfer of the extensor hallucis longus (Fig. 20-33). Their procedure is a substitute for the modified Jones' procedure, which they feel has the following disadvantages: (1) The original tendinous arrangement may be reestablished postoperatively; (2) the distal phalanx may become flexed; and (3) in children it is difficult to obtain fusion of the interphalangeal joint.

Reduction of hammered middle three toes. The following procedure for reduction of the hammered middle three toes is recommended.

1. Make a spindle-shaped transverse incision over the joint prominence extending from one side of the joint to the opposite side (Fig. 20-34, A).
2. Remove the skin and subcutaneous tissue.
3. Expose the tendon and joint capsule.
4. Remove a section of tendon and capsule along the outline of the original incision (Fig 20-34, B).
5. Expose the head of the proximal phalanx; if the distal joint is involved (mallet toe), expose the head of the middle phalanx.
6. Free the head of the proximal phalanx (or middle phalanx in the case of the distal joint) by incising the capsule on both sides of the joint (Fig. 20-34, C).
7. Amputate the head across the sulci that are present on each side of the head of the bone (Fig. 20-34, D).
8. Smooth the cut surface with a rasp.
9. Suture the margins with a mattress suture so that the base of the stitch includes the capsule and tendon and

the apex includes only the skin (Fig. 20-34, E and F). A bolster of Telfa or rubber tubing is incorporated in the suture to prevent strangulation (Fig. 20-35).

10. It is sometimes necessary to suture one side of the incision.
11. Occasionally a tenotomy and capsulotomy at the metatarsophalangeal joint are necessary so that the toe will lie flat.
12. Splint the toe to the adjacent toes by a cradle-gauze dressing (Fig. 20-36).

The same procedure is followed for mallet toe, except that the operation is done over the distal interphalangeal joint.

Of academic interest is the case illustrated in Fig. 20-37 in which complete regeneration of the head of a phalanx occurred within 5 years after an amputation for hammertoe (DuVries and Shogren, 1962). Franklin (1968) described a similar regeneration phenomenon in a patient on whom he performed three operations for contracted toes. Scheck (1968) reported the presence of degenerative changes in the metatarsophalangeal joints of three patients who had surgical correction of severe hammertoe deformities.

Reduction of hammered fifth toe. A hammered fifth toe may be corrected in the following manner:

1. Make a longitudinal incision over the dorsum of the involved toe.
2. Excise the head of the proximal phalanx.
3. Section the dorsal tendon and the metatarsophalangeal capsule if they are contracted, as they are in a high percentage of cases. This step alone often corrects the disability.

A rotation skin graft is recommended in the DuVries procedure for reduction of the hammered fifth toe with severe dorsal skin contracture.

1. Make a transverse incision over the fourth and fifth metatarsophalangeal joints (Fig. 20-38, A).
2. Plantar flex the fourth and fifth digits

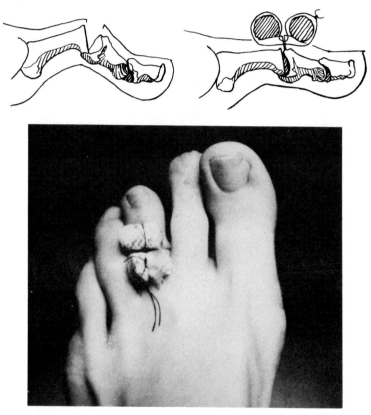

Fig. 20-35. Inclusion of bolsters in vertical mattress stitch to avoid strangulation of skin by surface portion of suture.

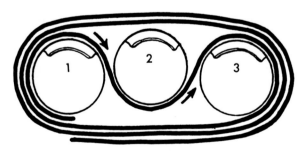

Fig. 20-36. Schematic drawing of immobilization of middle toe by means of cradle-gauze bandaging.

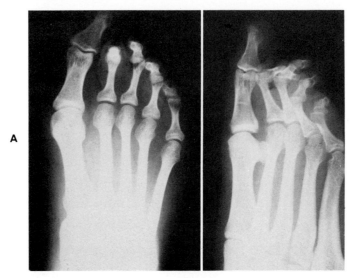

Fig. 20-37. Roentgenograms showing complete regeneration of head of phalanx. This occurred within 5 years after amputation for hammertoe. **A,** Hammertoe deformity shown in roentgenograms in September 1956. **B,** Amputation of head in March 1957. **C,** Roentgenograms in August 1961. The regenerated head is showing.

in a position of overcorrection. This forms a proximal and distal skin puckering; the incision is diamond shaped.

3. Section the tendon and capsule over the fifth metatarsophalangeal joint (Fig. 20-38, *B*).
4. Excise the triangular skin pucker (Fig. 20-38, *C*); rotate and fit it into the diamond-shaped wound after the proximal and distal skin incisions have been sutured (Fig. 20-38, *D*).
5. Control the bleeding so that a clot will not form under the graft and prevent its adherence.
6. Hold the fourth and fifth digits in mild plantar flexion with adhesive strapping for about 6 weeks.

Reduction of mallet toe

The procedure for reduction of mallet toe is essentially the same as for hammertoe (see p. 535) except that the incision is made over the distal interphalangeal joint and the head of the middle phalanx is excised. In cases in which the deformity occurs on the fourth toe, the distal end of the toe occasionally also underlaps the

third toe. In such cases the dorsal spindle-shaped skin incision should be made slightly fibularward in order to help straighten the toe.

Surgical treatment of clawtoe

Frank and Johnson (1966) described the use of an extensor shift procedure in a series of twenty-two feet, with excellent results in nine, satisfactory results in eleven, and no improvement in two. Sandeman (1967) stated that in the correction of clawtoes, structures on both the dorsum and the lateral aspects of the metatarsophalangeal joints must be adequately tenotomized to make full reduction possible.

Recommended technique. In most cases of clawtoe tendon transfer of the great toe (see Fig. 20-31) and hammertoe reduction of the lesser toes (Fig. 20-34) with sectioning of the long extensor tendons and the contracted dorsometatarsophalangeal joint capsules to the lesser toes usually produce good results (Fig. 20-39). Occasionally, when the lesser toes do not flatten into a normal position at the time of surgery, arthrodesis of the proximal interphalangeal

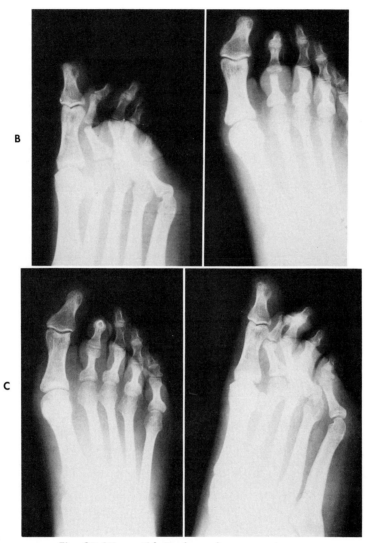

B

C

Fig. 20-37, cont'd. For legend see opposite page.

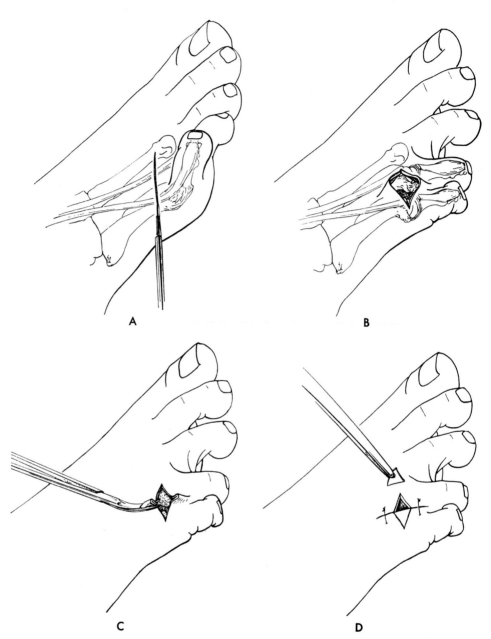

Fig. 20-38. DuVries' technique for reduction of hammered toe with severe skin contracture. **A,** Transverse incision over dorsum of fourth and fifth metatarsophalangeal joints just behind metatarsal necks. **B,** Dorsal tendon and capsule of fifth metatarsophalangeal joint sectioned. All other subdermal adhesive fibers are severed. The fourth and fifth toes are plantar flexed to form a diamond-shaped incision. The transverse axis is narrowed. The middle of both skin margins is puckered. **C,** Skin puckering excised. The pucker forms a triangular section of skin. **D,** Rotation of the triangular pieces of skin. The skin fits perfectly into the defect and is sutured in that position.

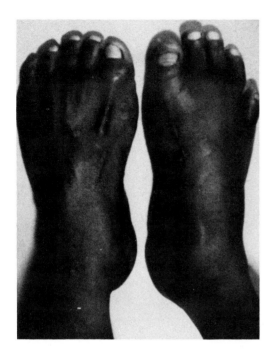

Fig. 20-39. Bilateral congenital clawtoe. *Left,* Uncorrected. *Right,* Reduced by Jones' tendon transfer and procedure used in reduction of hammered toes.

joints will correct the deformity. In the few cases in which the hindfoot is deformed to a degree that requires major stabilization, the aforementioned procedure is a valuable adjunct to the restoration of a well-functioning foot.

Surgical treatment of overlapping toes

Overlapping fifth toe. The following procedures have been used to correct overlapping fifth toe.

Lapidus' procedure. In 1942 Lapidus described a radical operation for the correction of fifth toe overlapping (Fig. 20-40), which consists of transferring the proximal end of the distal terminal portion of the extensor digitorum longus tendon of the fifth toe into the tendon of the abductor digiti quinti. The procedure is performed through two incisions, one extending from the dorsal surface of the middle phalanx of the fifth toe to the lateral side of the fifth metatarsophalangeal joint, and the other placed over the middle third of the fifth metatarsal. Through the second incision the extensor digitorum longus tendon is severed, and the distal end of the tendon is

extracted through the first incision; then it is sutured to the lateral side of the fifth metatarsophalangeal joint.

Lantzounis' procedure. Lantzounis (1940) divides the tendon of the extensor digitorum longus of the fifth toe at a point over the shaft of the proximal phalanx and drills a tunnel behind the head of the fifth metatarsal, through which the proximal end of the severed tendon is threaded and sutured to itself.

Wilson's procedure. Wilson (1953) advocated a procedure consisting of a **V**-shaped incision over the base of the fifth proximal phalanx. The extensor tendons and the dorsal capsule of the fifth metatarsophalangeal joint are sectioned and the fifth digit is plantar flexed. This pulls the tongue of the incision distally, now forming a **Y**-shaped incision. The skin is sutured in the **Y** shape (Fig. 20-41).

Recommended technique for correction of fifth toe overlapping in cases in which skin is not involved. The dorsal skin is not involved in maintaining the deformity if the fifth toe can be forcibly held in a plantar-flexed position without the skin be-

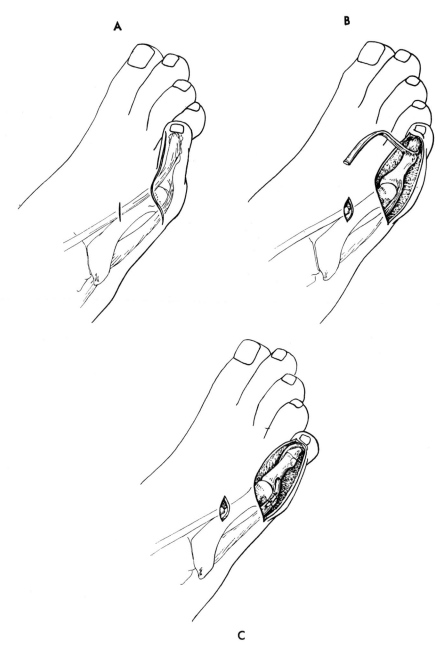

Fig. 20-40. Lapidus' technique for correction of overlapping fifth toe. **A,** Hockeystick incision over dorsum of fifth toe. A second incision is made over the middle of the shaft of the fifth metatarsal. **B,** Sectioning of extensor digitorum longus tendon to fifth toe at second incision. The distal portion is retracted. **C,** Threading of freed tendon through drill hole in proximal phalanx from tibial to fibular side. There it is sutured to the abductor digiti quinti tendon.

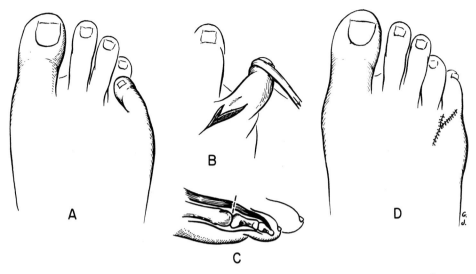

Fig. 20-41. Wilson's technique for correction of overlapping fifth toe. **A,** Overlapping toe. **B,** Y-shaped incision over fifth metatarsophalangeal joint. **C,** Sectioning of dorsal tendon and capsule of metatarsophalangeal joint. **D,** Correction of deformity and suturing of skin.

coming very tight; in such a case, the following procedure is recommended:

1. Make an incision about 2 cm. in length on the tibial side of the fifth metatarsophalangeal joint.
2. Section the tendon and capsule over this joint with a tenotome. At times the sectioning of the capsule needs to be carried to the sides of the joint until the toe maintains itself in a normal position.
3. Close the skin.
4. Place the toe in an overcorrected position. This position is held with adhesive tape for about 6 weeks.

Recommended technique for correction of fifth toe overlapping in cases in which dorsal skin is moderately contracted. DuVries' technique for correction of overlapping of the fifth toe is recommended:

1. Make a longitudinal incision over the fourth metatarsal interspace, beginning in the web between the fourth and fifth toe and extending over the dorsum to about the proximal third of the metatarsal shafts.

2. Carry the incision to a depth sufficient to sever all adhesive fibers holding the toe in deformity.
3. Perform tenotomy and capsulotomy of the dorsum of the fifth metatarsophalangeal joint if necessary so that the toe can lie in a normal position by its own weight (Fig. 20-42, A).
4. Stretch the fibular skin margin distally and the tibial margin proximally by plantar flexing the fifth toe, forming a pucker ("dog ear") at both ends of the incision. The puckered portion is excised (Fig. 20-42, B).
5. Suture the skin margins in the new position. Also suture the small transverse incision left by excision of the pucker (Fig. 20-42, C).
6. Place the toe in an overcorrected position with adhesive tape for about eight weeks. In cases in which the skin is severely contracted, the procedure described in Fig. 20-38 is indicated.

Correction of second toe overlapping. In second toe overlapping, the second toe

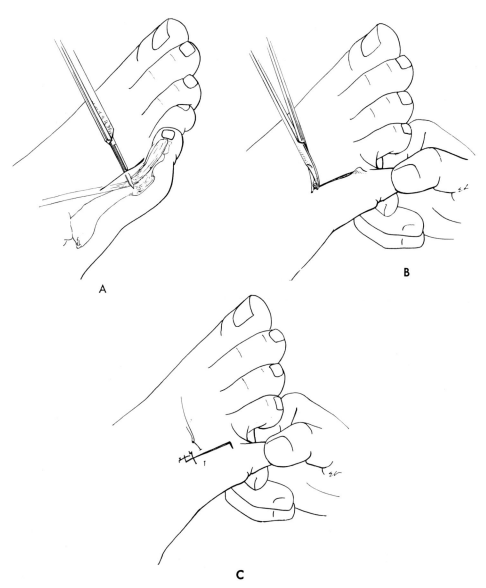

Fig. 20-42. DuVries' technique for overlapping fifth toe with moderate skin contracture. (For severe skin contracture, see Fig. 20-38, A-C.) **A,** Longitudinal incision made over fourth metatarsal interspace. Tenotomy and a capsulotomy over the fifth metatarsophalangeal joint are then performed. **B,** Fifth toe plantar flexed to force fibular margin of incision distally and tibial margin proximally. This forms a fold at each end of the incision. The folds are then excised. **C,** Incision sutured in new position.

usually overlaps the great toe. In most cases this deformity is static and is accompanied by hallux valgus. These two conditions must be reduced simultaneously (see Figs. 4-25 and 4-26).

Overlapping in the flaccid foot may be reduced when dislocation of the metatarsophalangeal joint is not present. This is accomplished by dorsal tenotomy and capsulotomy of the second metatarsophalangeal joint. The toe is then fixed with adhesive tape in an overcorrected plantar attitude and maintained in that position for 6 to 8 weeks.

REFERENCES

Blosser, J.: Fascia lata lacing for hallux valgus. Personal communication, 1964.

Borg, I.: Operation for hammer-toe, Acta Chir. Scand. 100:619-625, 1950.

Brandes, M.: Zur operativen Therapie des Hallux valgus, Zentralbl. Chir. 56:2434-2440, Sept. 1929.

Clayton, M. L.: Surgery of the forefoot in rheumatoid arthritis, Clin. Orthop. 16:136-140, 1960.

Cleveland, M., and Winant, E. M.: An end-result study of the Keller operation, J. Bone Joint Surg. 32-A:163-175, Jan. 1950.

DuVries, H. L., and Shogren, C. V.: Spontaneous restoration of the head of a proximal phalanx following amputation: A case report, J. Amer. Podiatry Assoc. 52:126-127, Feb. 1962.

Forrester-Brown, M. F.: Tendon transplantation for clawing of the great toe, J. Bone Joint Surg. 20:57-60, Jan. 1938.

Fowler, A. W.: The surgery of fixed claw toes, J. Bone Joint Surg. 39-B:585-586, Aug. 1957.

Fowler, A. W.: A method of forefoot reconstruction, J. Bone Joint Surg. 41-B:507-513, Aug. 1959.

Frank, G. R., and Johnson, W. M.: The extensor shift procedure in the correction of clawtoe deformities in children, South. Med. J. 59:889-896, Aug. 1966.

Franklin, L.: Regeneration of resected phalangeal heads, J. Amer. Podiatry Assoc. 58:511-513, Dec. 1968.

Galland, W. I., and Jordan, H.: Hallux valgus, Surg. Gynec. Obstet., 66:95-99, Jan. 1938.

Girdlestone, G. R., and Spooner, H. J.: A new operation for hallux valgus and hallux rigidus, J. Bone Joint Surg. 19:30-35, Jan. 1937.

Hawkins, F. B., Mitchell, C. L., and Hedrick, D. W.: Correction of hallux valgus by metatarsal osteotomy, J. Bone Joint Surg. 27:387-394, July 1945.

Hoffmann, P.: An operation for severe grades of contracted or clawed toes, Amer. J. Orthop. Surg. 9:441-448, 1912.

Hueter, C.: Klinik der Gelenkkrankheiten mit Einschluss der Orthopädie, Leipzig, 1870-1871, F. C. W. Vogel.

Jones, R.: Notes on military orthopedics, London, 1917, Cassel & Co.

Joplin, R. J.: Sling procedure for correction of splay-foot, metatarsus primus varus, and hallux valgus, J. Bone Joint Surg. 32-A:779-785, Oct. 1950.

Kates, A., Kessel, L., and Kay, A.: Arthroplasty of the forefoot, J. Bone Joint Surg. 49-B:552-557, Aug. 1967.

Keller, W. L.: The surgical treatment of bunions and hallux valgus. N. Y. Med. J., 80:741-742, Oct. 1904.

Keller, W. L.: Further observations on the surgical treatment of hallux valgus and bunions, N. Y. Med. J. 95:696-698, Apr. 1912.

Kirk, A. A., Kunkle, H. M., and Waive, H. J.: Ledge tenodesis of the extensor hallucis longus: A substitution for the Jones operation, J. Bone Joint Surg. 53-A:774-776, June 1971.

Krida, A.: A new operation for metatarsalgia and splay-foot, Surg. Gynec. Obstet. 69:106-107, July 1939.

Lantzounis, L. A.: Congenital subluxation of the fifth toe and its correction by periosteocapsuloplasty and tendon transplantation, J. Bone Joint Surg. 22:147-150, Jan. 1940.

Lapidus, P. W.: Operative correction of metatarsus varus primus in hallux valgus, Surg. Gynec. Obstet. 58:183-191, Feb. 1934.

Lapidus, P. W.: Operation for correction of hammer-toe, J. Bone Joint Surg. 21:977-982, Oct. 1939.

Lapidus, P. W.: Transplantation of the extensor tendon for correction of the overlapping fifth toe, J. Bone Joint Surg. 24:555-559, July 1942.

Levine, M. A.: An operative technique for hallux valgus, J. Bone Joint Surg. 20:923-925, Oct. 1938.

Lorenz, H.: Zur operativen Therapie des Hallux valgus, der Hammerzehe und unerträglicher Clavi, Wien. Med. Wochenschr. 79:713-715, May 1929.

McBride, E. D.: A conservative operation for bunions, J. Bone Joint Surg. 10:735-739, 1928.

McBride, E. D.: The conservative operation for "bunions": End results and refinements of technic, J.A.M.A. 105:1164-1168, Oct. 1935.

McBride, E. D.: Hallux valgus, bunion deformity: Its treatment in mild, moderate and severe stages, J. Int. Coll. Surg. 21:99-105, Jan. 1954.

McElvenny, R. T., and Thompson, F. R.: A clinical study of one hundred patients subjected to simple exostosectomy for the relief of bunion pain, J. Bone Joint Surg. 22:942-951, Oct. 1940.

Marmor, L.: Surgery of the rheumatoid foot, Surg. Gynec. Obstet. **119**:1009-1012, Nov. 1964.

Mayo, C. H.: The surgical treatment of bunion, Ann. Surg. **48**:300-302, Aug. 1908.

Michele, A. A., and Krueger, F. J.: Operative correction for hammertoe, Milit. Surg. **103**:52-53, July 1948.

Mitchell, C. L., Fleming, J. L., Allen, R., Glenney, C., and Sanford, G. A.: Osteotomy-bunionectomy for hallux valgus, J. Bone Joint Surg. **40-A**:41-60, Jan. 1958.

Moynihan, F. J.: Arthrodesis of the metatarsophalangeal joint of the great toe, J. Bone Joint Surg. **49-B**:544-551, Aug. 1967.

Rix, R. R.: Modified Mayo operation for hallux valgus and bunion—a comparison with the Keller procedure, J. Bone Joint Surg. **50-A**:1368-1378, Oct. 1968.

Sandeman, J. C.: The role of soft tissue correction of claw toes, Brit. J. Clin. Pract. **21**:489-493, Oct. 1967.

Scheck, M.: Degenerative changes in the metatarsophalangeal joints after surgical correction of severe hammer-toe deformities: A complication associated with avascular necrosis in three cases, J. Bone Joint Surg. **50-A**:727-737, June 1968.

Schein, A. J.: Keller operation—partial phalangectomy in hallux valgus and hallux rigidus: Report of 55 operations in 32 cases, Surgery **7**:342-355, Mar. 1940.

Seeburger, R. H.: Surgical implants of alloyed metal in joints of the feet, J. Amer. Podiatry Assoc. **54**:391-396, June 1964.

Selig, S.: Hammer-toe: A new procedure for its correction, Surg. Gynec. Obstet. **72**:101-105, Jan. 1941.

Sgarlato, T. E.: Transplantation of the flexor digitorum longus muscle tendon in hammertoes, J. Amer. Podiatry Assoc. **60**:383-388, Oct. 1970.

Silver, D.: The operative treatment of hallux valgus, J. Bone Joint Surg. **5**:225-232, Apr. 1923.

Soresi, A. L.: The radical cure of hallux valgus (bunion): Subarticular resection of the head of the metatarsal bone, Surg. Gynec. Obstet. **52**:776-777, Mar. 1931.

Stanley, L. L., and Breck, L. W.: Bunions, J. Bone Joint Surg. **17**:961-964, Oct. 1935.

Taylor, R. G.: An operative procedure for the treatment of hammer-toe and claw-toe, J. Bone Joint Surg. **22**:608-609, July 1940.

Thomas, F. B.: Keller's arthroplasty modified, J. Bone Joint Surg. **44-B**:356-365, May 1962.

Tierney, A.: Hammer-toe: The cup and ball procedure. In Pauchet, V., editor: La pratique chirurgicale illustrée, ed. 2, Paris, 1937, G. Doin & Co.

Wagner, L. C.: The operative correction of extreme flexion contraction of the great toe, J. Bone Joint Surg. **16**:914-918, Oct. 1934.

Wilson, J. N.: V-Y correction for varus deformity of the fifth toe, Brit. J. Surg. **41**:133-135, July-Aug. 1953.

Wilson, J. N.: Oblique displacement osteotomy for hallux valgus, J. Bone Joint Surg. **45-B**:552-556, Aug. 1963.

Wilson, J. N.: Cone arthrodesis of the first metatarsophalangeal joint, J. Bone Joint Surg. **49-B**:98-101, Feb. 1967.

Young, C. S.: An operation for the correction of hammer-toe and claw-toe, J. Bone Joint Surg. **20**:715-719, July 1938.

Index

A

Abnormalities; *see* Anomalies
Abrasions, 176-191
   treatment, 191
Abscess, Brodie's, 374-375
   metatarsal, 374
   phalanx, 375
   tibia, 374
   treatment, 375
Achilles bursa; *see* Bursa, Achilles
Achilles tendon; *see* Tendon, Achilles
Adolescent, plantar fibromatosis in, 387
Adventitious bursa; *see* Bursa, adventitious
Ainhum disease, 349
Allis forceps, 334-335
Amputations, 443-456
   forefoot, weight bearing in, 446
   in hallux valgus, base of proximal phalanx, 510-511, 516-519
      Keller technique, 510-511, 516-517, 518
      Lapidus technique, 518
      McBride technique, 519, 520
      Silvers technique, 517, 519
   in hallux valgus, subcapital type, 508-510, 511-515
      end results of, 512
      Mayo technique, 511
   indications for, 443-444
   levels, 446-447
   metatarsal, 451-452
      transmetatarsal, 452-453
   at metatarsophalangeal joint
      hallux, 450-451
      of lesser toes, 449-450
   operative principles, 444-445
   operative technique, 447-455
   phalanx
      distal, 448
      distal, of hallux, 447-448
      phalangeal joint of hallux, 448-449
   plantar flap with, 449
   Syme's; *see* Syme's amputation
   toes, 451
      second, causing hallux valgus, 220
   transmetatarsal, 452-453
Anesthesia, 438-439
   ankle block, technique, 438
   postoperative, 441-442
   precautions, 438-439
Aneurysm, traumatic, 440-441

Angioma, 389-390
Angiosarcoma, 390, 391
Ankle
   anatomy of, 120
   anomalies, 23-24
   approaches to, 457-470
      anterior, 462-463
      anterolateral, 462-463
      anterolateral, Jergesen's, 460
      lateral, 460-461
      lateral, simple, 460
      medial, 458-460
      medial, anterior, 459
      medial, to medial malleolus, by osteotomy, 460
      medial, to posterior malleolus, 460
      medial, simple, 458-459
      posterior, 462
      posterolateral, Gatellier and Chastang's, 460-461
      posterolateral, Henry's, 461
      posteromedial, Colonna and Ralston's, 459-460
      posteromedial, Jergesen's, 459
   in arthritis, rheumatoid, 283, 285
   arthrodesis; *see* Arthrodesis, ankle
   arthrography; *see* Arthrography
   axis, 12-17
      estimating location of, 31
      obliquity of, 16
      obliquity of, estimation, 15
      variations in inclination of, 14
   ball-and-socket ankle joint, 273
   biomechanics of, 3-22
   block anesthesia, technique, 438
   degrees of stability of, methods, 127
   disorders of
      soft-tissue procedures, 475-482
      surgical procedures for, 471-482
   examination; *see* Examination, foot and ankle
   fracture-dislocation; *see* Fracture-dislocations, ankle
   fractures; *see* Fractures, ankle
   ligaments; *see* Ligaments, ankle
   sprains; *see* Sprains, ankle
   strappings; *see* Strappings, ankle
   in stressed position, 180
Anomalies
   ankle, 23-24

Anomalies—cont'd
  in arthritis, rheumatoid; *see* Arthritis, rheumatoid, deformities in
  arthrogryposis multiplex congenita causing, 107
  calcaneocavus, crescentic osteotomy of calcaneus for, 271
  calcaneus, 251
  in cerebral palsy; *see under* Cerebral palsy
  foot; *see* Foot, anomalies
  lower extremity, 28
  metatarsal, 73-74, 84
  metatarsophalangeal joint, first, 206-239
  nails, 353-368
  phalanges, 84
  recurrence after surgery, 440
  sesamoid, 74, 78-80
  talonavicular, 85
    planovalgus due to, 259
  toes; *see* Toes, anomalies of
Aponeurosis
  plantar, 33
    palpation, 34
    windlass mechanism of, 254
Apophysis, calcaneal, osteochondrosis of, 378-380
Apophysitis, 376
Appliances, 428-430, 445-446
  leather, 428-429, 430
  metal, 429-430
    hallux valgus and, 515
  orthopaedic, for rheumatoid arthritis, 285
  orthotic, 430
  for varus and valgus forefoot, 432
Arm swing, symmetry of, 26
Arthritis
  gouty, 287
  psoriatic, 286
  rheumatoid, 282-286
    ankle in, 283, 285
    clinical course of, 284
    deformities in, ankle, 285
    deformities in, forefoot, 285-286
    deformities in, hindfoot, 285
    diagnostic procedures, 47
    in hallux valgus; *see* Hallux valgus, in rheumatoid foot
    metatarsophalangeal joints, 283
    in skeletal specimen, 284
    surgical procedures, limited, 286
    tarsus, 283
    treatment, 283-286
    treatment, medical, 283-285
    treatment, surgical, 285
  traumatic
    first metatarsal-first cuneiform articulation, 398
    hallux rigidus and, 228
    metatarsophalangeal joint, 398
Arthrodesis
  ankle, 472-475
    compression type, 474-475
    grafts in, anterior tibial, 473-474, 475
    grafts in, intra-articular bone, 472-473
    osteotomies in, malleolar, 473, 474
  calcaneus fractures and, 139-140
  in flatfoot, 499, 500-501
  Grice, 274, 484
  in hallux flexus, 234

Arthrodesis—cont'd
  in hallux valgus, 506-507
    Girdlestone and Spooner's technique, 508
  Hoke, 483
  in metatarsus adductus and varus, 99, 101
  in paralytic foot deformities, 485
  tarsus
    combined talonavicular, talocrural, and pantalar, 484
    extra-articular, 486-487
    pantalar, 484, 486
    subtalar, 482-484
    triple, 482-484
Arthrography
  ankle, 181
    ligaments, 181, 182
    showing extravasation of dye along medial malleolus, 182
Arthrogryposis multiplex congenita, 107
Arthroplasty for keratosis under metatarsal heads, 337
Aseptic necrosis; *see* Necrosis, aseptic
Astragalectomy, 484, 487-489
Ataxia, Friedreich's, 275
Athletic trauma; *see* Trauma, athletic
Atrophy
  bone, localized; *see* Osteoporosis
  Sudeck's, 406, 407
    with metatarsal march fracture, 408
Avulsion
  fractures; *see under* Fractures
  ligaments, ankle, collateral, 184, 187-189
    treatment, 184, 187-189
  nail, for ingrown nail, 358, 361

B

Bacteria tests, 47
Ball-and-socket ankle joint, 273
Bandages
  cradle-gauze, 541
  Gelocast, 187
  sponge rubber, 525
Banks and Laufman's exposure
  ankle, by medial malleolus osteotomy, 460
  calcaneus
    lateral, 465
    posterior, 465-466
Barograph, 21
Betts' approach to digital nerves for perineural fibroma removal, 469
Bimalleolar fracture, 122-123
Bimalleolar fracture-dislocation, 122-123
  closed reduction of, 126
Biopsy, 45-46
Birthmark, 349-350
Bolster in hammertoe reduction, 541
Bones
  accessory, 52-58
  affections of, local, 371-412
  atrophy, localized; *see* Osteoporosis
  block, posterior, 475, 476
  cancer, 402-404
  cyst; *see* Cyst, bone
  excision in hallux valgus, methods, 507
  forceps, double-action, 436
  infarct, 380-381
  infectious disorders of, 371-375

Bones—cont'd
  nonunion, 442
  tumor, 390-402
  tumorous conditions of, 385-404
  vascular disorders, 375-384
Bow strapping, 432
Brockman's approach to plantar structures, 467
Brodie's abscess; *see* Abscess, Brodie's
Broomhead's approach to malleolus, 460
Brown grasping forceps, 436
Bunion, 206-239
  dorsal; *see* Hallux flexus
  tailor's, 236-239
    DuVries' correction of, 238
    etiology, 236
    fifth metatarsal head in, 237, 239, 240
    postoperative complications, 241
    symptoms, 236, 238
    treatment, 238-239
Bunionette; *see* Bunion, tailor's
Burns, 168-170
  calcaneal tuberosity destruction in, 169
  classification, 168-169
  toes, causing plantar contracture, 169
  treatment, 169-170
Bursa
  Achilles, approaches to, 466
    posterior, 466
    posterolateral, 466
  adventitious
    under metatarsal head, 311-313
    under metatarsophalangeal joint, fifth, 313
    under weight-bearing surfaces, 313
  formation with hallux valgus, 221
Bursitis, 307-309, 310-313
  gout causing, 288
  retrocalcaneal, 307-309
    etiology, 308
    treatment, 308-309
  septic, acute, 307
  serous, chronic, 311
  simple, acute, 311

C
Calcaneocavus deformity, calcaneus osteotomy for, 271
Calcaneocuboid articulations, 33-34
Calcaneocuboid joint, sprain of, 191
Calcaneocuboid ligaments, 191
Calcaneofibular ligaments, 178
  tear of, 187
Calcaneonavicular bar, excision in pes planus, 498
Calcaneonavicular ligament, plantar, 33
Calcaneonavicular synchondrosis, 262
Calcaneonavicular synostosis, 108
  spastic flatfoot and, 262
Calcaneus
  anatomy, 131, 132
  anomalies
    in cerebral palsy, 271
    posterior tuberosity, 251
  apophysis, osteochondrosis of, 378-380
  approaches to, 465-466
    circumferential heel incision, 465-466
    lateral, 464, 465
    medial, 465

Calcaneus—cont'd
  approaches—cont'd
    posterior, 465-466
    split heel, 466
  burns and, 169
  cyst of, solitary, 392
  disorders of, acquired nontraumatic, 250-256
  fractures of; *see* Fractures, calcaneus
  hyperconvex, 251
  hypoconvex, 251
  osteotomy of; *see* Osteotomy, calcaneus
  sarcoma, Ewing's, in children, 404
  shape variations, 251
  spurs; *see* Spurs, calcaneal
  surgical procedures, 489-495
  tendon; *see* Tendon, Achilles
  tuberosity, 33
  variation in angles of posterosuperior tuberosity, 252
Calcification and tendo achillis fibromatosis, 388
Callus, 325-326
  etiology, 325-326
  under heel, 326
  march fractures and, 158
  under metatarsal head
    fifth, 326
    first, 326
    middle three, 326
Cancer
  bone, 402-404
  soft tissues, 390
Carcinomas, 351-352
Casts, equinus, and calcaneus fracture, 139
Causalgia, 419-421
  etiology, 419
  symptoms, 419
  treatment, 419
Cell
  giant; *see* Giant cell tumors
  palisade arrangement in neurofibroma, 414
  reticulum cell sarcoma, 404
Cellulitis, 305
  clostridial, and gas gangrene, 308, 309
Cerebral palsy, 269-275
  characteristics, 269-275
  deformities in
    calcaneus, 271
    dorsal bunion, 274
    equinus, 270-271
    valgus, 271-275
    valgus, hallux, 272
    varus, 271-275
    varus, spastic hallux, 274
Cerebrovascular accidents, 268-269
Chandler elevator, 436
Charcot-Marie-Tooth disease, 275
Charcot's joint in syphilis, 301
Cheilectomy for hallux rigidus, 228, 232
Chilblains, 171
Children
  adolescent, plantar fibromatosis in, 387
  ankle examination in, 24-35
  exostosis in, subungual, 401
  foot anomalies, 88-89
  foot examination in, 24-35
  fractures in, metatarsal, 159
  infant; *see* Infant

Children—cont'd
  myopathies in, 280
  sarcoma in calcaneus, Ewing's, 404
Chip fractures; *see under* Fractures
Chondroblastoma, 401
Chondroma, 400-401
Chondromalacia, 411
Chondromyxoid fibroma, 401-402
Chondromyxoma, phalanges, 401
Chondromyxosarcoma, 403
Chondrosarcoma, 403
Chopart's joint dislocations, 160
Clavus; *see* Corn
Clawfoot, 103-105, 263-264
  etiology, 103-104
  osteotomy for, 493
    midtarsal, 498
  symptoms, 104
  treatment, 104-105, 497
Clawtoes, 241-249
  etiology, 248-249
  joints in, 245
  Jones' tendon transfer for, 545
  muscle action in, 246, 247
  pathogenesis, 249
  treatment, 249, 542, 545
Clayton's approach to metatarsal heads, 469
Clayton's correction of hallux valgus in rheuma-
    toid foot, 530-531
Cleft foot, 110, 111-112
  bilateral, 112
  treatment, 111-112
Clostridial cellulitis and gas gangrene, 308, 309
Clubfoot; *see* Talipes, equinovarus
Clubnail, 355
Coccidioides immitis, 301-302
Colonna and Ralston's approach to ankle, 459-460'
Compression arthrodesis, ankle, 474-475
Compression dressings for calcaneus fracture, 139
Condylectomy
  for corns, 320-322
    DuVries' technique, 320
  for hallux valgus
    modified type, 506
    osteotomy and; *see* Osteotomy, step-down, and
      condylectomy for hallux valgus
    simple type, 506
    Stanley and Breck's technique, 508
  plantar, for keratosis under metatarsal heads,
    337
  for wide first metatarsal head, 209
"Confusion" test, dorsiflexion, 270
Contracture
  Dupuytren's, 386-387
  plantar, and burns, 169
  skin, and overlapping fifth toe, DuVries' cor-
    rection, 544, 548
  Volkmann's ischemic, 201-202
Contusions, 176-191
  treatment, 191
Corn, 318-325
  condylectomy for; *see* Condylectomy, for corns
  etiology, 318-319
  fifth toe, lateral side, 319-320
    operative treatment, 319-320
    phalanx head excision for, 320
  great toe, tibial side, 324

Corn—cont'd
  metatarsals and, 324-325
  neurovascular, 325
    treatment, 325
  soft
    excision, Haboush and Martin's technique, 323
    on lesser toes, 322-324
    in web between fourth and fifth toes, 320-322
  treatment, 319-325
Cotton's fracture, 471-472
Cradle-gauze bandaging, 541
Crush injury
  foot, 200
  heel, 200
Cryoglobulinemia, diagnostic procedures, 47-48
Cuboid
  calcaneocuboid; *see* Calcaneocuboid
  cyst of, solitary, 392
  dislocation, 141, 160
  displacement of plantar surface, 142
  fractures; *see* Fractures, cuboid
  osteochondrosis of, 381
  transference for metatarsus adductor and varus,
    100, 101
Cultures, 45
Cuneiform
  anomalous medial, 59
  bifurcated first, 84
  bifurcated medial, 58
    horizontal, 59
  joint, first, high dorsum of base of, 83
    treatment, 83
Cuneonavicular articulation, 33-34
Cyst
  bone, 390-402
    aneurysmal, 393
    simple, 393
  calcaneus, solitary, 392
  cuboid, solitary, 392
  epidermal, 346-349
    ball of foot, 347
    inclusion, beneath nail, 402
    large, 347
    over metatarsophalangeal joint, first, 348
    toes, 348
  epidermoid; *see* Cyst, epidermal
  ganglionic, and hallux valgus, 221
  inversion; *see* Cyst, epidermal
  metatarsal, aneurysmal, 394

D

Deformities; *see* Anomalies
Dehiscence, wound, 440
Denis Browne splint for talipes equinovarus, 94
Dermatitis from shoe irritants, 346
Dermatologic procedures, 45-47
Dermatophytosis, 345-346
  toes, 346
Diabetes mellitus, 288-293
  diagnostic procedures, 47
  gangrene in, 292-293
    treatment, 292-293
  neuropathy in; *see* Neuropathy, diabetic
  sesamoid necrosis secondary to, 409-410
  ulcer in, 293
    under metatarsal head, 294

Diagnostic procedures
  ancillary, 44-48
  dermatologic, 45-47
Diastasis, tibiofibular syndesmosis, 179
Dickson's pie technique for intractable keratosis,
  331
Digit; *see* Toe
Disarticulation; *see* Amputation
Dislocations, 158-163
  Chopart's joint, 160
  cuboid, 141, 160
  fracture-; *see* Fracture-dislocations
  hallux, 153-154
  Lisfranc's joint, 161
  metatarsophalangeal joint, 162-163
  metatarsophalangeal joint, second, 239-241
    complete static, 242, 243
    etiology, 240
    hallux valgus and, 526
    symptoms, 240
    treatment, 240-241
  midtarsal joint, 160
  peroneal, sulcus deepening in, 482
  phalanges, 162-163
  subtalar joint, 158-160
  tarsometatarsal joint, 160-162
  tendon, ankle, 481-482
"Dorsiflexion confusion test," 270
Dressings
  compression, and calcaneus fracture, 139
  for hallux valgus, postoperative, 525
  materials for, 437
Dropfoot, 264-265
  etiology of, 264
  paralytic, treatment, 476
  stabilization operations, 265
  symptoms of, 264
  treatment of, 264-265, 476
Drug therapy in rheumatoid arthritis, 284
Dupuytren's contracture, 386-387
DuVries'
  approach
    to digital nerves for perineural fibroma re-
      moval, 469
    to plantar structures, 467
  modification
    bone forceps, 436
    Jones' tendon transfer for hammered great
      toe, 537
    Sistrunk scissors, 436
  technique
    condylectomy of corn on fifth toe, 320
    deltoid ligament reconstruction, 480
    hallux valgus reduction, 521-523
    overlapping fifth toe with skin contracture,
      544, 548
    plastic reduction of hypertrophy of ungual-
      abia, 364, 365, 366
    tailor's bunion correction, 238
DuVries-Dickson correction of hallux valgus in
    rheumatoid foot, 531-533, 535
Dwarfism, metatarsal, 113
Dwyer's approach to calcaneus, 465
Dysmelia, 23-24
Dystrophy
  muscular, 280
  reflex, 406, 407

E

Eccrine poroma, 350-351
Electrode, galvanic, 361
Elevation for calcaneus fracture, 139
Elevator
  Chandler, 436
  Frost, 361
Enzymes in calcaneus fracture, 139
Epidermal cyst; *see* Cyst, epidermal
Epidermoid cyst; *see* Cyst, epidermal
Epiphysitis, definition, 375-376
Epithelioma, 351
Equinus
  casts and calcaneus fractures, 139
  deformity in cerebral palsy, 270-271
Ewing's sarcoma, 403-404
  calcaneus, in children, 404
  toe, 404
Examination
  foot and ankle, 23-43
    in adults, 24-35
    in children, 24-35
    in infant, preambulatory, 23-24
    ligamentous structures, 33
    muscular structures, 33
    in newborn, 23-24
    ranges of motion, 30-33
    roentgenographic, 44
    sequence of, 25-30
    in toddler, 24
  leg surface, 29-30
  shoes, 26-27
Excrescences, 318-342
Exostosis, 393, 394-395
  cartilaginous, and chondrosarcoma, 403
  metatarsal, 399
  sesamoid, 80
  subungual
    anvil-shaped, 396
    in children, 401
    great toe, 394
    phalanges, 397, 400
  talus, 399
Extensors, paralysis, causing hallux flexus, 234
Extremities, lower, abnormalities, 28

F

Fascia, plantar
  fibromatosis of, in adolescent, 387
  sprains, 191
Fasciitis, plantar, 310
  strappings for, 430, 432
  treatment, 310
Fatigue fractures; *see* Fractures, fatigue
Feet; *see* Foot
Felon, 305-307
  great toe, 306
  osteomyelitis of phalanx after, 306
  treatment, 306-307
Felt pads, 428, 429, 432
  hammertoe and, 433
Fibroma, 385
  chondromyxoid, 401-402
  neurofibroma, 388, 414
  perineural; *see* Nerves, digital, approaches for
    removal of perineural fibromas

Fibromatosis
  plantar, 386-388
    in adolescent, 387
    excision, technique, 387-388
    recurrent massive, 386
    treatment, 387
  tendo achillis, 342
    calcification and, 388
    ossification in, 314
Fibrosarcoma, 390
Fibrosis, tendo achillis, 315
Figure-of-eight ankle wrap, 187
Flail toes from phalangectomy, 321
Flaps
  keratosis under metatarsal heads and, 339
  plantar, in amputations, 449
Flatfoot, 256, 258-263
  arthrodesis for, 499, 500-501
  calcaneonavicular bar excision in, 498
  examination, 24
  forefoot eversion and abduction and, 258
  hallux valgus and, 211-214
  osteotomy for, calcaneus, 490
    displacement type, 491
  peroneal spastic, 143, 259-263
    etiology, 260-261
  rigid, 24
    congenital, 105-107
    congenital, treatment, 107
  symptomatic flexible, 258-259
    tendo achillis in, 260
  symptomatic severe, 261
  treatment, 261, 263, 497-501
  types of, 27, 28, 29
Flexor hallucis brevis tendon ossification, 316
Foot
  absence of part of, 111-112
  anomalies of, 23-24
    acquired nontraumatic, 204-267
    during childhood, 88-89
    congenital, major, 88-118
    congenital, minor, 51-87
    during infancy, 88
    paralytic, arthrodesis, 485
  approaches to, 457-470
  biomechanics of, 3-22
  bizarre, congenitally, 112
  bones, accessory, 52-58
  clawfoot; see Clawfoot
  cleft; see Cleft foot
  clubfoot; see Talipes, equinovarus
  cyst, epidermal, 347
  disorders of
    cause of, 204-206
    incidence of, 204-206
  dropfoot; see Dropfoot
  examination; see Examination, foot and ankle
  flatfoot; see Flatfoot
  forefoot; see Forefoot
  hindfoot; see Hindfoot
  hollow; see Clawfoot
  immersion, 171-172
  ligaments of, 177
  lobster-claw; see Cleft foot
  Madura, 302-303
  metabolic disorders affecting, 282-288
  nerves of, plantar, 414

Foot—cont'd
  neuromuscular diseases, 268-281
  ossification centers of, 89
  pronation during early stance phase, 26
  rocker-bottom, 261
  splayfoot, and hallux valgus, 529
  split; see Cleft foot
  strappings; see Strappings, foot
  suppurating sinuses of; see Sinuses, suppurating,
    of foot
  vascular disorders affecting, 288-289
    differential diagnosis, criteria for, 297
Forceps
  Allis, 334-335
  bone, double-action, 436
  Brown grasping, 436
Forefoot
  amputations, weight bearing in, 446
  approaches to, 467-469
    dorsal, 468
  in flatfoot, 258
  in male, 205
  in rheumatoid arthritis, 285-286
  shoes and, 428
    ill-fitting, 206
  sprain, 191
  surgical procedures, 506-550
  valgus, orthotic appliances for, 432
  varus, orthotic appliances for, 432
Foreign bodies, 172-176
  glass as, 173, 175
  gunshot particles as, 176
  hair as, exogenous, 173, 176
  localization of, 172
  needles as, 173, 174
Fowler and Philip's approach to Achilles bursae,
    466
Fracture(s), 119-167
  ankle, 120-127
    classification, 120-121
    comminution and instability with, 124, 125
    compound type, 123-124
    physical therapy, 433
    reduction of, open, 471-472
    traction for, fixed, 125
  calcaneus, 131-140
    anterior process of, 134, 135
    arthrodesis and, primary, 139-140
    beak type, 135
    classification, 131-138
    classification, Rowe's, 133
    comminuted type, 132
    compression dressings in, 139
    elevation in, 139
    enzymes in, 139
    equinus casts and, 139
    fatigue type, 160
    grafting for, 489
    horizontal, 137
    navicular fracture with, 143
    pins in, 139
    reduction of, open, 139, 489
    tendo achillis and, 136, 137
    traction for, 139
    treatment, 138-140
    treatment, conservative, 138
    treatment, historical approach to, 138

Fracture(s)—cont'd
  Cotton's, 471-472
  cuboid, 130, 140, 141-142
    chip type, 142
    comminuted type, 141
    comminuted type, compression, 141
  -dislocations; *see* Fracture-dislocations
  fatigue, 152, 158, 159, 160
    calcaneus, 160
    comminuted, with callus formation and asep-
      tic necrosis, 158
    metatarsal; *see* Fracture, metatarsal
  malleolus, 121-122
    bimalleolar, 122-123
    fibular, 121
    fixation of, internal, 126-127
    internal, open reduction of, 471
    isolated, 121
    lateral, open reduction of, 471
    lateral, with posterior displacement of proxi-
      mal fibular fragment, 124, 126
    medial, 122
    reduction of, closed, 126
    reduction of, open, 471-472
    tibial, 121
    trimalleolar, 123
    trimalleolar, open reduction of, 471-472
    trimalleolar, and talus displacement, 123
    types of, 121
  march; *see* Fracture, fatigue
  metatarsal, 147-148, 149, 150-151
    avulsion type, 146
    base of, 150
    base of, fifth, 147
    base of, and plaster boot, 150
    comminuted type, 146
    concomitant type, 151
    fatigue type, 158
    fatigue type, in children, 159
    fatigue type, and Sudeck's atrophy, 408
    malunited, 149
    neck of, 148
    neglected, 151
    oblique, 146, 149
    old, 151
    spiral type, 146
    spontaneous, in children, 159
    transverse, 146
    transverse, with displacement, 146
    types of, 146
    ununited, 149
  navicular, 140, 143-145
    chip type, 144
    comminuted type, 145
    neck of, and calcaneus fracture, 143
    neck of, without displacement, 143-144
    transverse, 145
  phalanx, 148-149, 151
    fifth proximal, 148
    fifth proximal, nonunion, 152
    hallux, 151
    hallux, avulsion type, 154
    hallux, comminuted type, 153-154
    hallux, impacted type, 153
    middle toes, 148-149, 151
  sesamoid, 151-152, 155-157
    fibular, comminuted type, 156-157

Fracture(s)—cont'd
  sesamoid—cont'd
    tibial, comminuted type, 155-156
    tibial, proximal portion of, 155-156
    tibial, transverse type, 155-156
  stress; *see* Fractures, fatigue
  talus, 127-131
    chip type, 129
    classification, 128-131
    comminuted type, 130-131
    complications, 128
    neck of, 130
    necrosis and, aseptic, 128, 130-131
    osteochondral, 131
    treatment, 131
  tibia lip
    distal, 123, 124
    reduction of, closed, 126
    reduction of, open, 471-472
    treatment, criteria for, 119-120
Fracture-dislocations, 119-167
  ankle, 120-127
    classification, 120-121
    compound, 123-124
    bimalleolar, 122-123
    closed reduction of, 126
  Lisfranc's joint, 161
  phalanx, fifth proximal, 152
  talus, 127-131
    classification, 128-131
    complications, 128
    treatment, 131
  tarsometatarsal joint, 161
  treatment, criteria for, 119-120
  trimalleolar, 123
    closed reduction of, 126
Freezing, 170-172
Freiberg's infraction, 378
  in active state, 378
  in static state, 379
Friction causing excrescences, 318-342
Friedreich's ataxia, 275
Frost elevator, 361
Frostbite, 170-171
  treatment, 170-171
Fungus, scraping for, 45

G
Gaenslen's split heel approach to calcaneus, 466
Galvanic electrode, 361
Ganglion, 389
  cyst, and hallux valgus, 221
  excision, 389
Gangrene
  diabetic, 292-293
    treatment, 292-293
  gas, 308, 309-310
    clostridial cellulitis and, 308, 309
    diagnosis, 309-310
    treatment, 310
Garré's osteomyelitis, 375, 376
  treatment, 375
Gas gangrene; *see* Gangrene, gas
Gatellier and Chastang's approach to ankle, 460-
    461
Gelocast bandage, 187
Germ plasm defect and talipes equinovarus, 92-93

Giannestras' step-down osteotomy
  in hallux valgus, 510
  in plantar keratosis, 338
Giant cell tumors
  bone, 402
  tendon sheath, 388-389
Gibney basket weave strapping, 186
Gill procedure for paralytic dropfoot, 476
Girdlestone and Spooner's correction of hallux val-
    gus, 508
Glass as foreign body, 173, 175
Glomus tumor, 350, 390
  beneath nail, 402
Goniometer measuring subtalar motion, 32
Gout, 286, 288
  arthritis and, 287
  bursitis from, 288
  categories of, 287-288
  diagnostic procedures, 47
  indications for surgery, 288
Grafts
  in ankle arthrodesis; *see* Arthrodesis, ankle,
    grafts in
  flap; *see* Flaps
  in fractures; *see under* Fractures
  pedicle skin, for crush injury of heel, 200
Granuloma, great toe, 302
Grice
  approach to sinus tarsi, 463-465
  arthrodesis, 274, 484
Griffith's procedure, calcaneal spurs, 495
"Growing paraplegic," 277
Gunshot particles as foreign bodies, 176

H

Haboush and Martin's excision of soft corn, 323
Haglund's disease, 250-252
  osteotomy for, 494
  surgery of, 491-494
Hair, exogenous, as foreign body, 173, 176
Hallux; *see also* Hallux valgus, Hallux varus
  accessory, 63-66
    bilateral, in infant, 64-65
    bizarre, first metatarsal, 64
    phalanx of, 63
    syndactyly and, 62
  amputations; *see under* Amputations
  anomalies, 84
  corn over, 324
  dislocation, 153-154
  exostosis of, subungual, 394
  extensus, 234, 236
  felon of, 306
  flexus, 232-234
    arthrodesis and, triple, 234
    in cerebral palsy, 274
    hallux rigidus causing, severe, 233
    paralysis of extensors causing, 234
    pathologic-anatomic appearance of, 235
    reduction of, Lapidus' technique, 235
  granuloma of, massive, 302
  hammered; *see* Hammertoes, great toe
  limitus; *see* Hallux, rigidus
  nail
    congenital double, 354
    lip, hypertrophied; *see* Hypertrophy, nail lip,
      hallux

Hallux—cont'd
  osteomyelitis of, 373
  phalanges fractures; *see* Fractures, phalanx,
    hallux
  rigidus, 226-232, 398
    acquired type, 227, 230-232
    arthritis and, 228
    cheilectomy for, 228, 232
    congenital, 73
    hallux flexus due to, 233
    metatarsal heads in, 229, 230
    shoe sole modification for, 427
    treatment, 228-232
    types of, 226-228
Hallux valgus, 209-223
  amputations causing, second toe, 220
  amputations for; *see* Amputations, in hallux val-
    gus
  arthrodesis for, 506-507
    Girdlestone and Spooner's technique, 508
  bone excision in, methods, 507
  bursa formation with, massive adventitious, 221
  cerebral palsy and, 272
  condylectomy for; *see* Condylectomy, for hallux
    valgus
  dislocation and, second metatarsophalangeal
    joint, 526
  dressings for, postoperative, 525
  DuVries' correction, 521-523
  etiology, 210-223
  ganglionic cyst and, 221
  interphalangeal, 73
  metatarsals in
    head of, peculiarly shaped, 216, 217
    length of, first, 214-215
  metatarsus primus varus and, 529
  metatarsus varus and, 214
  muscle variation in, 215-216
  overlapping second toe and, 70
  pathologic anatomy of, 222
  pes planus and, 211-214
  plantar sling for, 507
    Joplin's technique, 509
  pronation of foot in, 211-213
  rapidly developing, 219
  in rheumatoid foot, 530-533, 535
    Clayton procedure, 530-531
    DuVries-Dickson procedure, 531-533, 535
  sesamoids in, 222
  shoes and, 210-211
    postoperative, 524
  splayfoot and, 529
  supination of foot in, 211-213
  surgical procedures for, 506-535
Hallux varus, 64-65, 223-226
  in cerebral palsy, 274
  congenital, 71-73
    bilateral, 72
    treatment, 73
  at interphalangeal joint, 73
  overlapping toes and, Keller procedure for, 224
  postoperative, 223-226
    bilateral, McBride procedure for, 223
    tendon shortening causing, abductor hallucis,
      223
    treatment of, 224-226
  sesamoid rotation in, 225

Hammertoes, 241-249
    congenital, 68, 69
    etiology, 248-249
    felt pads and, 433
    fifth toe, reduction of, 540, 542
    foot strappings for, 430, 433
    fourth toe, 244
    great toe, 69, 243
        Jones' tendon transfer for; *see* Jones' tendon
            transfer, in hammered great toe
        reduction of, 535-538, 540
    middle three, correction of, 534, 539-543
        cradle-gauze bandaging and, 541
    pathogenesis, 249
    second toe, 69, 244
        surgical procedures, 536
    shoes and, 248
    third toe, 244
    treatment, 249, 535-542, 543
Hansen's disease; *see* Leprosy
Hawkins-Mitchell osteotomy for hallux valgus, 510
Hawkins osteotomy for hallux valgus, 509
Healing, delayed, 439-440
Heel
    callus under, 326
    crush injury to, 200
    "hugger," 273
    inverted, osteotomy in, 493
    shoe; *see* Shoe, heel
    sinus tracts, draining, 303
    ulcers under, traumatic, 341
    verruca plantaris on, 344
Heloma; *see* Corn
Hemiplegia, spastic, 268-269
    treatment, 268-269
Hemorrhagic tenosynovitis, 194-195
Hemostat with Penrose drain as tourniquet, 437
Henry's approach
    to ankle, posterolateral, 461
    to plantar structures, 466-467
Heredity and talipes equinovarus, 92
Heyman, Herndon, and Strong correction of con-
        genital metatarsus varus, 101-103
Hindfoot
    deformity in rheumatoid arthritis, 285
    tendon transfers about, 478, 480-481
Hoffmann's approach to metatarsal heads, 468-469
Hoke arthrodesis, 483
Hollow foot; *see* Clawfoot
Hostler's toe, 355-356
Hygroma, 311
Hyperkeratosis, 343
    under fibular sesamoid, 327
Hyperplasia, 353
Hypertrophy
    nail lip, 357
        advanced, 362-363
        avulsion of nail causing, 358
        hallux, advanced, 362-363
        hallux, correction of, 359-365
        hallux, postoperative care, 363, 365
        overlapping and, 359
    scars, 353
    sesamoids; *see* Sesamoids, distorted and hyper-
        trophied
    tendo achillis skin and soft tissues, 342

I
Immersion foot, 171-172
Infant
    accessory hallux in, 64-65
    ankle examination in, 23-24
    foot anomalies, 88
    foot examination in, 23-24
    metatarsal fractures in, 159
    metatarsus varus in, 98
    talipes equinovarus in, 90
Infarct, 375
    bone, 380-381
Infections
    bones and, 371-375
    postoperative, 439-440
Infectious disorders, 299-310
Inflammatory diseases, noninfectious, 310-316
Infraction; *see* Freiberg's infraction
Ingrown nails; *see* Nails, ingrown
Injury; *see* Trauma
Instructions to surgical patient, 435-436
Instruments, surgical, 436-438
Intrauterine pressure, abnormal, causing talipes
        equinovarus, 92

J
Jergesen's approach to ankle
    anterolateral, 460
    medial, 459
    posteromedial, 459
Joints
    calcaneocuboid, sprain of, 191
    Charcot's, in syphilis, 301
    Chopart's, dislocations of, 160
    knee, in syphilis, 301
    Lisfranc's, dislocations of, 160-162
    metatarsophalangeal;   *see*   Metatarsophalangeal
        joint
    midtarsal, dislocations of, 160
    subtalar; *see* Subtalar joint
    talocrural; *see* Ankle
    talonavicular; *see* Talonavicular joint
    tarsometatarsal; *see* Tarsometatarsal joint
Jones' tendon transfer
    in clawtoe, 545
    in hammered great toe, 535-538, 540
        DuVries' modification, 537
        Kirk's modification, 538
Joplin's plantar sling technique for hallux valgus,
    509
Joseph nasal rasp, 436

K
Kaplan's approach to digital nerves for perineural
        fibroma removal, 469
Kaposi's sarcoma, 390, 391
Keller procedure
    hallux valgus, 510-511, 516-517, 518
    hallux varus and overlapping toes, 224
Keloids, 352-353, 385-386
Keratosis
    hyperkeratosis, 343
        under sesamoid, 327
    plantar, distribution of lesions in 139 cases, 330
    under metatarsal heads
        Dickson's pie technique for, 331

Keratosis—cont'd
  under metatarsal head—cont'd
    excision, coaptation of skin margins after, 339
    fifth, 331
    first, 327-329
    middle three, 329-331
    procedures for, 331-337, 338, 339
    roentgenograms, 332-333
    types of, 330
Kirk's modification of Jones' tendon transfer for hammered great toe, 538
Kirschner wires in tarsometatarsal fracture-dislocation, 161
Knee joint in syphilis, 301
Kocher's approach to subtalar and talonavicular joints, 463
Köhler's disease, 377-378

L

Lantzounis' procedure for overlapping fifth toe, 545
Lapidus' procedure
  hallux flexus reduction, 235
  hallux valgus correction, 518
  overlapping fifth toe correction, 545, 546
Leather appliances, 428-429, 430
Leg examination, 29-30
Leprosy, 304
  effects on feet, 304
  intermediate, 304
  lepromatous, 304
  lesions in, 304
  tuberculoid, 304
Lifts; see Shoe, lifts
Ligaments
  ankle
    arthrography, 181, 182
    collateral, avulsion of, 184, 187-189
    collateral, lateral, reconstruction, 476-477, 478-479
    deltoid, reconstruction of, 477-478, 480
    examination, 33
    lateral side, 178
    ruptures of; see Ruptures, ligament, ankle
    surgical repair of, 475-478
  calcaneocuboid, 191
  calcaneofibular, 178
    tear of, 187
  calcaneonavicular, plantar, 33
  foot, 177
    examination, 33
  malleolar; see Trauma, malleolar ligaments
  talofibular
    anterior, 178
    anterior, disruption of, 190
    tear of, 187
  tibiofibular, tear of, 179, 187
  weakness, congenital, 112, 115
Limp, 25-26
Lipoma, 388
Lipping at talonavicular joint; see Talonavicular joint, lipping at
Lisfranc's joint dislocations, 160-162
Lobster-claw foot; see Cleft foot
Locomotion; see also Walking
  kinetics of, 7-12
Locomotor system, 4-5

Louisiana heel lock strapping, 186
Lymphangitis, 305
  treatment, 305

M

Macrodactyly, 67-68
Madura foot, 302-303
Malformations; see Anomalies
Malignancy; see Cancer
Malleolus
  fracture; see Fractures, malleolus
  fracture-dislocations; see under Fracture-dislocations
  ligaments; see Trauma, malleolar ligaments
  osteotomy; see Osteotomy, malleolar
  posterior, approach to, 460
  ulcer over, varicose, 295
Mallet
  mastoid, 436
  toe, 241-249
    etiology, 248-249
    pathogenesis, 249
    shoes and, 248
    treatment, 249, 542
Maltz rasp, 436
March fractures; see Fractures, fatigue
Mastoid mallet, 436
Mayo operation for hallux valgus, 511
McBride procedure
  hallux valgus, 519, 520
  hallux varus, bilateral postoperative, 223
McKeever's approach to digital nerves for perineural fibroma removal, 469
McLaughlin and Ryder's lateral approach to ankle, 460
Megalodactylia, 67-68
Melanoma, malignant, 351-352
Metabolic disorders affecting foot, 282-288
Metal appliances, 429-430
  hallux valgus and, 515
Metatarsal(s); see also Metatarsus
  abscess of, Brodie's, 374
  accessory
    bizarre, 61
    polydactylia with, 60
  amputation of, 451-453
  anomalies, 73-74, 84
  bars, 427
  callus and; see under Callus
  corns and, 324-325
  cyst of, aneurysmal bone, 394
  dwarfism, 113
  exostosis of, 399
  first
    grating into second, 84
    length of, and hallux valgus, 214-215
  fractures of; see Fractures, metatarsal
  fusion, 74
  glass in, 175
  head
    approaches for resection, 468-469
    approaches for resection, Clayton's, 469
    approaches for resection, Hoffmann's, 468-469
    bursa under, adventitious, 311-313
    fifth, in tailor's bunion, 237, 239, 240
    first, congenitally wide, 207-209

Metatarsal(s)—cont'd
  head—cont'd
    first, congenitally wide, condylectomy for, 209
    first, congenitally wide, reduction technique, 208-209
    first, congenitally wide, symptoms of, 207-208
    flat type of, 217
    in hallux rigidus, 229, 230
    keratosis under; *see* Keratosis, under metatarsal heads
    lesions under, intractable, 326-337
    osteochondritis of, 383
    osteochondrosis of; *see* Freiberg's infraction
    shapes of, 208, 217
    ulcers under, diabetic, 294
    ulcers under, traumatic, 341
    windlass mechanism of, 254
  intermetatarsal joint mobilization for metatarsus adductus and varus, 101-103
  necrosis of, aseptic, 84
  short, 74, 75-76
  synostosis of, 84
  transmetatarsal amputation, 452-453
  tuberculosis of, 300
Metatarsalgia, 34-35
Metatarsophalangeal break, 19-22
  location of, 20
Metatarsophalangeal joint
  amputations at; *see* Amputations, at metarsophalangeal joint
  anatomy, 207
  in arthritis
    rheumatoid, 283
    traumatic, 398
  bursa under, adventitious, 313
  cyst over, epidermal, 348
  deformities of, 206-239
  dislocations; *see* Dislocations, metatarsophalangeal joint
  neuropathy of, diabetic, 290, 291
  sprains, first, 191
  surgical procedures, 506-535
  trophic destruction of, 276
Metatarsus; *see also* Metatarsals
  adductus, 90, 98, 99-103
    arthrodesis in, 99, 101
    etiology, 99
    tendon transfer in, 100, 101
    treatment, 99-103
  primus varus, 73-74
    hallux valgus and, 529
  proximus, 74, 77
  varus, 99-103
    arthrodesis in, 99, 101
    etiology, 99
    hallux valgus and, 214
    Heyman, Herndon and Strong correction, 101-103
    in infant, 98
    resistant, treatment, 103
    tendon transfer in, 100, 101
    treatment, 99-103
Microscopic examination, direct, 45
Midtarsus
  joint dislocation, 160

Midtarsus—cont'd
  osteotomy, 498
    pes cavus and, 498
  surgical procedures, 495-501
Mole, 349-350
Morton's syndrome, 249-250
Mosaic plantar wart, 345
Multiple sclerosis, 275
Muscle(s)
  ankle, examination, 33
  in clawtoes, 246, 247
  dystrophy, 280
  foot, examination, 33
  neuromuscular diseases, 268-281
  variation causing hallux valgus, 215-216
  weakness, congenital, 112, 115
Musculoneurogenesis, prenatal, and talipes equinovarus, 92
Mycetoma, 302-303
Myelodysplasia, 275-279
Myopathies, childhood, 280

N
Nails
  clubnails, 355
  cutting of, consequence of, 359
  cysts, epidermoid inclusion, 402
  deformities of, 353-368
  diseases of, 353-368
  great toe, congenital double, 354
  groove, occlusion of, 357
  incurvated, 365-367
  ingrown, 356-365; *see also* Hypertrophy, nail lip
    avulsion of nail for, 358, 361
    etiology, 358
  inverted, 365-367
  involuted, 365-367
  lip
    hypertrophy; *see* Hypertrophy, nail lip
    panhypertrophy, 363, 365, 366
  ram's horn, 355-356
  tumors involving, 356, 402
    glomus, 402
Navicular
  absence of, congenital, 112, 114
    bilateral, 113
  accessory, 54-58
    symptoms, 57
    treatment, 57-58
    types of, 55-56
  calcaneonavicular; *see* Calcaneonavicular
  cuneonavicular articulation, 33-34
  fractures of; *see* Fractures, navicular
  necrosis of, avascular, 382
  osteochondrosis of, 377-378
  talonavicular; *see* Talonavicular
Necrosis
  aseptic, 375, 380-381
    march fracture and, 158
    metatarsal, 84
    talus fractures and, 128, 130-131
  avascular, 380-381
    navicular, 382
    phalanx, 381
  sesamoids; *see* Sesamoids, necrosis of
  syphilis and, 301
  ulcer and, 293-294

Needles
  as foreign bodies, 173, 174
  suturing, 437
Neoplasms; *see* Tumors
Nerve(s)
  digital, approaches for removal of perineural fi-
      bromas, 469
    dorsal, longitudinal, 469
    plantar, longitudinal, 469
    plantar, transverse, 469
  diseases, 413-424
  entrapment syndrome; *see* Tarsal-tunnel syn-
      drome
  foot, plantar, 414
  peripheral, examination, 35
  plantar, third branch of, 416
Neurofibroma, 388, 414
Neuroma, interdigital plantar, 413-419
  diagnosis, 415-416
  etiology, 415
  operative technique, 417-419
  symptoms, 415
  treatment, 416-419
Neuromuscular diseases, 268-281
Neuropathy
  diabetic, 288-292
    etiology, 288-289
    of metatarsophalangeal joints, 290, 291
    pathogenesis, 289
    symptoms, 289
    of tarsometatarsal articulations, 290, 291
    treatment, 289, 292
  syphilitic, 300-301
Neurovascular corns, 325
  treatment, 325
Nevus, 349-350
Newborn, foot and ankle examination in, 23-24
Nocardia, 303

O

Ober's approach to plantar structures, 467
Occlusion, nail groove, 357
Office procedures, 425-434
  surgical, 435
Ollier's approach to subtalar joint, 465
Onychauxis, 355
Onychia, 354
Onychocryptosis; *see* Nails, ingrown
Onychogryposis, 355-356
Onychoma, 356
Operative considerations, 438-439
Operative principles and requirements, 435-442
Orthopaedic appliances for rheumatoid arthritis,
    285
Orthotic appliances, 430
  for valgus and varus forefoot, 432
Os peroneum, osteochondritis of, 410
  dissecans, 59
Os trigonum, 52-54
  diagnosis, 52
  removal procedure, 52-54
Os vesalianum, 54
Ossicles, accessory, 58
Ossification
  centers of foot, 89
  tendon, 313-316
    Achilles, 313-316

Ossification—cont'd
  tendon—cont'd
    Achilles, and fibromatosis, 314
    Achilles, due to Z-plasty lengthening, 314
    flexor hallucis brevis, 316
Osteoblastoma, 398, 400
Osteochondritis, 381-384, 385
  definition, 376
  deformans juvenilis, 411
    definition, 376
  dissecans, 384
    of os peroneum, 59
  juvenile deforming tarsal, definition, 376
  metatarsal head, 383
  os peroneum, 59, 410
  trochlear surface of talus, 385
Osteochondroma, 393-394
  phalanges, 395, 396
  tendo achillis, 315
Osteochondrosis, 377-380
  definition, 376
  calcaneal apophysis, 378-380
  cuboid, 381
  metatarsal head; *see* Freiberg's infraction
  of tarsal navicular, 377-378
Osteoclastoma, 402
Osteogenic sarcoma, 402-403
Osteoid osteoma, 395, 397
Osteoma
  calcaneal spurs and, 257
  osteoid, 395, 397
Osteomyelitis, 371-375
  acute, 371-373
    treatment, 372-373
  chronic, 373-374
    treatment, 373-374
  Garré's, 375, 376
    treatment, 375
  hallux, 373
  phalanges, 372
    after injury, 306
  sesamoids, nonpyogenic type, 409
  types of, 374-375
Osteoporosis, 404-406
  postmenopausal, 405
  postoperative, 440
Osteosarcoma, 402-403
Osteosclerosis and calcaneal spurs, 256, 257
Osteotome, 496
  Stille, 436
Osteotomy
  calcaneus, 489-495
    crescentic, for calcaneocavus deformity, 271
    for flatfoot correction, 490
    for flatfoot correction, displacement osteot-
        omy, 491
    for Haglund's disease, 494
    for inverted heel, 493
    for pes cavus, 493
    for spurs, Griffith's osteotomy, 495
    for spurs, Steindler's osteotomy, 496
    for talipes equinovarus, 96-97
  Giannestras'; *see* Giannestras' step-down osteot-
      omy
  malleolar
    in ankle arthrodesis, 473, 474
    for surgical exposure of ankle, 460

Osteotomy—cont'd
  midtarsal, 498
    for pes cavus, 498
    step-down, and condylectomy for hallux valgus,
      507-508
      Hawkins, 509
      Hawkins-Mitchell, 510
  for talipes equinovarus, 96-97
    calcaneal osteotomy, 96-97
    rotational osteotomy, 97
Overlapping toes, 68-71
  bilateral, 69
  fifth, 545-547
    Lantzounis' procedure, 545
    Lapidus' procedure, 545, 546
    skin contracture and, DuVries' technique, 544,
      548
    Wilson's procedure, 545, 547
  hallux valgus and, 70
  hallux varus and, Keller procedure for, 224
  second, correction of, 547, 549
  surgery of, 545-549

P

Pads, felt, 428, 429, 432
  hammertoe and, 433
Palsy; see Cerebral palsy
Panhypertrophy of nail lip, 363, 365, 366
Papilloma wart; see Verruca plantaris
Paralysis
  extensors, causing hallux flexus, 234
  in foot anomalies, arthrodeses, 485
Paraplegic, "growing," 277
Paresthesia, postoperative, 441-442
Paronychia, 354
Patch test, 46
Patient, surgical, instructions to, 435-436
Pedicle skin graft for crush injury of heel, 200
Pelvic tilt, 27-28
Penrose drain with hemostat as tourniquet, 437
Peritendinitis; see Tenosynovitis, traumatic
Perniones, 171
Peroneal spastic flatfoot, 143, 259-263
  etiology, 260-261
Pes cavovarus; see Clawfoot
Pes cavus; see Clawfoot
Pes planus; see Flatfoot
Pes valgus; see Talus, vertical congenital
Phalangectomy
  flail toes produced by, 321
  subtotal, 447-448
  total, 448
Phalanges
  abscess, Brodie's, 275
  accessory distal, of hallux, 63
  amputations; see under Amputations
  chondromyxoma of, 401
  delta, 63
  dislocations, 162-163
  exostosis of, 397
    subungual, 400
  fracture; see Fractures, phalanx
  fracture-dislocations, fifth proximal, 152
  metatarsophalangeal; see Metatarsophalangeal
  necrosis of, avascular, 381
  osteochondroma, 395, 396

Phalanges—cont'd
  osteomyelitis, 372
    after injury, 306
  proximal, abnormal, 84
  sesamoids under; see Sesamoids, under phalanx
Physical therapy
  ankle
    fractures, 433
    sprains, 433
  tendo achillis, 433-434
  toes, 433
Pigmented villinodular synovitis, 389
Pins in calcaneus fractures, 139
Planovalgus due to talonavicular anomaly, 259
Plantar
  aponeurosis, 33
    palpation of, 34
  calcaneonavicular ligament, 33
  contractures, and burns, 169
  fascia; see Fascia, plantar
  fasciitis; see Fasciitis, plantar
  flap in amputations, 449
  nerves, 414
  sling in hallux valgus, 507
    Joplin's technique, 509
  structures, medial approaches to, 464, 466-467
    Brochman's 467
    DuVries', 467
    Henry's, 466-467
    Ober's, 467
  surface, glass in, 176
  wart, mosaic, 345
Plaster boot for metatarsal fracture, 150
Poliomyelitis, 279-280
Polydactylia, 58, 60-63, 84
  accessory metatarsal and, 60
  bilateral, 60
  treatment, 62-63
Polyonchia, 354
Poroma, eccrine, 350-351
Postoperative care, 439
Preoperative considerations, 435-436
Pressure
  excrescences due to, 318-342
  ulcers, 341
Pridie's split heel approach to calcaneus, 466
Prostheses; see Appliances
Psoriatic arthritis, 286
"Pump bump," 194
Pyogenic infections, 305-310

R

Radiation, diagnostic
  in ankle injuries, 179-180
  foot, 44
Ram's horn nails, 355-356
Rasp
  Joseph nasal, 436
  Maltz, 436
Ray resection, 451-452
Reflex dystrophy, 406, 407
Rest and rheumatoid arthritis, 284-285
Rete malpighii, 343
Reticulum cell sarcoma, 404
Retractor, Weitlander self-retaining, 436
Rheumatoid arthritis; see Arthritis, rheumatoid
Rocker-bottom foot, 261

Rodent ulcer, 352
Roentgenography; *see* Radiation
Rowe's classification, calcaneus fractures, 133
Ruptures
  ligament, ankle
    collateral, lateral, 184-185
    deltoid, 184-185
  tendon, Achilles, 137, 198, 199
  tendon, traumatic subcutaneous, 196-199
    Achilles, 198, 199
    peroneus longus, 198-199
    tibialis anterior, 196-198
    tibialis anterior, treatment, 197, 198

S

Sarcoma
  angiosarcoma, 390, 391
  chondromyxosarcoma, 403
  chondrosarcoma, 403
  Ewing's; *see* Ewing's sarcoma
  fibrosarcoma, 390
  Kaposi's, 390, 391
  osteogenic, 402-403
  osteosarcoma, 402-403
  reticulum cell, 404
  synovial, 390, 391
Saw, nasal, 436
Scaphoid, tarsal; *see* Navicular, accessory
Scar, hypertrophic, 353
Schoolfield's technique, deltoid ligament recon-
    struction, 480
Scissors, Sistrunk, 436
Sclerosis
  multiple, 275
  osteosclerosis and calcaneal spurs, 256, 257
  tuberous, 275
Scraping for fungus, 45
Septic bursitis, acute, 307
Sesamoid(s)
  abnormalities of, 74, 78-80
  accessory, 81
  diseases of, 406, 408-411
  distorted and hypertrophied, 74, 78
    symptoms, 78, 80
    treatment, 80
  exostosis, 80
  fractures of; *see* Fractures, sesamoid
  in hallux valgus, 222
  in hallux varus, 225
  hyperkeratosis under, 327
  inconstant, 80-82
  necrosis of
    aseptic, after diabetes mellitus, 409-410
    avascular, 411
  osteomyelitis of, nonpyogenic, 409
  under phalanx, first proximal, 82-83
    characteristics, 82-83
    treatment, 83
  tibial, congenital absence of, 80
Sesamoiditis
  acute, foot strappings in, 430
  simple, 408-411
Sever's disease, 378-380
Shoes
  examination of, 26-27
  hallux valgus and, 210-211, 524
  hammertoe and, 248

Shoes—cont'd
  heel
    height of, 26
    lifts, 426
    modifications, 425-426
    Thomas, 425-426, 428
    widened, 426
  ill-fitting, and forefoot, 206
  irritants causing dermatitis, 346
  lifts
    heel, 426
    sole, and Thomas heel, 428
  mallet toe and, 248
  modifications of, 425-430
  rotary slippage of, 26
  shank of, 426
  sole, 426-427, 428
    modification for hallux rigidus, 427
  type of, 26
Silver's correction of hallux valgus, 517, 519
Sinus(es)
  draining sinus tracts of heel, 303
  suppurating, of foot, 338, 340
    etiology, 338
    site of, 338, 340
    treatment, 340
  tarsi, approach to, lateral, 463-465
Sistrunk scissors, 436
Skeletal structures, appraisal of, 30
Skin
  contracture and overlapping fifth toe, DuVries'
    correction, 544, 548
  disorders of, 318-370
  incisions of foot, 439
  over tendo achillis, hypertrophy of, 342
Sling
  for hammertoe, 433
  plantar, for hallux valgus, 507
    Joplin's technique, 509
Soft tissues
  affections of, local, 371-412
  cancer, 390
  over tendo achillis, hypertrophy of, 342
  trauma to, 168-203
  tumorous conditions of, 385-404
  tumors of, 385-390
  vascular disorders, 375-384
Sole
  of foot; *see* Plantar
  shoe, 426-427, 428
    modification for hallux rigidus, 427
Spina bifida, lumbosacral vertebra defects in, 276
Splayfoot and hallux valgus, 529
Splints, Denis Browne, 94
Split foot; *see* Cleft foot
Sponge rubber bandages after hallux valgus opera-
    tion, 525
Sprains, 176-191
  anatomy, 176-177
  ankle
    physical therapy, 433
    recurrent, 190-191
  calcaneocuboid joint, 191
  forefoot, 191
  mechanism, 177-191
  metatarsophalangeal joint, first, 191
  plantar fascia, 191

Spurs, calcaneal
 foot strappings and, 430, 432
 osteosclerosis of posterior tuberosity and, 256, 257
 osteotomy for
  Griffith's, 495
  Steindler's, 496
 surgery, 494-495, 497
 of tuberosity, plantar, 252-256
  diagnosis, 254
  etiology, 252-254
  inflammation and, 253
  osteolytic changes causing, 256
  treatment, 254-256
  unusually shaped, requiring special evaluation, 255
 of tuberosity, posterior, 257
Stabilization procedures, 499
 for dropfoot, 265
Stanley and Breck's correction of hallux valgus, 508
Staple, 436
Stapler, 436
Steinberg's trephine, 360
Steindler's rotation osteotomy for heel spur, 496
Steroids and rheumatoid arthritis, 284-285
Stille osteotome, 436
Strappings
 ankle, 186
  figure-of-eight, 187
  Gibney basket-weave, 186
  Louisiana heel lock, 186
 foot, 430, 432-433
  bow, 432
  calcaneal spurs and, 430, 432
  hammertoe and, 430, 433
  after injury, 430
  plantar fasciitis and, 430, 432
  in sesamoiditis, 430
Stress fractures; see Fractures, fatigue
Strokes, 268-269
Subtalar articulations, approaches to, 462-465
Subtalar joint
 approaches to
  lateral, 463-465
  Ollier's, 465
 axis of, 17-19
 dislocations of, 158-160
 motion in, goniometer measuring, 32
 stability of, 28-29
Sudeck's atrophy, 406, 407
 with metatarsal march fracture, 408
Sulcus deepening preventing peroneal tendon dislocations, 482
Suppurating sinuses; see Sinuses, suppurating
Surgical procedures, complications of, 439-442
Suturing
 importance of, 439
 materials for, 437
  reactions to, 440
 needles, 437
Syme's amputation, 453-455
 complications, 455
 postoperative care, 455
Symphalangism and syndactyly, 85
Synchondrosis, calcaneonavicular, and spastic flatfoot, 262

Syndactyly, 66-68
 accessory hallux and, 62
 symphalangism and, 85
 treatment, 67-68
Syndesmosis, tibiofibular, diastasis of, 179
Synostosis
 calcaneonavicular, 108
  spastic flatfoot and, 262
 metatarsals, 84
Synovectomy, 481
Synovioma, 390, 391
Synovitis, pigmented villinodular, 389
Syphilis, 300-301
 Charcot's joint in, 301
 knee joint in, 301
 necrosis in, 301
 neuropathy in, 300-301

T

Tailor's bunion; see Bunion, tailor's
Talectomy, 484, 487-489
Talipes
 calcaneovalgus, 97, 99
  treatment, 97, 99
 deformity, types of, 90
 equinovarus, congenital, 91-97
  development and, 92
  etiology, 92-93
  germ plasm defect causing, 92-93
  heredity causing, 92
  in infant, 90
  intrauterine pressure causing, abnormal, 92
  osteotomy for; see Osteotomy, for talipes equinovarus
  prenatal musculoneurogenesis causing, 92
  reshaping procedures for, 97
  retarded rotation causing, 93
  splint for, Denis Browne, 94
  tendon lengthening for, Achilles, 95
  tendon transplantation for, 95
  treatment of, conservative, 93-94
  treatment of, surgical, 94-97
 valgus, 90
 varus, 90
Talocrural joint; see Ankle
Talofibular ligaments; see Ligaments, talofibular
Talonavicular articulation, 33-34
Talonavicular joint
 anomalies, 85
  planovalgus due to, 259
 approach to, 463
 lipping at, 109-111
  etiology, 110
  symptoms, 110-111
Talus
 displacement with trimalleolar fracture, 123
 exostosis, 399
 fracture; see Fractures, talus
 fracture-dislocations; see Fracture-dislocations, talus
 osteochondritis, 385
 vertical congenital, 105-107
  treatment, 107
Tarsal(s); see also Tarsus
 articulations, transverse, 19
  approaches to, 462-465

Tarsal(s)—cont'd
  coalition, 107-109
    diagnosis, 108-109
    symptoms, 108
    treatment, 109
  scaphoid; *see* Navicular, accessory
  tunnel, anatomy of, 420
  -tunnel syndrome, 419-421
    diagnosis, 420
    etiology, 419-420
    symptoms, 420
    treatment, 420-421
Tarsometatarsal articulations, diabetic neuropathy
    of, 290, 291
Tarsometatarsal joint
  dislocations of, 160-162
  fracture-dislocations of, 161
  mobilization for metatarsus adductus and varus,
    101-103
Tarsus; *see also* Tarsal(s)
  arthritis of, rheumatoid, 283
  arthrodesis; *see* Arthrodesis, tarsus
  midtarsus; *see* Midtarsus
  surgical procedures, 482-495
Tendon
  abductor hallucis, shortening, causing hallux
    varus, 223
  Achilles
    calcaneus fractures and, 136, 137
    exposure of, 466
    fibromatosis; *see* Fibromatosis, tendo achillis
    fibrosis of, 315
    in flatfoot, symptomatic flexible, 260
    hypertrophy of skin and soft tissues of, 342
    lengthening for talipes equinovarus, 95
    osteochondroma, 315
    physical therapy and, 433-434
  ankle, subluxation, 481-482
  calcaneal; *see* Achilles *above*
  dislocations, ankle, 481-482
  luxation, 199
    treatment, 199
  ossification of; *see* Ossification, tendon
  ruptures; *see* Ruptures, tendon
  sheath, giant cell tumors of, 388-389
  transfers
    for clawtoe, 249
    for hammertoe, 249
    about hindfoot, 478, 480-481
    Jones'; *see* Jones' tendon transfer
    for mallet toe, 249
    for talipes equinovarus, 95-96
    tibialis anterior, for metatarsus adductus and
      varus, 100, 101
  trauma to, 193-199
Tenosynovitis
  infectious, 307
    acute, 307
    chronic, 307
  traumatic, 193-195
    hemorrhagic, 194-195
    peroneal tendon, 196
    process, 193-194
    symptoms, 193-194
    treatment, 193-194

Tenotomy
  for clawtoes, 249
  for hammertoes, 249
  for mallet toe, 249
Therapy
  conservative, 425-434
  physical; *see* Physical therapy
Thomas heel, 425-426
  lateral sole lift and, 428
Tibia
  Brodie's abscess of, 374
  fractures; *see* Fractures, tibia
Tibiofibular ligament tears, 179, 187
Tibiofibular syndesmosis, diastasis of, 179
Tilt board, 189
Tinea infection of toes, 341
Tissues; *see* Soft tissues
Toe(s)
  absence of, congenital, 113
  amputations; *see under* Amputations
  anomalies of, 58-73
    great toe, 71-73, 84
    surgical procedures for, 535-549
  clawtoes; *see* Clawtoes
  corns on; *see* Corns
  cysts of, epidermal, 348
  dermatophytosis of, 346
  flail, from phalangectomy, 321
  great; *see* Hallux
  hammered; *see* Hammertoes
  hostler's, 355-356
  -in, degree of, 26
  mallet; *see* Mallet, toe
  middle, phalanx fractures, 148-149, 151
  movements when rising on, 28
  necrosis, in syphilis, 301
  nerves; *see* Nerves, digital
  -out, degree of, 26
  overlapping; *see* Overlapping toes
  physical therapy and, 433
  sarcoma of, Ewing's, 404
  tinea infection of, 341
  ulcers over, traumatic, 341
  underlapping, congenital, 71
Toenails; *see* Nails
Tourniquets, 437-438
  Penrose drain with hemostat as, 437
Traction in fractures
  ankle, fixed, 125
  calcaneus, 139
Transmetatarsal amputation, 452-453
Trauma
  aneurysm and, 440-441
  athletic, 191-193
    differentiation, 191-193
    sites of, 192
    treatment, 192-193
  crush injury; *see* Crush injury
  foot strapping after, 430
  malleolar ligaments, lateral, 178-184
    classification, 178
    diagnosis, 178-183
    diagnosis, roentgenograms in, 179-180
    symptoms, 178
    treatment, 183-184
  malleolar ligaments, medial, 189
    treatment, conservative, 189

Trauma—cont'd
  osteomyelitis of phalanges after, 306
  soft tissues, 168-203
  tendon, 193-199
  tenosynovitis; *see* Tenosynovitis, traumatic
  ulcer; *see* Ulcer, traumatic
Trephine, Steinberg's, 360
Trimalleolar fracture; *see* Fractures, malleolus
Trimalleolar fracture-dislocations, 123
  closed reduction of, 126
Tuberculosis, 299-300
  metatarsal, 300
  osseous, 299-300
Tuberous sclerosis, 275
Tumors
  bone, 390-402
    giant cell, 402
  glomus, 350, 390
    beneath nail, 402
  malignant; *see* Cancer
  nail, 356, 402
  soft tissues, 385-390
  tendon sheath, giant cell, 388-389
Tyloma; *see* Callus
Tzanck test, 46-47

U

UC-BL inserts, 430
  sizes of, 431
  for valgus after cerebral palsy, 273
Ulcer
  diabetic, 293
    under metatarsal head, fourth, 294
  indolent, 294-295
    over medial malleolus, 295
  malignant, 352
  necrotic, 293-294
  pressure, 341
  rodent, 352
  traumatic, 200-201, 340-342
    under heel, 341
    under metatarsal heads, 341
    toes, 341
  varicose, 294-295
    over medial malleolus, 295
  vascular deficiency causing, 293-295
Underlapping toes, 71

V

Valgus
  in cerebral palsy, 271-275
  forefoot, orthotic appliances for, 432
  hallux; *see* Hallux valgus
  heel, heel wedge for, 426
  planovalgus, 259
Varicose ulcer, 294-295
  over medial malleolus, 295
Varus
  in cerebral palsy, 271-275
  forefoot, orthotic appliances for, 432
  hallux; *see* Hallux varus
  heel, heel wedge for, 426

Verruca plantaris, 342-345
  diagnosis, 344
  etiology, 344
  on heel, 344
  microscopic section of, 343
  treatment, 344-345
Vertebra defects, lumbosacral, and spina bifida, 276
Vessels
  cerebrovascular accidents, 268-269
  deficiency, causing ulcers, 293-295
  disorders affecting bones, 375-384
  disorders affecting foot, 288-298
    differential diagnosis, criteria for, 297
  disorders affecting soft tissues, 375-384
  neurovascular corns, 325
    treatment, 325
  peripheral vascular disease, 295-298
    symptoms, 296-298
Volkmann's ischemic contracture, 201-202

W

Walking
  displacements of the body during
    horizontal, 6-7
    lateral, 7, 8
    vertical, 5-6
  intervals of
    first, 9-10
    second, 10, 11
    third, 10-12, 13
  kinematics of, 5-7
Wart
  mosaic plantar, 345
  papilloma; *see* Verruca plantaris
Weight
  bearing
    in equinus casts for calcaneus fracture, 139
    faulty, causing excrescences, 318-342
    in forefoot amputations, 446
    surfaces, adventitious bursa under, 313
      after surgery, 439
  distribution, postoperative, 439
Weitlander self-retaining retractor, 436
Westin and Hall's approach to sinus tarsi, 463
Wilson's procedure for overlapping fifth toe correction, 545, 547
Windless action, 28, 30
  of aponeurosis and metatarsal heads, 254
  diagrammatic representation of, 14
Wires, Kirschner, and tarsometatarsal fracture-dislocation, 161
Wound dehiscence, 440

X

X-ray; *see* Radiation

Z

Zadek's approach to Achilles bursae, 466
Z-plasty lengthening causing tendo achillis ossification, 314